# UNDERSTANDING THE U.S. HEALTH SERVICES SYSTEM

# UNDERSTANDING THE U.S. HEALTH SERVICES SYSTEM

## Third Edition

Phoebe Lindsey Barton

Health Administration Press, Chicago, Illinois
AUPHA Press, Washington, DC

AUPHA
HAP

Your board, staff, or clients may also benefit from this book's insight. For more information on quantity discounts, contact the Health Administration Press Marketing Manager at (312) 424-9470.

11  10  09  08  07    5  4  3  2  1

**Library of Congress Cataloging-in-Publication Data**
Barton, Phoebe Lindsey
    Understanding the U.S. health services system /
Phoebe Lindsey Barton—3rd ed.
      p. cm.
    Includes bibliographical references and index.
    ISBN-13: 978-1-56793-263-8
    ISBN-10: 1-56793-263-0 (alk. paper)
    1. Medical care—United States.   2. Medical policy—United
States.   3. Medical economics—United States.   I. Title.
    RA395.A3B27 2006
    362.10973—dc22                                                     2006043637

The paper used in this publication meets the minimum requirements of American National Standard for Information Sciences—Permanence of Paper for Printed Library Materials, ANSI Z39.48-1984.™

Production: Putman Productions; Cover design: Betsy Perez;
Acquisitions editor: Audrey Kaufman

Health Administration Press          Association of University Programs
A division of the Foundation            in Health Administration
  of the American College of          2000 N. 14th Street
  Healthcare Executives               Suite 780
One North Franklin Street             Arlington, VA 22201
Suite 1700                            (703) 894-0940
Chicago, IL 60606-3424
(312) 424-2800

*In loving memory of*
*Doctors Milton and Ruth Roemer*
*and their seminal work on health care systems.*

# BRIEF CONTENTS

# CONTENTS

# LIST OF ACRONYMS AND ABBREVIATIONS

| | |
|---|---|
| AAPCC | adjusted average per capita cost |
| AARP | American Association of Retired Persons |
| ACS | American Cancer Society |
| ADA | Americans with Disabilities Act of 1990 |
| ADL | activities of daily living |
| AFDC | Aid to Families with Dependent Children |
| AHA | American Heart Association |
| AHA | American Hospital Association |
| AHCs | academic health centers |
| AHCPR | Agency for Health Care Policy and Research |
| AHP | Association Health Plan |
| AHRQ | Agency for Healthcare Research and Quality |
| ALA | American Lung Association |
| ALOS | average length of stay |
| AMA | American Medical Association |
| APA | Administrative Procedures Act |
| APACHE | Acute Physiological and Chronic Health Evaluation |
| APHA | American Public Health Association |
| APNs | advanced practice nurses |
| | |
| BHO | behavioral health organization |
| BIA | Bureau of Indian Affairs |
| | |
| CABG | coronary artery bypass graft |
| CAH | critical access hospital |
| CAM | complementary and alternative medicine |
| CBO | Congressional Budget Office |
| CCMC | Committee on the Costs of Medical Care |
| CDC | Centers for Disease Control and Prevention |
| CFR | Code of Federal Regulations |
| CHAMPUS | Civilian Health and Medical Program of the Uniformed Services |
| CHP | Comprehensive Health Planning Act |

| CMS | Centers for Medicare and Medicaid Services |
| COBRA | Consolidated Omnibus Budget Reconciliation Act |
| COGME | Council on Graduate Medical Education |
| CON | certificate of need |
| CPOE | computerized physician order entry |
| CQI | continuous quality improvement |
| CRO | contract research organization |
| DALYs | disability-adjusted life years |
| DEA | Drug Enforcement Agency |
| DEFRA | Deficit Reduction Act |
| DGME | direct graduate medical education (payment) |
| DHEW | U.S. Department of Health, Education, and Welfare |
| DME | durable medical equipment |
| DOD | U.S. Department of Defense |
| DRGs | diagnosis-related groups |
| EACH | essential access community hospital |
| EAP | employee assistance programs |
| ECFMG | Education Commission for Foreign Medical Graduates |
| EMCRO | Experimental Medical Care Review Organization |
| EMIC | Emergency Maternal and Infant Child Care Program |
| EMTALA | Emergency Medical Treatment and Active Labor Act |
| EPA | Environmental Protection Agency |
| EPO | exclusive provider organization |
| ERISA | Employee Retirement Income Security Act |
| ESP | Economic Stabilization Program |
| ESRD | end-stage renal disease |
| EU | European Union |
| FDA | Food and Drug Administration |
| FDCA | Food, Drug, and Cosmetic Act |
| FEHBP | Federal Employee Health Benefits Program |
| FMG | foreign medical graduate |
| GDP | gross domestic product |
| GME | graduate medical education |
| GMENAC | Graduate Medical Education National Advisory Committee |
| GNP | gross national product |
| HCBS | home- and community-based service |
| HCFA | Health Care Financing Administration |

| | |
|---|---|
| HEDIS | Health Plan Employer Data and Information Set |
| HI | Hospital Insurance, Part A of Medicare |
| HIAA | Health Insurance Association of America |
| HIE | Health Insurance Experiment (RAND) |
| HIPAA | Health Insurance Portability and Accountability Act of 1996 |
| HIPC | health insurance purchasing cooperative |
| HMO | health maintenance organization |
| HPSA | health professional shortage area |
| HRSA | Health Resources and Services Administration |
| HSA | Health Savings Account |
| HSA | Health Systems Agency |
| HSA | Health Security Act of 1993 |
| HHS | U.S. Department of Health and Human Services |
| | |
| IADL | instrumental activities of daily living |
| ICF | intermediate care (nursing) facility |
| ICFMR | intermediate care facility for mentally retarded |
| IHS | Indian Health Service |
| IME | indirect medical education (payments) |
| IMG | international medical graduate |
| IND | investigational new drug |
| IOM | Institute of Medicine |
| IPA | independent practice association |
| | |
| JCAHO | Joint Commission on Accreditation of Healthcare Organizations |
| | |
| LCME | Liaison Committee on Medical Education |
| | |
| MCO | managed care organization |
| MDUFMA | Medical Device User Fee and Modernization Act |
| MedPAC | Medicare Payment Advisory Commission |
| METs | multiple employer trusts |
| MEWA | multiple employer welfare arrangements |
| MHSS | Military Health Services System |
| MMA | Medicare Prescription Drug Improvement and Modernization Act |
| MRI | magnetic resonance imaging |
| MSA | metropolitan statistical area |
| MSO | management services organization |
| MUA | medically underserved area |

| | |
|---|---|
| NCHSR | National Center for Health Services Research |
| NCQA | National Committee on Quality Assurance |
| NDA | new drug application |
| NHI | national health insurance |
| NHIS | National Health Interview Survey |
| NHSC | National Health Service Corps |
| NIH | National Institutes of Health |
| NIMBY | "not in my backyard" |
| NMES | National Medical Expenditures Survey |
| NP | nurse practitioner |
| NPC | nonphysician clinicians |
| NPP | nonphysician providers |
| NQF | National Quality Forum |
| | |
| OBRA | omnibus budget reconciliation act |
| OECD | Organization for Economic Cooperation and Development |
| OHTA | Office of Health Technology Assessment |
| OSHA | Occupational Safety and Health Administration |
| OTA | Office of Technology Assessment (in the U.S. Congress) |
| OTC | over-the-counter drugs |
| | |
| P4P | pay for performance |
| PA | physician assistant |
| PACE | Program of All-Inclusive Care for the Elderly |
| PCA | personal care attendant |
| PDUFA | Prescription Drug User Fee Act |
| PET | positron-emissions tomography |
| PGPs | prepaid group practices |
| PHO | physician hospital organization |
| PHS | Public Health Service |
| PhysPRC | Physician Payment Reform Commission |
| PMC | patient management categories |
| PPRC | Physician Payment Reform Commission |
| PORT | patient outcome research team |
| POS | point-of-service plan |
| PPI | producer price index |
| PPO | preferred provider organization |
| PPS | prospective payment system (Medicare) |
| PROs | peer review organizations |
| PROPAC | Prospective Payment Assessment Commission |
| PSN | provider-sponsored network |
| PSO | provider-sponsored organization |

PSRO            professional standards review organization

QALYs           quality-adjusted life years
QIOs            quality improvement organizations
QMB             qualified Medicare beneficiaries

RBRVS           resource-based relative value scale
RMP             regional medical program
RPCH            rural primary care hospital

SCHIP           State Child Health Insurance Plan
SES             socioeconomic status
SHCC            Statewide Health Coordinating Council
SHMO            social health maintenance organization
SHPDA           State Health Planning and Development Agency
SIP             sickness impact profile
SMI             Supplemental Medical Insurance (Medicare Part B)
SNF             skilled nursing facility
SRO             single room only
SSA             Social Security Act
SSDI            Social Security Disability Insurance
SSI             Supplemental Security Income

TANF            Temporary Assistance to Needy Families
TEFRA           Tax Equity and Fiscal Responsibility Act
TQM             total quality management
TRICARE         Health insurance program for military dependents
                and retirees

UCR             usual, customary, reasonable charge
USMG            U.S. medical graduate
USUHS           Uniformed Services University of the Health Sciences

VA              Department of Veterans Affairs

WHO             World Health Organization
WIC             Women's, Infants' and Children's nutrition program

YLL             years of life lost

# LIST OF FIGURES AND TABLES

## Chapter 7

## Chapter 8

## Chapter 9

## Chapter 10

## Chapter 17

## Chapter 18

## Chapter 19

## Chapter 20

# PREFACE

The U.S. health services system is constantly changing. The notion that its dynamic nature can be captured in a static freeze-frame provokes a range of reactions—from amusement to skepticism to curiosity.

This third edition of *Understanding the U.S. Health Services System* captures this moving target at one moment in time to provide the most up-to-date snapshot possible. At the same time, this edition offers a policy context that identifies change agents and issues to help the reader assess this dynamic system.

## Capturing a Moving Target

Our changing world continues to shape the U.S. health services system. The economic downturn that followed the strong economy of the late 1990s is unquestionably changing the financing of health services. An employer's ability to offer health insurance will be affected by increases in insurance premiums. An employee's ability to influence greater provider or other choices in employer-sponsored health insurance is strong in a tight labor market, but weak to nonexistent in a labor market with higher unemployment rates. Retiree health benefits may be eroded or even terminated if a company goes bankrupt. The proportion of the population without private or public health insurance may climb. Safety-net programs, ever more needed in constrained economic circumstances, not only experience resource losses but also face pressures to provide services to more people. We can conclude that change will continue as uncertainty abounds. The directions and magnitude of change are less well known.

## Obtaining Timely and Consistent Data

In addition to the uncertainties facing the U.S. health services system, obtaining consistent data and information about it, in a timely manner, remains a challenge. No central repository of health services data exists.

Data on health services expenditures are centralized in the National Health Accounts maintained by the Centers for Medicare and Medicaid Services. These data are collected from multiple sources, have to be reconciled for reportage in a uniform time period, and currently require at least a two-year lag period for processing, reconciliation, and reporting. Various governmental units collect other types of data, including utilization data from the National Health Interview Survey and nursing home and other long-term care data from several sources. Some of these data collection and reporting activities occur at regular intervals; others are unevenly spaced, often directly related to the lack of resources to maintain their currency. This text also relies on data from scientific studies reported in the juried literature. In many instances, the study is a one-time project and will not be updated or replicated. Thus, one has to decide for how long a one-time data point maintains its relevance.

All of these data challenges add to the difficulty in pinpointing the beginning of a trend or the end of an era. From today's vantage point, we can more fully consider the "backlash" against managed care that was first reported in the late 1990s; we cannot, however, say that this trend began, for example, in June 1997, or at any other specific point in time.

## Accounting for Multiple Perspectives and Identifying Emerging Topics

The pluralistic and complex U.S. health services system is the result of many viewpoints and perspectives. It could be argued that the social model of care, as well as the medical model, merits consideration in a systems text. The greater openness with which complementary and alternative medicine providers are being viewed calls for examination and analysis. Other issues currently below the health services radar will rise to detection before the next edition is released. How to strike the right balance in coverage of key issues remains a challenge.

## New Emphases in the Third Edition

Chapter 1 provides an in-depth overview of how this book is organized, what is new in this edition, and how best to use this book. Data on health services financing, services utilization, health insurance coverage (including changes in the uninsured population), trends in morbidity and mortality, and other aspects of the U.S. system have been updated and, where possible, displayed graphically. In addition, this third edition features up-to-date coverage in the following areas:

- known and anticipated change agents, and the policy issues deriving from them;
- changes in access to services, costs of and expenditures for services, and the resulting quality of care received;
- the changing role of managed care and the apparent movement away from some of its more restrictive tenets; and
- challenges facing the system as the baby boom population reaches the age of Medicare eligibility.

## Aids to the Reader

An end-of-book Glossary of Key Terms provides current definitions of health services terms. Another reader aid is the helpful, quick-to-consult alphabetical List of Acronyms and Abbreviations on page xv. Lists of key words at the end of each chapter help the reader to identify the chapter's important concepts, and numerous tables and graphs illustrate and clarify key features of the U.S. health services system.

*Phoebe Lindsey Barton*

# INTRODUCTION

**1**

# INTRODUCTION TO THE U.S. HEALTH SERVICES SYSTEM

## Introduction

A country's health services system—the combination of resources, organization, financing, and management that culminates in the delivery of health services to a population—is an important, though not the sole, determinant of a population's health status (Roemer 1991). A health services system is shaped by the country's economic, political, and cultural values. In addition to affecting the health of its population, a country's health services system may also be an important sector of the economy in terms of employment, research and development, and exports, such as drugs, devices, and other medical technologies.

Milton I. Roemer, whose extensive contributions to our understanding of these systems have brought him international renown, has identified several classes of health services systems, based on each country's economic and political system (see Table 1.1).

The health services system in the United States is a market-based system in an affluent, industrialized economy, which nevertheless lacks universal access. In this book, the discussion of the U.S. system is structured around how health services are organized and managed, how resources such as the health workforce and technology are developed and deployed, what types of economic support drive the system, and how services are delivered. Limited historical information is provided to illuminate discussions of the system's evolution; the principal emphases, however, are on the current system, the range of proposals for changing parts or all of the current system, and the implications of these potential reforms.

This third edition updates all health services expenditure and utilization information; expands the discussion of the public health sector, adding a discussion on health disparities in Chapter 3; provides additional information on the current status of and proposed changes to Medicare and Medicaid; looks at the changing role of the hospital; augments the discussion on the growing interest in complementary and alternative medicine; and examines the continuing evolution of managed care and managed care organizations.

Despite the failure to enact systemic reform such as that proposed in the 1993 Health Security Act, incremental reforms—particularly in the

TABLE 1.1
Types of
National
Health
Systems,
Classified by
Economic
Level and
Health Systems
Politics

| | Health System Policies (Market Intervention) | | | |
|---|---|---|---|---|
| Economic Level (GNP per Capita) | Entrepreneurial and Permissive | Welfare-Oriented | Universal and Comprehensive | Socialist and Centrally Planned |
| Affluent and Industrialized | United States | West Germany* Canada Japan | Great Britain New Zealand Norway | Soviet Union* Czech Republic |
| Developing and Transitional | Thailand Philippines South Africa | Brazil Egypt Malaysia | Israel Nicaragua | Cuba North Korea |
| Very Poor | Ghana Bangladesh Nepal | India Myanmar | Sri Lanka Tanzania | China Vietnam |
| Resource Rich | | Libya Gabon | Kuwait Saudi Arabia | |

SOURCE: Adapted from Roemer 1985.

*NOTE: Changes since 1991 in political systems in Germany and the Soviet Union and perhaps other countries may affect their classification.

way health services are financed and delivered—are rapidly changing the face of the U.S. health services system. A renewed focus on managing the system—including the provider's ordering and delivery of services, patients' utilization of services, and the associated expenses to all parties—is precipitating significant and constant change. Capturing this moving target presents a major challenge. This chapter provides a model developed by Dr. Roemer for analyzing the current system, from which future changes can be assessed. Three dominant values of care in the U.S. system—access to, costs of and expenditures for, and quality—are examined.

## Overview of the U.S. Health Services System

The U.S. health services system is a study in contradictions. Per capita expenditures for health services ($6,280 in 2004) are the highest of any health services system in the world, and yet as much as 20 percent of the U.S. population may not have financial access to health services during a year, or for the entire year. Approximately 20 percent of the population accounts for 80 percent of all health expenditures (described by some as the "20:80 rule") in the U.S. system. Although we are accustomed to referring to our health services system, which suggests the universal availability of a con-

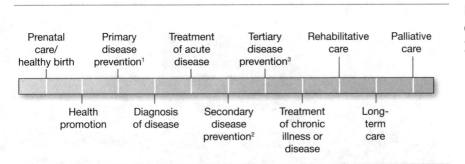

FIGURE 1.1
Continuum of
Health Services

NOTES: 1. Primary disease prevention is preventing agents from causing disease or injury. 2. Secondary disease prevention is early detection and treatment to cure and/or control the cause of disease. 3. Tertiary disease prevention is ameliorating the seriousness of disease by decreasing disability and the dependence resulting from it.

tinuum of care from health promotion to palliative care (Figure 1.1), the majority of services rendered focus on the treatment of illness and disease. For this reason, some refer to our "disease treatment system" or "illness system," rather than to our health services system.

Part I of this book focuses on the nature of the U.S. health services system, addressing such questions as:

- What factors influence health status?
- What factors influence the seeking of care?
- What are the effects of health services utilization on health status?
- Who has access to health services?
- Is access to health services a right?

## The Roemer Model of a Health Services System

The U.S. health services system can be analyzed from many perspectives. For example, an historical approach would examine the emergence of the health services system as the economic and political systems of the country evolved. Another approach would analyze the development of the continuum of health services. A third would consider the roles of various system participants—the patient or care seeker, the provider, the insurer or third-party payer, the public or government unit that manages the system, and the employer that provides health insurance—in shaping the system.

This book uses a systems model developed by Dr. Roemer (1984) to discuss the organization of programs and their management, the production of resources that support the system, the sources of economic support, and how services are delivered. The system is driven by health needs or problems to produce health results or outcomes. The model provides not only

**FIGURE 1.2**
National
Health System:
Components,
Functions,
and Their
Interdependence

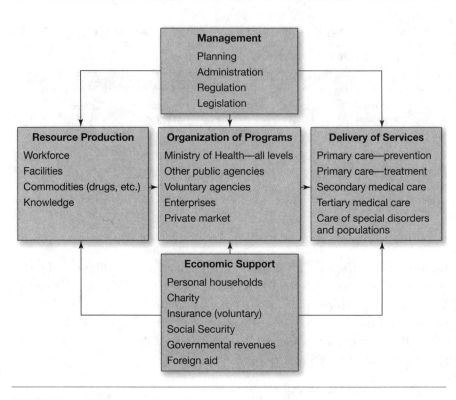

SOURCE: Roemer 1985.

a systematic way of examining any one system, but also a method for comparing health services systems across the more than 149 developed countries in the world. Figure 1.2 displays Dr. Roemer's five-part model of a health services system. Dr. Roemer defines a health service as an activity whose primary objective is health—its maintenance, its improvement, or, if it is failing, its recovery. Because of the complexity of the U.S. system, our application of the model begins with the central component: the organization of programs.

## Organization of Health Services

The U.S. health services system is an ever-shifting mixture of public or government sector, private sector, and voluntary or charitable services. The government's role in health, once limited primarily to protecting the public from epidemics of infectious diseases, has expanded to that of:

1. a major payer for care through large public-sector programs such as Medicare and Medicaid;

2. a major provider of health services to special populations such as the military and their dependents, veterans of military services, and indigenous populations; and

3. a major supporter of the education and training of many types of care providers.

The delivery of health services occurs primarily in the private sector, but the once-clear delineation of public and private sectors is becoming increasingly blurred. The voluntary sector is small but provides many services that may not be fully realized through either the public or the private sectors, including a focus on the prevention or cure of specific diseases, such as heart disease and cancer, and the championing of the care needs of special populations, such as children, people with mental illnesses, or persons living with AIDS. Part II of this book addresses the organization of U.S. health services.

## Management of a Health Services System

Management of the U.S. health services system, which includes planning, administration, legislation, and regulation, is addressed in Part III of this book. Although these functions occur in both the public and private sectors, the focus in Part III is on management in the public sector. Private-sector management issues are integrated into the discussion of the delivery system in which the private sector dominates. The public health system also receives special attention in Part III.

## Economic Support of Health Services

Economic support for the U.S. health services system is addressed in Part IV. Three types of health services organizations—those in the public, the private, and the voluntary sectors—influence the ways in which health services are financed in the United States. How the health services system is financed dictates which populations receive care and the kinds of care they receive. From this, it is possible to deduce the populations likely to receive little or no care, because the U.S. system lacks universal coverage. The primary financing mechanisms—private and public health insurance—are examined for their effects on access to, costs of, and expenditures for care.

## Production of Health Services Resources

In addition to financial support, the provision of health services requires resources, such as a trained workforce, the availability of appropriate levels of facilities in which services can be provided, biomedical research to balance the art and the science of care, and medical technology, including drugs, devices, and advances in medical and surgical procedures. Part V discusses the development and deployment of health resources in the U.S. system.

### Delivery of Health Services

Four components of the Roemer model—organization, management, economic support, and resource production—all contribute to how health services are delivered, which is the focus of Part VI. The effects of managed care, broadly defined as care provided in a system that integrates the financing and delivery of health services, are emphasized in that section as well.

## System Values: Access, Cost and Expenditures, and Quality

Health services analysts frequently assess access to, costs of and expenditures for, and quality of care. These values of the U.S. health services system have been recognized in legislation such as the National Health Planning and Resources Development Act of 1974 (PL 93-641) and the enabling legislation for the Agency for Healthcare Research and Quality (AHRQ, formerly the Agency for Health Care Policy and Research) and serve as the foundation for health services research. Access to health services has many dimensions, including geographic, physical, cultural, temporal, and economic. In a country that values social justice but provides neither uniform nor universal health services coverage, access is a particularly important consideration. Chapter 3 focuses on issues of access to care and their relationship to expenditures for care.

The cost of care—driven by inflation, the increased volume of services due to population demographics, health insurance coverage, and the increased intensity of services—has resulted in expenditures that in 2004 absorbed 16 percent of the gross domestic product (GDP). U.S. government expenditures for health are surpassed only by expenditures for Social Security; they significantly exceed expenditures for education, transportation, agriculture, and other government services (with the exception of defense, for the first time in several decades). Private expenditures for health services have shown commensurate growth, stimulating ongoing proposals for changing the ways in which health services are financed and delivered. The effects of costs of and expenditures for health services are examined in depth in Part IV and are discussed elsewhere in this book.

As we learn more about the outcomes of health services, quality of care becomes an increasingly important consideration. The examination of quality explores such questions as:

• How effective is an intervention?
• How appropriate is a particular intervention and under what conditions?
• Do the benefits of an intervention exceed its costs?

Chapter 19 is devoted to quality-of-care issues.

Access to, costs of and expenditures for, and quality of care are often inextricably linked. Increasing access to care, as occurred through the passage of Medicare and Medicaid legislation in 1965, inexorably leads to increases in utilization, and thus to increases in the costs of and expenditures—both public and private—for care. Unprecedented expenditure increases prompt decision makers to look for ways to reduce them, such as instituting controls on utilization and constraining provider payments. Increases and decreases in utilization bring quality of care into focus. Too many or too few services can compromise the quality of care, and poor quality of care can ultimately result in higher expenditures to correct the problem. Achieving a satisfactory balance among these values remains a major challenge as the U.S. health services system continues to change.

## Organization of the Book

Dr. Roemer's model of a health services system serves as the organizing principle for this book. Part I focuses on the needs or problems that drive the system, including access to care. How the U.S. health services system is organized and the roles of its public and private sectors constitute Part II. Part III addresses the management of the system, including its planning, administrative, legislative, and regulatory functions. How the system is financially supported and the significance of health insurance as the principal financing mechanism are discussed in Part IV. Part V examines the production of resources essential to the successful operation of a system, including the workforce, health facilities, knowledge, and biotechnology. How these various model components result in the delivery of care is the focus of Part VI. The results or outputs of this model are many and varied; Part VII addresses one way in which we measure results—by examining the quality of care that is delivered. Finally, Part VIII broadly summarizes the current and anticipated changes in the U.S. health services system.

### Data on U.S. Health Services

The complexity of the U.S. health services system is exemplified in the data that describe it. No central source for health services data exists. Lags between data collection and reporting affect the currency of the data. Data on various components of the system (e.g., resources and economic support) are collected by different agencies using different time frames. This text uses the most recent data available to describe the U.S. health services system, but the use of incomplete and sometimes fragmented data increases the potential for gaps and possible inconsistencies. Every graph and figure that could be updated with more recent data has been revised in this edition.

Some graphs and figures, used with permission from the juried literature, could not be updated but have been retained if they contribute to the understanding of the concepts presented.

### Aids to Understanding the Complexity of the U.S. Health Services System

A language of specialty terms and acronyms accompanies the complex U.S. health services system. Three aids are included in this text to enhance understanding of the system:

1. The key words and concepts in each chapter are listed at the chapter's end for ready reference and review.
2. A lexicon of acronyms and abbreviations is provided at the beginning of the text.
3. A glossary defining the most frequently encountered terms (key words) precedes the bibliography at the end of the book.

---

## Key Words

| | |
|---|---|
| access to care | hospital planning councils |
| Agency for Healthcare Research and Quality (AHRQ) | managed care |
| | Medicaid |
| continuum of care | Medicare |
| costs of/expenditures for care | private sector |
| gross domestic product (GDP) | public sector |
| health care outcomes | universal access or universal coverage |
| health care reform | |
| Health Security Act of 1993 | utilization of health services |
| health service | voluntary sector |

---

## References

Roemer, M. I. 1991. *National Health Systems of the World, Vol. I.* New York: Oxford University Press.

———. 1985. *National Strategies for Health Care Organization: A World Overview.* Chicago: Health Administration Press.

———. 1984. "Analysis of Health Services Systems—A General Approach." In *Reorienting Health Services,* edited by C. O. Pannenborg, A. van der Werff, G. B. Hirsch, and K. Barnard, 47–59. New York: Plenum Press.

# AN OVERVIEW OF THE U.S. HEALTH SERVICES SYSTEM AND ITS USERS

## Introduction

A general characterization of a health services system and the people who use it creates a context in which the component parts can be examined and better understood. This chapter provides an overview of the U.S. health services system and the demographics and health services utilization patterns of the U.S. population. Following the overview of the system, this chapter addresses such system characteristics as:

- distinguishing health from illness and disease;
- the cultural, economic, genetic, and perceived health status factors that influence care-seeking behaviors; and
- the utilization of health services by subpopulation groups.

The chapter concludes with an overview of the effects on health status of receiving, or not receiving, health services.

## An Overview of the U.S. Health Services System

The $1.9 trillion U.S. health services system is a unique amalgam of public-, private-, and voluntary-sector programs. Elements of a health services system can be traced to the colonial and early Federalist periods. Public health programs, first organized at the local level, originated to protect the public from communicable diseases and unsanitary living conditions. One of the first public health programs was the U.S. Marine Hospital Service, established in 1798 to provide care to merchant seamen who transported goods—and sometimes diseases—from port to port.

Major forces in the development of health services in the private sector include the growing population, the population's increasing mobility, the commensurate demand for services, and the resulting expansion of the health workforce. The provision of health services began as a private transaction between the provider and the recipient and remained primarily on that basis until the growth of private health insurance during and immediately following World War II.

The voluntary health services sector, which often addresses issues unclaimed by either the public or private sectors, has its origins in the establishment of almshouses for the care of the indigent during the American colonial period. Almshouses were antecedents of today's hospitals, many of which were founded by charitable organizations.

### The Organizational Component

The post–World War II economy spurred the conversion of a health services cottage industry into what has been described as the medical-industrial complex (Relman 1980). Growth occurred in all components of the system. Within the organizational component, a cabinet-level department—the U.S. Department of Health, Education, and Welfare (DHEW), now the U.S. Department of Health and Human Services (HHS)—was established in 1953 to administer the nation's health programs. Attention to the safety of food and drugs increased. The government's role in biomedical research blossomed. Public health programs expanded to address a range of environmental health issues, to serve as the collector of vital event data (i.e., births, deaths, marriages, divorces, adoptions, and abortions), and to provide leadership on such diverse health issues as immunizations, sexually transmitted diseases, and violence affecting the health of populations.

The private sector was growing too, fueled by an increasingly industrialized economy in which employers began to offer health insurance as a benefit of employment. Demand for more health services stimulated growth in the health workforce; the establishment of additional hospitals, nursing homes, and other health facilities; and technology development.

Filling the gaps created by the two other sectors, the voluntary sector met the challenge of both well-known and new diseases by forming such organizations as the March of Dimes for polio, the American Heart Association for coronary disease, the American Lung Association for respiratory diseases, and the American Cancer Society for malignancies.

### The Management Component

The growth of public-sector and private-sector programs in a market economy increased the need for program management, including the functions of planning, administration, legislation, and regulation. Planning for health services was instituted at the national level with the 1966 Comprehensive Health Planning (CHP) Act (PL 89-749) and at the local level by hospital planning councils. Important health services legislation preceded World War II: the 1935 Social Security Act (SSA) (PL 74-271) included a number of titles authorizing health services for children, people with disabilities, and others. The SSA became the umbrella in the mid-1960s for other significant health legislation, including Medicare and Medicaid. A spate of additional health legislation was authorized independently of the SSA; these programs stimulated the development of multiple regulations for their full implementation.

## The Economic Support Component

The growth of a health services system depends on the level of economic support available to it. Thirty-five percent of the economic support for the U.S. system in the year 2004 came from private health insurance, 45 percent came from the federal government in the form of tax-generated revenue and trust funds and from state revenues, 13 percent came from individual out-of-pocket payments, and 7 percent came from foundations and other charitable sources.

## The Resources Component

Other resources, such as a workforce and facilities, are essential to a health services system. The health workforce continues to grow. Between 1960 and 1990, the supply of U.S. physicians increased 55 percent (Aiken and Salmon 1994). By the mid-1970s, the United States had doubled its capacity to train physicians in an effort to meet perceived workforce shortages (Cooper 1995; Mullan, Politzer, and Davis 1995). Over 871,000 physicians were licensed to practice in the United States in 2003. The number of nurses has remained relatively constant at about 2.2 million, yet many work settings continue to experience a nurse shortage. Growth in these and other professions has been aided by governmental support to expand educational opportunities. New professions have emerged to meet new needs: the number of billing and reimbursement specialists and business-trained administrators is growing to keep pace with the increasingly contractual nature of the U.S. health services industry.

The development of health facilities reflects the growing and changing health services system. Beginning in 1946, the growth in the number of hospitals and other kinds of health facilities was assisted by federal funds. Hospitals, until recently the hub of the system, grew in number and size until the 1980s. In the increasingly competitive 1990s through 2005, however, the overall number of hospitals declined, the number of licensed beds decreased, and the development of outpatient services and facilities mushroomed to reflect the changing delivery system. However, increases in hospital spending for both inpatient and outpatient services and also in Medicare hospital spending suggest that the hospital sector is once again growing.

## The Delivery System Component

Much of the change in the U.S. system is occurring in the delivery system component. The growth of the health services system, the increasing expenditures required to sustain it, the significant number of people without access to care, and the projections of increased demand from an aging population are stimulating changes in both the financing and delivery systems.

The most pervasive change has been the shift away from the fee-for-service delivery system to managed care, with indications as early as 1998 of a backlash against managed care that portends further system changes (Blendon et al. 1998; Levit et al. 2002). Managed care, once considered the alternative delivery system, was recommended as early as 1932 in a report by the Committee on the Costs of Medical Care and has its modern origins in the 1973 Health Maintenance Organization Act, which encourages the integration of the financing and delivery of health services to achieve more efficient and cost-effective care.

Achieving a health services system that provides both equity and efficiency—two competing values in U.S. society—becomes a major challenge in a market economy; the struggle to balance these values is reflected in the unevenness of the U.S. health services system. Although great strides have been made to increase the equity in access to care, many may not have financial access to care at any given time. The majority of the uninsured, who often lack financial access to care, are in the U.S. workforce or are dependents of someone who is in the U.S. workforce but has been unable to secure health insurance.

### Proposed Changes to the U.S. Health Services System

Although the U.S. health services system is the most costly and one of the most advanced in the world, recognition is growing that it is unbalanced and, in the view of some, out of control. This recognition has resulted in calls for reform from many quarters: the public, the providers, the payers for care (i.e., the government, the employer, or the individual), and politicians. Proposed wide-scale reforms have largely failed in their attempts to expand access to health services to the entire population, reduce costs of and expenditures for care, alter the incentives for provider payment, and change the ways in which health services are delivered.

Despite the failure to effect systemic reform, the health services system is changing significantly and continuously. Current changes that this book addresses are the:

- changing emphases on managed care and its multiple effects on the delivery system through the 1990s, and recent pressures from patients, providers, and others to effect yet another swing in the pendulum;
- recent initiatives to expand access to care, especially for expectant mothers and their children;
- continued pressures to reduce the costs of and expenditures for care;
- efforts to deal with workforce supply and distribution, including shortages in the work complement of nurses and a reorientation to

primary care in the 1990s, with recent skepticism about the success of that movement; and

• movement away from the hospital as the center of the U.S. health services system to care provided in outpatient and ambulatory settings.

To better understand each component and its interrelationship with the others, we first consider the distinctions between health and disease, review ways in which health status is measured, and explore factors such as population demographics that affect care-seeking behavior. A snapshot of current patterns of health services utilization provides a basis for understanding the interactions between the design of a health services system and its users.

## Distinguishing Health from Illness and Disease

The purpose of a health service is to positively affect one's health—its maintenance, its improvement, or its recovery. But what does *health* mean? The World Health Organization (WHO) defines health as not merely the absence of disease but as a state of physical, mental, and social well-being. This comprehensive definition provides a gold standard, but it is worthy to note that the U.S. health services system focuses largely on physical health. The First International Conference on Health Promotion, held in Ottawa, Canada, in 1986, provided another definition of *health*: health is a resource for living. What is now called the Ottawa Charter for Health Promotion identifies the fundamental conditions and resources for health as peace, shelter, education, food, income, a stable ecosystem, sustainable resources, social justice, and equity (WHO 1999).

Despite the general belief that the receipt of health services is one of the major influences on health status, other factors are of equal or greater importance. Figure 2.1 displays some of the determinants of health, including physical and social environments; personal traits; physical, mental, and social well-being; and access to a continuum of health services.

### Measuring the Health of a Population

A health provider using a range of indicators can measure an individual's health status, or health status can be self-assessed. One standard self-assessment measure is an individual's report of his or her health status, using a scale of excellent, very good, good, fair, or poor. Many studies have documented the strong correlation between perceived and measured health status (LaRue et al. 1979; Wolinsky and Johnson 1992; Kaplan and Camacho 1983). Studies have also documented what seems a truism: people with perceived poorer health status are likely to utilize health services more often (Anderson and Knickman 1984; Blaum, Liang, and Liu 1994).

**FIGURE 2.1**
Determinants
of Health

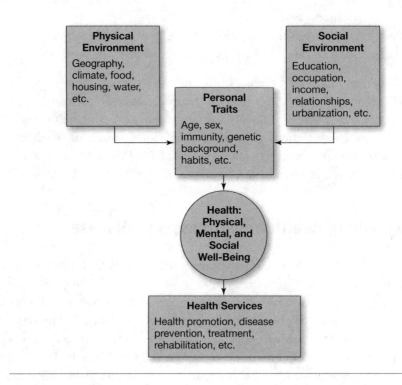

SOURCE: Roemer 1985.

The health status of a population can also be described and measured in several ways. Common indicators used to assess and compare the health status of populations include fertility and natality, life expectancy, morbidity, disability days, years of productive life lost, and mortality. Each individual measure provides one dimension of the health status of a population; collectively, along with other measures beyond the scope of this discussion, they indicate the general health status of a population. Cultures may value these indicators differently: In one culture, high fertility and natality rates may be perceived as indicators of good health and general well-being in a population; in another culture, these same indicators may suggest diminished health status, poverty, or lack of population control measures.

### Fertility and Natality

Figure 2.2 shows U.S. fertility rates according to live birth order for selected years between 1950 and 2003. The total fertility rate has declined by nearly 43 percent in the 53 years represented in Figure 2.2. The crude birth rate for 2003 was 14.1 live births per thousand women, and the fertility rate for that same year was 66.1 per thousand women (USDHHS 2005).

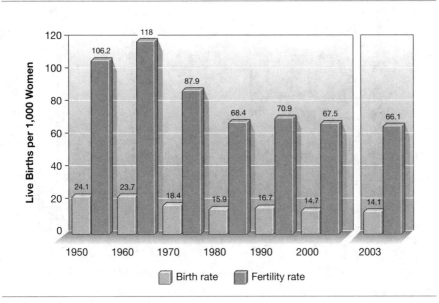

FIGURE 2.2
U.S. Crude
Birth Rates
and Fertility
Rates, All
Races
(Select Years,
1950–2003)

SOURCE: USDHHS 2005.

NOTES: Crude birth rate is live births per thousand population. The fertility rate is the total number of live births regardless of age of mother per thousand women 15–44 years of age.

## Life Expectancy

Life expectancy at birth in the United States is shown in Figure 2.3. In this century, life expectancy has grown significantly, with people born in 2002 having 28 to 31 years of additional life expectancy over the 1900 cohort. Females continue to have several more years of life expectancy per cohort than males. Data for 2002 show that U.S. life expectancy at birth is 77.3 years, at age 65 is 18.2 years, and at age 75 is 11.5 years, all slight increases over the data for 2000 (USDHHS 2005).

## Birth Weight

Birth weight is an indicator of a population's health, with low-birthweight and very low birthweight babies at higher risk of both immediate and longer-term health problems. Figures 2.4 and 2.5 show the percentage of low-birthweight and very low birthweight babies, respectively, among live births for all mothers, white mothers, and black mothers for the year 2003. Black mothers are at higher risk of having both low-birthweight and very low birthweight babies. While the proportion of low-birthweight babies of black mothers has remained relatively stable for the past two decades, the proportion of very low birthweight babies to this group of mothers has increased. (See also Figures 2.29 and 2.30, which depict levels of prenatal care.)

**FIGURE 2.3**
U.S. Life
Expectancy at
Birth, Age 65,
and Age 75
(Select Years,
1950–2002)

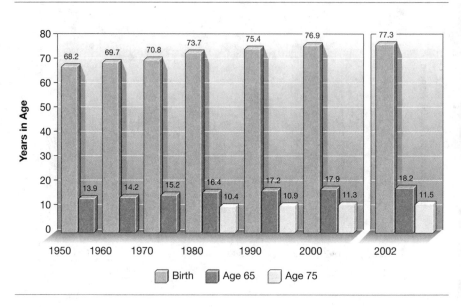

SOURCE: USDHHS 2005.

**FIGURE 2.4**
U.S. Low-
Birthweight
(<2,500
grams) Babies,
by Mother's
Race or
Ethnicity
(2003)

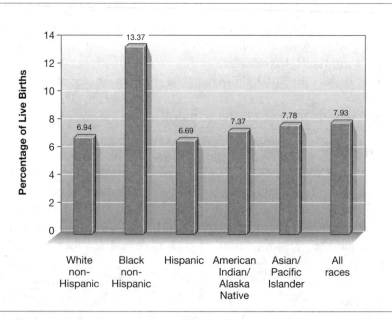

SOURCE: USDHHS 2005.

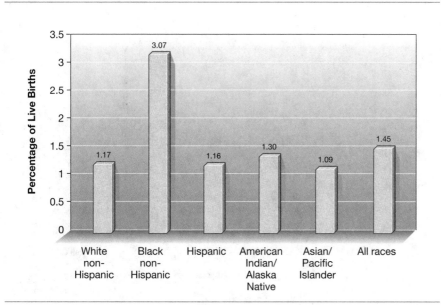

FIGURE 2.5
U.S. Very Low
Birthweight
(<1,500
grams) Babies,
by Mother's
Race or
Ethnicity
(2003)

SOURCE: USDHHS 2005.

## Morbidity

One measure of morbidity (the effects of disease in a population) involves the limitations caused by chronic conditions. Figure 2.6 shows the percentage of the U.S. population, by age group, with activity limitations. As one may expect, the percentage reporting more severe or complete limitations increases with age. Disability days, not shown here, are another morbidity measure. Health services researchers often use quality-adjusted life years (QALYs) to measure the health status of individuals or populations. Another measure that incorporates aspects of both morbidity and mortality is the disability-adjusted life year (DALY). The loss of life from premature deaths is assessed by evaluating all deaths in a year and using them to estimate years of life lost (YLL) for each disease category. This measure has been helpful in making comparisons between and among countries (Merson, Black, and Mills 2001).

## Mortality

Mortality or death rates are calculated separately for infants as an indicator of a population's health status. Figure 2.7 shows mortality rates for infants (children younger than one year), neonates (younger than 28 days), early neonates (younger than 7 days), and for children in the post-neonatal period (28 to 365 days) for select years between 1950 and 2002. The total infant death rate in 2002 is 24 percent of what it was in 1950, a witness to overall increases in health status, due to improved environmental and living

**FIGURE 2.6**
Limitations
Caused by
Chronic
Conditions,
U.S. Population
by Age Group
(2002)

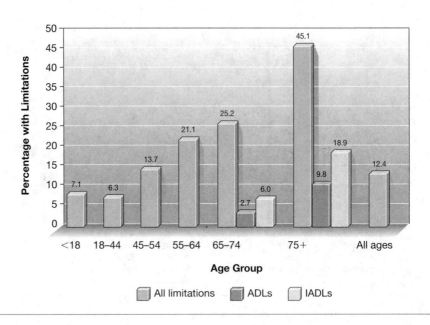

SOURCE: USDHHS 2004.

NOTES: ADLs = activities of daily living; IADLs = instrumental activities of daily living.

**FIGURE 2.7**
U.S. Infant
Mortality
Rates, Fetal
Death Rates,
and Perinatal
Mortality
Rates, All Races
(Select Years,
1950–2002)

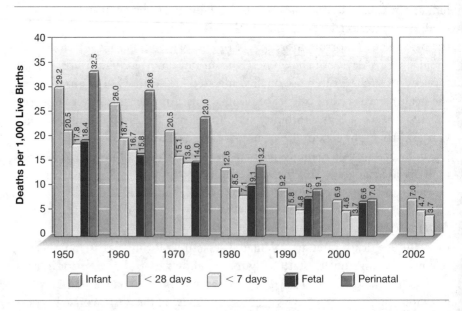

SOURCE: USDHHS 2005.

NOTES: Infant = one year; neonatal = <28 days; early neonatal = <7 days; perinatal = number of late fetal deaths plus infant deaths within seven days of birth per thousand live births plus late fetal deaths.

| Cause of Death | Number of Deaths |
|---|---|
| All causes | 2,443,387 |
| Diseases of the heart | 696,947 |
| Malignant neoplasms | 557,271 |
| Cerebrovascular disease | 162,672 |
| Chronic lower respiratory disease | 124,816 |
| Unintentional injuries | 106,742 |
| Diabetes mellitus | 73,249 |
| Pneumonia and influenza | 65,681 |
| Alzheimer's disease | 58,866 |
| Nephritis, nephrotic syndrome, and nephrosis | 40,974 |
| Septicemia | 33,865 |

TABLE 2.1
Leading
Causes of
Death, All
Races and
Both Genders,
U.S. Rank
Order and
Number of
Deaths (2002)

SOURCE: USDHHS 2005.

conditions and advanced technologies to save newborns. Data for 2002 show 7.0 infant deaths per thousand live births, 4.7 neonatal deaths per thousand live births, 2.3 post-neonatal deaths per thousand live births, 4.7 deaths per thousand live births in those younger than 28 days, and 3.7 deaths per live births for those younger than 7 days (USDHHS 2005).

Table 2.1 shows the leading causes of death and the number of deaths in 2002 for all races and both genders. Heart disease, malignant neoplasms (cancers), and cerebrovascular disease continue to be the dominant causes of death. Examining cause of death by age group, gender, and race or ethnic origin gives a better understanding of mortality in a population. Tables 2.2 and 2.3 show eight leading causes of death for males and females, respectively, by race and/or Hispanic origin. Heart disease is the number one cause of death of males in all but American Indian and Alaska Native racial and ethnic groups (with no report for the Hispanic male population), and the number one cause of death for females in all racial and ethnic groups (with no report for the Hispanic female population). The second and third leading causes of death—malignant neoplasms and cerebrovascular disease—remain relatively constant across both genders and all racial and ethnic groups. Real differences in rank order of causes of death across racial and ethnic groups appear among other leading causes of death, particularly

**TABLE 2.2**
Leading
Causes of
Death for U.S.
Males, by Race
and/or
Hispanic
Origin (2002)

| Rank | Diseases of the Heart | Rank | Malignant Neoplasms |
|---|---|---|---|
| 1 | White | 2 | White |
| 1 | Black | 2 | Black |
| 2 | American Indian/Alaska Native | 3 | American Indian/Alaska Native |
| 1 | Asian/Pacific Islander | 2 | Asian/Pacific Islander |
| NR | Hispanic | NR | Hispanic |

| Rank | Cerebrovascular Disease | Rank | Chronic Lower Respiratory Disease |
|---|---|---|---|
| 4 | White | 5 | White |
| 4 | Black | 9 | Black |
| 5 | American Indian/Alaska Native | NR | American Indian/Alaska Native |
| 4 | Asian/Pacific Islander | 7 | Asian/Pacific Islander |
| NR | Hispanic | NR | Hispanic |

| Rank | Unintentional Injuries | Rank | Diabetes |
|---|---|---|---|
| 3 | White | 9 | White |
| 3 | Black | 10 | Black |
| 1 | American Indian/Alaska Native | 10 | American Indian/Alaska Native |
| 3 | Asian/Pacific Islander | 10 | Asian/Pacific Islander |
| NR | Hispanic | NR | Hispanic |

| Rank | Pneumonia and Influenza | Rank | Homicide |
|---|---|---|---|
| 6 | White | NR | White |
| 7 | Black | 5 | Black |
| 7 | American Indian/Alaska Native | 6 | American Indian/Alaska Native |
| 5 | Asian/Pacific Islander | 8 | Asian/Pacific Islander |
| NR | Hispanic | NR | Hispanic |

SOURCE: USDHHS 2005.

NOTE: NR = no report.

deaths from chronic obstructive pulmonary disease (COPD) and homicide. Gender differences in causes of death are particularly observable for diabetes mellitus.

Age-adjusted death rates are also useful indicators of a population's health status. Figure 2.8 shows the U.S. age-adjusted death rates for selected causes for all races for select years between 1950 and 1999. Figure 2.9 concentrates on age-adjusted death rates from natural causes, including the top three—heart disease, malignant neoplasms, and cerebrovascular disease—as well as pneumonia and influenza and chronic lower respiratory disease.

| Rank | Diseases of the Heart | Rank | Malignant Neoplasms |
|------|----------------------|------|---------------------|
| 1 | White | 2 | White |
| 1 | Black | 2 | Black |
| 1 | American Indian/Alaska Native | 2 | American Indian/Alaska Native |
| 1 | Asian/Pacific Islander | 2 | Asian/Pacific Islander |
| NR | Hispanic | NR | Hispanic |

| Rank | Cerebrovascular Disease | Rank | Chronic Lower Respiratory Disease |
|------|------------------------|------|-----------------------------------|
| 3 | White | 8 | White |
| 3 | Black | NR | Black |
| 5 | American Indian/Alaska Native | NR | American Indian/Alaska Native |
| 3 | Asian/Pacific Islander | NR | Asian/Pacific Islander |
| NR | Hispanic | NR | Hispanic |

| Rank | Unintentional Injuries | Rank | Diabetes |
|------|-----------------------|------|----------|
| 4 | White | 6 | White |
| 4 | Black | 5 | Black |
| 3 | American Indian/Alaska Native | 6 | American Indian/Alaska Native |
| 4 | Asian/Pacific Islander | 5 | Asian/Pacific Islander |
| NR | Hispanic | NR | Hispanic |

| Rank | Pneumonia and Influenza | Rank | Homicide |
|------|------------------------|------|----------|
| 5 | White | NR | White |
| 7 | Black | 8 | Black |
| 7 | American Indian/Alaska Native | 10 | American Indian/Alaska Native |
| 7 | Asian/Pacific Islander | 9 | Asian/Pacific Islander |
| NR | Hispanic | NR | Hispanic |

**TABLE 2.3**
Leading Causes of Death for U.S. Females, by Race and/or Hispanic Origin (2002)

SOURCE: USDHHS 2005.

NOTE: NR = no report.

## U.S. Health Status Compared to Other Industrialized Countries

To create a context in which to evaluate the overall health status of the U.S. population, comparing its health status with other industrialized countries is helpful. Table 2.4 compares infant mortality, life expectancy at birth, and life expectancy at age 65 for both males and females for select countries among the 24 member countries in the Organization for Economic Cooperation and Development (OECD), an entity that includes European countries, Australia,

**FIGURE 2.8**

U.S. Age-Adjusted Death Rates, Selected Causes, All Races (Select Years, 1950–1999)

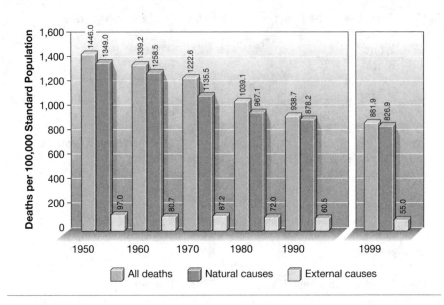

SOURCE: USDHHS 2001.

NOTES: Rates for 1999 are preliminary. External causes include unintentional injuries (including motor vehicle injuries), suicide, and assault (homicide).

**FIGURE 2.9**

U.S. Age-Adjusted Death Rates, Natural Causes, All Races (Select Years, 1950–2002)

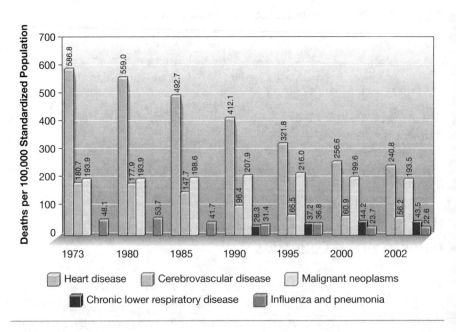

SOURCE: USDHHS 2005.

NOTE: Data intervals are irregular.

| Country | Ranking of Infant Mortality (Deaths/1,000 Live Births) | Life Expectancy at Birth, Males (Years) | Life Expectancy at Birth, Females (Years) | Life Expectancy at Age 65, Males (Years) | Life Expectancy at Age 65, Females (Years) |
|---|---|---|---|---|---|
| Australia | 17 | 77.0 | 82.4 | 17.2 | 20.7 |
| Canada | 23 | 77.1 | 82.2 | 17.1 | 20.6 |
| France | 8 | 75.5 | 82.9 | 16.9 | 21.3 |
| Germany | 11 | 75.6 | 81.3 | 16.0 | 19.6 |
| Japan | 4 | 78.1 | 84.9 | 17.8 | 22.7 |
| United Kingdom | 21 | 76.0 | 80.6 | 16.1 | 19.2 |
| United States | 28 | 74.4 | 79.8 | 16.4 | 19.4 |

**TABLE 2.4**
Health Outcome Measures in Select OECD Countries (1997–2002)

SOURCE: USDHHS 2005.

NOTES: OECD = Organization for Economic Cooperation and Development. Twenty-four countries provide data to the OECD database (www.oecd.org). United Kingdom = England and Wales.

Canada, Japan, the United States, and other countries in its databases. In the United States, the infant mortality rate is higher than in those select countries shown, and the United States ranks higher than other countries shown. Life expectancy at birth for U.S. males and females is lower than for their counterparts in the select countries shown. Life expectancy at age 65 for U.S. males and females is lower than for their counterparts in most other countries.

The lower health status for the United States along some of these measures is not due to lower overall spending or lower per capita spending on services. The United States allocates a greater proportion of its gross domestic product (GDP) to health than do other countries—nearly twice that of the United Kingdom and of Japan. The United States spends more than double the amount per capita on health services than does Australia, Japan, and the United Kingdom, yet it does not provide universal coverage, as do most of the other countries shown in Table 2.4.

Although maintaining or regaining health is the purpose of a health services system, the assessment of health and the focus of many health services systems is on the deviations from health—that is, on illness and disease. *Illness* is a relative term, generally used in the lay community to represent an individual response to a set of psychologic and physiologic stimuli. A *disease* state indicates the presence of pathology and is precisely defined by the provider community (May 1993). The extent of one's illness or disease can be measured by a Sickness Impact Profile (SIP) or by various

measures of severity of illness. The SIP assesses sickness-related dysfunction in the following areas: sleep and rest, eating, work, home management,
recreation and pastimes, ambulation, mobility, body care and movement,
social interaction, alertness behavior, emotional behavior, and communication (Patrick and Erickson 1993). A number of severity-of-illness measures, including the Acute Physiological and Chronic Health Evaluation
(APACHE), MedisGroups, Computerized Severity Index (CSI), disease
staging, Patient Management Categories (PMCs), and the acuity index
method, have been developed to improve the classification of hospital patients
(Thomas and Ashcraft 1991).

## Factors That Affect Care-Seeking Behavior

People enter the health services system for a variety of reasons. The person who is ill or injured seeks treatment; the person with a chronic disease seeks regular monitoring; the pregnant female seeks prenatal care to
protect her health and that of her fetus; and the person with a terminal
condition seeks relief from pain through palliative care. People also seek
health services to prevent the occurrence of diseases, such as measles and
influenza, and to detect and ameliorate the effects of other illnesses and
diseases.

A number of factors govern care-seeking behaviors, including perceived health status, ease of access to providers, and risk factors affecting
health. Perceived health status is a major reason why people seek services.
People who perceive that their health status is fair or poor are much more
likely to seek and use health services than those who rate their health status higher. Included in this group are the "worried well"—people whose
measured health status is good but whose concerns about illness or disease
result in their potential overutilization of services. Figure 2.10 shows the
respondent-assessed health status for 2003, focusing on the proportion of
the population that rates its health status as fair or poor. Poorer health status is associated with age, gender, and race. As people age, more of them
report fair or poor health status.

As is discussed in Chapter 3, the multiple dimensions of access—
geographic, physical, temporal, cultural, and financial—also affect care-
seeking behavior.

Certain genetic, behavioral, and other traits known to increase the
risk of poor health are referred to as risk factors. Common risk factors that
inform the study of health status include hypertension, obesity, lack of physical activity, and smoking.

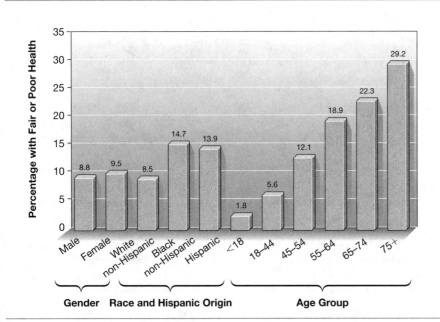

**FIGURE 2.10**
U.S. Respondent-Assessed Health Status, According to Select Characteristics (2003)

SOURCE: USDHHS 2005.

# Utilization of Health Services

The study of health services utilization reveals not only who does and does not access care, but also what types of care are accessed, with what frequency, and under what circumstances. The study of utilization also provides insight into costs of and expenditures for health services. Demographic factors, such as gender, age, race and ethnicity, and socioeconomic status, as well as risk factors and other variables affect health services utilization.

## Gender
Gender affects care-seeking behavior. Females, especially in their reproductive years, use more health services than do males in the same age groups. Females have a longer life expectancy than do males and as a group may use more health services. Figure 2.11 shows the distribution of gender in the U.S. population.

## Age
Age affects utilization of health services. Very young people may be frequent users of preventive and routine checkup services. Utilization of services increases with age, as physical and mental health deteriorates and chronic

**FIGURE 2.11**
U.S.
Population by
Gender (2003)

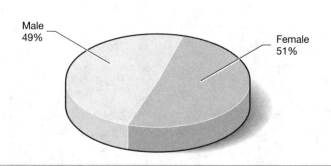

SOURCE: USDHHS 2005.

NOTE: Total population: 290,811,000. Estimates of the 2003 population are projected from the 2000 census.

**FIGURE 2.12**
U.S. Population
by Age Group
(2003)

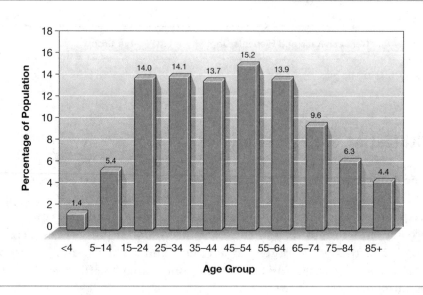

SOURCE: USDHHS 2005.

NOTE: Based on total population of 290,811,000.

conditions progress. Figure 2.12 shows the age distribution of the U.S. population for 2003. Of major concern is the aging of a significant proportion of the U.S. population as baby boomers (those born between 1946 and 1964 in the post–World War II population explosion) reach older age categories and increase the demand for health services. The total population is expected to grow by 0.6 percent each year until the year 2020, but the elderly population will grow three times as much: 1.8 percent annually. The oldest old (people age 85 and older) will grow at the fastest rate of all: 2.9 percent annually over the next 30 years (USDHHS 1990).

## Race and Ethnicity

Race and ethnicity may affect health services utilization in several ways. Some diseases are specific to or more prevalent in certain populations—for example, Tay-Sachs in people of Ashkenazic (central-eastern Europe) Jewish ancestry and sickle-cell anemia in African Americans. People with these conditions are likely to utilize the health services system because of their particular needs for treatment. Cultural beliefs associated with race or ethnicity may also affect utilization. For example, females from some cultures may be reluctant to seek health services from male providers. People from some cultures may be reluctant to obtain organ transplants or to serve as organ donors.

In addition, the ways in which health services are provided to members of certain racial or ethnic groups may differ. Studies have documented the differences in rates of angiography, angioplasty, and coronary artery bypass grafts among racial and ethnic groups, for example, that do not appear to be directly related to physiologic differences among these groups (Carlisle, Leake, and Shapiro 1995). Recognition of the differences in utilization, some of which may be traced to differences in access to health services among special populations, has led to a national focus on reducing disparities in health status (see Chapter 3). Several sources of federal funding for program development and research give preference to proposals that specify how such disparities can be reduced or eliminated.

Figure 2.13 shows the racial and ethnic composition of the U.S. population. About 13.7 percent of the total population is of Hispanic ethnicity; Hispanic people may be of any race.

## Socioeconomic Status

Socioeconomic status (SES) affects utilization of health services. People with limited income and financial resources, particularly the uninsured, are likely to seek fewer health services. Figure 2.14 shows the proportion of the U.S. population, by race and ethnicity, whose family income is below the 2003 poverty threshold of $18,769 for a nonfarming family of four. The proportion of black and Hispanic families below the poverty level is more than twice that of white families. People with incomes below the poverty level are not necessarily precluded from obtaining services. Some of them may be Medicaid enrollees or have access to other health services. Nevertheless, a higher proportion of people at lower income levels may report poorer health status than other income groups and may, as a result of their socioeconomic status and other factors, be at a higher risk for health problems. People with higher educational levels, and thus typically at higher employment and income levels, are more likely to have health insurance or be able to obtain health services—particularly dental, mental health, and other preventive services—than people with lower educational levels.

**FIGURE 2.13**
U.S. Population
by Race (2003)

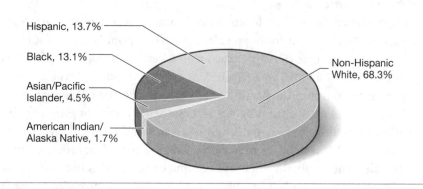

Hispanic, 13.7%

Black, 13.1%

Asian/Pacific
Islander, 4.5%

American Indian/
Alaska Native, 1.7%

Non-Hispanic
White, 68.3%

SOURCE: USDHHS 2002.
NOTE: Total population: 290,811,000.

**FIGURE 2.14**
Percentage of
U.S. Persons
and Families
below Poverty
Level, by Select
Characteristics
(Select Years,
1973–2003)

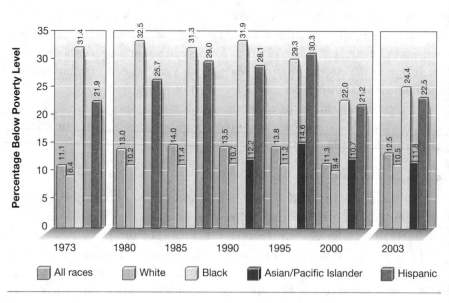

SOURCE: USDHHS 2005.

## Models of Health Services Utilization

Models to explain care-seeking behavior and the utilization of health services have been developed by Aday, Andersen, and Fleming (1980); Rosenstock (1974); and others. The health behavior model of services utilization
developed by Aday, Andersen, and Fleming, shown in Figure 2.15, analyzes

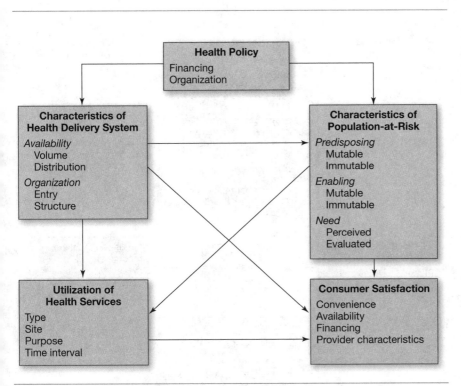

SOURCE: Aday, Andersen, and Fleming 1980. Reprinted by permission of Sage Publications, Inc.

**FIGURE 2.15**

Expanded Health Behavior Model

utilization in a health services system based on health policy factors, the characteristics of the population at risk, the characteristics of the services delivery system, and consumer satisfaction with health services. In the population characteristics component, predisposing characteristics include general health beliefs, attitudes, and knowledge, as well as demographics and employment status. Enabling characteristics include family income and place of residence. The model of access to care in Chapter 3 is based on this health behavior model.

The health belief model (Figure 2.16) suggests that utilization of health services is stimulated by one's set of beliefs about disease and the effectiveness of a health services system in preventing and treating disease. Individual perceptions and modifying factors, such as demographic, sociopsychological, and structural variables, affect the likelihood of one's action in seeking care and treatment.

These and other models draw attention to the complexities of analyzing utilization where some variables are explicit and measurable and others are highly specific to the individual and thus more difficult to measure.

**FIGURE 2.16**

Expanded
Health Belief
Model

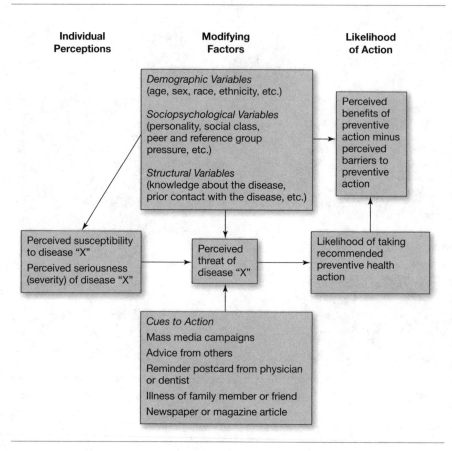

| Individual Perceptions | Modifying Factors | Likelihood of Action |
|---|---|---|

*Demographic Variables*
(age, sex, race, ethnicity, etc.)

*Sociopsychological Variables*
(personality, social class,
peer and reference group
pressure, etc.)

*Structural Variables*
(knowledge about the disease,
prior contact with the disease, etc.)

Perceived
benefits of
preventive
action minus
perceived
barriers to
preventive
action

Perceived susceptibility
to disease "X"

Perceived seriousness
(severity) of disease "X"

Perceived
threat of
disease "X"

Likelihood of taking
recommended
preventive health
action

*Cues to Action*

Mass media campaigns

Advice from others

Reminder postcard from physician
or dentist

Illness of family member or friend

Newspaper or magazine article

SOURCE: Rosenstock 1974. Reprinted with permission from the Society for Public Health Education, Washington, DC, 1998.

## Rates of Health Services Utilization

**Physician Visits and Contacts**

Figures 2.17 through 2.28 provide data on the utilization of major health services, such as physician contacts, hospital discharges, and nursing home residency. Figures 2.17 through 2.22 show the per capita contacts to physicians by number of visits, demographic characteristics (i.e., age, gender, race, and income), health insurance, poverty status, and site of the contact or visit (i.e., physician's office, home visit, hospital emergency department, or hospital outpatient department). The number of physician contacts per year is related to age, health status, financial access (such as health insurance coverage), and possible nursing home or other institutionalization for the oldest age group. Nearly 40 percent of those who report fair or poor health status have ten or more home visits and visits to physicians' offices and emergency departments per year, whereas only 11 percent of those who report their health status as good to excellent have ten or more visits per year to these providers (Figure 2.17). The number of physician contacts, including hospital outpatient department and hospital emergency department visits, increases with age (Figure 2.18).

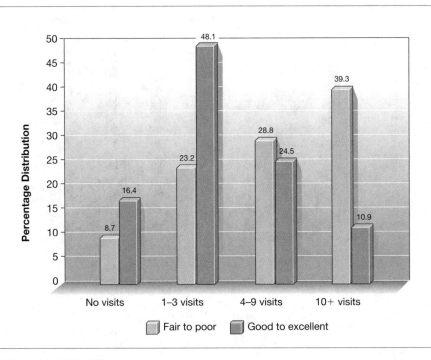

**FIGURE 2.17**
Health Services
Home Visits
and Visits to
Physicians'
Offices and
Emergency
Departments
Within the Past
12 Months, by
Self-Assessed
Health Status
(2003)

SOURCE: USDHHS 2005.

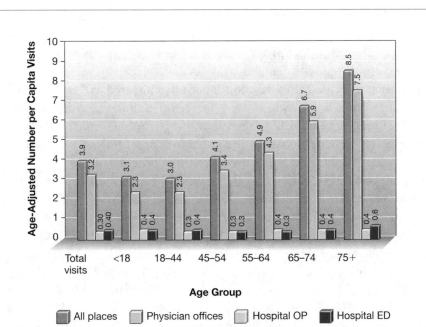

**FIGURE 2.18**
U.S.
Ambulatory
Visits to
Physicians'
Offices,
Hospital
Outpatient
Departments,
and Emergency
Departments,
by Age Group
(2003)

SOURCE: USDHHS 2005.

NOTES: ED = emergency department; OP = outpatient.

FIGURE 2.19

Health Services
Home Visits
and Visits to
Physicians'
Offices and
Emergency
Departments
Within the Past
12 Months, by
Gender and
Race/Ethnicity
(2003)

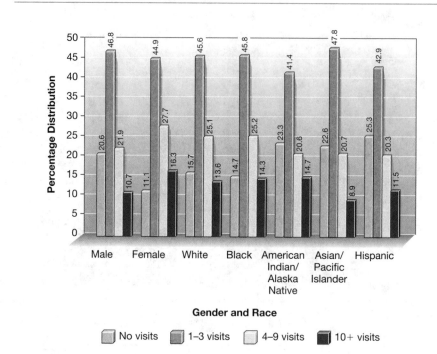

SOURCE: USDHHS 2005.

All other racial and ethnic groups generally have fewer physician contacts in the "4–9 visits" category in a 12-month period than do whites (Figure 2.19). A higher proportion of males have no visits in a 12-month period, compared with females, and a higher proportion of females have more than three visits in a 12-month period, compared with males. Health insurance status and financial status affect the number of visits. In Figure 2.20*a*, nonpoor persons have the lowest proportions in the "no visits" and "10+ visits" categories and the highest proportions in the "1–3 visits" and "4–9 visits" categories. Forty-two percent of people younger than age 65 who are poor and uninsured do not have a physician's office visit or other physician contact in a 12-month period, compared with only 13 percent of the population who are nonpoor and insured (Figure 2.20*b*).

Most physician contacts occur in physicians' offices, although some occur in hospital emergency departments and hospital outpatient departments. Figure 2.21 shows ambulatory care visits to physicians' offices, hospital outpatient departments, and emergency departments by gender and race. Females have more visits to all locations than do males. Whites have more visits to all sites overall and more to physicians' offices, whereas blacks have more visits per 100 persons to hospital outpatient departments and emergency departments.

(a)

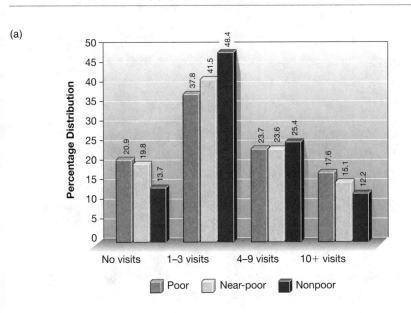

(b)

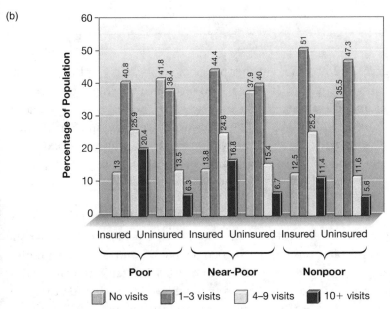

**FIGURE 2.20**
Health Services
Home Visits
and Visits to
Physicians'
Offices and
Emergency
Departments
Within the Past
12 Months
(2003)
(*a*) By poverty
status. (*b*) By
health insurance
status and
poverty status,
under age 65.

SOURCE: USDHHS 2005.

FIGURE 2.21
Ambulatory
Care Visits to
Physicians'
Offices,
Hospital
Outpatient
Departments,
and Emergency
Departments,
by Gender and
Race (2003)

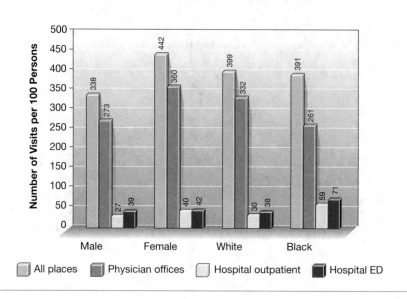

SOURCE: USDHHS 2005.

NOTE: ED = emergency department.

Figure 2.22 provides another perspective on visits to physicians—by type of insurance coverage (including no insurance coverage) for both the population under age 65 and that over age 65. The majority of the latter group is entitled to Medicare, the social insurance program, if they meet Medicare's eligibility criteria (see Chapter 3). As one would expect, a higher proportion of those with health insurance have physician contact in a 12-month period than those who are uninsured.

**Hospital Utilization**

Figures 2.23 through 2.26 show hospital utilization by age group, gender, race/ethnicity, income, and insurance status. One person in 13 under the age of 65 is hospitalized each year; people age 65 and older have higher hospitalization rates due to chronic conditions and failing health. More females than males, and more blacks than whites per thousand are hospitalized each year. As was true for physician contacts, people in lower income categories have higher rates of hospitalization than do those in higher income categories.

**Home Health Care Utilization**

Home health care has permitted many people with chronic illnesses and short- or long-term disabilities to avoid institutionalization by receiving health services in their homes. Until recently, home health care was the fastest growing Medicare-reimbursed service. Figure 2.27 shows home

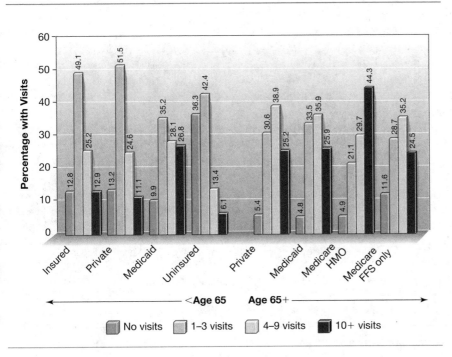

**FIGURE 2.22**
Health Care
Home Visits
and Visits to
Physicians'
Offices and
Emergency
Departments
Within the Past
12 Months, by
Health
Insurance
Status and Age
(2003)

SOURCE: USDHHS 2005.
NOTE: FFS = fee-for-service.

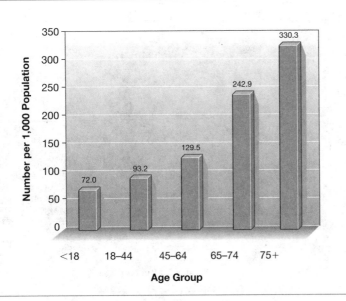

**FIGURE 2.23**
Discharges
from U.S.
Short-Stay
Hospitals, by
Age Group
(2003)

SOURCE: USDHHS 2005.

FIGURE 2.24
Discharges
from U.S.
Short-Stay
Hospitals, by
Age, Gender,
and Race/
Ethnicity
(2003)

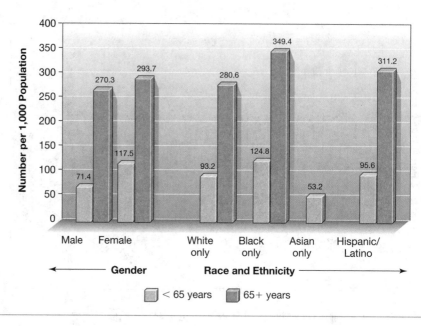

SOURCE: USDHHS 2005.

NOTE: Data for the Asian/Pacific Islander group are available only for the under-65 age group.

FIGURE 2.25
Discharges
from U.S.
Short-Stay
Hospitals, by
Poverty Status
and Age (2003)

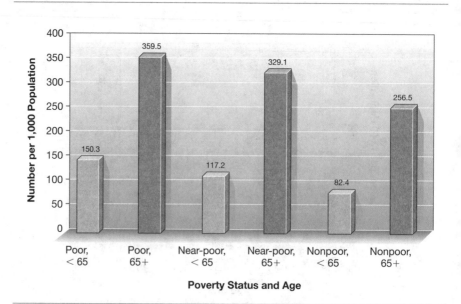

SOURCE: USDHHS 2005.

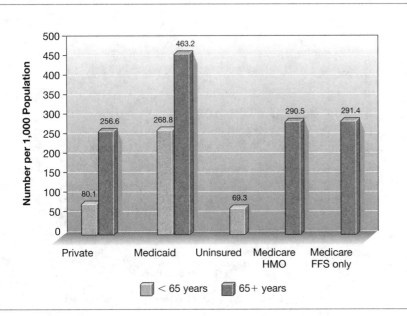

**FIGURE 2.26**
Discharges
from U.S.
Short-Stay
Hospitals, by
Insurance
Status and Age
Group (2003)

SOURCE: USDHHS 2005.

NOTE: FFS = fee-for-service.

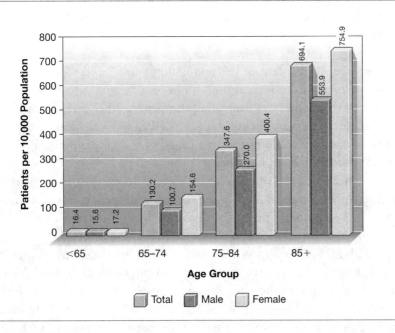

**FIGURE 2.27**
U.S. Home
Health Care
Patients,
According to
Age and
Gender (2000)

SOURCE: USDHHS 2002.

NOTES: Total home health care patients = 1,355,290. Group <65 is crude rate; other groups are age-adjusted.

FIGURE 2.28
U.S. Nursing
Home
Residents Age
65+, by
Gender and
Race (1999)

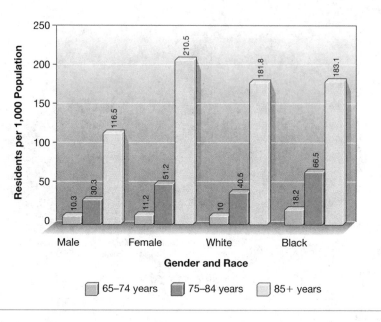

SOURCE: USDHHS 2001.

health care utilization in 2000, by age group and gender. More females
than males utilize home health services, due in part to females' greater
longevity.

**Nursing Home Utilization**

An estimated 4.5 percent of the population age 65 and older is in a nursing or personal care home, although not all of them remain there for the
duration of their lives (U.S. Bureau of the Census 2002). The sixth National
Nursing Home Survey was conducted in 1999 by the National Center for
Health Statistics (within the Centers for Disease Control and Prevention
[CDC]). Survey results indicate that the average length of stay for a discharge was 272 days (Jones 2002). Figure 2.28 shows the proportion of
the elderly, by age group, gender, and race, who were residents of nursing
or personal care homes in 1999. A seventh version of the survey was conducted in 2004, with data to be released sometime in 2006.

Although these aggregated data provide important encounter information, they neither inform of the range of physician visits per person, for
example, nor the number of rehospitalizations included in the hospital
utilization figure. More importantly, these data reflect only the usage of
services; they cannot inform of the unmet need for services due to access

or other barriers that people who needed services but could not obtain them faced.

## The Effects on Health Status of Receiving Health Services

Receiving health services is assumed to have an ameliorative effect on health status. For those services proven to be effective, positive outcomes are likely. Timely prenatal care, for example, is known to improve birth outcomes. Figure 2.29 shows the percentage of live births to mothers who began prenatal care in their first trimester of pregnancy for all mothers, white mothers, black mothers, and Hispanic-origin mothers for select years between 1970 and 2003. Figure 2.30 shows the percentage of mothers, by race, who either did not begin receiving care until the third trimester of their pregnancies or who received no care at all. Lower utilization of prenatal care in all trimesters of pregnancy is correlated with a lower percentage of live births.

Despite the significant advances in medical care, however, much remains to be learned. Long-recognized diseases such as polio, for example, are taking on new manifestations as the polio victim ages. Recently identified diseases such as HIV and the Ebola virus are not yet fully understood. We know little about the long-range effects of some interventions, and we still know too little about the patient outcomes for many therapies and treatments in current use. The number of studies of the outcomes of care is growing to expand our knowledge of the effects of health services on health status.

Receiving health services may, in certain instances, have pejorative effects on health status. Hospitalized patients may acquire nosocomial infections as a direct result of their hospitalizations. Patients may also develop iatrogenic illnesses, such as drug interactions, as a result of the treatments they receive.

It is important to remember that the receipt of health services is only one factor affecting health status. Roemer's determinants-of-health model shown in Figure 2.1 lists other factors, including genetic heritage, demographics, an individual's living and working environments, and the safety of the physical environment. Some posit that the overall health of a population, as well as individual health status, would be more improved by the provision of a guaranteed minimum income than by the provision of more health services. The effects of lifestyle and behavior, including violent behavior, on health status—many of which are outside the domain of the health services system—must also be acknowledged.

**FIGURE 2.29**
Prenatal Care
for U.S. Live
Births, by Race
and Hispanic
Origin of
Mother
(Select Years,
1970–2003),
First Trimester

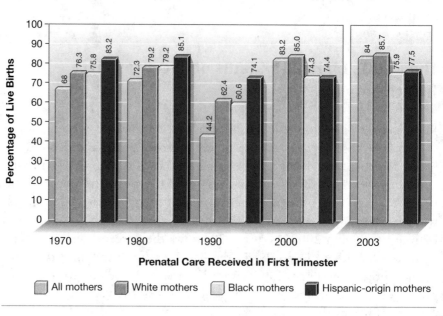

SOURCE: USDHHS 2005.

**FIGURE 2.30**
Prenatal Care
for U.S. Live
Births, by Race
and Hispanic
Origin of
Mother
(Select Years,
1970–2003),
Third Trimester

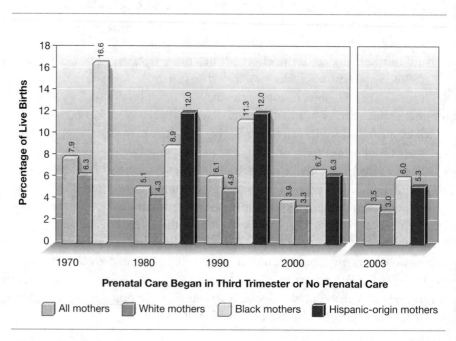

SOURCE: USDHHS 2005.

## Summary

Many factors affect the health of individuals and populations, including demographic factors (e.g., age, gender, and socioeconomic status), as well as access to and utilization of services. The U.S. population's health status, as measured by crude birth rates and fertility rates, birth weight, life expectancy, morbidity, and mortality, is graphed and, where possible, compared with status reported for other countries. Two models that attempt to explain health services utilization—the health belief model and the health behavior model—are explained, and the U.S. utilization of key health services is graphed. Although appropriate health services utilization can be important in maintaining personal health, it is possible to overutilize services in a way that can negatively affect health status.

## Key Words

acuity index
Acute Physiological and Chronic
    Health Evaluation (APACHE)
almshouses
baby boomer
Committee on the Costs of Medical
    Care (CCMC)
Comprehensive Health Planning
    (CHP) Act
Computerized Severity Index
determinants of health
disability-adjusted life years (DALYs)
disability days
disease
disease staging
fee-for-service delivery system
gross domestic product (GDP)
health
health behavior model
health belief model
health maintenance organization
    (HMO)
health outcomes
health status
iatrogenic illness

illness
life expectancy
managed care
Medicaid
medical-industrial complex
Medicare
morbidity
nosocomial infection
Organization for Economic Cooperation
    and Development (OECD)
Patient Management Categories (PMC)
poverty level
quality-adjusted life years (QALYs)
risk factors
self-assessed health
severity of disease
Sickness Impact Profile (SIP)
Social Security Act (SSA)
socioeconomic status (SES)
U.S. Department of Health,
    Education, and Welfare (DHEW)
U.S. Department of Health and
    Human Services (HHS)
World Health Organization (WHO)

# References

Aday, L. A., R. Andersen, and G. V. Fleming. 1980. *Health Care in the U.S.: Equitable for Whom?* Thousand Oaks, CA: Sage Publications.

Aiken, L. H., and M. E. Salmon. 1994. "Health Care Workforce Priorities: What Nursing Should Do Now." *Inquiry* 31 (3): 318–29.

Anderson, G., and J. R. Knickman. 1984. "Patterns of Expenditures among High Utilizers of Medical Care Services." *Medical Care* 22 (2): 143–49.

Blaum, C. S., J. Liang, and X. Liu. 1994. "The Relationship of Chronic Diseases and Health Status to the Health Services Utilization of Older Americans." *Journal of American Geriatrics Society* 42 (10): 1087–93.

Blendon, R. J., M. Brodie, J. M. Benson, D. E. Altman, L. Levit, T. Hoff, and L. Hugick. 1998. "Understanding the Managed Care Backlash." *Health Affairs* 17 (4): 80–94.

Carlisle, D. M., B. D. Leake, and M. F. Shapiro. 1995. "Racial and Ethnic Differences in the Use of Invasive Cardiac Procedures among Cardiac Patients in Los Angeles County, 1986 through 1988." *American Journal of Public Health* 85 (3): 352–56.

Cooper, R. A. 1995. "Perspectives on the Physician Workforce to the Year 2020." *Journal of the American Medical Association* 274 (19): 1534–43.

Jones, A. 2002. "The National Nursing Home Survey: 1999 Summary." *Vital Health Statistics* 13 (152): 1–116.

Kaplan, G. A., and T. Camacho. 1983. "A Nine-Year Follow-Up of the Human Population Laboratory Cohort." *American Journal of Epidemiology* 117 (3): 292–304.

LaRue, A., L Bank, L. Jarvik, and M. Hetland. 1979. "Health in Old Age: How Do Physicians' Ratings and Self-Ratings Compare?" *Journal of Gerontology* 34 (5): 687-91.

Levit, K., C. Smith, C. Cowan, H. Lazenby, and A. Martin. 2002. "Inflation Spurs Health Spending in 2000." *Health Affairs* 21 (1): 172–81.

May, L. A. 1993. "The Physiologic and Psychological Bases of Health, Disease, and Care Seeking." In *Introduction to Health Services,* 4th ed., edited by S. J. Williams and P. Torrens, 31–45. New York: Delmar.

Merson, M. H., R. E. Black, and A. J. Mills. 2001. *International Public Health: Diseases, Programs, Systems, and Policies.* Gaithersburg, MD: Aspen Publications.

Mullan, F., R. M. Politzer, and C. H. Davis. 1995. "Medical Migration and the Physician Workforce: International Medical Graduates and American Medicine." *Journal of the American Medical Association* 273 (19): 1521–27.

Patrick, D. L., and P. Erickson. 1993. *Health Status and Health Policy.* New York: Oxford University Press.

Relman, A. S. 1980. "The New Medical Industrial Complex." *The New England Journal of Medicine* 303 (17): 963–70.

Roemer, M. I. 1985. *National Strategies for Health Care Organization: A World Overview.* Chicago: Health Administration Press.

Rosenstock, I. M. 1974. "Historical Origins of the Health Belief Model." *Health Education Monograph* 2: 344.

Thomas, J. W., and M. L. Ashcraft. 1991. "Measuring Severity of Illness: Six Different Systems and Their Ability to Explain Cost Variations." *Inquiry* 28 (1): 39–55.

U.S. Census Bureau. 2002. "Older Americans Month Celebrated in May." [Online article or information (CB02-FF.07); retrieved 1/19/06.] www.Census.gov/Press-Release/www.releases/archives/facts_for_features_special_edition.

U.S. Department of Health and Human Services. 2005. *Health, United States, 2005.* Pub. No. (PHS) 2005-1232. Hyattsville, MD: USDHHS.

———. 2004. *Health, United States, 2004.* Pub. No. (PHS) 2004-1232. Hyattsville, MD: USDHHS.

———. 2002. *Health, United States, 2002.* Pub. No. (PHS) 2002–1232. Hyattsville, MD: USDHHS.

———. 2001. *Health, United States, 2001.* Pub. No. (PHS) 2001–1232. Hyattsville, MD: USDHHS.

———. 1990. *Seventh Report to the President and Congress on the Status of Health Personnel in the United States.* Pub. No. HRS-P-OD-90-3. October. Washington, DC: USDHHS.

Wolinsky, F. D., and R. J. Johnson. 1992. "Perceived Health Status and Mortality in Older Men and Women." *Journal of Gerontology* 47 (6): 5304–12.

World Health Organization/Health Promotion. 1999. "Ottawa Charter for Health Promotion." [Online information; retrieved 1/27/03.] www.who.int/hpr/archive/docs/ottawa.html.

# ACCESS TO HEALTH SERVICES

## Introduction

Until the breakup of the Soviet Union, only two major industrialized countries—South Africa and the United States—did not provide universal access to health services. Neither South Africa nor the United States has a national health system such as Canada's or a national health service such as Great Britain's to provide a basic set of services to their entire populations. In the free-market economy of the United States, health services are among many goods and services that individuals are generally expected to provide for themselves. Despite years of debate about whether its citizens have a right to health services, the U.S. system assures only the right to emergency care in most hospitals under certain circumstances. Medicare beneficiaries are also entitled to inpatient hospital care, hospice services, and home health care.

This chapter discusses how people in the United States, in the absence of a national health system or service, obtain access to care and also focuses on the care seeker's access to a provider. Issues of access among providers also exist (e.g., a generalist's access to a specialist, or a provider's access to backup support, rehabilitation, or long-term care services for patient referrals) but are beyond the scope of this book.

## Defining Access

The term *access* connotes different things to analysts of health services. To Penchansky and Thomas (1981), access is the measure of fit between characteristics of providers and health services, and characteristics and expectations of clients, incorporating five reasonably distinct dimensions: availability, accessibility, accommodation, affordability, and acceptability.[1] Access may describe the entry into or use of services. Access may also be defined by factors influencing entry or use of services. For purposes of this discussion, the latter definition of access is employed.

Access to care has a direct bearing on the two other important dimensions of the health services system: cost/expenditures and quality. Increasing access to health services can actually decrease unit costs in some instances but inevitably increases expenditures. Limited or no access to care can

FIGURE 3.1

Dimensions of
Access to
Health Services

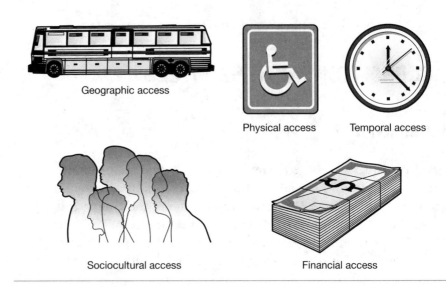

Geographic access

Physical access          Temporal access

Sociocultural access          Financial access

decrease a person's health status and quality of life, but excessive access can also be detrimental.

As Figure 3.1 indicates, access to care has many dimensions: geographic, physical, temporal, sociocultural, and financial. *Geographic access* is influenced by where the care seeker lives in relationship to where the provider practices. A full range of medical services is unlikely to be available in a coastal village in Alaska, a mountain mining town in Nevada, or a rural farming community in the Midwest, even though physician-to-patient ratios suggest that physician supply is adequate to serve the population. Medical care is most likely to be found where a population base and related services to support it exist. Those who live outside such areas may have to travel considerable distances, often over difficult terrain and through imposing weather, to reach care. Transportation is a factor in geographic access. Public transportation systems do not serve all areas where people live, and private transportation may not be available to the care seeker.

*Physical access* to care is influenced by the care seeker's physical mobility and mental competence in reaching a provider, as well as by the ease of access to the provider's facility. Today's system of health services usually requires that the care seeker be present to the provider. In-home services, while growing, still do not typically include home visits by physicians for routine care. The ease of access to a provider's facility has been assisted by the Americans with Disabilities Act (ADA) of 1990, which recommends appropriate access and imposes sanctions for noncompliance. Another potential way to increase access to a provider is through the use of telemedicine and through remote monitoring of chronic diseases. Such mechanisms have not yet begun to reach their full potential (Freed and Grigsby 2002).

*Temporal access* may be inhibited when, because of an inflexible work schedule, the unavailability of care for young and old dependents, or other time constraints, a care seeker is unable to obtain care during the hours it is provided. Temporal barriers may also include waiting or queue times between the request for an appointment and the provider's availability.

Multicultural societies such as the United States experience *socio-cultural* barriers to access. The provider and care seeker may speak different languages or may come from differing cultures that value health services in quite disparate ways and employ conflicting customs and beliefs. These differences may inhibit an individual from seeking needed care because of the frustrations inherent in communicating or may prevent the care seeker from obtaining the full benefits of the recommended treatment because of the potential for misunderstandings.

*Financial access* to health services in the United States is largely governed by the individual's access to health insurance coverage—either private insurance or public or social insurance.[2] Health insurance, addressed more fully in Chapter 6, became the dominant payment mechanism for health services in the last half of the twentieth century. This trend stems from the growth of private health insurance coverage during and immediately following World War II and the establishment of public or social health insurance in the mid-1960s. In addition to private and public health insurance, financial access to health services is attained by private payment, by qualifying for government-sponsored programs, or through the provision of charity care.

Given these varying dimensions of access, what factors affect an individual's ability to access health services in the U.S. system? This question is explored by examination of the model in Figure 3.2. This model was adapted from one developed by the congressional Office of Technology Assessment (OTA), based on work done by Ron Andersen, LuAnn Aday, and other researchers in the utilization of health services.[3] Factors affecting health that may not be influenced by access to personal health services are considered briefly. Three types of factors—predisposing, need, and enabling—that potentially affect access are then examined. Finally, the potential adverse health outcomes associated with both lack of access to care and unconstrained access to care are considered.

## Factors Affecting Access to Health Services

Some factors affecting an individual's health status may not be influenced by access to personal health services. Figure 3.2 identifies three such factors: (1) individual factors, (2) the physical environment, and (3) the social environment. Individual factors include inherited (i.e., genetic) characteristics and individual behaviors that reflect a person's beliefs, attitudes, and

**FIGURE 3.2**

Factors
Affecting
Access to
Health Services

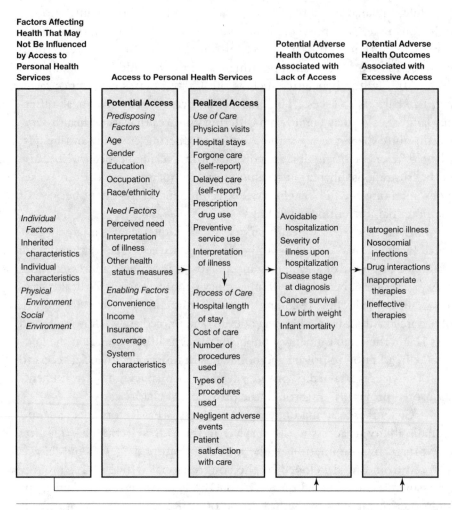

SOURCE: Adapted from OTA 1992.

values. Physical environmental factors include air and water quality, as well as the presence or absence of disease vectors. A person's friends and social relationships are examples of societal environmental factors that may not be influenced by access to personal health services.

### Predisposing Factors

As shown in Figure 3.2, predisposing, need, and enabling factors affect potential access. These factors vary in their importance in affecting access, and they do not operate independently; rather, their effect is interactive in influencing access.

Predisposing factors are an individual's demographic characteristics: age, gender, education, occupation, and race/ethnicity. The two ends of the age spectrum—the young and the old—often require increased access to services. Because these age groups are often dependent on others to secure their care, access may be directly affected by their ability to get assistance in obtaining care.

Gender also influences access to care. For example, females of child-bearing age are likely to access health services more frequently than their male counterparts. Gender may also affect participation in clinical research studies. Criticism has been directed at the National Institutes of Health (NIH) for supporting large-scale research studies that limited their investigations to male subjects, even though the studied condition affected both genders (Finnegan 1996). NIH has made strides in correcting this imbalance.

Educational levels influence access. People with higher educational levels more frequently access health services.

A person's occupation may affect access in several ways. First, a hazardous occupation, such as mining, puts one at greater risk for injuries and some types of illness (e.g., black lung disease), requiring more frequent contact with the health services system. Second, a person's occupation has a direct influence on income and health insurance status, two enabling factors covered later in this discussion.

Finally, a person's race and ethnicity may affect access in several ways. Some diseases—Tay Sachs or sickle-cell anemia, for example—affect only certain racial or ethnic groups. Racial and ethnic groups may also face cultural barriers or discriminatory practices that affect their ability to access health services.

## Need Factors

A range of need factors—perceived health, interpretation of illness, and other health status measures—affect access to care. Numerous studies have shown that individuals who perceive their health status as fair or poor are more likely to access care (McCall et al. 1991; Short and Lair 1994/95), assuming they have the financial means to do so. A patient's understanding and interpretation of his or her illness affects access. Health status measures such as levels of disability and functioning also affect access to care.

## Enabling Factors

The third category of factors affecting potential access—the enabling factors—constitutes the major focus for the remainder of this section. Enabling factors include convenience, income, insurance coverage, and system characteristics. Convenience embodies temporal, geographic, and physical dimensions of access, as discussed earlier. Individuals' income directly affects their financial access and frequency of access to health services, and also influences whether they have private health insurance coverage. Private and public insurance coverage is the major route of financial access to health services in the United States. Although health insurance is explored comprehensively in Chapter 6, an overview of its effects on access follows. This section concludes with a discussion of other characteristics of the U.S. health services system affecting access—principally, the availability of governmental and other programs that provide access to special populations. Following the discussion of these enabling factors, the problems of people who lack financial access to care are addressed.

## Financial Access to Health Services

Private insurance and public or social insurance are first discussed as means of financial access to health services. Private payment (out-of-pocket payment) for health services is then addressed. Finally, the important role of government-sponsored programs, such as the U.S. Department of Veterans Affairs (VA) system and the military system of health services, is described.

### *Private Health Insurance*
Private health insurance is the greatest source of health insurance coverage for people under age 65. Medicare, discussed in the next section, provides public or social insurance for the majority of people who are age 65 and older, as well as for people with certain types of disabilities, including end-stage renal disease (ESRD). In 2003, 68.9 percent of the population under the age of 65 reported some form of private health insurance coverage (U.S. Department of Health and Human Services [USDHHS] 2005). Figure 3.3 shows the percentage of the population with private health insurance by age, gender, race/ethnicity, and various poverty levels. Children under age 18 below the federal poverty level had the lowest insurance coverage rates of any of these demographic groups.

Two types of private health insurance are available in the United States: individually purchased policies, which are usually limited in coverage and relatively expensive to purchase, and insurance provided as one of the benefits of employment. Employer-sponsored insurance is generally more comprehensive in scope because the risk of insuring is spread over a group of employees and because those in the workforce are generally healthier than those of working age who are not in the workforce and are not the dependents of an insured worker. Group insurance is thus less expensive per person than individual policies. In most cases, employers and employees

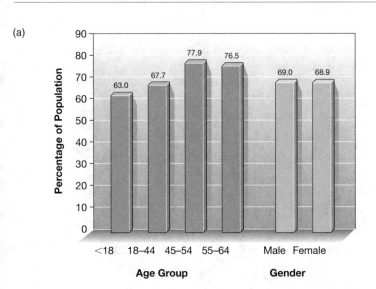

(a)

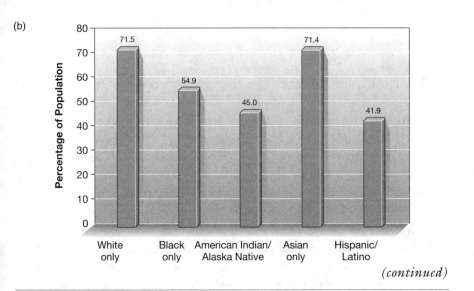

(b)

(continued)

**FIGURE 3.3**
Private Health
Insurance
among Persons
<65 Years of
Age (2003)
(*a*) By age
group and
gender. (*b*) By
race/ethnicity.
(*c*) By federal
poverty level
(FPL).

share the cost of this insurance. Many employers are beginning to shift a greater proportion of these costs to their employees.

Individual policies are purchased by people who can afford them, who may be self-employed, who work in industries such as mining or fishing in which insurance is difficult to obtain, or who otherwise do not have access to a group health insurance policy. Individual high-deductible policies may also be purchased by people who do not anticipate much utilization of health

FIGURE 3.3
Continued

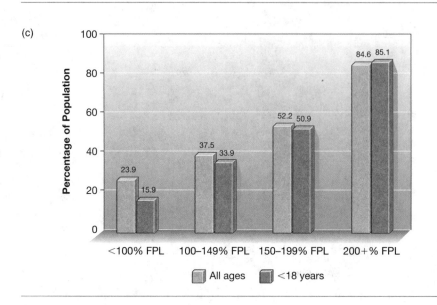

(c)

SOURCE: USDHHS 2005.

services but want the security of catastrophic coverage. Individual policies often impose stringent limitations for preexisting conditions.

About 63 percent of the nonelderly who have health insurance are likely to have insurance as a benefit of employment, either as the employee or as the dependent of an insured employee. Health insurance provided as a benefit of employment varies by size of firm, type of industry, the employee's work status (full-time or part-time), and other factors. Midsize to larger firms (100 or more employees) typically offer one or more types of health insurance coverage to their full-time workers, whereas smaller firms (25 or fewer employees) may not offer health insurance as a benefit. Certain industries, such as farming, logging, floral businesses, and interior design—viewed as high risk by insurers because of the potential for physical injury or the perceived high-risk lifestyles of the employees—may typically not offer health insurance as a benefit (U.S. Bipartisan Commission 1990). Many employers, regardless of firm size, do not offer health insurance to contingent, seasonal, or part-time workers.

Private health insurance coverage for the nonelderly varies by race/ethnicity: a greater proportion of whites than nonwhites are more likely to be insured (Figure 3.4), and a greater proportion are likely to have employment-related insurance (66 percent versus 52 percent). As a bridge to the next section on public health insurance, Figure 3.5 shows the percentage of the U.S. population that had any kind of health insurance coverage in 2004.

(a)

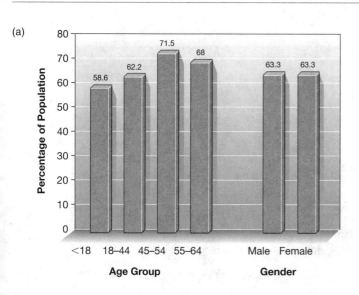

(b)

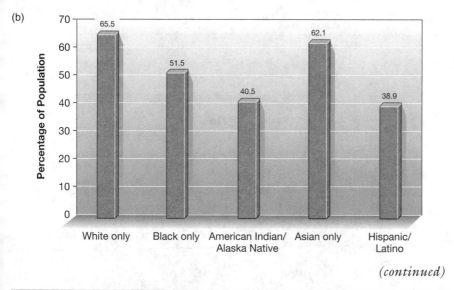

*(continued)*

**FIGURE 3.4**
Private Health
Insurance
Obtained
Through the
Workplace,
<65 Years of
Age (2003)
*(a)* By age
group and
gender. *(b)* By
race/ethnicity.
*(c)* By federal
poverty level
(FPL).

## Public or Social Health Insurance

Many consider Medicare and Medicaid, two government-supported programs initiated as amendments to the Social Security Act (SSA, titles XVIII
and XIX, respectively) in 1965 and implemented the following year, to be
public insurance programs. Both are entitlement programs, meaning that
eligible individuals have a legislative entitlement to all the covered services
they require. Only the Medicare program really fits an insurance model and
was designed to conform to the structure of private health insurance. Because

**FIGURE 3.4**
Continued

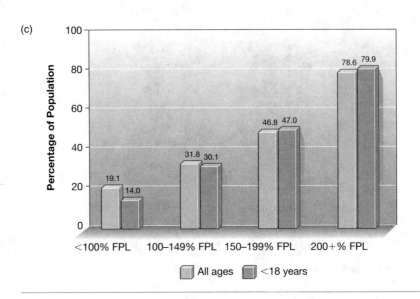

SOURCE: USDHHS 2005.

**FIGURE 3.5**
Health
Insurance
Coverage, All
Ages (2004)

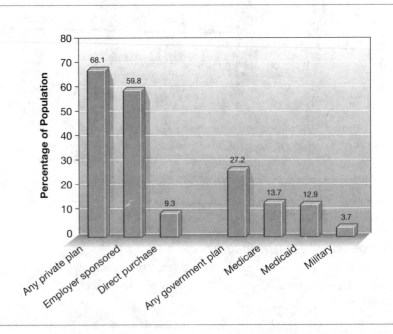

SOURCE: U.S. Census Bureau 2005.

the programs are so frequently compared—and confused—both are discussed in this section.

The Medicare and Medicaid programs, a legacy of President Lyndon Johnson's Great Society, resulted from compromises following the failure to enact some form of national health insurance (Anderson 1968). Medicare was intended to provide mandatory hospitalization benefits (Part A) to qualified beneficiaries, and optional physician services and outpatient coverage (Part B) to beneficiaries who could afford the monthly premium. Medicare beneficiaries initially were persons age 65 and over, which was retirement age in that era; later amendments included people with ESRD (1972) and long-term disabilities (1973).

The Medicaid program, a welfare program, was established to pay for a mandated set of health services to low-income children and their caretakers who were the recipients of, or eligible to receive, public assistance funds from the Aid to Families with Dependent Children (AFDC) program or the Supplemental Security Income (SSI) program.[4] The Medicaid program has been amended over time to include people who have developmental disabilities (1972) and to expand eligibility to other low-income groups, including children, pregnant women, and the elderly. The Personal Responsibility and Work Opportunity Reconciliation Act (PL 104-93) of 1996 replaced the AFDC program with the Temporary Assistance for Needy Families (TANF) program.

Although the Medicare and Medicaid programs were established in the same congressional session and were intended to provide health services access to the two ends of the population spectrum—the elderly and children with their adult caretakers—the programs differ widely in their requirements for eligibility, covered benefits, financing, and proportion of the population each covers. These differences are illustrated in Table 3.1 and discussed in more detail in Chapter 6.

## Private Payment for Health Services

Private, out-of-pocket payment for health services is another way in which a person obtains financial access to care. Private out-of-pocket payment includes payment for all health services expenditures by uninsured people who can afford to do so. It also includes payment for health services not covered by private, public, or social health insurance and payment for the deductibles, copayments (set dollar amounts), and co-insurances (percentages of total charges) that various insurance companies require. (Premiums are not usually considered out-of-pocket payments in the calculation of the National Health Accounts.) Out-of-pocket payments constitute an important revenue source for financing health services. In 2004, 13 percent of health services revenues came from private out-of-pocket payments (see Chapter 7).

TABLE 3.1
Comparison
of Medicare
and Medicaid
Programs

|  | Medicare | Medicaid |
|---|---|---|
| *Eligibility* | Age 65+<br>Disabled persons<br>End-stage renal disease<br>Retired railroad employees | Categorical welfare<br>  (AFDC, SSI)*<br>Persons living with AIDS<br>Low-income pregnant women<br>Low-income children<br>Low-income elderly |
| *Financing* | Part A:<br>  Employer/employee<br>    contributions<br>  Copayments and deductibles<br><br>Part B:<br>  Premiums<br>  Deductible<br>  General revenue (federal funds)<br>Part C: Medicare Advantage<br>    (formerly Medicare+Choice)<br>  Capitation payment funded by<br>    Part A Trust Fund and Part B account<br>Part D: Outpatient prescription<br>    drug coverage<br>  Premiums and general revenue<br>    (federal funds) | 50% federal funds<br>  (at minimum)<br>50% or less state funds<br>Limited copayments<br>  (cost sharing) |
| *Benefits* | Part A:<br>  Hospital inpatient<br>  Skilled nursing facility care<br>  Home health care<br>  Hospice<br>Part B (optional):<br>  Physician services<br>  Outpatient services<br><br>Part C: Medicare Advantage<br>    (formerly Medicare+Choice)<br>Part D: Outpatient prescription<br>    drug coverage | Hospital (inpatient and<br>  outpatient)<br>Rural health clinic<br>Laboratory<br>X-ray<br>Skilled nursing facility,<br>  age 21+<br>Home health care<br>EPSDT<br>Physician services<br>Family planning<br>Nurse midwife (where<br>  permitted) |
| *Population Covered* | 39 million persons, including<br>  5 million persons with disabilities | 40.6 million persons |
| *Means Test* | None required | Income and asset limits |

*Medicaid eligibility may differ from state to state, depending on how the state redefines the linkage between welfare programs and Medicaid eligibility as a result of the Personal Responsibility and Work Opportunity Reconciliation Act of 1996.

NOTES: AFDC = Aid to Families with Dependent Children; EPSDT = Early and Periodic Screening, Diagnosis, and Treatment Program; SSI = Supplemental Security Income.

## Government-Sponsored Programs That Provide Access to Health Services

A range of government-supported health programs provide direct access to health services for special populations. A select set of these programs, including the U.S. Department of Veterans Affairs system, Department of Defense programs (including TRICARE), the Indian Health Service, and the prison health services system, are discussed in the sections that follow.

The U.S. Department of Veterans Affairs (VA) health services system, established in 1921 as the U.S. Veterans Bureau (Shonick 1995) to provide inpatient, outpatient, and long-term care services to veterans with military-service–connected conditions, provides care through a system of 172 hospitals and 381 community-based outpatient clinics (Maciejewski and Chapko 2002). Some states have several VA hospitals; others, such as Alaska, have none.

    VA health services facilities provide care to an important segment of the U.S. population and serve as training sites for medical students and residents. In 1972, in what was perceived as an era of physician shortages, the VA linked with other organizations to establish eight new medical schools to increase the supply of physicians.

    Congress, given the declining number of eligible veterans and the unused capacity at many VA hospital facilities, periodically questions the future of the VA system. Proposals to expand VA services to include dependents of veterans, to serve other community members, or to dismantle the VA system have been discussed at the congressional level but have not yet reached legislative status. With the advancing technologies to treat war wounds and injuries, the VA system has a new focus in treating veterans of military actions in Afghanistan and Iraq.

**U.S. Department of Veterans Affairs System**

The Department of Defense (DOD) is an important provider of health services to active military members and their dependents. The army, navy, and air force each operates its own medical services, and the DOD operates eight "tri-service" joint medical facilities that serve the army, air force, and navy. TRICARE serves more than nine million beneficiaries in 76 military hospitals and 460 clinics around the world that are referred to as military treatment facilities (MTFs) (TRICARE 2002; U.S. Government Accountability Office [USGAO] 2005a). Contractual services are negotiated with the private sector in places where no military facilities exist. A medical school to train physicians for military service—the Uniformed Services University of the Health Sciences—was established in 1972.

    Military dependents and retirees, and their dependents and survivors, receive health services through TRICARE, formerly known as the Civilian

**Department of Defense Health Services**

Health and Medical Program of the Uniformed Services (CHAMPUS), an insurance program whose origins date back to the Emergency Maternal and Infant Child Care Program (EMIC) established in 1943 (Shonick 1995). The DOD requires considerable cost sharing of its TRICARE enrollees and uses managed care as one way to project and better manage expenditures for military dependents and retirees.

**Indian Health Service**

The Indian Health Service (IHS), first established as a unit of the War Department in 1802 (Shonick 1995), and now a part of the U.S. Department of Health and Human Services (HHS), provides health services to an estimated 1.5 million of the estimated 2.6 million American Indians and Alaska Natives enrolled in more than 557 tribes, villages, bands, and pueblos throughout the United States. IHS maintains 49 hospitals and 364 health centers in a number of states for its beneficiaries, but may also contract with the private sector for provision of services to individuals who live outside the service areas of these facilities (IHS 2002; USGAO 2005b). Through the Indian Self-Determination Act of 1975, many tribal authorities have assumed responsibility for the provision of health services, contracting with IHS for the funds to support the development and implementation of tribal-specific health plans.

**Prison Health Services**

No group within the U.S. population has a constitutionally established right to health services. Prison inmates, however, are described by some as having the nearest thing to a constitutional right to care of any population group. This description stems from the provision of services that has resulted from inmate lawsuits claiming the right to care under the auspices of the Eighth Amendment to the U.S. Constitution, which prohibits "cruel and unusual punishment."

Inmates in federal and state prison systems receive government-funded health services that vary in extent and coverage by individual facility.[5] Prisons may have staff physicians on site, contract for physician services on an as-needed basis with nearby communities, maintain on-site clinics staffed by midlevel practitioners, provide care through the use of telemedicine, or arrange for health services in other ways. Few prisons maintain full-scale inpatient hospital facilities; they obtain such services from nearby communities on an as-needed basis. Dental services may also be provided according to a variety of arrangements.

Correctional facility administrators are concerned about the increasing demand and expenditures for health services due to the aging of the prison population, with more inmates receiving and serving longer sentences. Additional concerns include the incidence of HIV positivity and

AIDS, the increase in tuberculosis and other communicable diseases, the prevalence of chronic diseases in an aging population, the prevalence of mental illnesses, and other serious health problems in an incarcerated population.

## Potential Adverse Outcomes Associated with Lack of Access or Unconstrained Access to Health Services

The access-to-health-services model (Figure 3.2) incorporates the potential adverse health outcomes associated with lack of access and excessive access. Having financial access to health services directly affects care-seeking behavior. A lack of health insurance is associated with reduced access to medical care, a lower prevalence of recommended preventive services, potentially avoidable hospitalizations, and subsequently higher mortality independent of other risk factors (Franks, Clancey, and Gold 1993). Uninsured adults and children have fewer provider visits than people with insurance. Uninsured adults use about one-half of the nonemergency ambulatory visits, two-thirds or fewer emergency department visits, and a much smaller fraction of inpatient hospital days—12 percent for men and 20 percent for women—than their insured counterparts. While uninsured children appear to use emergency care on a par with insured children, they still use only 70 percent as much nonambulatory care and are only 25 percent as likely as children with insurance to enter a hospital (Spillman 1992). Children with health insurance gaps are at increased risk of having more than one care site (Kogan et al. 1995), thus jeopardizing continuity of care. They are less likely to receive medical care from a physician, even when it seems reasonably indicated, and are at risk for substantial avoidable morbidity (Stoddard, St. Peter, and Newacheck 1994).

Table 3.2, taken from a 1993 study by Davis et al. (1995), shows that 71 percent of those without insurance postponed seeking care and 34 percent went without care because of financial reasons, in contrast to 23 percent of people with insurance postponing care and 9 percent with insurance going without care because of financial reasons. In a 1992 report, the OTA reported that the uninsured are more than three times as likely as those with private insurance to experience a lower utilization of services, potentially worse health services, and adverse outcomes. The OTA also reported that people with public insurance (Medicaid in particular) are up to two and one-half times more likely than those with private insurance to experience potentially inadequate health services and four times more likely to have an adverse outcome.

Since these seminal studies were reported, others have continued to document the effects of lack of health insurance on health status. A

TABLE 3.2
Effects of
Insurance on
Obtaining
Health Services
(1993)

| | Percentage Insured | Percentage Uninsured | Percentage Total U.S. Population |
|---|---|---|---|
| Postponed seeking care | 23 | 71 | 30 |
| Going without care because of financial reasons | 9 | 34 | 13 |

SOURCE: Davis et al. 1995.

study by Ayanian et al. (2000) showed that a significantly higher proportion of those who were uninsured for more than one year could not see a physician because of the cost and had no routine checkup within the last two years compared to those who were uninsured less than one year or who had not lost insurance. The Institute of Medicine (IOM) is currently examining the issue and has issued three of a planned series of six reports on the problems of the uninsured in the United States. Members of an expert panel are examining findings from more than 130 research studies. In the report "Care Without Coverage: Too Little, Too Late," issued in May 2002, the IOM reported that adult health status changes when adults remain uninsured: adults in late middle age (especially between ages 55–65) and adults with low incomes are especially susceptible to deteriorating health if they never had or they lost health coverage (IOM 2002). A study by Baker et al. (2002) corroborates the IOM findings: adults ages 51–61 who lost all health insurance were at increased risk of major declines in overall health and had increased risks of developing a new mobility difficulty within two years of their health insurance coverage losses.

Although it seems a smaller problem when compared to the magnitude of the uninsured population whose access to care is limited, unconstrained access to care may also contribute to, rather than alleviate, health problems. Iatrogenic (physician-induced) illness and nosocomial (hospital-acquired) infections may occur as a result of treatment. Adverse drug interactions are more likely when a patient's treatment by a range of providers is not coordinated. Despite their widespread use, not all therapies have been proven to be effective. Between one-quarter and one-third of care given to insured people in the United States falls in the inappropriate or equivocal area in which medical benefit does not exceed its risk (Brook 1991). Andrew Booth, with contributions from others, provides a resource guide that analyzes 18 studies to assess what proportion of medical practice is evidence-based (www.shef.ac.uk/scharr/ir/percent.html).

## Access to Health Services for the Uninsured

An estimated 96 percent of people age 65 and older have financial access to health services through the Medicare program, and nearly 84 percent of the population younger than 65 access health services through private health insurance, Medicaid, Medicare (for people with disabilities under age 65 and those with ESRD), private out-of-pocket payments, or government-sponsored programs such as the VA system (USDHHS 2002; Iglehart 2002).

How do people not covered by these programs—an estimated 16 percent of the population younger than 65—get health services when they need them? Who are the uninsured? What are some reasons why people are uninsured? This section addresses these questions.

People who have no health insurance, limited ability to pay out-of-pocket, and limited or no access to other governmental health programs may access care from public hospitals and clinics; neighborhood, community, or migrant health centers; or clinics established by charitable organizations or other volunteers that provide low-cost or no-cost care. Although many of these facilities and the providers who staff them offer comprehensive care, patients may not always be able to avail themselves of it. Thus, such sites may serve as stopgaps, providing urgent or emergency outpatient care, rather than the comprehensive care that a person with insured access to the system can experience. Individuals seeking care in hospital emergency departments are likely to get such care if their situations are truly emergent or to be referred to more appropriate care, in large part because hospitals participating in the Medicare program are required to provide emergency care, regardless of the patient's ability to pay. Such patients constitute a significant economic burden to hospitals, particularly public hospitals, whose provision of charity care (also called uncompensated care or bad-debt care) may jeopardize their ability to remain financially viable.

Physicians and other providers often provide free or pro bono care to a limited number of patients. Clinics, particularly in inner-city areas, may be established as "free clinics," providing basic care to all who seek their services, to the extent that their resources permit them to do so. Such clinics may be staffed by volunteer providers, with supplies and other services donated by community members or underwritten by community institutions. Helpful as these free clinics are, they cannot begin to replace a regular source of care for everyone who needs it.

### Demographic Characteristics of the Uninsured

Who are the uninsured? Figure 3.6 shows the proportion of the population that is uninsured, by age, gender, race/ethnicity, and poverty level status. The 18- to 44-year-old age group has the highest proportion of uninsured persons. American Indians and Alaska Natives have the highest proportion of uninsured

**FIGURE 3.6**
No Health
Insurance
Coverage
among Persons
<65 Years
(2003)
(*a*) By age
group and
gender. (*b*) By
race/ethnicity.
(*c*) By federal
poverty level
(FPL).

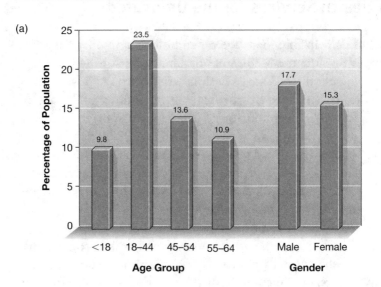

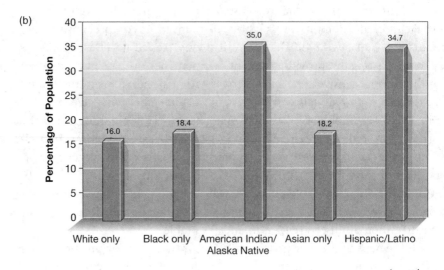

(*continued*)

persons (35 percent), followed closely by those of Hispanic/Latino ethnicity at 34.7 percent. Rates of uninsurance decrease with increases in income.

### Reasons Why People Lack Health Insurance

Individuals lack health insurance for many reasons. They may not have access to employer-sponsored health insurance either because their employer does not offer it or because they are not in the workforce. They may not be able to afford the premiums of an individual health insurance policy. They may

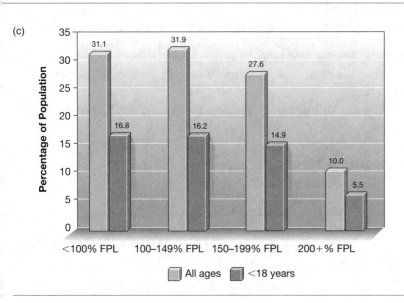

FIGURE 3.6
Continued

(c)

SOURCE: USDHHS 2005.

not qualify for Medicare or Medicaid or be eligible for other government-supported health programs, such as military care.

One sometimes-overlooked reason that individuals lack health insurance is that they decline employer-sponsored coverage. Cooper and Schone (1997) found an 8.2 percentage point decrease in the number of workers who accepted health insurance between 1987 and 1996. They attribute this decline to a number of factors, including declining real incomes, especially among workers who are the least likely to have coverage (e.g., healthy young males in the workforce); increasing costs of insurance; rising employee contributions to health insurance premiums; and expansions in Medicaid coverage.

### Initiatives to Expand Financial Access to Health Services

Despite the fact that arranging for financial access to health services has largely been left to the individual, with the exception of Medicare beneficiaries who have assured access, the public periodically expresses concern that more than one-sixth of the U.S. population has no health insurance and thus has limited access to care. Recommendations for national health insurance were introduced as early as the Roosevelt administration in 1935 (Litman and Robins 1991) and again in 1993 with the unsuccessful Health Security Act (HSA). Such proposals failed for a variety of reasons—not the least of which is the likely increase in federal expenditures to support them.

A range of other proposals, each of which is briefly described in the sections that follow, have been offered in the last several decades, including:

- expanding the Medicare program to include other beneficiaries;
- expanding the Medicaid program to include even more of the uninsured;
- providing health insurance coverage to special populations, such as children;
- creating a single-payer system similar to that in Canada;
- creating risk pools for the uninsurable; and
- establishing statewide health insurance programs.

At the federal level, the Medicaid program has been expanded to cover more of the uninsured (see Appendix 6.2 in Chapter 6), the State Children's Health Insurance Program was established in 1997, some states have created risk pools for the uninsurable, and a number of states have established statewide health insurance programs. These changes are addressed in Chapter 6.

**Expanding Medicare**    The 1993 HSA was one of several proposals to expand eligibility to Medicare. The HSA proposed adding a Part C to Medicare that would provide coverage to many of the uninsured. Expenditure projections and a distaste for a larger governmental role in health services contributed to the defeat of this bill. A different Part C, the Medicare+Choice plan (discussed in Chapters 6 and 19), was added to Title XVIII by the 1997 Balanced Budget Act and has since been replaced by the Medicare Advantage program established by the 2003 Medicare Prescription Drug Improvement and Modernization Act (MMA).

**Expanding Medicaid**    Although a broader expansion of Medicaid eligibility has been discussed at the national level, the only action on this idea is occurring at the state level. After years of grassroots development, the state of Oregon was granted a waiver from the Health Care Financing Administration (HCFA—now the Centers for Medicare and Medicaid Services [CMS]) to initiate the Oregon Health Plan, which enrolls people whose incomes are below 100 percent of poverty into the Medicaid program, even if they are not categorically eligible. Oregon proposed even more comprehensive coverage through its state plan, but Oregon voters rejected this expansion in the fall 2002 elections. In January 1994, the state of Tennessee replaced its Medicaid program with TennCare to cover more of the low-income uninsured. Managed care organizations (MCOs) and behavioral health organizations (BHOs) provided care to enrollees through three products: TennCare Medicaid, TennCare Standard, and TennCare Assist (TennCare 2003). The Oregon and Tennessee programs are examples of Medicaid expansions; a number of other states have established similar expansions or are piloting such expansions.

In 1997 Congress added Title XXI to the Social Security Act, creating the State Children's Health Insurance Program (SCHIP), which provided $40 billion in matching funds to states over ten years to support health insurance coverage for children. States could choose to expand their Medicaid programs, start or augment a separate insurance program for children, or devise a hybrid of these strategies (Demkovich 1997).

**Providing Health Insurance Coverage for Children**

Twenty-one states chose to expand their Medicaid programs, 12 to have separate SCHIP programs, and 21 to operate combination programs. Despite slow enrollment starts in many SCHIP programs, by the end of March 2005, 4.4 million children had been enrolled in the SCHIP program at some point during the prior fiscal year (CMS web site). Since 1997, Congress has changed how the SCHIP funds are allocated; between 2002 and 2004, states experienced a 26 percent decline in the amount of federal funds available to them (Ryan 2002).

Canada's health services system, in which the government serves as the single payer for care, has been proposed as a model for the U.S. system to emulate. The Canadian system achieves a comparable—and some would claim a higher—health status at significantly lower per capita expenditures. The likelihood of the United States following Canada's lead seems slim for several reasons. One reason is the difference in roles that the health insurance industry holds in the two systems: in the United States, the health insurance industry has been a dominant influence on how the system has developed, whereas the Canadian system has no major counterpart to the U.S. industry. Additionally, the Canadian system, under considerable pressure to change because of increasing expenditures and an oversupply of physicians, imposed controls on physician training and practice sites, the availability of hospital beds, and other services in the late 1990s. More recently, an improving economy and belt tightening by the Canadian federal government has led to the development of budget surpluses. Workforce planning has shifted to programs that encourage increasing the education slots available for nursing and medical students (Canadian Institute for Health Care 2002).

**Creating a Single-Payer System**

The unsuccessful 1993 HSA proposed several reforms to the health insurance industry, including the establishment of uniform billing and the streamlining of other administrative procedures. Although Congress did not enact the sweeping reforms proposed by the HSA, incremental changes in the industry are occurring. The 1996 Health Insurance Portability and Accountability Act (HIPAA) makes retaining coverage easier for insured people when they leave a job (portability); establishes federal insurance requirements for carriers offering coverage in the individual, small-group, and large-group markets; and imposes specific insurance reforms on self-funded health insurance plans (see Chapter 6).

**Reforming the Health Insurance Industry**

**Creating Risk Pools for Uninsurables**

Thirty states have established subsidized health insurance plans for people with chronic conditions or other risk factors that have made them uninsurable (Gates 2002). Health insurance from a state risk pool is likely to be limited in scope and more expensive. It is less likely to cover dependents than private health insurance but fills a crucial health insurance need for those who can afford it.

**Establishing Statewide Insurance Programs**

Several states have established or are considering the establishment of statewide health insurance programs. Washington's Basic Health Plan, established in 1988, began as a three-county demonstration insurance plan for low-income residents and expanded statewide in 1993. As of 2002, approximately 124,000 people had enrolled in the basic health plan, with additional slots available for small employer groups that had never before been offered health insurance (Health Care Authority 2003). Massachusetts is the most recent state to establish a health insurance plan. The 2006 Massachusetts legislature passed a universal insurance program that the governor signed into law.

**Other Proposals**

New proposals for group purchasing—HealthMarts, association health plans (AHPs), health insurance purchasing cooperatives (HIPCs), and multiple employer welfare arrangements (MEWAs)—are emerging (see Chapter 6). How these proposed new products will survive in a complex market remains to be seen. Analysts suggest that these new products warrant cautious and careful consideration but are not likely to produce a significant overall reduction in premiums or an increase in insurance coverage (Hall, Wicks, and Lawlor 2001). Many of these products appear to be eclipsed by newer initiatives, including the interest in consumer-directed health plans (see Chapter 6).

## A Focus on Health Disparities

Individuals have differences in health status for a variety of reasons. The determinants of health (see Chapter 2) affect each person differently. Income differences are believed by some to be the most influential factor in differences in health status, or health disparities. Other factors that might influence disparities in health status include demographic factors, such as race/ethnicity and age.

A national focus on health disparities centers on those disparities that can be corrected through improved access or other interventions. The Healthy People 2010 objectives (and prior versions of the objectives) aim to reduce disparities that are amenable to change (USDHHS 2000).

This chapter has focused principally on disparities related to financial access to health services. Figure 3.6 is particularly telling regarding the part of the U.S. population that is uninsured.

## Summary

Access to health services has several dimensions—geographic, physical, temporal, sociocultural, and financial—that can ensure or inhibit access to care. Potential access is affected by predisposing factors (age, gender, education, occupation, and race/ethnicity); need factors (perceived health, interpretation of illness, and other health status measures); and enabling factors (convenience, income, insurance coverage, and system characteristics). Of the enabling factors, financial access to care in the United States is usually predicated on insurance coverage, either private or public, or personal income (ability to make out-of-pocket expenditures for care). For those who do not have health insurance, government health programs, such as those sponsored by the Department of Veterans Affairs, Department of Defense, and the Indian Health Service, provide care to eligible populations. People ineligible for health insurance or these governmental health services programs may be able to access care through low-cost or no-cost clinics.

As much as 20 percent of the U.S. population may have limited or no financial access to health services in a given year. This population is at greater risk of morbidity and mortality and frequently presents on an emergency basis with poorer health status than those people who have no financial impediments to receiving care.

Major changes in health insurance, the primary health services financing mechanism in the United States, seem unlikely, given the defeat of the Health Security Act. Instead, incremental reforms, such as those incorporated in the Health Insurance Portability and Accountability Act of 1996, appear to be the most likely to effect change.

## Notes

1. Penchansky and Thomas (1981) define the dimensions of access as follows: Availability is the relationship of the volume and type of services (and resources) to the client's volume and type of needs. It refers to the adequacy of the supply of physicians, dentists, and other providers; of facilities such as clinics and hospitals; and of the specialized programs and services, such as mental health and emergency care. Accessibility is the relationship between the location of

clients, taking account of client transportation resources, travel time, and cost. Accommodation is the relationship between the manner in which the supply resources are organized to accept clients (including appointment times, hours of operation, walk-in facilities, and telephone services), the client's ability to accommodate to these factors, and the client's perceptions of their appropriateness. Affordability is the relationship between prices of services and providers' insurance or deposit requirements to the client's income, ability to pay, and existing health insurance. The client's perception of worth relative to total cost is a concern here, as is the client's knowledge of prices, total cost, and possible credit arrangements. Acceptability is the relationship between clients' attitudes about personal and practice characteristics of providers to the actual characteristics of existing providers, as well as to provider attitudes about acceptable personal characteristics of clients.

2. Insurance coverage does not, however, guarantee access to care. If providers are unavailable or if they will not accept the insurance company's payment for services, an insured individual still may not have access to health services.

3. The OTA's version of the chart, which did not include the final column on potential adverse outcomes associated with excessive access, was based on Aday, Andersen, and Fleming (1980), Weissman and Epstein (1992), Mechanic (1989), and studies reviewed for the interim report.

4. The Supplemental Security Income (SSI) program is a federal cash assistance program for low-income aged and disabled people that has standard eligibility requirements. It was established to replace state-provided cash assistance programs to low-income and aged and disabled people.

5. The focus of this discussion is on prisoners with long-term sentences. Jail inmates who may be awaiting trial or a hearing or who are serving out a short sentence may not be eligible for other than emergency services.

## Key Words

Aid to Families with Dependent
    Children (AFDC)
Americans with Disabilities Act
    (ADA) of 1990
association health plans (AHPs)
bad-debt care
behavioral health organizations
    (BHOs)
Centers for Medicare and Medicaid
    Services (CMS)
charity care
Civilian Health and Medical Program
    of the Uniformed Services
    (CHAMPUS)
co-insurance
copayments
Emergency Maternal and Infant Child
    Care Program (EMIC)
end-stage renal disease (ESRD)
entitlement programs
Health Care Financing Administration
    (HCFA)
Health Insurance Portability and
    Accountability Act (HIPAA)
health insurance purchasing
    cooperatives (HIPCs)
HealthMarts
Health Security Act (HSA) of 1993
iatrogenic illness
Indian Health Service (IHS)
Indian Self-Determination Act of 1975
Institute of Medicine (IOM)

managed care organizations (MCOs)
Medicaid
Medicare (Parts A and B)
Medicare+Choice plans
Medicare Prescription Drug
    Improvement and
    Modernization Act (MMA)
multiple employer welfare
    arrangements (MEWAs)
nosocomial infection
Office of Technology Assessment
    (OTA)
Oregon Health Plan
out-of-pocket payment
portability of health insurance
preexisting condition
private health insurance
public/social health insurance
single payer system
Supplemental Security Income (SSI)
TennCare
uncompensated hospital care
Uniformed Services University of the
    Health Sciences (USUHS)
uninsurable
uninsured
U.S. Department of Defense (DOD)
U.S. Department of Health and
    Human Services (HHS)
U.S. Department of Veterans Affairs
    (VA)
Washington Basic Health Plan

## References

Aday, L. A., R. Andersen, and G. V. Fleming. 1980. *Health Care in the U.S.: Equitable for Whom?* Thousand Oaks, CA: Sage Publications.

Anderson, O. W. 1968. *The Uneasy Equilibrium: Public and Private Financing of Health Services in the United States, 1875–1965.* New Haven, CT: College and University Press.

Ayanian, J. Z., J. S. Weissman, E. C. Schneider, J. A. Ginsburg, and A. M. Zaslavsky. 2000. "Unmet Health Needs of Uninsured Adults in the United States." *Journal of the American Medical Association* 284 (16): 2061–69.

Baker, D. W., J. J. Sudano, J. M. Albert, E. A. Borawski, and A. Dor. 2002. "Loss of Health Insurance and the Risk for a Decline in Self-Reported Health and Physical Functioning." *Medical Care* 40 (11): 1126–31.

Booth, A., B. Djulbegovic, B. Guthrie, M. Perleth, D. Sackett, S. Endersly, D. Jenkins, S. Richardson, C. Taylor, T. Dent, and M. Enkin. "What Proportion of Health Care Is Evidence-Based?" Resource Guide. [Online information; retrieved 12/15/05.] www.shef.ac.uk/scharr/ir/percent.html.

Brook, R. H. 1991. "Health, Health Insurance, and the Uninsured." *Journal of the American Medical Association* 265 (22): 2998–3002.

Canadian Institute for Health Care. 2002. "Health Care in Canada 2002." [Online information; retrieved 2/3/03.] http://secure.cihi.ca/cihiweb/dispPage.jsp?cw_page=AR_43_E&cw_topic=43.

Centers for Medicare and Medicaid Services. "Welcome to the State Children's Health Insurance Program." [Online information; retrieved 10/13/05.] www.cms.hhs.gov/schip/about-SCHIP.asp.

Cooper, P. F., and B. S. Schone. 1997. "More Offers, Fewer Takers for Employment-Based Health Insurance: 1987 and 1996." *Health Affairs* 16 (6): 142–49.

Davis, K., D. Rowland, D. Altman, K. S. Collins, and C. Morris. 1995. "Health Insurance: The Size and Shape of the Problem." *Inquiry* 32 (2): 196–203.

Demkovich, L. 1997. "$24 Billion Question: Which Child Health Options Will States Choose?" *State Health Notes* 18 (264): 1, 6.

Finnegan, L. P. 1996. "The NIH Women's Health Initiative: Its Evolution and Expected Contributions to Women's Health." *American Journal of Preventive Medicine* 12 (5): 292–93.

Franks, P., C. M. Clancey, and M. R. Gold. 1993. "Health Insurance and Mortality." *Journal of the American Medical Association* 270 (6): 737–41.

Freed, M. J., and J. Grigsby. 2002. "Telemedicine and Remote Patient Monitoring." *Journal of the American Medical Association* 288 (4): 423–25.

Gates, V. S. 2002. *State of the States: State Coverage Initiatives.* Washington, DC: Academy for Health Services Research and Health Policy.

Hall, M. A., E. K. Wicks, and J. S. Lawlor. 2001. "HealthMarts, HIPCs, MEWAs, and AHPs: A Guide for the Perplexed." *Health Affairs* 20 (1): 142–53.

Health Care Authority. 2003. "Basic Health." [Online information; retrieved 4/21/03.] www.basichealth.hca.wa.gov/bhhistory.shtml/.

Iglehart, J. K. 2002. "Changing Health Insurance Trends." *New England Journal of Medicine* 347 (12): 956–62.

Indian Health Service. 2002. "Indian Health Service Introduction." [Online information; 3/27/03.] www.ihs.gov/PublicInfo/PublicAffairs/ Welcome—Info/ThisFacts.asp.

Institute of Medicine. 2002. *Care Without Coverage: Too Little, Too Late.* Washington, DC: National Academy of Sciences Press.

Kogan, M. D., G. R. Alexander, M. A. Teitelbaum, B. W. Jack, M. Kotelchuck, and G. Pappas. 1995. "The Effect of Gaps in Health Insurance on Continuity of a Regular Source of Care among Preschool-Aged Children in the United States." *Journal of the American Medical Association* 274 (18): 1429–35.

Litman, T. J., and L. S. Robins. 1991. *Health Politics and Policy,* 2d ed. New York: Delmar.

McCall, N., T. Rice, J. Boismier, and R. West. 1991. "Private Health Insurance and Medical Care Utilization: Evidence from the Medicare Population." *Inquiry* 28 (3): 276–87.

Maciejewski, M., and M. Chapko. 2002. "Community-Based Outpatient Clinics Improve Access to Care and Patient Satisfaction, HSR&D Evaluation Shows." *Forum* (October): 4, 8.

Mechanic, D. 1989. "Medical Sociology: Some Tensions among Theory, Method, and Substance." *Journal of Health and Social Behavior* 30(2):147-60.

Office of Technology Assessment. 1992. *Does Health Insurance Make a Difference? A Background Paper.* OTA-BP-H-99. Washington, DC: U.S. Government Printing Office.

Penchansky, R., and J. W. Thomas. 1981. "The Concept of Access: Definition and Relationship to Consumer Satisfaction." *Medical Care* 19 (2): 127–40.

Ryan, J. M. 2002. "SCHIP Turns 5: Taking Stock, Moving Ahead." National Health Policy Forum Issue Brief No. 781. Washington, DC: The George Washington University.

Shonick, W. 1995. *Government and Health Services.* New York: Oxford University Press.

Short, P. F., and T. J. Lair. 1994/95. "Health Insurance and Health Status: Implications for Financing Health Care Reform." *Inquiry* 31 (4): 425–37.

Spillman, B. C. 1992. "The Impact of Being Uninsured on Utilization of Basic Health Care Services." *Inquiry* 29 (4): 457–66.

Stoddard, J. J., R. F. St. Peter, and P. W. Newacheck. 1994. "Health Insurance
      Status and Ambulatory Care for Children." *New England Journal of
      Medicine* 330 (20): 1421–25.

TennCare. 2003. "What Is TennCare?" [Online information; retrieved 2/5/03.]
      www.state.tn.us/tenncare/whatis.

TRICARE. 2002. "Stakeholders' Report. Volume IV." [Online information;
      accessed 6/19/02.] www.TRICARE.osd.mil/onestop/index.html.

U.S. Bipartisan Commission on Comprehensive Health Care. 1990. *A Call for
      Action: The Pepper Commission Final Report.* Washington, DC: U.S.
      Government Printing Office.

U.S. Census Bureau. 2005. *Income, Poverty, and Health Insurance Coverage in
      the United States, 2004.* Washington, DC: U.S. Department of
      Commerce.

U.S. Department of Health and Human Services. 2005. *Health, United States,
      2005.* Pub. No. (PHS) 2005-1232. Hyattsville, MD: USDHHS.

———. 2002. *Health, United States, 2002.* Pub. No. (PHS) 2002–1232.
      Hyattsville, MD: USDHHS.

———. 2000. *Healthy People 2010.* Washington, DC: U.S. Government
      Printing Office.

U.S. Government Accountability Office. 2005a. *Defense Health Care:
      Implementation Issues for New TRICARE Contracts and Regulatory
      Structure.* GAO-05-773. July. Washington, DC: USGAO.

———. 2005b. *Indian Health Service; Health Care Services Are Not Always
      Available to Native Americans.* GAO-05-789. August. Washington, DC:
      USGAO.

Weissman, J., and A. M. Epstein. 1992. "The Relationships among Insurance
      Coverage, Access to Services, and Health Outcomes: A Critical Review
      and Synthesis of the Literature." Contractor paper prepared for the Office
      of Technology Assessment. Washington, DC: U.S. Congress.

# SYSTEM ORGANIZATION

# ORGANIZATION OF THE U.S. HEALTH SERVICES SYSTEM

## Introduction

The central component of the Roemer model of a health services system is the system's organization. It includes the Ministry of Health, other public agencies, voluntary agencies, enterprises (which in this context means the health programs and services provided directly by private businesses), and the private market (refer back to Figure 1.3). Unlike the centralized health services systems in many other industrialized countries, the U.S. system is decentralized. The Ministry of Health counterpart in the U.S. system—the Department of Health and Human Services (HHS)—regulates and finances many health services, but the delivery of services occurs primarily in the private sector. This chapter focuses on the public sector of the U.S. system and opens with a discussion of public health roles and functions. Voluntary agencies and enterprises are addressed as well. The private market receives little attention here because it is the predominant focus of Part VI of this book, which discusses the delivery system.

## Public Health Roles and Functions

In contrast to the private health services delivery system, which provides care at the individual level, public health focuses on the health of populations. Public health, therefore, emphasizes the prevention of disease, the promotion of health, the reporting and control of communicable diseases, the responsibility for environmental factors such as air and water quality that affect the public's health, and the collection and analysis of vital event data to provide indicators of the public's health. Although some public health departments directly deliver some personal health services—for example, immunizations and diagnosis and treatment of sexually transmitted diseases—public health departments are generally careful to avoid direct competition with the private sector.

The functions initially performed by public health agencies included quarantines against known contagious diseases and, as germ theory became better understood, the introduction and enforcement of sanitation principles.

In 1946 a committee sponsored by the American Public Health Association (APHA) issued the Emerson Report, outlining six public health functions that both state and local health departments were expected to perform: vital statistics, public health education, environmental sanitation, laboratory services, prevention and control of communicable diseases, and maternal and child health services (Table 4.1).

Public health departments have provided these population-based services for decades. Concern exists, however, that concentration on this limited set of services has contributed to a lack of public health leadership and loss of the sight of public health goals. An Institute of Medicine (IOM) committee on the future of public health concluded in 1988 that "this nation has lost sight of its public health goals and has allowed the system of public health activities to fall into disarray" (Committee for the Study of the Future of Public Health of the Institute of Medicine 1988). The committee defined the mission of public health as "fulfilling society's interest in assuring conditions in which people can be healthy." It recommended a three-part governmental role in public health: (1) assess the health of the community, (2) develop comprehensive public health policy, and (3) ensure the provision of needed health services (see Table 4.1).

In 2002 the IOM issued an update on the state of public health, focusing on a widespread need for training the workforce. IOM surveys had disclosed that as much as three-quarters of the public health workforce—from entry-level positions to top-line administrators—had never been trained in public health. The IOM group that studied this issue recommended both short- and long-term solutions for academia and the government to undertake (IOM 2002).

The Public Health Service (PHS) has defined, among other functions, essential public health services to include monitoring health status, identifying and solving community health problems, diagnosing and investigating health problems and health hazards in the community, and enforcing laws and regulations that protect health and ensure safety (see Table 4.1).

## Ministry of Health

In the Roemer model, the Ministry of Health is the major governmental or public agency responsible for a country's health services system; in the United States, the HHS is the equivalent of the Ministry of Health and has cabinet status in the executive branch of government. Although pieces of a health services system have existed since the country's founding, a ministry- or cabinet-level focus on health has existed only since 1953, when the Eisenhower administration established the U.S. Department of Health, Education, and Welfare (DHEW). All but the education function became the

| | | |
|---|---|---|
| **Emerson Report, 1946** | • Vital statistics<br>• Public health education<br>• Environmental sanitation<br>• Public health laboratories, if private facilities are not available<br>• Prevention and control of communicable diseases<br>• Hygiene of maternity, infancy, and childhood, if private facilities are not available | **TABLE 4.1**<br>The Roles of<br>Public Health |
| **Institute of Medicine Report, 1988** | • Assess the health of the community<br>• Develop comprehensive public health policy<br>• Assure the provision of needed health services | |
| **Essential Public Health Services, 1995** | • Monitor health status to identify and solve community problems<br>• Diagnose and investigate health problems and health hazards in the community<br>• Inform, educate, and empower people about health issues<br>• Mobilize community partnerships and action to identify and solve health problems<br>• Develop policies and plans that support individual and community health efforts<br>• Enforce laws and regulations that protect health and ensure safety<br>• Link people to needed personal health services and assure the provision of health care when otherwise unavailable<br>• Ensure a competent public health and personal health care workforce<br>• Evaluate effectiveness, accessibility, and quality of personal and population-based health services<br>• Research for new insights and innovative solutions to public health problems | |

HHS in 1980. The following discussion first considers the development of the U.S. Public Health Service, a central unit of the HHS, and then addresses the other health responsibilities within the HHS. Figure 4.1 provides an organization chart of the HHS.

## Public Health at the National Level

The Public Health Service at the national level had its origins in the Marine Hospital Service (MHS), which was established in 1798 to provide medical

**FIGURE 4.1**
U.S.
Department
of Health
and Human
Services
Organization
Chart

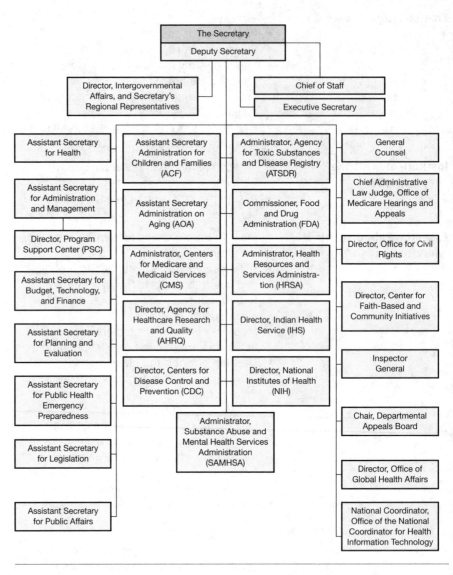

SOURCE: USDHHS 2006.

care to merchant seamen. In 1902 the MHS changed its name to the U.S. Public Health and Marine Hospital Service to reflect its expanded mission to provide medical care for specified additional people and to continue to quarantine as a protection against diseases introduced via the seaports. The agency's name was shortened to the U.S. Public Health Service (PHS) in 1913, and the PHS was housed in the Treasury Department. Congress began to funnel funds through the PHS to local agencies for field investigations and research into such public health problems as typhoid fever and rural sanitation. The Public Health Service Act was established in 1944 to consolidate all public health service authorities into a single statute and to continue the programs of assistance to state and local health departments, some of which were established by the 1935 Social Security Act (SSA) (Shonick 1995). The SSA also provided for a commissioned corps of PHS officers, headed by the surgeon general, to provide public health leadership and services in major federal offices, such as the Centers for Disease Control and Prevention (CDC).

The PHS today encompasses the CDC, the Food and Drug Administration (FDA), the Health Resources and Services Administration (HRSA), the National Institutes of Health (NIH), the Substance Abuse and Mental Health Services Administration (SAMHSA), and the Agency for Healthcare Research and Quality (AHRQ) (Figure 4.1).

Although PHS-commissioned corps members may directly deliver some primary care services, the focus of the PHS is not on service delivery but on shaping the nation's public health system to promote health and to prevent disease. The PHS also provides guidance for the development of a health services delivery system aimed at preventing unnecessary disability and disease and at achieving a better quality of life for all Americans. This guidance originated with the 1979 publication *Healthy People: The Surgeon General's Report on Health Promotion and Disease Prevention* (USDHEW 1979); its most current issue is *Healthy People 2010: National Health Promotion and Disease Prevention Objectives* (USDHHS 2000).

The mission of the Centers for Disease Control and Prevention (CDC), located in Atlanta, Georgia, is to promote health and quality of life by preventing and controlling disease, injury, and disability. In addition to national programs in immunization, global health, public health practice, and women's health, the CDC has centers that work with state and local health departments, academic centers and programs, and others to fulfill its mission in the following areas:

**Centers for Disease Control and Prevention**

- Birth defects and developmental disabilities
- Chronic disease prevention and health promotion
- Environmental health
- Health statistics
- HIV, STD, and TB prevention
- Infectious diseases
- Injury prevention and control

The CDC also has a national immunization program, a National Institute for Occupational Safety and Health (NIOSH), and several other special offices.

**Food and Drug Administration**

The Food and Drug Administration (FDA), created in 1906 by the Food and Drug Act, was originally housed in the Department of Agriculture but was transferred to the Federal Security Agency, the predecessor of the DHEW, in 1940. FDA responsibilities include monitoring the safety of food (i.e., meat, butter, canned food, and seafood regulation); the safety of cosmetic products; the safety and efficacy of drugs, both prescription and over-the-counter; and the safety and efficacy of medical devices such as pacemakers. The FDA role in drug and device assessment is described in Chapter 10.

**Health Resources and Services Administration**

The Health Resources and Services Administration (HRSA) is responsible for supporting the development of a strong health services workforce. The HRSA administers training grants for a range of health professions, including medicine, nursing, and public health, and provides funding for some physician residency programs, such as those in preventive medicine. The HRSA is the home agency of the National Health Service Corps (NHSC), which provides both scholarships and loan forgiveness for physicians, dentists, pharmacists, and those in other health professions who agree to practice in underserved and health workforce shortage areas.[1] The HRSA also maintains the National Practitioner Databank, a database of malpractice actions filed against physicians.

**National Institutes of Health**

The National Institutes of Health (NIH), created in 1930, is the major arm of federally supported biomedical research and is made up of 19 research institutes, the National Library of Medicine, and seven specialty centers (Table 4.2). The institutes are organized according to specific diseases such as cancer, or specific organ systems such as heart, lung, and blood. The NIH supports both intramural and extramural research. Through its consensus development conferences, it provides technology assessments of new medical and surgical procedures (see Chapter 10).

**Substance Abuse and Mental Health Services Administration**

The Substance Abuse and Mental Health Services Administration (SAMHSA) provides leadership in policy, services, and knowledge transfer for mental illness and substance abuse treatment and prevention. Through the provision of research grants, SAMHSA supports studies of treatment improvement methods, demonstrates effective treatment approaches, and trains substance abuse treatment and mental health practitioners. SAMHSA also supports health services delivery programs that assist homeless people.

**Indian Health Service**

The Indian Health Service (IHS) has been a part of the PHS since 1955 but has a much longer history. As early as 1806, the War Department was assigned responsibility for the limited health services provided to indigenous populations. This assignment was transferred to the Department of

| | | TABLE 4.2 |
|---|---|---|
| **Institutes** | National Cancer Institute (1937) | National |
| | National Heart, Lung, and Blood Institute (1948) | Institutes of |
| | National Institute of Diabetes and Digestive and Kidney Diseases (1948) | Health |
| | National Institute of Allergy and Infectious Diseases (1948) | |
| | National Institute of Child Health and Human Development (1962) | |
| | National Institute on Deafness and Other Communication Disorders (1988) | |
| | National Institute of Dental and Craniofacial Research (1948) | |
| | National Institute of Neurological Disorders and Stroke (1950) | |
| | National Eye Institute (1968) | |
| | National Institute on Aging (1974) | |
| | National Institute of Arthritis and Musculoskeletal and Skin Diseases (1986) | |
| | National Institute on Drug Abuse (1973) | |
| | National Institute of Mental Health (1949) | |
| | National Human Genome Research Institute (1989) | |
| | National Institute on Alcohol Abuse and Alcoholism (1970) | |
| | National Institute of Environmental Health Sciences (1969) | |
| | National Institute of General Medical Sciences (1962) | |
| | National Institute of Nursing Research (1986) | |
| | National Institute of Biomedical Imaging and Bioengineering (2000) | |
| **Libraries** | National Library of Medicine (1956) | |
| **Centers** | NIH Clinical Center (1953) | |
| | John E. Fogarty International Center (1968) | |
| | Center for Information Technology (1964) | |
| | National Center for Research Resources (1990) | |
| | Center for Scientific Review (1946) | |
| | National Center for Complementary and Alternative Medicine (1992) | |
| | National Center on Minority Health and Health Disparities (1993) | |

SOURCE: National Institutes of Health 2006.

the Interior in 1849. In 1873 a new Division of Education and Medicine was organized with the Bureau of Indian Affairs (BIA) to provide health services to American Indians (Shonick 1995). Today, the IHS is available to the 1.34 million American Indians and Alaska Natives who qualify for IHS services. As a result of self-determination policies, members of the more than 545 federally recognized American Indian tribes, bands, pueblos, and villages have the option to staff and manage IHS programs in their communities.

**Agency for Healthcare Research and Quality**

The Agency for Healthcare Research and Quality (AHRQ)—formerly known as the Agency for Health Care Policy and Research (AHCPR) and before that as the National Center for Health Services Research (NCHSR)—is an independent agency established under the PHS umbrella by the 1989 Omnibus Budget Reconciliation Act (OBRA, PL 101-239). The broad mission of the AHRQ is to analyze the functions of the U.S. health services system and how it addresses access, affordability, and quality of care. The effectiveness of medical treatment and the measurement of outcomes of the provision of medical care are major AHRQ foci. AHRQ has supported patient outcome research teams (PORTs) to explore a range of treatments or interventions for breast cancer, dialysis care, medical testing prior to cataract surgery, back pain, and cesarean sections, among others. AHRQ is the home of several national databases, including the National Medical Expenditure Survey (NMES) database. In recent years, AHRQ has added medical safety, including the prevention of adverse outcomes, and evidence-based medicine and health care to its research agenda.

**Other Department of Health and Human Services Responsibilities**

Two additional major programs within the HHS are the Administration for Children and Families (ACF) and the Centers for Medicare and Medicaid Services (CMS), formerly know as the Health Care Financing Administration (HCFA). The ACF supports the development of programs for special populations, including children, youth, families, people with developmental disabilities, and American Indians. The ACF is also responsible at the national level for assisting in child support enforcement, family assistance programs, and refugee resettlement.

The CMS administers Medicare, the social insurance program for the elderly and people with disabilities, and Medicaid, the program that pays for health services to qualifying low-income people. The CMS also maintains the National Health Accounts database, discussed in Chapter 7.

One major program was removed from the HHS umbrella. The Social Security Administration (SSA), in existence since 1935, was a part of the HHS or its predecessor organizations until 1995, when it became a separate agency. The HHS budget declined sharply after the SSA, which constituted a major budget component, became a separate agency.

### Public Health at the State Level

The emergence of a major health problem that affected a significant proportion of a state's population often galvanized the establishment of state health authorities, including boards of health and state health departments. A yellow fever outbreak may have stimulated the establishment of the first board of health in Louisiana in 1855. Massachusetts claims the distinction of being the first state to convert its board of health into a permanently established governmental entity in 1869. By 1909 all states had organized a type of state board of health (Shonick 1995).

State boards of health and health departments varied widely in the range of services provided to their populations. In an effort to bring uniformity to public health services offerings, the American Public Health Association (APHA) sponsored a study of state and local health departments under the chairmanship of Haven Emerson. As noted in Table 4.1, the 1946 Emerson Report identified six core public health functions that both state and local health departments should perform (Shonick1995):

1. vital statistics;
2. public health education;
3. environmental sanitation;
4. public health laboratories, if private facilities are not available;
5. prevention and control of communicable diseases; and
6. hygiene of maternity, infancy, and childhood, if private facilities are unavailable.

Functions 1, 2, 3, and 5 clearly affect the health of the entire population. The remaining two functions—public health laboratories and maternal and child health programs—involve the direct provision of services and have the qualifier "if private facilities are not available." The qualifier was intended to clearly delineate the public from the private sector and to discourage any incursion of the public into the private sector. Public health departments sometimes serve as safety-net providers, making some primary care services available to people who have no other access to care. The extent to which state, and more particularly, local health departments directly provide services in competition with the private sector remains a point of considerable sensitivity to private providers in a community and to governmental agencies.

All states today have state public health departments whose authority stems from the health powers of the state constitution. Health departments may be organized either as separate governmental units, sometimes called single state agencies, or as part of a human services umbrella agency that may include the state's mental health program (e.g., state-owned psychiatric hospitals, substance abuse treatment programs, or social services). One of the greatest areas of variability across state health departments is their responsibility for environmental health. Although some health departments have retained responsibility for environmental health, others have lost this function to a separate agency.

An IOM report (Committee for the Study of the Future of Public Health of the Institute of Medicine 1988) recommends that state health departments be responsible for:

- assessing health needs in the state based on statewide data collection;
- ensuring an adequate statutory base for health activities in the state;
- establishing statewide health objectives, delegating power to localities as appropriate and holding them accountable;
- ensuring appropriate organized statewide efforts to develop and maintain essential personal, educational, and environmental health services;
- providing access to necessary services;
- solving problems inimical to health;
- guaranteeing a minimum set of essential health services; and
- supporting local service capacity, especially when disparities in local ability to raise revenue or administer programs require subsidies, technical assistance, or direct action by the state to achieve adequate service levels.

The funding for state health departments comes from state general (tax-based) funds; federal grants and contracts; fees for licenses, permits, and copies of vital records; and other sources. Much federal funding comes through four major block grants that Congress created in 1980 to consolidate many discrete programs. These block grants provide program support for public health activities in prevention, maternal and child health, alcohol and drug abuse, mental health, and primary care.

Not all state health departments are governed by a board of health. As of 2000, 16 states did not have boards of health. In the states with boards of health, some boards may appoint the director of the state health department, but in most states, the director of the state health department is likely to be a gubernatorial appointee. Thus, the state health department is equivalent to a ministry of health at the subnational level. Nearly all states once required that the state health department director be a physician, but many states have eliminated this requirement.

### Public Health at the Local Level

As a part of the U.S. health services system, public health originated at the local level with the establishment of city, multicity, county, or multicounty local health boards to protect the public's health through quarantine and sanitation. Local health departments began to include in their areas of responsibility such services as immunizations, communicable disease control, laboratory services, and vital event data collection. With the wave of immigration that began in 1892, local health boards and departments began providing some personal-care services to meet the multiple health services and social needs of burgeoning populations crammed into marginal living conditions (Shonick 1995).

An IOM report (Committee for the Study of the Future of Public Health of the Institute of Medicine 1988) recommends that local health departments perform the following functions:

- assess, monitor, and provide surveillance of local health problems and needs, and of resources for dealing with them;
- develop policy and leadership that foster local health involvement and a sense of ownership, that emphasize local needs, and that advocate equitable distribution of public resources and complementary private activities commensurate with community needs; and
- ensure that high-quality services, including personal health services, needed for the protection of public health in the community are available and accessible to all people; that the community receives proper consideration in the allocation of federal and state as well as local resources for public health; that the community is informed about how to obtain public health, including personal health services, or how to comply with public health requirements.

The availability of local public health departments varies widely across states. Following World War II, Assistant Surgeon General Joseph W. Mountin and his associates surveyed all counties to determine the number and scope of local health departments, issuing their findings in 1945. Mountin reported that 1,851 of the nation's nearly 3,000 counties had local health departments and that at least 60 cities with populations greater than 10,000 had a type of full-time official public health organization (Shonick 1995).

Today, nearly 3,000 organized local health departments exist in the United States (NACCHO 2002). Those organized at the city level generally report to the mayor or city manager, and those at the county level report to county commissioners or other county officials. Local health department funding comes from tax revenues, such as property taxes, the sale of permits and licenses, and fees for inspections and other services; the state; federal funds that may come directly to the local health department or are passed through the state health department; and other sources. Not all of the nation's 3,044 counties or its sizable cities have local health departments. Some states, such as Colorado, support a public health nurse and a sanitarian in counties lacking organized local health departments. Other states have established public health regions or districts that incorporate multiple counties in their service areas. The relationship between state and local health departments varies by state. It may include the state providing direct financial support of local health departments, and programmatic and personnel linkages between them, or the relationship may be much more distant, with the state serving only as a pass-through for certain funds to the local health department.

## Other Ministry-Level Health Functions in the U.S. System

Although the HHS is the major ministry-level governmental unit responsible for parts of the U.S. health services system, health program responsibilities are also scattered among other cabinet-level departments and governmental units. The Department of Defense (DOD), for example, administers the health services programs for active-duty military personnel and their dependents and for military retirees. The Department of Veterans Affairs (DVA) oversees the nationwide system of hospitals, clinics, and nursing homes that provide health services to military veterans. The Department of Justice (DOJ) administers the correctional health services system in the nation's prisons. The Drug Enforcement Agency (DEA) within the DOJ governs the use of narcotic prescription drugs (i.e., controlled substances). The Department of Agriculture (DOA) administers the Special Supplemental Nutrition Program for Women, Infants, and Children (WIC), which does not provide direct health services but is closely linked to programs that provide or pay for health services to low-income recipients. The Department of Labor (DOL) oversees the Occupational Safety and Health Administration (OSHA), which enforces regulations to ensure healthy and hazard-free workplaces. The Environmental Protection Agency (EPA) has national-level responsibility for the protection of the environment, including air and water quality, and for cleaning up sites contaminated by toxins and pollutants.

The passage of legislation in the fall of 2002 to establish a cabinet-level agency—the Department of Homeland Security—may affect the organization and delivery of some federal-government–supported health services. The new department has assumed some responsibilities and drawn part of its workforce from as many as 20 current federal departments and agencies. This new department's effects on the landscape of health organizations in the U.S. system are not yet fully known.

## Quasi-Governmental Organizations

A brief review of quasi-governmental organizations adds one more dimension to the U.S. health services system. The term *quasi-governmental* is sometimes used to describe organizations that perform statutorily mandated services under contract to the government. Such agencies are generally organized as private, not-for-profit corporations, but their sole or primary function is to carry out a legislatively specified scope of work. Quality improvement organizations (QIOs), formerly called peer review organizations (PROs), were established by the 1982 Tax Equity and Fiscal Responsibility Act (TEFRA) as successors to the professional standards review organizations (PSROs). QIOs may be considered quasi-governmental because they are under contract with the CMS to review the quality of care provided to Medicare beneficiaries and to evaluate the outcomes of care. Some QIOs may contract with state Medicaid programs and even with private insurers to provide similar services for their enrollees and subscribers.

## Voluntary Agencies in the U.S. Health Services System

A variety of voluntary agencies meet needs unfilled by the public and private sectors; these generally focus on a specific disease, population, or health issue.

Disease-specific voluntary agencies, such as the American Cancer Society (ACS), the American Heart Association (AHA), and the American Lung Association (ALA), raise funds to support research, concentrate on public education about the risk factors for these diseases, and may provide funds for diagnosis and treatment of the disease in certain populations.

Population-specific voluntary agencies focus their energies on subsets of the population. The Children's Defense Fund lobbies for programs to improve the health and well-being of children, provides data on the health status of children, and supports public and legislative education about children's needs. AARP, the stand-alone acronym for the American Association of Retired Persons, concentrates on health, social services, and other needs at the opposite end of the age spectrum. A wide range of voluntary agencies have specific health functions. The American Red Cross, for example, assists in disaster relief, procuring health services, food, shelter, and other services for victims of natural disasters and war.

Professional health associations are another type of voluntary health agency and include such bodies as the American Public Health Association (APHA), the American Hospital Association (AHA), and the American Medical Association (AMA). Religious groups may also establish voluntary agencies to meet special health services needs, such as clinics to provide health services to low-income people or homeless people who do not have regular providers.

Philanthropic foundations may sponsor a range of health-related activities, including community development aimed at strengthening the health services system, the support of health services delivery to needy populations, and research into health problems and issues.

## Enterprises in the U.S. Health Services System

Enterprises, which are defined in the Roemer model as health services functions sponsored by nonhealth businesses, are usually found in larger businesses where the volume of workers warrants their development or in workplaces such as major mining or construction operations where an on-site clinic is essential to the treatment of work-related injuries or occupationally induced illnesses. Enterprises may include occupational health clinics, wellness and fitness centers that are a part of the workplace and readily accessible to employees, and employee assistance programs (EAPs) that offer aid to employees with behavioral health problems, including substance abuse.

## The Private Market in the U.S. Health Services System

Although every country's health services system has unique features, the U.S. system, with its combination of public and private sectors, has no true counterparts among other industrialized countries. The majority of U.S. health services are delivered in the private sector, with the exception of the health services that governmental agencies provide to special populations, such as the military, veterans, indigenous populations, and inmates in federal and state prisons. Part VI focuses on how health services are delivered in the U.S. system.

The private market has aspects other than the delivery of personal health services that warrant brief discussion here. Those aspects include the manufacture of medical equipment and devices; the production of pharmaceuticals and supplies; the health insurance industry, including claims processing and fiscal intermediaries; and the education and training of the health workforce.

### Manufacture of Medical Equipment and Devices

The production of the latest generation of durable medical equipment and devices has long been a hallmark of the U.S. health services system. In 2004, $23 billion out of $1.87 trillion was expended for medical durables, devices, and vision equipment products in the United States.

### Pharmaceuticals and Supplies

The production of pharmaceuticals and supplies is an important component of the private market in the U.S. health services system. In 2004, 10 percent of expenditures for health services were for the development, production, and purchase of pharmaceutical supplies. Prescription drug sales were one of the fastest growing categories of national health expenditures, increasing 8.2 percent over prescription drug expenditures for 2003, but home health care resumed its place as the service with the greatest percentage increase, as home health care expenditures grew 13.3 percent from 2003 to 2004.

## The Health Insurance Industry

The health insurance industry is a significant and growing component of the private market in the U.S. system, with more than one-third of the 1.1 million employees in the insurance industry focused on hospital and medical insurance (Health Insurance Association of America 2002). The health insurance industry includes the marketing and sale of policies and the claims processing and settlement business. Insurance companies may also act as fiscal intermediaries for the Medicare and Medicaid programs, reviewing and settling claims for service.

## Health Professional Training

The responsibility for producing the health workforce is shared between the public and private sectors (see Chapter 8). The federal government provides direct financial assistance for the basic training of some health professions and subsidizes the graduate training of physicians and, to a lesser extent, nurses through Medicare payments to teaching hospitals. States, through their university and college systems, support the education and training of a wide range of health professionals. Private universities also educate and train the health workforce.

## Summary

The organization of U.S. health services is spread across governmental agencies at the federal, state, and local levels and in voluntary agencies, enterprises, and the private market. Although many federal agencies have responsibilities for providing some health services, the Department of Health and Human Services (HHS) serves as the Ministry of Health unit in the Roemer model. The national responsibility for public health resides within the Public Health Service (PHS); state and local governments have established health departments to deliver and regulate public health services. Voluntary agencies such as the American Heart Association, the Children's Defense Fund, the American Red Cross, the American Public Health Association, and religious and philanthropic foundations have organized to meet discrete health services needs not addressed by the public or private sectors. Larger businesses may have health enterprises such as on-site clinics, fitness centers, or employee assistance programs to meet the health needs of their workforces. The private market, in addition to serving as the major site of health services delivery, also includes the manufacture of medical equipment and devices, the production of pharmaceuticals and supplies, the health insurance industry, and the training of the health workforce.

In summarizing the organization of the U.S. health services system, it is easier to describe what the system is not. The organization of the U.S. health services system is not centralized, although a recognizable Ministry of Health entity—the HHS—exists. The organization does not resemble a hierarchy. The public and private sectors are not always clearly delineated, nor do they, in combination, provide all the health services needs of the population. Voluntary agencies may fill in some of the gaps between the two sectors; other gaps, such as access to care for the working uninsured or the uninsurable, currently remain unfilled.

## Note

1.  A primary care health professional shortage area (HPSA) may be a distinct geographic area (such as a county), a specific population group within the area, or a specific public or nonprofit facility (such as a prison). The HPSA designation is used to determine whether an area has a critical shortage of physicians available to serve the population and was first used in 1978 in designating National Health Service Corps practice sites. A medically underserved area (MUA) is defined as a geographic area or a population with shortages of health services. An MUA is defined not only by the availability of health services providers but also by population characteristics, such as the infant mortality rate, the poverty rate, and the percentage of the population age 65 and older. The MUA designation is used to identify areas eligible for federally funded community health centers (U.S. General Accounting Office [now known as the U.S. Government Accountability Office—USGAO] 1995).

## Key Words

Administration for Children and
    Families (ACF)
Agency for Health Care Policy and
    Research (AHCPR)
Agency for Healthcare Research and
    Quality (AHRQ)
American Association of Retired
    Persons (AARP)

American Cancer Society (ACS)
American Heart Association (AHA)
American Hospital Association (AHA)
American Lung Association (ALA)
American Medical Association (AMA)
American Public Health Association
    (APHA)
block grants

Bureau of Indian Affairs (BIA)
Centers for Disease Control and
    Prevention (CDC)
Centers for Medicare and Medicaid
    Services (CMS)
Children's Defense Fund
Drug Enforcement Agency (DEA)
Emerson Report
Environmental Protection Agency
    (EPA)
Federal Security Agency
Food and Drug Administration (FDA)
Health Care Financing
    Administration (HCFA)
health professional shortage area
    (HPSA)
Health Resources and Services
    Administration (HRSA)
Healthy People 2000 Objectives
Indian Health Service (IHS)
Institute of Medicine (IOM)
Marine Hospital Service
medically underserved area (MUA)
Medicaid
Medicare
Mountin Report
National Center for Health Services
    Research (NCHSR)
National Health Accounts database
National Institutes of Health (NIH)

National Medical Expenditure Survey
    (NMES)
National Practitioner Databank
Occupational Safety and Health
    Administration (OSHA)
patient outcome research teams
    (PORTs)
peer review organizations (PROs)
professional standards review
    organizations (PSROs)
Public Health Service (PHS)
quality improvement organizations
    (QIOs)
quasi-governmental organizations
safety-net provider
single state agencies
Social Security Act (SSA)
Special Supplemental Nutrition
    Program for Women, Infants,
    and Children (WIC)
surgeon general
U.S. Department of Agriculture (DOA)
U.S. Department of Defense (DOD)
U.S. Department of Health and
    Human Services (HHS)
U.S. Department of Justice (DOJ)
U.S. Department of Labor (DOL)
U.S. Department of Veterans Affairs
    (DVA)

# References

Committee for the Study of the Future of Public Health of the Institute of
    Medicine. 1988. *The Future of Public Health.* Washington, DC: National
    Academy Press.

Health Insurance Association of America (HIAA). 2002. *Source Book of Health
    Insurance Data 2002.* Washington, DC: HIAA.

Institute of Medicine. 2002. *Who Will Keep the Public Healthy?* Washington, DC:
    National Academy of Sciences Press.

National Association of City and County Health Officials (NACCHO). 2002.
    "About NACCHO." [Online information; retrieved 8/26/02.]
    www.nacho.org/about.cfm.

National Institutes of Health. 2006. "Institutes, Centers, and Officers." [Online information; retrieved 6/3/06.] www.nih.gov/icd.

Shonick, W. 1995. *Government and Health Services.* New York: Oxford University Press.

U.S. Department of Health, Education, and Welfare. 1979. *Healthy People: The Surgeon General's Report on Health Promotion and Disease Prevention.* Pub. No. (PHS) 79-55071. Washington, DC: DHEW.

U.S. Department of Health and Human Services. 2006. "USDHHS Organizational Chart." [Online information; retrieved 5/2/06.] www.dhhs.gov/about/orgchart.html.

———. 2000. *Healthy People 2010: National Health Promotion and Disease Prevention Objectives.* Washington, DC: U.S. Government Printing Office.

U.S. Government Accountability Office (formerly the U.S. General Accounting Office). 1995. *Health Care Shortage Areas: Designations Not a Useful Tool for Directing Resources to the Underserved.* GAO/HEHS-95-200. September. Washington, DC: USGAO.

# SYSTEM MANAGEMENT

# MANAGEMENT OF THE U.S. HEALTH SERVICES SYSTEM

## Introduction

The management component of the Roemer model of a health services system incorporates four major functions: planning, administration, legislation, and regulation. Legislation is the sole purview of the public sector. Although planning, administration, and regulation occur in both the public and private sectors, the focus of this chapter is on management in the public sector. These functions, as they apply to the private sector, will be included in discussions of the delivery system in Part VI.

## Planning

Planning occurs at several levels within a health services system—at the level of a project, program, or organizational unit or subunit, for example. For the purposes of this chapter, we consider planning at the system level and concentrate on planning that occurs at a national level within the public sector. Specifically, we consider national-level health planning.

Only the heartiest of optimists would argue that the U.S. health services system shows evidence of national-level planning. The way in which the U.S. system is organized, with its mix of services provided by both public and private sectors, presents a substantial planning challenge. No central authority exists from which planning might emanate. In a market economy, services develop in response to demand, which may or may not correspond to service needs identified through a comprehensive assessment and planning process. The public sector exercises some control over developments in the private sector but can neither influence nor control the entire sector.

Despite these challenges to health planning, two major national initiatives were mounted: the 1966 Comprehensive Health Planning Act (PL 89-749) and the 1974 National Health Planning and Resources Development Act (PL 93-641). The first planning program grew out of the Great Society era in which community development and consumer participation in that development were national priorities. The second planning program developed as a result of consciousness-raising about the growing expenditures for health and the need to rationalize the development of health services. The second program was also intended to correct the flaws of the first.

### Comprehensive Health Planning

The 1966 Comprehensive Health Planning (CHP) Act created a state CHP-A agency and local CHP-b agencies charged with developing a statewide, comprehensive plan for the delivery of health services in each state. Each agency had a governor-appointed advisory board with required participation from consumers of health services. Consumer involvement was intended to provide a strong community voice about what the health services system should be and to protect against health services providers dominating the system.

Local "b" agencies were established to recognize the importance of regional differences and the preferences for local control. With their boards, "b" agencies were responsible for assessing the health services needs of the populations in their designated areas, evaluating the availability of health resources, and formulating a plan that specified what was required to meet the population's needs. The "A" agency would then combine the various "b" agency plans into a comprehensive plan intended to guide state allocation of resources as well as the development of services and facilities in the private sector.

The CHP program succeeded in bringing together community members and health services providers to discuss the area's health services system. States generated massive planning documents, but their success in implementing these plans varied. Success was contingent on several assumptions:

1. that resources to meet identified needs would be forthcoming;
2. that consumers and providers could achieve a collaborative process and formulate a plan that was generally supported and could feasibly be implemented; and
3. that all participants would voluntarily abide by the plan, even if it meant the denial of an institutional development for the greater good of the community.

Experience with the CHP program has shown that not all of these assumptions were viable. Although the Great Society era was a time of significant growth in governmental programs, and discretionary funds were far more readily available than they are now, the CHP program had no resource development component. Resources to meet the community's identified needs were not assured and had to be sought outside the CHP program.[1] Consumers and providers proved that they could work together, but the potential for one co-opting the other was omnipresent. Additionally, it proved to be difficult for either party to give up a potential service or resource for their community or institution in favor of having the development occur elsewhere. Territoriality often proved a stronger force than the impetus for collaboration.

## The 1974 National Health Planning and Resources Development Act

As optimism about the community planning process turned to disappointment and Congress became increasingly concerned about the growing federal expenditures for health services, the CHP program was replaced in 1974 by another national health planning program. The replacement program outlined by the 1974 National Health Planning and Resources Development Act established three levels of organization: the Statewide Health Coordinating Council (SHCC), the State Health Planning and Development Agency (SHPDA), and Health Systems Agencies (HSAs). The SHCC was governor-appointed and charged with approving and implementing the state health plan developed by the SHPDA. The SHPDA was a unit of state government, usually located within the state's health department, but in a few cases located either in the governor's office or created as a separate state agency. The SHPDA provided staff support to the SHCC, developed the state health plan, and carried out the regulatory functions of the act. HSAs were local organizations with community boards, designed much like their predecessor CHP-b agencies. HSAs were charged with the development of local health plans to be compiled by the SHPDA into a state health plan.

As was true of the CHP program, the new health planning program required consumer participation. The National Health Planning and Resources Development Act, however, was far more prescriptive about the composition of the SHCC and the HSA boards: the maximum numbers and types of each category of member were specified, and, in an effort to avoid conflicts of interest, spouses of providers could not be considered as consumer members. HSAs in particular, but to a certain extent the SHCCs as well, spent so much time establishing the appropriately constituted boards that their ability to assess community needs and develop plans was sometimes compromised.

Recognizing that the voluntary CHP program had failed to control the expansion of the health services system, the 1974 planning legislation required the development of national health planning standards that states were expected to meet. Among the standards established was a hospital bed-to-population ratio of 4:1,000. States with a higher number of hospital beds were expected to deny requests for the development of additional beds until the desired ratio had been achieved.

The regulatory stick that required states to act on proposals for changes in health services was the certificate of need (CON) program. The CON program, administered by the SHPDA with input from the HSAs, required that proposed changes in services costing above a certain threshold, originally $150,000, required an application to the SHPDA and could not proceed without SHPDA approval. Failure to obtain approval could result in the loss of Medicare and other funding to the offending developer.

Administration of the CON program became one of the most contentious aspects of the 1974 National Health Planning and Resources Development Act and contributed to its repeal in 1986. Providers resented the need to submit their proposed changes in service to the review and action by "outside" parties, and were frustrated at the delays incurred by their plans. The territoriality problem that the CHP program had been unable to resolve continued to be a problem for the new planning program as well. Frustration led to litigation to the extent that the planning act was sometimes referred to as the "full employment act for attorneys."

Despite the frustration that many states experienced with the CON program, some have retained their programs as one way to regulate the development of services and facilities that they deem to be unnecessary. Although 12 states immediately dropped their CON programs when the national law was repealed (Hackey 1993), many retained and modified their CON programs, increasing the expenditure threshold as one way to control the state's Medicaid reimbursement for capital development expenditures. Thirty-six states and the District of Columbia had CON statutes on the books in 1997; all of these states regulate nursing home care, and more than half of them regulate home health care (Demkovich 1997).

No new national health planning programs have replaced the CHP and 1974 planning acts. The Health Security Act of 1993 proposed changes to remedy the escalating health services expenditures and the lack of health insurance coverage for part of the population, but Congress did not enact this proposed legislation.

## Administration

Administration is defined in the Roemer model as "the decision making of program leaders and the supervision, controls, and other actions to ensure satisfactory performance and attain certain goals" (Roemer 1991). Both public and private health services programs depend on efficient administrative capacity to remain viable. Dimensions of an administrative capacity include:

- *organizing* a program into manageable units to accomplish the required tasks;
- *staffing* with appropriate personnel and *budgeting* for adequate resources to perform the work;
- *supervising* the workforce and *consulting* with employees to achieve the program's goals;
- *procuring* necessary supplies and materials;

- *maintaining* appropriate records and *establishing* reporting systems;
- *coordinating* activities; and
- *evaluating* the unit's efforts.

## Legislation

All governmental units have legislative authority to enact laws and ordinances to aid in governing. Roemer identifies six types of legislation that govern a health services system:

1. *authorizing* or *enabling* legislation to provide governmental authority to carry out a program or activity;
2. legislation that *facilitates resource production* to train the workforce or develop health services facilities;
3. *social financing of health services,* either through the direct provision of services by government employees or the reimbursement of providers from government funds;
4. *quality surveillance* to ensure that the health services and products offered meet established quality standards;
5. legislation that *prohibits injurious behavior,* including environmental protection laws; and
6. legislation that *protects individual rights,* such as laws regarding the informed consent of patients prior to the receipt of services.

Table 5.1 lists examples of these categories of national health services legislation.

At the national level, the U.S. Congress enacts legislation in several ways. Congress may act on a discrete, single-purpose bill, or it may amend or repeal an existing law. Additionally, Congress may enact legislation as part of the comprehensive annual budgeting process that results in an omnibus budget reconciliation act (OBRA). The budgeting process has been the major vehicle for health services legislation in recent years.

## Regulation

The regulatory process provides control mechanisms to authoritative bodies to ensure that programs or services are provided in the prescribed manner. Regulation can operate through command and control incentives or through the alteration of market incentives (Eisenberg 1994). In a free-market economy, regulatory provisions may be invoked when voluntary, collective-societal behavior does not accomplish the desired ends.

**TABLE 5.1**

Examples of
U.S. Health
Services
Legislation

| | |
|---|---|
| **Authorizing or Enabling Legislation** | **1935** Social Security Act (PL 74-271) included assistance to public health departments and funded health services for special populations. |
| | **1973** Health Maintenance Organization (HMO) Act (PL 93-277) provided assistance to establish and expand HMOs. |
| **Facilitating Resource Production** | **1946** Hospital Survey and Construction (Hill-Burton) Act (PL 79-725) supported construction and modernization of hospitals and other health care facilities. |
| | **1963** Health Professions Education Assistance Act (PL 88-129) provided health professional scholarships and loans, and assistance in the construction of educational facilities. |
| **Financing of Health Care** | **1962** Health Services for Agricultural Migrant Workers Act (PL 97-692) provided federal support for clinics that care for migratory workers and their dependents. |
| | **1965** Titles XVIII (Medicare) and XIX (Medicaid) of the Social Security Act paid for health care for elderly and disabled persons and for low-income children and their caretakers, respectively. |
| | **1992** Prescription Drug User Fee Act (PDUFA) allowed the FDA to augment its budget (and thus add staff to speed up the review process) by charging user fees to drug developers. |
| | **1997** Title XXI (State Children's Health Insurance Plan—SCHIP) of the Social Security Act provided federal funds to states to establish programs to cover uninsured children. |
| | **2000** Benefits Improvement and Protection Act (BIPA) increased the disproportionate share hospital (DSH) allotments for 2001 and 2002 and made other changes to DSH provisions that resulted in increased costs to the Medicaid program. |
| | **2002** Medical Device User Fee and Modernization Act (MDUFMA) provided the FDA with additional resources to ensure prompt approval or clearance of applications for marketing medical devices and licensing biological products. |

Governmental intervention through regulatory means in a free-market economy remains much debated in many areas, including the health services area. Argument continues over whether a fully competitive market can most efficiently produce health services or whether regulation is needed to ensure equity and other values of the U.S. health services system. Deregulation of major industries such as communications and transportation has produced divided camps of proponents and opponents. Proposals to deregulate the health services industry—to free hospitals from antitrust provisions, for example—continue to be met with mixed reactions.

The regulatory process takes several forms. Enabling legislation may include regulatory provisions. Regulations for the implementation of specific programs may be issued. Governing bodies may impose licensure, certification, or registration requirements on health facilities or health providers. Accreditation by a national body is an additional, and usually voluntary, form of regulation.

|  |  | TABLE 5.1 |
|---|---|---|
|  |  | Continued |

|  |  |
|---|---|
|  | **2003** Medicare Prescription Drug Improvement and Modernization Act (MMA) provided, among many other provisions, coverage of outpatient prescription drugs for Medicare beneficiaries, beginning January 1, 2006. |
| **Quality Surveillance** | **1906** Pure Food and Drug Act (PL 59-348) ensured the safety of food and cosmetics and the safety and efficacy of prescription drugs and medical devices (as amended). |
|  | **1972** Consumer Product Safety Act (PL 92-573) regulated hazardous substances, flammable fabrics, and poison prevention. |
|  | **1982** Tax Equity and Fiscal Responsibility Act (TEFRA) established peer review organizations (PROs) to replace professional standards review organizations (PSROs) to review the quality of care provided to Medicare beneficiaries. |
|  | **1986** Emergency Medical Treatment and Active Labor Act (EMTALA) allowed patients whose insurance or financial status was unclear to receive emergency medical treatment; intended to protect against patient dumping. |
| **Prohibition of Injurious Behavior** | **1963** Clean Air Act (PL 88-206) established federal enforcement in interstate air pollution and assistance to state and local governments in controlling air pollution. |
|  | **1965** Federal Cigarette Labeling and Advertising Act (PL 89-92) warned smokers about the health hazards of cigarette use. |
| **Protection of Individual Rights** | **1974** Child Abuse Prevention and Treatment Act (PL 93-247) provided assistance to develop programs to identify and treat child abuse. |

NOTE: PL stands for Public Law, and the first number following the PL designates the congressional session in which the law was enacted.

## Specific Program Regulations

Regulations are frequently required to fully implement a piece of legislation. Regulations spell out how one is to comply with the law and also specify any sanctions and penalties for noncompliance. The Administrative Procedures Act (APA) of 1946 provides for a rule-making process in which proposed regulations are printed and widely disseminated in the *Federal Register*. This process generally provides for a period of public comment and possibly public hearings as well. Following consideration of public input, final regulations with an effective date are issued and become part of the *Code of Federal Regulations*. Participation in the development of regulations by those to be regulated is an important aspect of the democratic process. It is also time consuming and often results in a lag between legislative authorization and implementation.

### Licensure

Licensure may be required for the operation of a facility or the ability to practice a profession. Licensure is generally the purview of state governments, although national standards are sometimes required to be incorporated into state licensure statutes. States license hospitals, nursing homes, and other health services facilities to ensure that they meet construction standards, have adequate numbers of appropriately trained personnel, have modern and safety-tested equipment, and provide services in a hazard-controlled environment.

States license many health professions, including physicians, nurses, pharmacists, and dentists. Professional licensure specifies, usually in a Practice Act, the scope of practice and provides sanctions, including loss of licensure, for misconduct and malpractice. Although some states permit reciprocity in licensure, most require specific licensure by that state before a professional may practice there. Licensure is a way to control entry into the marketplace—a form of franchising—and professionals, such as chiropractors or optometrists, for example, may seek licensure to control the size of the workforce.

Interest in licensure for public health workers has blossomed in the last several years. Studies by Lichtveld et al. (2001) show that as much as 80 percent of the public health workforce has received little or no education or training in public health, and this lack of education and training is pervasive throughout the workforce, from the leadership to the entry-level worker. The Institute of Medicine's (IOM) 2002 report, *Who Will Keep the Public Healthy?*, addresses licensure and certification issues. The Centers for Disease Control and Prevention (CDC) has taken a leadership role by convening, in 2000, an Expert Panel on the Public Health Workforce to address both public health education and public health research. Although the CDC continues its work on this issue, the terrorist attacks of September 2001 required it to focus on issues of bioterrorism and emergency preparedness.

### Certification

Certification may also be required for a facility or a profession, or it may be voluntary but sought as an indicator of advanced practice and professionalism. Hospitals, nursing homes, and certain other facilities must be certified by the Medicare program as meeting its quality standards before Medicare will reimburse for care in those facilities. State health facility licensure agencies, usually located within state departments of health, generally conduct the Medicare certification process in conjunction with their own on-site facility licensure inspection and review.

Certain professions offer certification in at least two instances. First, professions that are not licensed may be certified to have met a standard set of skills and competencies. Second, professions that are licensed may offer certification of advanced training and specialization. Physicians, for example, seek board certification as evidence of their additional training and increased competency in specialty areas of medicine. The Association of Schools of Public Health (ASPH) is currently preparing a certification examination process that it plans to implement in 2007, aimed at certifying the competency of students who graduate from an accredited school or program with a Master in Public Health (MPH) or equivalent graduate degree.

## Accreditation

Accreditation, though usually voluntary, is an additional way to ensure that facilities and programs meet certain national standards. Hospitals and other facilities may seek accreditation by the Joint Commission on Accreditation of Healthcare Organizations (JCAHO) as evidence that their facilities and services meet national standards. Health maintenance organizations (HMOs) and other managed care organizations seek accreditation by the National Committee for Quality Assurance (NCQA) as proof to providers, consumers, and payers of their ability to provide high-quality services. Educational programs seek accreditation by the appropriate professional bodies as evidence of their advanced standing among their counterparts. Medical schools seek accreditation through the Liaison Committee on Medical Education (LCME), and schools of public health and public health programs in other academic settings seek accreditation by the Council on Education for Public Health (CEPH). Accreditation ensures the users of a facility or a program—be they patients, students, faculty members, or the public—that the program or facility meets specified operational standards.

## Summary

Effective management of a health services system incorporates the functions of planning, administration, legislation, and regulation. In the public-private U.S. health services system, legislation is the domain of the public sector. Both sectors perform the other three functions, which may be explicitly delineated or implicit but less readily identifiable in an organization or a program. Of these management functions, regulation may be the cause of the most controversy, regarding both the extent of regulatory activities and also whether regulation is needed at all. A significant body of literature explores whether the U.S. health services system should be managed through regulation or competition (Wallack, Skwara, and Cai 1996; Fuchs 1988; Altman and Rodman 1988). The majority opinion, however, is that at least some regulation is required to protect the integrity of a health services system and its users.

## Note

1.  Potential resources for program development under CHP planning were the nation's 56 regional medical programs (RMPs) that were established in 1965 to decrease the lag time between health technologic developments and their general application to patients. Because RMPs focused their developmental efforts on the leading causes of death—heart disease, cancer, and stroke—their utility as a funding source for CHP program needs was essentially limited to these areas.

### Key Words

accreditation
Administrative Procedures Act (APA)
board certification
certificate of need (CON) program
certification
Code of Federal Regulations (CFR)
Comprehensive Health Planning
    (CHP) Act
Council on Education for Public
    Health (CEPH)
discretionary funds
Federal Register
Great Society
health maintenance organization
    (HMO)
health planning
Health Security Act of 1993

Health Systems Agency (HSA)
Institute of Medicine (IOM)
Joint Commission on Accreditation
    of Healthcare Organizations
    (JCAHO)
Liaison Committee on Medical
    Education (LCME)
National Committee for Quality
    Assurance (NCQA)
omnibus budget reconciliation act
    (OBRA)
proposed rule making
regional medical program (RMP)
Statewide Health Coordinating
    Council (SHCC)
State Health Planning and
    Development Agency (SHPDA)

## References

Altman, S. H., and M. A. Rodman. 1988. "Halfway Competitive Markets and Ineffective Regulation: The American Health Care System." *Journal of Health Politics, Policy, and Law* 13 (2): 323–29.

Demkovich, L. 1997. "CON and Managed Care: Can the Concepts Coexist?" *State Health Notes* 18 (249): 1–2

Eisenberg, J. M. 1994. "If Trickle-Down Physician Workforce Policy Failed, Is the Choice Now Between the Market and Government Regulation?" *Inquiry* 31 (3): 241–49.

Fuchs, W. R. 1988. "The 'Competition Revolution' in Health Care." *Health Affairs* 7 (3): 5–24.

Hackey, R. B. 1993. "New Wine in Old Bottles: Certificate of Need Enters the 1990s." *Journal of Health Politics, Policy and Law* 18 (4): 927–35.

Institute of Medicine. 2002. *Who Will Keep the Public Healthy?* Washington, DC: National Academy of Sciences Press.

Lichtveld, M. Y., J. P. Cioffi, E. L. Baker, Jr., K. Gebbie, J. V. Henderson, D. L. Jones, R. F. Kurz, S. Margolis, K. Miner, L. Thielen, and H. Tilson. 2001. "Partnership for Front-Line Success: A Call for a National Action Agenda on Workforce Development. *Journal of Public Health Management and Practice* 7 (4): 1–7.

Roemer, M. I. 1991. *National Health Systems of the World*. Vol. I. New York: Oxford University Press.

Wallack, S. S., K. C. Skwara, and J. Cai. 1996. "Redefining Rate Regulation in a Competitive Environment." *Journal of Health Politics, Policy and Law* 21 (3): 489–510.

# ECONOMIC SUPPORT

# HEALTH INSURANCE: THE MAJOR FINANCING MECHANISM FOR THE U.S. HEALTH SERVICES SYSTEM

## Introduction

Beginning with the second half of the twentieth century, health insurance became the major financing mechanism for health services in the United States. Both private and public (or social) insurance had origins in the nineteenth century, but neither covered a substantial proportion of the general population for other than work-related injuries until after World War II. The origins of the private health insurance industry can be traced to the mid-nineteenth century; public health insurance originated with workers' compensation laws that individual states began to enact shortly after 1900.

Significant changes are occurring in the U.S. health insurance industry, just as they are in the remainder of the health services sector. Capturing this moving target presents a major challenge. In recent years, the role of the insurance industry has been more visible, and in the view of many, more powerful. Efforts to redistribute this power, or to reduce or eliminate the role of the health insurer, are being proposed by employers who provide health insurance as an employee benefit, by legislators, and by other health services providers.

This chapter presents an overview of insurance concepts, a discussion of health insurance–specific concepts, and a description of the evolution of insurance as a major funding mechanism for health services. Private health insurance is discussed first, public or social insurance is explored next, and then other types of health insurance, such as workers' compensation, are described. The regulation of health insurance is also considered. The chapter closes with a discussion of the pending and proposed reforms for health insurance, including the policy implications of insurance reform.

Although prepaid group practices (PGPs), health maintenance organizations (HMOs), and other models of managed care combine the functions of health insurer and service deliverer, they are not comprehensively addressed in this chapter; these topics are included in discussions of the delivery system in Chapter 19. It is important to note, however, that HMOs serve about 14 percent of people who have health insurance (U.S. Department of Health and Human Services [USDHHS] 2005), and other forms of managed care serve the majority of those with health insurance in the United States.

## General Insurance Concepts

In the purest sense, insurance is a mechanism to protect against unpredictable loss (Wilensky, Farley, and Taylor 1984). The basic function of insurance is to spread infrequent, large losses over a wide base (Light 1992). Insurance, by way of a contractual relationship (an insurance policy) is intended to bear and transfer risk from insured individuals to insurers. Risk is a central component of insurance. The insurer assesses, as accurately as possible, the risk it will bear for covering an individual or a group against specified types and extents of losses (the risk assessment function of insurance). Insurers establish their extent of risk in two ways: (1) through the underwriting process, in which actuaries assess the likelihood of events in a certain population (or structures, or vehicles, or whatever is being insured) and adjust accordingly for the risk; and (2) through experience rating, in which an insurer uses prior claims experience to predict future utilization and claims.

The risk assessment process may be subject to selection bias, in which the insurer seeks to insure only the most favorable risks—those individuals or groups likely to present the fewest claims. This practice is sometimes called *cream skimming* or *cherry picking*. Selection bias may also be a part of the potential insured's decision making, in which the person seeking insurance chooses the policy most likely to be beneficial for his or her circumstances, not all of which may be known to the insurer. When people in poor health are disproportionately concentrated in richer-benefit plans, this is known as *adverse selection*.

As part of the contractual relationship established by an insurance policy, the insurer sets a premium, to be paid monthly, annually, or on another basis, to cover the specific set of losses against which it is insuring the individual or group. The established premium includes an amount to cover the administrative load, which encompasses the cost of insuring, including risk assessment, marketing, and claims processing. The insurer varies this premium to cover the risk it determines it is incurring (the risk adjustment function of insurance).

Risk adjustment depends on the pool of individuals or groups over which the risk is spread—thus, the term *risk pooling*. Insurers may adjust their risk through *redlining,* in which the insurer determines that geographic areas, population groups, or types of businesses are too high-risk and thus ineligible for insurance.

The insurance policy may also require a deductible—an amount the insured must incur before coverage becomes effective. The insurer's goal is to achieve a favorable loss ratio: the amount it returns to the insured as benefits does not exceed the premium paid. The ratio enables the insurer to retain some of the premium as profit. This is known as the *retention rate*.

## Concepts Specific to Health Insurance

Unlike most other industrialized countries in the world, the United States does not have national health insurance (NHI) or an alternative system of universal coverage. Individuals have financial access to U.S. health services through private or public health insurance, or through other government-sponsored programs. The private health insurance market is closely linked to employment because health insurance is usually provided as a benefit of full-time employment in mid-size (100 to 499 employees) and large (500 or more employees) firms. Those employed by smaller firms (fewer than 100 employees) or who are self-employed may have more limited access to private health insurance. Public health insurance, such as Medicare, was enacted to close some of the coverage gaps that employment-based private health insurance created.

Health insurance initially was limited to inpatient hospitalization, an infrequent and usually large loss that is often unpredictable. One out of 13 nonelderly people in the United States experiences a hospitalization in any given year (Swartz 1994), whereas older people have a higher rate of hospitalization. Many hospitalizations are for serious or terminal conditions, but a significant number of hospitalizations for nonelderly females are related to childbirth. The hospital discharge rate for deliveries is higher than for any other diagnosis for either gender in every age group under 65 (USDHHS 1995a).

In the last several decades, the concept of health insurance has expanded to embrace the majority of interactions with the health services system, including physicians' services, and mental health, dental, and vision services. Health insurance has therefore become more of a financial function for predictable costs than a risk transference function for unexpected costs (Hall 1992). This expansion of insurance to nonrandom, noncatastrophic events changes the nature of insurance and how it functions within the health services system. Shonick (1995) attributes this change to the tension between the commercial purpose of insurance, which is to reduce the utilization of insured services as much as possible, and the social purpose of health insurance, which is to advocate health insurance for populations that have poor access to thereby increase their use of insured services.

### Risk Assessment

As is generally true of insurance, health insurance includes risk assessment—the process of modeling and calculating the expected expenses of one group of people relative to others. Risks are commonly stated as the deviation from the average risk, which is defined as equal to one (Bowen 1995). Assessing the risk of utilizing health services in a population provides special challenges because health status varies by age, gender, and socioeconomic, genetic, and other factors, and because a small proportion of insureds account for the majority of utilization. Studies of risk assessment in the health services market indicate that in a typical health plan, 35 percent of the subscribers have never had a paid claim, and 5 percent of the subscribers account for the majority of claims (Gauthier, Lamphere, and Barrand 1995). This finding is consistent with work by Monheit and Berk (1992), which shows that 5 percent of the users of the U.S. health services system account for 58 percent of all health expenditures (see Chapter 7).

To differentiate the high utilizers from average or low utilizers, health insurers assess risk through a range of medical screening approaches, including requiring workers in firms applying for health insurance to complete a questionnaire about their health history; obtaining health history information from an attending physician or the Medical Information Bureau, an organization that maintains data on negative answers to health screening questions asked on health and life insurance applications (Glazner, Braithwaite, and Hull 1995); or requiring an applicant to pass a physical examination administered according to insurance company criteria. These assessments may identify preexisting conditions that the insurer excludes from coverage.

Exclusion of preexisting conditions varies by type of insurance. A study by the U.S. General Accounting Office (now known as the U.S. Government Accountability Office [USGAO] 1995c) found that 59 percent of indemnity plans, 70 percent of preferred provider organizations (PPOs), and 56 percent of point-of-service (POS) plans had preexisting clauses. HMOs typically did not. The Health Insurance Portability and Accountability Act (HIPAA) of 1996 and its subsequent amendments established a series of constraints about the use of preexisting conditions in insurance offerings to make insurance more readily accessible. Employers may choose not to cover a new employee for a preexisting condition, but that exclusion can last no longer than 12 months.

Insurance coverage organized on an indemnity basis reimburses the insured for medical expenses at a predetermined rate (e.g., per day, or by type of procedure) but not necessarily for the entire bill. Under a PPO plan, employees have lower cost sharing if they choose an employer-specified panel of providers. In POS plans, subscribers to a managed care plan can select among different delivery systems (e.g., fee-for-service or HMO) when a service is obtained, rather than choosing one system at the time of enrollment.

### Direct and Indirect Risk Adjustment

Risks may be adjusted directly or indirectly (Light 1992). Direct risk adjustment includes medical underwriting and redlining. Insurers use medical underwriting to determine to whom, under what conditions, and for what price a policy is issued. Medical underwriting techniques include tier rating and durational rating. Tier rating stratifies groups according to their members' particular health risks and their industry's claims experience. Durational rating offers a low rate at first but then imposes large increases in subsequent years after the predictive effects of the initial medical screening begin to dissipate and workers are no longer protected under preexisting exclusion periods (Hall 1992).

For employer-sponsored health insurance, medical underwriting is often used for smaller businesses and experience rating for larger businesses. Some analysts have observed an underwriting six-year cycle, in which three years of rising profitability is followed by three years of falling profitability, with premium increases lagging the falling cycle by about two years (Feldstein and Wickizer 1995; Iglehart 1992). A study by Glazner, Braithwaite, and Hull (1995) provides evidence that medical underwriting may not be that definitive in identifying a group's risk. The study examined the claims history of two employed populations covered by a large insurer, one screened and the other not screened. It found no significant differences in the amounts claimed by the two populations over six years. This study suggests that medical underwriting could be eliminated in the small-group market without an increase in premiums. Rosenblatt (2004) suggests that six factors caused the underwriting cycle between 1965 and 1991: (1) claims payment time cycle, (2) renewal dates and processes, (3) growth versus profit objectives, (4) the role of the actuary, (5) rate regulation, and (6) reimbursement methods. According to her analysis, the six-year cycle has not fit the health insurance industry well since 1991. She suggests that this cycle may continue to apply to some—but not all—insurers.

Redlining, the second method of direct risk adjustment, denies insurance coverage to certain individuals or groups because of the hazardous nature of their employment, presumed high-risk lifestyles, a history of excessive claims, a propensity toward litigation, or other potential risks. Some insurers will not insure employees of commercial fisheries, barber and beauty shops, physicians' offices, or law firms because they contend that the risk of utilization and claims is excessive. Table 6.1 lists examples of industries ineligible for health insurance under select insurance plans.

Indirect risk adjustment methods include instituting copayments for certain services; limiting the benefit package by excluding certain procedures, tests, or pharmaceuticals from coverage; and placing caps or ceilings on the level of services or total expenditures (per coverage period or per lifetime) that the insurer will cover (Light 1992). Health insurers may also indirectly adjust for risk by requiring a waiting period of 30 days or longer before the insurance becomes effective. Risk adjustment exemplifies the tension between forces of economic efficiency and of equity in the U.S. health

TABLE 6.1

Examples
of Industries
Ineligible
for Health
Insurance
under Selected
Insurer Plans

| | |
|---|---|
| Amusement parks | Hotels/motels |
| Aviation | Insurance agencies |
| Auto dealers | Janitorial services |
| Barber and beauty shops | Junkyard/refuse collectors |
| Bars and taverns | Law firms |
| Car washes | Liquor stores |
| Commercial fishing | Logging/mining |
| Construction | Moving companies |
| Convenience stores | Parking lots |
| Domestic help | Physicians' practices |
| Entertainment/athletic groups | Restaurants |
| Exterminators | Roofing companies |
| Foundries | Security guard firms |
| Grocery stores | Trucking firms |
| Hospitals and nursing homes | |

SOURCE: American Hospital Association 1988.

services system. Risk adjustment, as currently practiced, permits the insurer to limit rather than spread the risk of insuring and thus introduces questions of equitable financial access to health services.

In ideal economical circumstances, and assuming that health insurance remains the primary financing mechanism in the U.S. health services system, risk adjustment would occur in a defined market with standardized benefit packages. Free and easy market entrances and exits would be controlled to protect against adverse selection in the market itself (Bowen 1995). Individuals would pay the same premium regardless of their health status, but the premium payments that the insurer received would be adjusted to reflect the differences in individuals' expected health services costs (USGAO 1994c). Such ideal economic circumstances do not exist in the U.S. system.

To move the U.S. system closer to these ideal circumstances, the GAO (1994c) proposes that health insurance risk adjustment should:

1. predict health services costs with accuracy;
2. treat participating HMOs reasonably and fairly;
3. be difficult for participating health plans to manipulate;
4. respect patient privacy and confidentiality;
5. create incentives for appropriate care; and
6. be feasible and inexpensive to administer.

Others suggest that an independent agency should administer risk adjustment on a national level. All insurers would use a form of community rating to establish premiums. In community rating, a health plan sets its premium in a specific geographic area to reflect its average cost for all subscribers (Luft 1986). This type of risk adjustment would provide payment to insurance plans commensurate with the risks of the populations they serve (Bowen 1995) and would eliminate the problem of selection bias for both the insurer and the insured.

## Evolution of Health Insurance as the Primary Mechanism for Financing Health Services

Although health insurance did not become the major financing mechanism for health services in the United States until World War II, the private health insurance industry originated a century earlier. In 1850, the Franklin Health Assurance Company of Massachusetts offered coverage for medical expenses for bodily injury that did not result in death, and in 1860, Travelers Insurance Company of Hartford began to offer medical expense coverage on a basis resembling the present form of health insurance. By 1866, another 60 insurance companies were writing health policies. These policies were predominantly loss-of-income policies and provided benefits for a limited number of diseases, such as typhus, typhoid, scarlet fever, smallpox, diphtheria, and diabetes (Health Insurance Association of America [HIAA] 1992).

The public or social insurance industry began at the state government level, with the emergence of workers' compensation (then called workmen's compensation) insurance shortly after 1900. Federal public health insurance programs introduced in the mid-1960s, Medicare in particular, have significantly altered the balance between private and public health insurance in the U.S. system. Figure 6.1 shows the proportion of the population that is covered by private insurance, Medicare, Medicaid, those who have both Medicare and Medicaid (the dually entitled, discussed later in this chapter), and the uninsured. Table 6.2 shows the percentage of the insured population by age group and type of insurance coverage.

### Private Health Insurance
Although private health insurance policies were available to some employed populations as early as the mid-1850s, private health insurance as a benefit of employment was not widely available until the World War II era. The concept of private health insurance was slow to spread for many reasons. The economy of the mid-1850s was still principally agrarian or extractive-resource based, and the workforce was only beginning to be industrialized. Labor unions had not yet materialized as a force to be reckoned with, and the concept of workers' rights was still embryonic. The medical care sector was equally unformed at this point, and the majority of care consisted of private transactions between physicians, or other providers, and patients. Physician training was not yet standardized, hospitals were not yet a significant force

**FIGURE 6.1**
Percentage
Distribution
of U.S.
Population,
by Health
Insurance
Coverage
(2003)

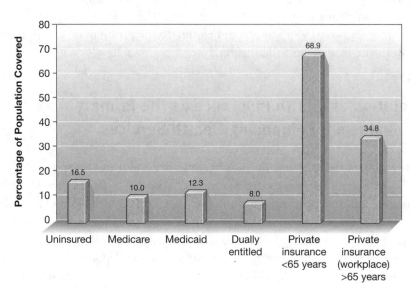

SOURCE: USDHHS 2005.

NOTE: These are not mutually exclusive categories. Individuals may have multiple coverage (e.g., both Medicare and private insurance).

**TABLE 6.2**
Percentage of
U.S. Population
Covered
by Health
Insurance,
by Age and
Type of
Coverage
(2003)

| Type of Insurance Coverage | < 65 Years | 65+ Years |
|---|---|---|
| Private health insurance | | |
|     Self-employed | 13.7 | NA |
|     Employer-sponsored/retiree | 63.3 | 34.8 |
| Public health insurance/vendor payers | | |
|     Medicare | 1.7 | 95.0 |
|     Medicaid | 12.3 | 8.0 |

SOURCES: USDHHS 2005; Liska, Brennan, and Bruen 1998.

NOTE: NA = not available.

in the delivery system, and the state of medical technology was rudimentary at best. There was, in short, little for which a patient could be insured, and the workforce was not organized to think about employee benefits.

By the 1920s, however, changes in the economy, in the sophistication of the medical care sector, and in the expectations of the workforce created a more favorable climate for the growth of private health insurance. Although the economy remained predominantly agrarian, industrialization was moving the workforce from the fields to the factories and into other business sectors. Hospitals were increasingly available to provide care to patients with serious injuries or illnesses. Workers and the public in general began to express concern about safer workplaces, and the Great Depression had begun.

Schoolteachers and Baylor University Hospital in Dallas, Texas, are credited with stimulating in 1929 the growth of employer-sponsored private health insurance. The hospital agreed to provide schoolteachers with room, board, and specified ancillary services for 21 days of hospital care per year at a predetermined monthly cost, annualized to a $6 premium (HIAA 1992; Starr 1982). Baylor University Hospital expanded this concept, which became known as Blue Cross, to other sizable employed groups, resulting in what Starr calls "the birth of the Blues." Soon, other area insurers were emulating this model. As the Depression took its toll on voluntary hospitals, they began to offer hospital service contracts to employed groups as one way to secure financial stability. Under a service contract, the insurer guarantees payment for services directly to the hospital, and the payment often covers the full bill. The major hospital trade association, the American Hospital Association (AHA), promoted the development of group hospitalization service plans that ultimately resulted in a network of Blue Cross plans blanketing most of the country. Blue Cross plans are linked to the Blue Cross Association by a licensing agreement (USGAO 1994b).

**Development of Blue Cross and Blue Shield**

Blue Cross plans differ from commercial insurers in several ways. First, Blue Cross plans were established as not-for-profit organizations, whereas other commercial insurers were generally established as proprietaries.

Second, Blue Cross offers only health insurance, whereas other insurers may offer health insurance as one of several lines (e.g., life, fire, or automobile). Health insurance may even be a "loss leader" for some insurers, used to secure other, more profitable lines.

Third, coverage is offered on a service basis, meaning that only the select hospital or hospitals under contract provide a designated set of benefits with the plan. In contrast, commercial insurance is often organized on an indemnity basis, giving the insured a choice of a range of hospitals from which to obtain care. Additionally, Blue Cross pays the hospital directly rather than reimbursing the patient for the cost of the hospitalization (HIAA 2002).

Fourth, Blue Cross plans typically use community rating to determine their premium structure. Commercial insurers use experience rating, basing the next year's premiums on the specific claims experience of an insured group in a prior year. Blue Cross plans also feature open enrollment and contractual relationships with physicians and hospitals, often with prospectively set rates (Iglehart 1992), whereas their commercial counterparts typically do not.

Additionally, Blue Cross plans often serve as an insurer of last resort, agreeing to insure populations or individuals other carriers will not insure. In recognition of this community service role and to offset costs associated with insuring all risks, Blue Cross plans and Blue Shield plans were given federal and state tax exemptions and other statutory benefits, such as discounts on hospital charges, not available to commercial insurers (USGAO 1994b).

By 1940, the 39 Blue Cross plans had more than six million subscribers (Starr 1982), and by 1955, the plans had about 45 percent of the private insurance market (Shonick 1995). The AHA maintained its close relationship with Blue Cross plans until 1972, when the AHA transferred the names, the marks (logos), and the plan approval program to the Blue Cross Association, and both organizations eliminated their overlapping board member requirements (Cunningham and Cunningham 1997).

Blue Shield plans, which insure subscribers for physician care, were first established in Michigan and California in 1939 and soon spread to other states (Iglehart 1992). State and local medical associations stimulated the development of Blue Shield plans, and like their Blue Cross hospital counterparts, they were organized as not-for-profits.

A trend among Blue Cross plans is the conversion from not-for-profit to proprietary status. Blue Cross plans in Colorado, Ohio, and other states have effected this change in recent years. The assets from the not-for-profit plans have, in some instances, become the corpus for educational and other philanthropic foundations that support health-related research and development. In the decade between 1993 and 2002, Blue Cross plans in 15 states, including California and New York, converted to for-profit status, and most of these merged into two large holding companies—Wellpoint and Anthem (Hall and Conover 2003)—which have since merged. Because Blue Cross plans hold such a significant market share, analysts have expressed concern about the continued likelihood of Blue Cross's traditional coverage as an insurer of last resort.

## Growth of Commercial Health Insurance

Although commercial insurers began offering indemnity coverage against hospital expenses on a group basis in 1934 and expanded this coverage to surgical bills four years later, provider-organized health insurance plans were dominant prior to World War II (Starr 1982). The war set into motion a series of forces that further stimulated the growth of commercial health insurance (see Chapter 7). Unlike the development of the Blue Cross and Blue Shield plans, which were provider-organized, the development of commercial health insurance was an outgrowth of disability insurance that insurers were marketing to the middle class (Starr 1982) and the advent of providers who established not-for-profit hospital service insurance companies (Shonick 1995). As was true with the development of Blue Cross plans, commercial health insurance still focused primarily on marketing group health plans to employees of larger businesses and their dependents to best spread their risk. Employees of small businesses, where risk may not so easily be spread, and those who were self-employed had more difficulty obtaining health insurance. By 1955, commercial health insurance also had about 45 percent of the total private health insurance market (Shonick 1995).

| Type of Industry Medium and Large Establishments | Full-Time Workers | Part-Time Workers |
|---|---|---|
| All workers | 76 | 21 |
| Professional, technical, and related workers | 79 | 29 |
| Clerical and sales workers | 78 | 20 |
| Blue-collar and service workers | 74 | 19 |

SOURCE: USDHHS 2005.

**TABLE 6.3**
Percentage of Workers with Employer-Sponsored Health Insurance, by Type of Industry (1997)

Table 6.3 shows the percentage of workers, by type of industry, that had employer-sponsored health insurance coverage in 1997. Employer-sponsored insurance is associated with size of industry: the larger the business or industry, the more likely it is to offer its employees health insurance as a benefit (Figure 6.2*a*). Figure 6.2*b* shows the percentage of firms, by firm size, offering employer-sponsored health insurance in 2003. Employer-sponsored insurance is also associated with the type of business or industry. Unionized businesses are most likely to offer health insurance, and service businesses—particularly smaller ones—are least likely to offer health insurance as a benefit. The link between employment and health insurance offered as a benefit was forged by the 1947 Taft-Hartley Act, which established health benefits as a "condition of employment" for which labor was entitled to negotiate (Cunningham and Cunningham 1997).

The type of health insurance that employers offer varies considerably. Large employers may offer a triple option: an indemnity plan, an HMO plan that combines insurance and service delivery functions, and a preferred provider organization (PPO) plan. Employees choose among health plans based, in part, on premium cost and the availability of preventive care for families (Feldman, Wholey, and Christianson 1989). Some employees choose a plan to obtain a specific service they anticipate needing, and some switch plans for the same reason. Such choices represent selection bias.

Although full-time employees in mid- to large-sized businesses have come to expect health insurance as a benefit of employment, employees in smaller firms (fewer than 100 employees) may not have health insurance as a benefit. Nearly one-half of the labor force works in firms of fewer than 100 employees (Kronick 1991), and more than 90 percent of U.S. firms have fewer than 150 employees (Wickizer and Feldstein 1995). Almost one-third of uninsured workers are the dependents of people who work for small businesses (USGAO 1991b), so the potential for being unable to obtain employer-sponsored health insurance is widespread in the workforce.

**Availability of Health Insurance in Small Businesses**

**FIGURE 6.2**

Percentage of
Workers, Ages
18–64, with
Health
Insurance, by
Size of Firm
*(a)* 1999.
*(b)* 2003.

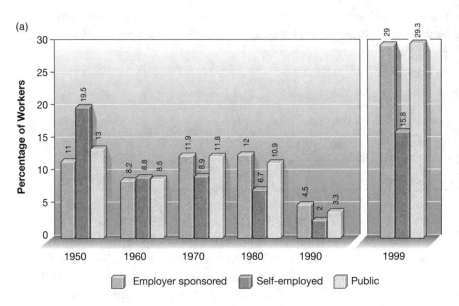

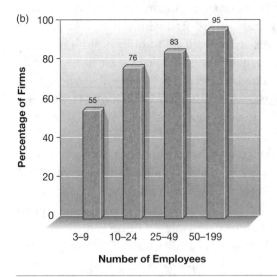

SOURCES: *(a)* Health Insurance Association of America 2002. Used with permission from America's Health
Insurance Plans (formerly the Health Insurance Association of America). *(b)* Robert Wood Johnson
Foundation 2004a. Used with permission.

       Health insurance may not be available in smaller firms for many
reasons:

1. The nature of the business, or the presumed lifestyle of its employees,
   is considered too high-risk (Table 6.1). In fact, about 15 percent of

small firms are in industries routinely redlined (Zellers, McLaughlin, and Frick 1992).

2. The premium becomes unaffordable when the risk is spread over a small group.
3. The workforce is largely part-time or contingent.
4. A catastrophic claim from one employee results in unsustainable premium increases for all employees.
5. Small firms have less potential to self-fund their health insurance programs and are thus subject to state regulation, premium taxation, and requirements to provide certain benefits if they do offer health insurance.

Providing employee health insurance to smaller firms is far more expensive than to larger firms. Health plan costs are 10 to 40 percent higher for smaller firms than for larger firms for comparable plans and benefits (USGAO 1992b). These higher costs are due in part to the higher administrative costs for smaller firms that insurers pass on through higher premiums. Figure 6.3 shows insurance company overhead by size of firm. In a small-group plan with one to four employees, insurers' overhead accounts for 40 percent of claims, whereas the administrative expense for a large-group plan with ten thousand or more employees is 5.5 percent of claims.

Both state and federal governments have instituted reforms to address two dimensions of the small business health insurance problem: (1) how to assist small firms to continue to provide health insurance, and (2) how to enable more small firms to offer health insurance.

Between 1990 and 1994, 40 states enacted small-group insurance regulations that include portability standards to permit employees to transfer their insurance from one place of employment to another (USGAO 1995c). Other state reforms address guaranteed issue, which requires insurers to offer plans to small employers, and guaranteed renewal, which requires insurers to renew coverage to small employers. Other reforms place limits on the exclusion of preexisting conditions.

At the federal level, HIPAA establishes national requirements for carriers offering coverage in the individual, small-, and large-group markets; provides for portability from group to individual plans; and limits preexisting condition waiting periods (Blue Cross/Blue Shield Association 1996).

Retiree health insurance has been an important benefit to some in the workforce, especially those working in larger companies of two thousand or more employees. Several kinds of insurance are included in the retiree health category: employer-sponsored group coverage, individually purchased Medisup policies, or publicly sponsored coverage such as Medicaid. This discussion focuses principally on changes that are occurring in employer-sponsored group coverage for retirees.

**Retiree Health Insurance**

FIGURE 6.3
Insurance
Company
Administrative
Expenses by
Size of Firm
(1991)

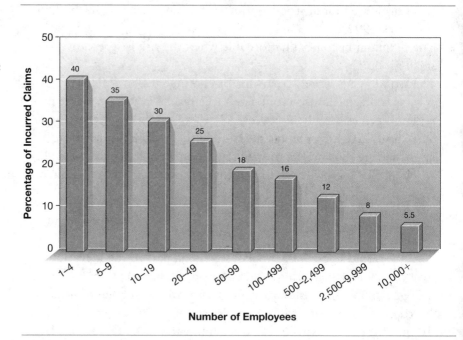

SOURCE: USGAO 1992b.

Getting a fix on the current extent of employer-sponsored retiree health insurance is complex. No one database reports these data; analysts must use multiple data sources and correct for the overlaps and gaps among them. It is estimated that more than one-third of all persons age 65 and older (about 11 million persons) had supplemental coverage from an employer in 2004 (Neuman 2004). The prevalence of employer-sponsored retiree health insurance has declined since the late 1980s and also since the implementation of Standard Financial Accounting Standard (SFAS) 106 in the early 1990s (McCormack et al. 2002a). SFAS 106 directed private-sector firms to include the present value of the costs of future retiree health benefits as a liability; public-sector firms, which are a substantial provider of retiree health benefits, are exempt.

Figure 6.4 shows the percentage of large firms that offered retiree health benefits through 2000. The Kaiser/HRET annual survey provides further insight into the decline in retiree health insurance benefits. In 1988, 66 percent of firms with over two hundred employees offered retiree health insurance, but by 2005, only 33 percent of such firms retained this coverage (Kiplinger's Retirement Report 2005). Many of the largest firms (over one thousand employees) have imposed caps on their future obligations for retiree health benefits, and many retirees with these benefits have or soon will reach these caps. Even more common than benefit terminations are increases in retiree contributions to premiums and cost-sharing arrangements (Neuman 2004).

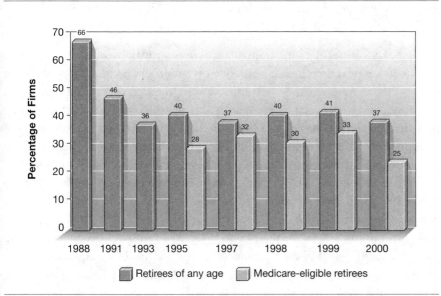

**FIGURE 6.4**
Large Firms
That Offered
Retiree Health
Benefits (Select
Years,
1988–2000)

SOURCE: McCormack et al. 2002a.

NOTES: Includes firms with two hundred or more employees. Data are weighted to reflect all employees nationally. Data intervals are irregular.

Neuman's report to Congress in May 2004 noted the following findings about retiree health insurance from a Henry J. Kaiser Family Foundation study:

- More than half of retirees ages 55–64 have employer-sponsored health benefits.
- One in three persons with Medicare also has employer-sponsored health benefits.
- Seniors with employer-sponsored drug coverage are less likely to skip medications due to cost.
- The share of employers offering health benefits has declined.
- Total retiree health costs increased on average by 13.7 percent between 2002 and 2003, an increase similar to that of other workers.
- Nearly half of large private-sector employers offering health benefits to retirees age 65 and older have caps on their firms' contributions.
- Seven in ten employers increased retiree premium contributions in the past year.
- One in ten employers terminated benefits for *future* retirees.
- Employers reported an increase in retirees' cost sharing for health benefits in the past year.
- Nearly nine in ten employers say that higher premium contributions are likely in the next three years. Two in ten say that termination of such benefits for future retirees is likely.

• Employers say that increases in cost sharing for retiree health benefits are likely in the next three years.

Several issues affecting retiree health insurance are worthy of note. First, the financing of retiree health insurance by employers became an issue in the mid-1980s, stemming from the failure, closure, merger, or acquisition of these businesses and the consequent jeopardy of benefits to which an employee may have made payroll contributions over time. Although businesses are now required to report how they will fund the future costs of retiree health benefits, the retiree whose former employer has gone out of business has little recourse.

Second, for the retiree with private insurance who is also eligible for Medicare, the matter of payer of first resort arises (i.e., which insurer has primary responsibility for paying for the retiree's health services). Three federal omnibus budget reconciliation acts (OBRAs) address this question. The 1982 Tax Equity and Fiscal Responsibility Act (TEFRA) made Medicare the secondary payer for active workers ages 65–69. The 1984 Deficit Reduction Act (DEFRA) made Medicare the secondary payer for insured workers under age 65 with a spouse age 65–69 who is covered by Medicare. The 1985 Consolidated Omnibus Budget Reconciliation Act (COBRA) extended the DEFRA provisions to workers age 69 and older (Monheit and Schur 1989).

Third, employers are seeking ways to increase the cost sharing among all groups they cover, including retirees. This may lead employers to move from a defined benefit to a defined approach (McCormack et al. 2002b). (See the discussion "Cost Sharing" later in this chapter.)

Fourth, passage of the Medicare Prescription Drug Improvement and Modernization Act (MMA) of 2003, which provides outpatient prescription drug coverage for Medicare beneficiaries, could affect retiree health benefits. Medicare coverage of outpatient prescription drugs could result in reduced employer outlays, permitting employers to maintain retiree health insurance programs (McCormack et al. 2002a). Even though the MMA has provisions to subsidize employers who retain prescription drug coverage as a part of their retiree health benefit packages, it is not yet clear how many such employers will seek this subsidy. The Kaiser Family Foundation and Hewitt Associates conducted a 2005 survey of three hundred of the nation's largest employers that indicates that 79 percent of businesses that now provide retiree health benefits with prescription drug coverage will accept the subsidy for 2006, but by 2010, only half of this employer group expects to maintain the coverage and accept the subsidy (Medical Study News 2005).

**Health Insurance as a Major Cost of Doing Business**

Far from being solely a fringe benefit used to attract a stronger workforce, the provision of employee health insurance is currently a major expense of doing business. Business health spending as a share of total labor compensation was 10.2 percent for state and local government and 6.8 percent for private industry in 2005, up from 2 percent in 1965 (USDHHS 2005).

The increase in business spending on health services is due, in part, to increasing premium rates, which are affected by increases in benefit payments, the extent of HMO market penetration, the deductible levels and co-insurance rates, and the increase in the number of mandated benefits state-licensed insurers must offer (Feldstein and Wickizer 1995). Between 1980 and 1990, premiums grew at an average annual rate of 20.6 percent (Feldstein and Wickizer 1995). Figure 6.5 shows the percentage increase in health insurance premiums for select years from 1988 through 2003. Premium growth rates dropped well below 20.6 percent in 1994 and 1995

(a)
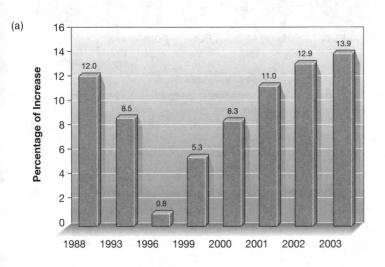

(b)
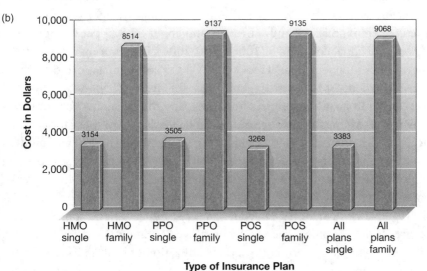

**FIGURE 6.5**
Increases in Health Insurance Premium Costs
*(a)* Percentage increases in insurance premiums (select years, 1988–2003).
*(b)* Average annual premium cost, by type of plan (2003).
*(c)* Average percentage of premium paid by employer, all types of plans (2003).

*(continued)*

**FIGURE 6.5**
Continued

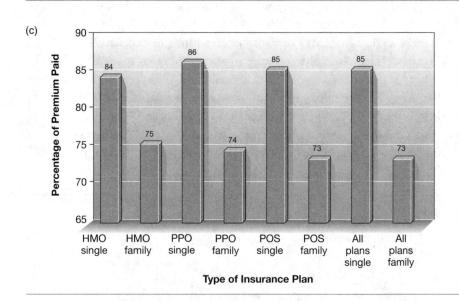

SOURCES: *(a)* Robert Wood Johnson Foundation 2004b. *(b)* and *(c)* Goff 2004.

NOTES: HMO = health maintenance organization; POS = point-of-service plan; PPO = preferred provider organization. In *(a)*, the data intervals are irregular.

(Levit, Lazenby, and Sivarajan 1996). Premiums continued their decline in 1996, increasing by less than 1 percent, according to Peat Marwick's survey of employers (Ginsburg and Pickreign 1997). At the same time, insurers' profitability was dropping. Ginsburg and Pickreign (1997) note that at some point, insurers will no longer be willing to raise premiums less than the increase in underlying cost, even if this means sacrificing market share.

The average employer spent $6,656 per employee per year on health insurance premiums for family coverage and about $2,875 per employee per year for individual coverage in 2003 (Goff 2004). This amount varies by the type of plan (conventional, HMO, PPO, POS) offered. Figure 6.6 shows that 75 percent of business expenditures for health services are directed toward paying health insurance premiums, and the balance is for contributions to the Medicare hospitalization fund, workers' compensation insurance, and the support of on-site clinics (enterprises, per the Roemer model).

Several factors account for the increasing cost to business of providing employee health insurance. To attract the desired workforce, employers—sometimes stimulated by negotiated labor agreements—offered first-dollar coverage plans. First-dollar coverage pays the full cost of the premium and requires little or no cost sharing by employees. Employees therefore have no incentive to monitor or control their utilization of health services. Insurance in this instance insulates employees from the true cost of health services because they may never see the provider's claims for reimbursement. In

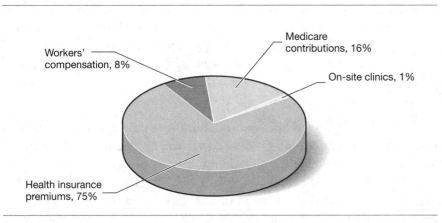

SOURCE: USGAO 1992b.

FIGURE 6.6
Components
of Business
Expenditures
on Health
(1992)

addition, the fee-for-service reimbursement system, until recently the dominant provider payment method, creates incentives to provide more discrete and separately billable services (often referred to as unbundled services) to the insured. With few constraints on the utilization or the provision of services, not surprisingly, utilization and expenditures increased. Employers who formerly considered the provision of employee health insurance as just another cost of business have been motivated by the significant increases in this expense to aggressively contain their health-related expenditures.

To contain the costs of and expenditures for providing health insurance, employers have instituted a number of measures, including employee cost sharing, reducing the scope of covered benefits, reducing or eliminating coverage for dependents, capping the total expenditures available per insured person, offering fewer fee-for-service and more managed care options, requiring authorizations before the use of services, and self-funding their own insurance programs. The following sections describe each measure.

**Measures to Contain the Costs of Expenditures for Health Insurance**

Employers instituted cost sharing as a way to control utilization of and thus expenditures for health services. Cost sharing may require the insured to pay part of the premium, pay a deductible before coverage becomes effective, make copayments of a fixed dollar amount for services such as prescription drugs, or pay co-insurance, a fixed percentage of the total costs.

*Cost Sharing*

The RAND Health Insurance Experiment (HIE) explored the effects of cost sharing on access to services in the late 1970s and early 1980s. This seminal health services research experiment found that:

> The more families had to pay out of pocket, the fewer medical services they used. . . . All types off service—physician visits, hospital admissions, prescriptions, dental visits, and mental health service use—fell with cost

sharing. There were no striking differences among these services in how their use responded to plan, with the exception of hospital admissions of children, which did not respond to plan. Another partial exception was demand for mental health services—which, the results indicate, would have been more responsive than other services to cost sharing had there been no cap on out-of-pocket expenditure (Newhouse 1993).

Cost sharing often does reduce utilization, though it is least likely to reduce children's utilization of services, particularly emergency department hospital services, because parents will not usually forego care that they perceive is needed for their children (Spillman 1992). Cost sharing reduces the use of many preventive services (Lurie, Manning, and Peterson 1987). It can have a negative effect on health status because the insured may not be able to distinguish between an urgently needed medication or service (e.g., hypertension drugs, which often treat asymptomatic disease) and a medication or service that may be less urgently needed but may provide more immediate and evident relief to the patient (Brook 1991; Rasell 1995). Cost sharing may also inhibit people with limited resources from obtaining needed services until their condition is far more serious—and more expensive to treat—than it would have been at the outset (Rasell 1995).

A 2005 survey of employer-sponsored health insurance high-deductible plans showed that employees enrolled in such plans were less likely to fill a prescription for certain types of drugs than were employees enrolled in non-high-deductible plans. For all drugs, 28 percent of those in a high-deductible plan did not fill prescriptions, compared to 13 percent in a non–high-deductible plan. For specific kinds of drugs, the proportions were even higher: for depression drugs, only 9 percent of enrollees in non–high-deductible plans did not fill these prescriptions, compared to 30 percent of enrollees in high-deductible plans; and for heart disease or hypertension drugs, only 8 percent of enrollees in non–high-deductible plans did not fill these prescriptions, compared to 18 percent of enrollees in high-deductible plans (Lee and Zapert 2005).

Increasingly, more of the costs of health services are being shifted to the beneficiaries through changes in the structure and generosity of health insurance plans (Monheit, Nichols, and Selden 1996). Table 6.4 shows the average monthly premium costs and the average percentage of the premium paid by the employee in 2003 for different types of health plans. Employees now typically pay 15 to 27 percent of the cost of their health insurance premiums, up from 10 percent in 1988 (USDHHS 2005). From 1992 through 1996, the dollar contributions of employees enrolled in employment-based insurance plans increased at an average annual rate of 7.2 percent, compared with premium increases that averaged 3.8 percent (Ginsburg and Pickreign 1997). The broader the choice of provider, the higher the employee's cost sharing is likely to be.

| Type of Plan | Average Annual Premium Cost | Average Percentage of Premium Paid by Employer |
|---|---|---|
| HMO single | $3,154 | 84 |
| HMO family | 8,514 | 75 |
| PPO single | 3,505 | 85 |
| PPO family | 9,137 | 74 |
| POS single | 3,268 | 85 |
| POS family | 9,134 | 73 |
| All plans single | 3,383 | 85 |
| All plans family | 9,068 | 73 |

**TABLE 6.4**
Employee Cost Sharing for Family Coverage, by Type of Plan, 2003

SOURCE: Goff 2004.

NOTES: HMO = health maintenance organization; PPO = preferred provider organization; POS = point-of-service plan.

*Limited Scope of Benefits*

Employers may limit or reduce the scope of benefits provided to an insured as another way to contain costs. The number of outpatient mental health visits an insured may obtain may be limited, for example, and certain services or procedures, such as heart-lung transplants, may not be covered by particular policies. Reducing or eliminating the health insurance coverage of an employee's dependents is another way of limiting the benefit package.

*Caps on Insurance Expenditures*

Employers may contain their expenditures by offering policies that have caps on the total expenditures for covered services for an individual in a specified coverage period or lifetime. Table 6.5 shows the percentage of maximum lifetime benefits covered by three types of plans: conventional, PPO, and POS. Although each plan offers maximum lifetime benefits of $1 million or more, or places no limits on the majority of its subscribers, a sizable percentage of each limits the maximum lifetime benefits. Insured people who exceed such caps may be dropped from coverage. The reason for exceeding the expenditure cap may be the expense of treating a chronic condition. In these situations, employees may find that they cannot easily obtain new insurance because the health problem constitutes a preexisting condition and thus is excluded from coverage, at least for a period of time, by a new insurer.

To contain costs and expenditures, employers may offer fewer insurance options or may require employees to join a managed care program in which utilization of services and choice of provider may be constrained.

| Type of Plan | Up to $250,000 | $250,001— $999,999 | $1+ million | None | Other |
|---|---|---|---|---|---|
| Conventional | 9 | 6 | 61 | 22 | 2 |
| PPO | 8 | 3 | 68 | 20 | 1 |
| POS | 4 | 0 | 58 | 0 | 38 |

SOURCE: Sullivan et al. 1992. Copyrighted and published by Project HOPE/*Health Affairs*. The published article is archived and available online at www.healthaffairs.org.

**Controls on Utilization of Services**

Directly controlling the utilization of services by requiring prior authorization, second opinions for surgery, or precertification for a nursing home stay (Chapter 15) are additional methods employers use to contain their health expenditures. By 1992, some type of utilization management governed the use of health services by more than 90 percent of employees covered by group health insurance (Wickizer and Feldstein 1995).

**Self-Funded Insurance**

Increasingly, employers who have a large enough workforce are choosing to self-fund their health insurance programs. In self-funded—sometimes referred to as self-insured—programs, the employer assumes the responsibility of defining a benefit package and paying directly for covered services, thus reducing or eliminating the need for an insurance company. Self-funding is possible under the provisions of the 1974 Employee Retirement Income Security Act (ERISA), which imposes federal requirements, administered by the Department of Labor, on all private and employment-based plans regarding reporting, disclosure, fiduciary obligations, and claims-filing procedures, whether self-funded or not (USGAO 1995b). Figure 6.7 shows the state and federal authority to regulate sources of private coverage under ERISA provisions. HIPAA preempts several ERISA provisions. The portability section of this act permits an employee who changes jobs to be protected against the preexisting conditions of the new insurer.

Self-funding offers a number of advantages to employers of larger workforces. ERISA exempts self-funded health insurance programs from having to offer benefits mandated by a state insurance commission of insurers licensed to do business in the state. Self-funded plans are exempt from paying state insurance premium taxes and are also exempt from any willing-provider laws (such laws require a health plan to include any provider who meets the plan's terms in its managed care network). They cannot be required to participate in funding state-created insurance programs for people deemed uninsurable through the commercial markets.

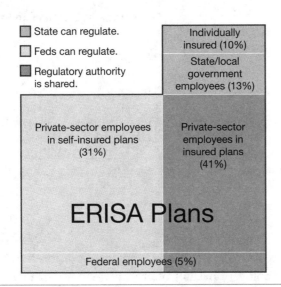

SOURCE: Butler 2000.

**FIGURE 6.7**
Americans with
Private Health
Coverage
(State and
Federal
Authority to
Regulate
Sources of
Private
Coverage)

Employers who self-fund may manage their own reserve funds. They do not pay a considerable up-front premium to insurers to cover services that may never be utilized. They pay only for services that are used and may also negotiate a discounted payment rate to providers. Self-funding also allows employers to maintain uniformity of plans in the 41 metropolitan areas that cross state boundaries (USGAO 1995b).

If a firm wishes to fund its employees' health insurance program but does not want to bear the entire financial risk, it may reinsure part of this risk with another insurer. In this instance, the firm can establish a stop-loss level—$25,000 per insured, for example—beyond which the reinsurer would bear the risk.

Similarly, if a firm wishes to fund its employees' health insurance program but does not want to handle all of the administrative functions (e.g., actuarial activities, benefit plan design, and claims processing), it may develop an administrative services only (ASO) agreement with an insurer for the provision of these services. Firms may also engage third-party administrators (TPAs) to maintain all records regarding the people covered under their plans. TPAs are outside people or firms and are not a party to the employer-employee health insurance relationship (HIAA 1992).

Table 6.6 shows the percentage of the population with employer-sponsored insurance that is covered by self-funded plans. Between 1997 and 2001, the percentage of employees in HMOs in self-funded, employer-sponsored plans dropped from 33 percent to 23 percent. During this same period, growth in enrollment in PPOs expanded from 31 percent to 48 percent (HIAA 2001).

TABLE 6.6
Enrollment
in Employer-
Sponsored
Health Plans,
by Type,
Select Years

| | Percentage of Enrollees in Each Plan Type | | |
|---|---|---|---|
| | *1997* | *1999* | *2001* |
| Conventional plans | 16 | 8 | 7 |
| HMO | 33 | 29 | 23 |
| PPO | 31 | 41 | 48 |
| POS | 17 | 22 | 22 |

SOURCE: HIAA 2002.

**Individual**
**Health**
**Insurance**
**Policies**

Individuals may not be covered by employer-sponsored health insurance because their employer does not offer it, they do not qualify for it, they are self-employed or not in the workforce, or for other reasons. These people may choose to purchase individual coverage. Individual policies can be purchased specifically for inpatient hospitalization, for catastrophic coverage, or for more complete coverage.

Individual policies are generally more expensive, less comprehensive in scope, and more sensitive to preexisting condition exclusions than group coverages are. Individual policies are more expensive because the insurer has no way to spread the risk, it is generally not feasible to include individuals in managed care organizations, and reimbursement is based on charges rather than discounted rates (Levit, Olin, and Letsch 1992). The administrative load for an individual policy may therefore be as high as 40 percent of the premium (Thorpe 1992), whereas it averages about 18 percent for firms of 50 to 99 employees, and 6 to 16 percent for larger firms (Monheit, Nicols, and Selden 1996).

More than half of those who have individual policies are people age 65 and older. These individual policies typically are Medisup/Medigap policies to complement their Medicare coverage, discussed later in this chapter.

Individuals who believe themselves to be in good health and/or who want to avoid paying increasing premiums and other cost sharing for group policies may choose to purchase individual policies. Such choices are, in part, predicated on a self-assessment of risk—namely, that no major illness or need for extensive health insurance coverage will occur.

The proportion of the population with privately purchased health insurance plans declined from 1980 to 1987 (18.2 percent to 16.6 percent) and from 1988 to 1991 (13.8 percent to 13.1 percent) (Levit, Olin, and Letsch 1992). From 1980 to 1995, the percentage of the population younger than 65 and covered by private health insurance decreased 9 percentage points, from 79.5 to 70.5 percent. The coverage of children, early retirees, and near-poor families declined faster than the coverage of the overall population. Rising premiums charged for those policies are a likely cause of the decline. Other causes include shifts in employment, low rates of growth in real family incomes, and indirect effects of expanded Medicaid coverage (USGAO 1997b).

Several special categories of private health insurance are worthy of note: "dread disease" policies, policies for specific services, and long-term care (LTC) insurance. "Dread disease" policies cover a specific disease type, such as cancer. Policies can also be purchased for specific services, such as prescription drugs. These policies are sold almost exclusively on an individual rather than group basis.

**Special Categories of Private Health Insurance**

LTC insurance is a relatively recent phenomenon in the U.S. market, first appearing in the 1970s. This first wave of LTC insurance, which ended in the mid-1980s, resulted in few sales of policies but established the form of LTC insurance: principally as a reimbursement-based product. The second wave of LTC insurance, although bolstered by such events as model legislation prepared by the National Association of Insurance Commissioners (NAIC), foundered a decade later, in part due to the delay in states passing legislation that would protect consumers (Desonia 2004). A third wave showed some gains in governmental interest and advocacy, but the number of policies in effect and the coverage they provide will not make a dent in the anticipated growth in LTC expenditures. The growing demand for and cost of LTC services are already straining federal and state budgets, and no solution is yet at hand for this increasingly significant problem (USGAO 2005).

*LTC Insurance*

Although some employers offer group LTC insurance as an employee benefit option, the majority of policies (97 percent) are still sold to individuals (Norton and Newhouse 1994). Because of a HIPAA provision, however, employers have an incentive to include LTC insurance benefits. As of January 1, 1997, employers can deduct from their taxes the cost of providing LTC coverage for employees. Individuals who purchase policies can deduct part of the premium from federal taxes if the total cost of medical and long-term care exceeds 7.5 percent of their income. This tax code provision does not appear to have markedly influenced growth in the sale (and retention) of LTC policies.

Although LTC insurance has been slow to gain a foothold in the U.S. health services system for several reasons. The insurance is most affordable to younger, healthier populations—the very groups who may not foresee the need for this coverage or for whom premium dollars compete with other basic needs, such as housing, education, and transportation. The average age of an LTC policy purchaser is 72 years, and the average age of nursing home entrance is 76 years (USGAO 1993b). LTC policies generally are structured as indemnity policies, in which a flat rate per nursing home day (or other covered service) is paid. Although some policies include an inflation factor, it is still difficult to predict what proportion of the prevailing rate the policy will cover when it is effected.

A high percentage of people who purchase LTC insurance do not retain their policies. In a study by the GAO (1993a) of five LTC insurance companies, an average of 20 percent of the policies lapsed in the first year of ownership, 50 percent lapsed within five years, and 65 percent lapsed in ten years. If a policy includes a nonforfeiture benefits clause, insurers are not required to return premiums on lapsed policies.

The reasons for lapsing LTC policies may include the use of an individual's resources for current needs as opposed to unknown future needs, the hope that a growing population of elderly will force the creation of additional governmental programs, or an awareness that the Medicaid program pays for nursing home care when an individual's other resources have been spent-down to Medicaid's level of eligibility.

**Private Health Insurance Summary**

Private health insurance finances the health services of nearly two-thirds of the U.S. population. The majority of this coverage occurs through group insurance, with larger employers being more likely than smaller ones to offer health insurance as a benefit. Some businesses also provide health insurance to their retirees. Offering health insurance as an employee benefit has become a significant cost of doing business. As a result, employers have instituted a number of measures to contain their expenditures for providing employee health insurance. People who are ineligible for employer-sponsored health insurance may, if they have the resources, purchase individual health insurance policies for full coverage or for specialized coverage, including long-term care.

### Public Health Insurance

Public health insurance, sometimes called social insurance, has been established to pay for health services to some populations that do not have or cannot obtain private health insurance. Private health insurance focuses largely on those in the workforce and their dependents and, in some instances, on retirees from the workforce. For the small proportion of the population that can afford them, individual health insurance policies are also part of the private health insurance market. People outside the workforce, because of age or health status, require other means of financial access to health services. This access is provided to some people through public health insurance. This section discusses the following seven major public insurance or vendor payment programs and considers the cost to the public of providing this care:

1. TRICARE, a health services program using military health care as the main delivery system (formerly known as CHAMPUS, the Civilian Health and Medical Program of the Uniformed Services);

2. Medicare;
3. Medicaid (a vendor payment program);
4. medically needy programs;
5. medically indigent programs;
6. state insurance programs for uninsurables; and
7. the State Children's Health Insurance Program.

The TRICARE program, Medicare, and Medicaid are entitlement programs. People who meet the statutorily defined eligibility criteria are entitled to all services that the program offers for the duration of their entitlement. Although the Medicaid program is not a true health insurance program (i.e., it has no premiums and the coverage is limited to certain categorically eligible groups and may be terminated if conditions of eligibility change), it is included in this discussion because it is frequently treated and labeled as a public insurance program.

Additionally, some states, such as Tennessee and Washington, have implemented statewide insurance programs. These programs are briefly discussed in Chapter 3.

**TRICARE**

The TRICARE program, which provides medical care to military dependents and retirees, originated from two governmental programs: the Emergency Maternal and Infant Care Program (EMIC) of 1943—a wartime measure to provide maternal and infant care benefits to the wives of active-duty servicemen—and its successor program, the Dependents Medical Care Program. In 1966, the Dependents Medical Care Program was expanded from its emphasis on obstetrical services to include outpatient and ambulatory care and a special program of medical care for dependents of active-duty military personnel. The CHAMPUS name was conferred in 1969 (Shonick 1995); the change to TRICARE occurred in 1994.

TRICARE is a health insurance program that is supplementary to the Military Health Services System (MHSS) and includes coverage for care either in the MHSS's worldwide system of 76 hospitals and 460 clinics or in civilian hospitals, by civilian physicians, and by other authorized professional providers (TRICARE 2002). TRICARE also pays for ambulatory services, prescription drugs, and authorized medical supplies and rental of durable medical equipment (Shonick 1995). TRICARE has approximately 8.4 million beneficiaries who are free to select providers and required to pay a deductible and copayment but have not had to pay premiums (USGAO 1995a; TRICARE 2002).

Because of escalating costs and government expenditures, the increasing administrative burden of running the military health program, and beneficiary dissatisfaction with it, the CHAMPUS Reform Initiative was established in the late 1980s to contain costs and improve services. One way to achieve these desired changes was to introduce aspects of managed care, including enrollment into specific plans, utilization management, assistance in referral to the most cost-effective providers, and reduced paperwork. In 1994, the Department of Defense began to restructure the entire MHSS program, including CHAMPUS, into 12 new service regions called TRICARE. For services that cannot be provided to military dependents and retirees by military medical facilities, contracts are awarded to civilian companies in the 12 health services regions (USGAO 1995a).

## Medicare

The Medicare program, created by Title XVIII of the Social Security Act, was established in 1965 and implemented the following year to pay for health services for people age 65 and older. Medicare was one of two compromises—the other was Medicaid—effected following the inability to secure national health insurance. Social health insurance was endorsed as early as 1912 by presidential candidate Teddy Roosevelt (Litman and Robins 1991) but had foundered on opposition from organized medicine, within Congress, and from other sources. (See Appendix 6.1 at the end of this chapter for an outline of national health insurance initiatives.) Initially aimed at the population age 65 and older—because age 65 was then the mandatory retirement age as well as the age for Social Security eligibility—Medicare was expanded in 1972 to include people of any age with end-stage renal disease (ESRD) and in 1973 to include people of any age who met Medicare's definition of disability.

### Eligibility for Medicare

Currently, people earn eligibility for Medicare principally by participating in the workforce and contributing to the Social Security system for 40 calendar quarters. The 1972 amendments to the Social Security Act, effective in July 1973, permit most people age 65 and older who are ineligible for hospital insurance to enroll voluntarily by paying a monthly premium (USD-HHS/HCFA 1990). For 2006, the monthly Part A premium for people who had 10 to 39 quarters of covered employment is $393. (Medicaid may pay this premium if the individual is a Medicaid enrollee.)

The majority of Medicare beneficiaries sign up for benefits upon reaching age 65. People with disabilities entitled to Social Security or railroad retirement cash benefits for at least 24 months become Medicare beneficiaries, as do most people with ESRD, regardless of their age.

Medicare beneficiaries who meet the age criterion of 65 retain their eligibility for life, regardless of their financial circumstances; Medicare does not employ a means test. Medicare beneficiaries who meet the disability criterion are also likely to retain their eligibility for life unless their disabling condition is ameliorated in some major way. ESRD Medicare beneficiaries may lose their Medicare eligibility if a kidney transplant, for example, improves their health status, thus removing their requirement for regular dialysis treatment.

| Medicare Program | Total Enrollees (in Millions) |
|---|---|
| Hospital Insurance (Part A) or Supplemental Medical Insurance (Part B) | 38.8 |
| Hospital Insurance (Part A) | 38.4 |
| Supplemental Medical Insurance (Part B) | 36.8 |

SOURCE: USDHHS 2005.

**TABLE 6.7**
Profile of Medicare Beneficiaries (2004)

Table 6.7 shows the distribution of Medicare beneficiaries by the Medicare program (hospital insurance and supplementary medical insurance) in which they are enrolled. Eighty-six percent of Medicare beneficiaries are age 65 and older; 14 percent are people with disabilities.

Medicare is organized into four major programs. Part A (hospital insurance, HI) covers inpatient hospital care, limited skilled nursing facility care, home health, and hospice care for all Medicare beneficiaries. Through its Part A HI plan, Medicare provides coverage for 90 days of inpatient hospital care in a benefit period (spell of illness). No limit exists for the number of benefit periods an individual may use. The program also provides a nonrenewable (lifetime) reserve of 60 days if a beneficiary exhausts the 90 days available in a benefit period. Part A also covers up to 100 posthospital days in a skilled nursing facility if the beneficiary is certified to require skilled nursing or rehabilitative care. Home health agency visits and hospice care are also covered by Part A. Beneficiaries pay an inpatient hospital deductible ($952 for 2006) for days 1 through 60 of each inpatient hospital benefit period, as well as co-insurance for hospital and skilled nursing facility stays.

*Medicare Parts A, B, C, and D*

Part B, supplementary medical insurance (SMI), covers physicians' and outpatient clinic services and is optional. Beneficiaries may choose to purchase this coverage for a monthly premium, which is $88.50 for 2006. Table 6.8 compares Parts A and B in terms of eligibility, covered benefits, program financing, and cost-sharing requirements.

Part C, the Medicare Advantage program (known as Medicare+Choice until the passage of the MMA in 2003), was established by the 1997 Budget Reconciliation Act to attract more Medicare beneficiaries into managed care plans. Many have judged the success of Part C to be mixed. Beneficiaries were slow to enroll; many providers, after experience in adding Medicare

**TABLE 6.8**
Comparison
of Medicare
Parts A (HI)
and B (SMI)
(2006)

| | Medicare Part A (Hospital Insurance) | Medicare Part B (Supplementary Medical Insurance) |
|---|---|---|
| Eligibility | All Medicare beneficiaries who met Medicare age (65) and/or disability criteria or are eligible for railroad retirement benefits | All Medicare beneficiaries who elect to purchase this optional coverage; some resident aliens |
| Covered Benefits | Inpatient hospital services, skilled nursing home coverage, hospice services, home health services | Services provided by a physician in any location, diagnostic tests, radiologic and pathologic services, drugs that cannot be self-administered |
| How It Is Financed | Trust fund supported by employer and employee payroll contributions, beneficiary cost sharing | Trust fund supported by monthly premiums (25% of total financing) and general revenue funds (75% of total financing) |
| Cost Sharing | Deductible $952 per benefit period | Monthly premium of $88.50, 20% copayment on all covered services |

SOURCE: CMS 2006.

beneficiaries to their plans, found them to be costly subscribers and have dropped Part C coverage under the Medicare+Choice option (Young 2001).

Medicare Part D was established by the 2003 MMA. The MMA has many provisions, including amending other sections of the Medicare legislation (as described earlier). Its principal focus was the establishment of outpatient prescription drug coverage for Medicare beneficiaries. Sign-up for the benefit began in the fall of 2005 and had to be completed by May 15, 2006 in order to avoid a financial penalty. Coverage became effective January 1, 2006.

Figure 6.8 shows the distribution of Medicare expenditures by type of service received for Parts A and B. Fifty-five percent of Medicare payments are directed to the HI (Part A) services of Medicare and 45 percent to the SMI (Part B) services of Medicare. Medicare does not cover several health services, such as routine eye examinations and certain preventive services, that Medicare beneficiaries widely use. Certain dental procedures are covered only if provided during an authorized hospital inpatient stay. Intermediate nursing care is not covered, and Medicare covers skilled nursing

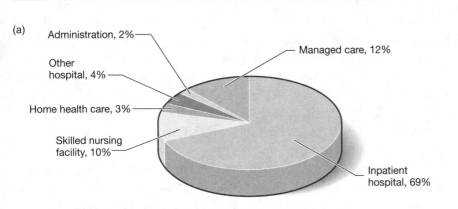

(a)
Administration, 2%
Other hospital, 4%
Home health care, 3%
Skilled nursing facility, 10%
Managed care, 12%
Inpatient hospital, 69%

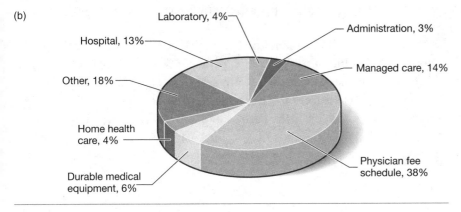

(b)
Laboratory, 4%
Hospital, 13%
Other, 18%
Home health care, 4%
Durable medical equipment, 6%
Administration, 3%
Managed care, 14%
Physician fee schedule, 38%

SOURCE: USDHHS 2005.

**FIGURE 6.8**
Distribution of Medicare Program Payments, by Type of Service (2003)
*(a)* Medicare Part A.
*(b)* Medicare Part B.

care only in the very limited circumstances described earlier. People who can afford insurance coverage for these services generally buy Medisup/Medigap and LTC insurance policies.

Medicare Part A is financed through payroll deductions and employer contributions and to a very limited extent by beneficiary deductibles and coinsurance payments. These contributions go into a trust fund, the long-term viability of which is periodically questioned. The stability of the trust fund is dependent on the size of the contributing workforce as well as the longevity of Medicare beneficiaries who use health services. The contributing workforce is diminishing. In 1960, five years before the Medicare program was authorized, five workers contributed to the Social Security system for each retiree; in 1995, the ratio was 3 to 1; and by 2020, when most baby boomers will have reached retirement age, the ratio is projected to be 2.2 to 1 (U.S.

Bipartisan Commission on Comprehensive Health Care 1990). As longevity increases due to technological advances against chronic diseases, beneficiaries have longer life spans in which to consume services, particularly inpatient hospital services, and thus further draw down the trust fund.

Medicare Part B is financed in part by the monthly premiums that beneficiaries pay, but about 75 percent of the funds come from federal general funds. Federal expenditures for Part B increase with the number of Medicare beneficiaries purchasing this coverage and their utilization of physician and outpatient services.

Part C is financed by beneficiary premiums, deductibles, and copayments, as well as by the Medicare trust fund described for Part A.

Part D is financed largely from federal general revenues, with varying levels of beneficiary cost sharing (copayments and deductibles), depending on the prescription drug plan the beneficiary chose.

*Medisup/*
*Medigap*
*Insurance*
*Policies*

The cost-sharing requirements of Parts A, B, C, and D of Medicare can require considerable out-of-pocket expenditures for the approximately 80 percent of beneficiaries who use health services in a given year (USDHHS 1995b). Figure 6.9 shows the percentage of beneficiary cost sharing for overall Medicare, as well as for Parts A and B. Because Part C is a managed

**FIGURE 6.9**
Medicare
Expenditures
by Type of
Expenditure
and Type of
Coverage
(2004)

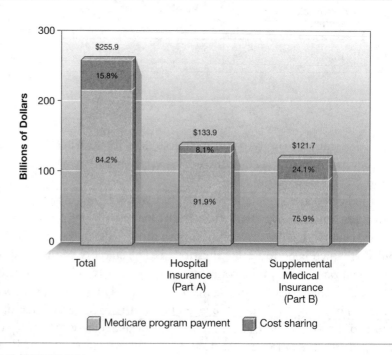

SOURCE: USDHHS 2006.

care option across varying plans, cost-sharing data are not readily available. Cost-sharing data for Part D will not be available for several years, inasmuch as this coverage was first available on January 1, 2006. On average, Medicare pays for less than half of the beneficiary's total health service expenditures (Reinhardt 1993). To reimburse for these out-of-pocket expenses, as well as to obtain coverage for optometry, dentistry, podiatry, and other services that Medicare does not cover, 61 percent of Medicare beneficiaries buy individual supplemental private health insurance. Premiums paid for Medisup policies in 1999 averaged $1,300 annually, with more than 20 percent going to administrative costs (USGAO 2002). The sale of such policies, formerly called Medigap and now called Medisup policies, came under federal regulatory control in 1988 to prevent further abusive sales and reimbursement practices to a particularly vulnerable population. As a result of the Baucus amendment to the Social Security Act, insurers may offer ten types of Medisup policies, labeled A through J. Federal regulations spell out the minimum coverage that each type of plan must offer (Table 6.9). States do not have to offer all ten types, and they may, under certain circumstances, approve innovative additional benefit plans. The premiums for Medisup policies vary by type of policy, by geographic area, and by demographic characteristics of the insured. Type A is the least comprehensive and least expensive, and Type J is the most comprehensive and most expensive. Figure 6.10 shows the distribution of Medisup enrollees, by plan

**TABLE 6.9**
Medisup/
Medigap
Benefits by
Plan Type

| Medisup/Medigap Benefits | A | B | C | D | E | F | G | H | I | J |
|---|---|---|---|---|---|---|---|---|---|---|
| Basic benefits | X | X | X | X | X | X | X | X | X | X |
| Part A hospital deductible | | X | X | X | X | X | X | X | X | X |
| Part A skilled national health co-insurance | | | X | X | X | X | X | X | X | X |
| Part B deductible | | | X | | | X | | | | X |
| Foreign travel emergency | | | X | X | X | X | X | X | X | X |
| At-home recovery | | | | X | | | X | | X | X |
| Part B excess physician charges 100% | | | | | | 100% | 80% | | 100% | 100% |
| Preventive screening | | | | | X | | | | | X |
| Outpatient prescription drugs | | | | | | | Basic | Basic | Extended | |

FIGURE 6.10
Distribution of
Medisup/
Medigap
Policies by Plan
Type (1999)

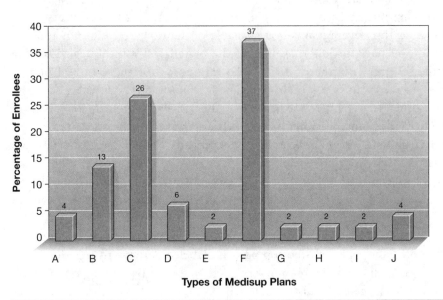

SOURCE: Health Insurance Association of America 2002. Used with permission from America's Health
Insurance Plans (formerly the Health Insurance Association of America).

type, for 1999. The nature of these plans and the benefits they cover will change as a result of the MMA of 2003.

A special type of Medicare supplemental policy, called Medicare SELECT, was authorized by OBRA 1990 and functions as a PPO. Beneficiaries who purchase Medisup/Medigap plans through the Medicare SELECT program get full coverage for their health services cost-sharing liabilities when they are treated by providers in the PPO network, but they are fully liable for cost sharing when treated by out-of-plan providers (Commerce Clearing House Medicare and Medicaid Guide 1995). Originally limited as a 15-state demonstration, Medicare SELECT was expanded to all states through 1998. Because it had until recently the status of a demonstration and is ongoing, little is yet available in the published literature about the program's effects. Further, provisions of the MMA of 2003 will likely alter this program.

Although many Medicare beneficiaries purchase Medisup/Medigap policies to help defray their out-of-pocket expenditures for health services, the increasing costs of such policies may soon restrict access to them by the oldest and sickest policyholders. A 1997 Lewin Group study found that nearly 70 percent of the 22 insurers with the largest Medisup/Medigap shares predicted double-digit annual rate increases in the future (Reichard 1997).

Medicare, the public insurer of health services for older Americans and those with certain disabling conditions, continues to be a major force in the growth of the U.S. health services system. Stimulated by faster growth in the Medicare-eligible population than in the general population, as well as by the increased need for health services in an aging population, the Medicare program faces significant challenges to remain solvent and to meet increasing demands. The difficulty in making hard decisions to reduce benefits that are viewed as entitlements should not be underestimated.

Like Medicare, the Medicaid program resulted from the failure of a national health insurance initiative in the mid-1960s. Medicaid was created to pay for a mandated set of health services to low-income children and their adult caregivers, and is known as a vendor payment program. Receipt of Medicaid payment for services was initially linked to eligibility for and/or the receipt of cash payments under the Aid to Families with Dependent Children (AFDC) program or the Supplemental Security Income (SSI) public assistance programs.[1] Medicaid eligibility was later expanded to low-income elderly people, people with developmental disabilities, pregnant women, and low-income children, even if their parents or caretakers were not eligible for or receiving public assistance from the AFDC or SSI programs.

**Medicaid**

The 1996 Personal Responsibility and Work Opportunity Reconciliation (PL 104-193) Act eliminated the AFDC program, replacing it with the Temporary Assistance to Needy Families (TANF) program. TANF provides states with grants to be spent on time-limited cash assistance, generally limits a family's lifetime cash welfare benefits to a maximum of five years, and permits states to impose a wide range of other requirements, including those pertaining to employment. Although most persons covered by TANF will receive Medicaid, PL104-193 does not require this coverage (USDHHS 2001).

Many states also made those people who receive general assistance or general public assistance (sometimes called general relief) eligible through a state-only program. Table 6.10 identifies the population groups that have mandatory and optional eligibility for Medicaid. Appendix 6.2 summarizes the expansions of Medicaid eligibility from 1984 to 1990.

Medicaid is a payer of health services for more than 13 percent of the U.S. population at any given time, but it is not a true health insurance program. Eligibility for Medicaid is still linked to the eligibility for and/or receipt of SSI public assistance funds for many enrollees and is usually means-tested (i.e., linked to an individual's income and assets). An improvement in an individual's personal financial circumstances often signals the termination of his or her Medicaid eligibility. Thus, eligibility for Medicaid is inconstant and episodic.

*Eligibility for Medicaid*

Because Medicaid pays for health services for people whose financial resources are most limited, it usually does not have premiums, and few programs have implemented deductibles. Individual Medicaid programs may institute limited cost sharing, which usually takes the form of

**TABLE 6.10**

Groups
Eligible for
Medicaid

| Mandatory Eligible Groups | Optional Eligible Groups |
|---|---|
| Families with children receiving AFDC or linked in specific ways to assistance through the AFDC program | Infants up to 1 year and pregnant women not-covered under the mandatory coverage but whose income is >100% FPL |
| Pregnant and/or postpartum women and children under age 6 whose family incomes do not exceed 133% FPL or a higher level if that level was used before the mandated 133% level. States are also required to extend eligibility until 19 years of age to children born after 8/30/83 in families at or below FPL. | Certain aged or disabled adults who have incomes above those requiring mandatory coverage but whose income is not >100% FPL |
| | Children under age 21, 20, 19, or 18 (state option) or groups of these children who meet income and resource requirements but are not otherwise eligible for AFDC |
| Recipients of adoption assistance and foster care under Title IV-E of the SSA | Caretaker relatives whose incomes and resources meet the AFDC income and resource requirements |
| Aged, blind, and disabled individuals receiving assistance from the federal SSI program or whose Medicaid eligibility is determined under state standards more restrictive than the standards for SSI | Institutionalized individuals with incomes and resources below specified limits |
| | Persons receiving care under home and community-based waivers |
| Medicare-eligible individuals whose incomes do not exceed the FPL and whose resources are at or below 2× the standard allowed under the SSI program; these are the QMBs.* | Pregnant women during a period of presumptive eligibility; this option allows states to make prenatal care available to these women based on a preliminary determination of eligibility done by a qualified provider |
| Special protected groups (usually individuals who lose cash assistance but who may keep Medicaid for a period because of some change in the cash program rules) | Aged, blind, and disabled recipients of state supplementary programs |
| People who are not citizens or nationals of the United States, or aliens lawfully admitted for permanent residence or permanently residing in the United States but who meet other Medicaid eligibility requirements, are eligible for treatment of emergency medical conditions | Tuberculosis-infected persons who meet SSI incomes and asset tests; benefits limited to those that are tuberculosis-related |

SOURCE:  USDHHS 2000.

*Two additional groups of Medicare beneficiaries may be eligible for some Medicaid benefits. See source document.

NOTES: AFDC = Aid to Families with Dependent Children; FPL = federal poverty level; QMB = qualified Medicare beneficiary; SSA = Social Security Act; SSI = Supplemental Security Income.

modest copayments (e.g., $1 to $2 per prescription) that may be waived if the Medicaid enrollee cannot pay. Cost sharing is also limited to certain types of services and certain Medicaid subpopulations. Some states have established copayments but make copayment collection the responsibility of the provider. Colorado's Medicaid program, for example, reduces the provider payment by the amount of the statutorily established copayment.

Participating state Medicaid programs must provide the following set of basic services:

*Medicaid Covered Services*

- hospital inpatient and outpatient;
- rural health clinic;
- laboratory;
- X-ray;
- skilled nursing care for people age 21 and older;
- home health care;
- early periodic screening, detection, and treatment (EPSDT) preventive services for children through age 21;
- physician services;
- family planning; and
- nurse midwife services where permitted by state practice acts.

States may limit the amount of coverage they provide for each service (e.g., states may cover only 15 days of inpatient hospitalization in a year or only a set number of family planning visits per year).

States may also provide an array of more than 30 optional services, shown in Table 6.11, to their Medicaid enrollees, depending on the Medicaid plan each state has developed. States may limit these services as well (e.g., states may establish a formulary to cover only certain kinds of prescription drugs or may limit the number of prescriptions per enrollee that it will cover).

The federal and state governments jointly finance the Medicaid program. Federal matching funds—at least 50 cents of every dollar (but no more than 83 cents of every dollar)—are based on the state's per capita income. Poorer states such as Mississippi have a higher federal match rate (76.8 cents in 2000) than states such as California and New York with higher per capita incomes. The Medicaid program is currently an open-ended program: enrollees receive covered services, and the federal and state governments pay their shares for total expenditures. Congress has considered capping the amount of federal funds available to Medicaid programs as one way of containing overall health services expenditures. The 1996 TANF program caps some Medicaid funds.

*Medicaid Financing*

**TABLE 6.11**

Medicaid
Optional
Services

States—depending on the Medicaid State Plan they have had approved by the Centers for Medicare and Medicaid Services (CMS), the unit of the U.S. Department of Health and Human Services (HHS), that administers the Medicare and Medicaid programs—may choose to offer some or all of the following services to their Medicaid enrollees. The services that are most commonly covered among state programs are designated by an asterisk (*).

Podiatrists' services

*Optometrists' services

Chiropractors' services

Other practitioners' services

Private duty nursing

*Clinic services

*Dental services

Physical therapy

Speech, hearing, and language disorder services

*Prescribed drugs

Dentures

*Prosthetic devices

*Eyeglasses

Other diagnostic, screening, preventive, and rehabilitative services

Inpatient hospital services (age 65+ in mental institution)

Nursing facility services (age 65+ in mental institution)

IMD (over age 65 or under age 21) and ICFMR services

Inpatient psychiatric hospital services (under age 21)

Christian Science nurses

Christian Science sanitoria

*Nursing facility services (under age 21)

Emergency hospital services

Personal care services

Transportation services

Case management services

Hospice services

Respiratory care services

Other services approved by the HHS secretary

SOURCE: Congressional Research Service 1993.

NOTES: ICFMR = intermediate care facility for the mentally retarded; IMD = institutions for mental

Figure 6.11 compares the categories of Medicaid enrollees—aged, blind, and disabled; low-income children; low-income adults; and others—with the proportion of expenditures directed to each group. Children constitute 46 percent of all Medicaid enrollees but absorb just over 16 percent of the Medicaid program expenditures.

*Medicaid Expenditures*

By contrast, low-income disabled people constitute 15 percent of Medicaid enrollees but absorb more than 43 percent of expenditures, and the aged constitute 8 percent of Medicaid enrollees but absorb 26 percent of expenditures. Medicaid enrollees also include low-income elderly people, known as the dually entitled or crossover populations. More than 14 percent of Medicare beneficiaries are also Medicaid enrollees and receive long-term care and other services through the Medicaid program (USDHHS 1995b).

A special group of Medicare beneficiaries, the Qualified Medicare Beneficiaries (QMBs), became eligible for some Medicaid services, exclusive of outpatient prescription drugs, in 1988. Many states also pay the Medicare Part B premiums for low-income Medicare beneficiaries, thus providing their access to physician and other outpatient services and making Medicare, rather than Medicaid, the payer of first resort for this population.

Figure 6.12 shows that 13.9 percent of Medicaid expenditures are for inpatient hospital care and 25.2 percent are for nursing home care for people

**FIGURE 6.11**
Medicaid Enrollees, by Medicaid Category and Expenditures per Category, 2002.

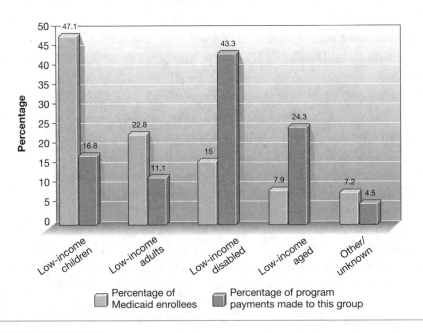

SOURCE: USDHHS 2006.

**FIGURE 6.12**

Distribution of
Medicaid
Payments by
Type of Service
(2001)

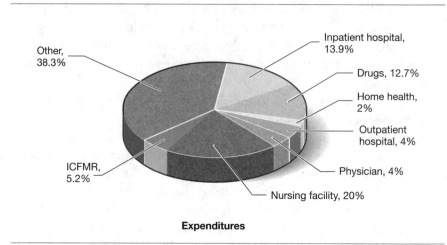

**Expenditures**

SOURCE: USDHHS 2005.

NOTE: ICFMR = intermediate-care facility for the mentally retarded.

with developmental disabilities, people with other disabilities, and the aged. Medicaid, in fact, is a major payer for nursing home care, directing a far greater proportion of its resources to this service than Medicare does.

**Medically
Needy
Programs**

States have the option to establish Medically Needy programs to pay for the health services of those who are categorically eligible for Medicaid but whose income and/or assets exceed the state's established levels. Thirty-eight states, the District of Columbia, and five territories have Medically Needy programs and receive federal matching funds for this population. States that offer a Medically Needy program must, at a minimum, provide coverage to the following groups:

- pregnant women who, except for income and assets or resources, would be eligible as categorically needy;
- individuals under age 18 who, except for income and resources, would be covered as mandatory categorically needy;
- all newborn children born on or after 10/1/84 to a woman who is eligible as medically needy on the date of the child's birth; and
- women who, while pregnant, applied for, were eligible for, and received Medicaid services as medically needed on the day that their pregnancy ends. The Medicaid agency must provide medically needy eligibility to these women for an extended period (60 days) following termination of pregnancy (Congressional Research Service 1993; Centers for Medicare and Medicaid Services [CMS] 2005).

Eligibility for Medicaid, originally established to pay for a basic set of health services to low-income children and their caretakers, has been expanded to other low-income groups and pays for health services for about 13 percent of the nation's population. In fiscal year 1999, federal Medicaid funds constituted nearly 44 percent of all federal revenues provided to states. States spend, on average, about 22 percent of their total budgets on their Medicaid programs (AcademyHealth 2006). Federal and state expenditures accounted for 6 percent of total federal expenditures and 20 percent of total state expenditures (USGAO 1997a).

State governments are spending an increasing slice of their budgets to pay for their share of Medicaid. Until a recent slowing of the annual Medicaid growth rate, the average annual growth rates in the early 1990s exceeded 20 percent (USGAO 1997a). Although Medicaid is an important safety net to provide health services to certain populations, it does not guarantee health services for most of them. The average span of eligibility for Medicaid is less than a year, although individuals may have multiple periods of eligibility.

Welfare reform, enacted at the state government level, is likely to have a significant but not fully known effect on eligibility for Medicaid and the resulting health status of needy people. The 1996 Personal Responsibility and Work Opportunity Reconciliation Act (PL 104-193), more widely known as welfare reform, repealed the AFDC, JOBS (Job Opportunity and Basic Skills Training), and emergency assistance programs and replaced them with a capped federal block grant called Temporary Assistance for Needy Families (TANF). As they revise their welfare programs, states are still determining the implications of welfare reform on access to health services for low-income people, including linkages between welfare programs and Medicaid. Determining the effect of welfare reform changes on Medicaid enrollment and utilization is difficult in strong economic conditions. As the economy weakens, however, and unemployment rates grow, demand for Medicaid will probably increase.

**Medically Indigent Programs**

States may also establish programs for the medically indigent that may cover similar benefits to those provided to Medicaid enrollees. State programs for the medically indigent do not receive federal Medicaid matching funds.

**State-Sponsored Health Insurance Programs for Uninsurables**

People with chronic, expensive-to-treat health conditions are sometimes unable to obtain private health insurance because insurers consider them to be high-risk. Since 1976, 32 states and the District of Columbia have developed pools of high-risk individuals and subsidized their coverage (AcademyHealth 2006). These state high-risk insurance plans are financed by premiums paid by the insured and often by an assessment on other insurance plans doing business in that state. Except in the first year or two of operation, most state high-risk pools lose money and require subsidization from other sources. More than 200,000 individuals nationwide who may not otherwise have been able to obtain coverage have been insured by these state programs between 1976 and mid-1995 (Stearns and Mroz 1996).

Although state programs provide an essential service to people who can afford the premiums, they are limited in scope. Most state programs set their premiums at 150 percent of the standard risk. State programs often require a waiting period of 6 to 12 months for conditions that were present 3 to 6 months prior to enrollment. Few state programs provide coverage to the insured's dependents. States have faced challenges in maintaining the risk pools because changes in the health insurance market are forcing carriers to leave the market (AcademyHealth 2002).

Disenrollment from state high-risk pools is high: 15 to 20 percent disenroll annually, and 40 to 70 percent disenroll within two years. Disenrollment is often a response to premium increases that either were implemented by the plan or occurred as enrollees aged into higher-risk categories. People choosing higher levels of deductibles are less likely to disenroll, and disenrollment declines with the increasing age of the enrollee (Stearns and Mroz 1996).

**State Children's Insurance Program**

The Balanced Budget Act of 1997 (PL 105-33) authorized the establishment of the State Children's Health Insurance Program (SCHIP) as Title XXI of the Social Security Act. This program authorizes federal matching funds to states to initiate and expand the provision of health assistance to uninsured, low-income children. To receive matching funds, states may expand their Medicaid programs to better meet the needs of uninsured children; start, or augment, a separate insurance program for children; or develop a hybrid, combining the prior two options. Federal funds may be used to increase coverage for children with family incomes less than 200 percent of the federal poverty level (FPL). Each state's allocation is determined by a formula based largely on the number of uninsured children under 200 percent of the FPL in the state (Weil 1997).

States have had difficulty in spending their federal allotments under SCHIP for a variety of reasons ("Three Years. . ." 2001). One important result of this inability to spend allocated funds was the slower-than-projected enrollment of eligible children, potentially compromising their abilities to obtain needed services. By 2003, however, monthly enrollments in SCHIP had increased to such an extent that state Medicaid programs and expenditures were growing as well. By the third quarter of 2003, 3.8 million children were enrolled in SCHIP (Kenney and Chang 2004). This growth occurred during the years (2002 through 2004) when the federal funds decreased by $1 billion. Thus, the jury remains out on the full effects of SCHIP enrollment on Medicaid expenditures (Gates 2002).

**Public Health Insurance Summary**

Public health insurance programs fill in some of the gaps left by private insurance, with 13 percent of the insured population covered by Medicare, 10 percent by Medicaid, and 4 percent by TRICARE. Other public insurance programs, such as state-sponsored health insurance programs for the uninsured, cover only a fraction of the population. Workers' compensation insurance covers people in the workforce for work-related injuries.

### Other Types of Health Insurance

Several other kinds of health insurance, including workers' compensation and viatical settlements, are important components of the U.S. health services system.

As the U.S. economy became more industrialized in the early part of the twentieth century, the number and extent of industrial accidents removed workers from the workforce and their livelihoods. By 1907, 26 states had passed employer liability acts declaring the employer's legal obligation to provide for safety in the workplace. The next year, the Federal Employers Liability Act was passed for the same purpose. Other federal acts were passed to cover specific industries, including the Federal Employees' Compensation Act to cover U.S. governmental employees, the Longshoremen and Harbor Workers Act to cover maritime workers other than seamen, and the black lung program to cover miners (Shonick 1995).

**Workers' Compensation Insurance**

Employer liability acts were soon followed by workers' compensation acts, with the state of New York passing the first workers' compensation statute in the early 1900s. By 1948, every state had a workers' compensation act that provided two types of benefits: cash payments to replace the loss of wages due to the inability to work and free medical care for conditions caused by work-related traumas. Employers in all states paid the entire premium for such coverage (Shonick 1995).

Workers' compensation insurance is significant not only for the scope of the nation's population it covers—albeit for work-related injuries only—but for the linkage it strengthened between employment and health insurance as an employment benefit. Workers' compensation insurance is also significant because of the growth in medical care payments. Figure 6.13 shows the growth in public-sector payments between 2001 and 2004 for personal health care services provided under the Workers' Compensation program. For 2004, expenditures for medical services were more than $25.5 billion dollars. These expenditures do not include the costs to administer the program or other costs that are not specifically for the provision of medical services.

Workers' compensation benefits are relatively generous, characterized by first-dollar coverage for all services and medications, with no copayments or deductibles. States, recognizing that their costs for workers' compensation have grown at a faster rate than many of their other health expenditures, have instituted some controls on utilization. All but seven states restrict workers' rights to select their initial health services providers and to change providers at any time (Himmelstein and Rest 1996). At least

**FIGURE 6.13**
Workers'
Compensation
Public Fund
Expenditures
for Personal
Health Care,
2001–2004

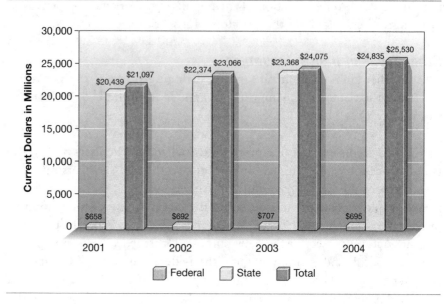

SOURCE: CMS 2004.

six states have mandated the use of managed care for some or all workers in their jurisdictions.

Proposals to overhaul the workers' compensation system focus on mandatory managed care and/or instituting "24-hour coverage," the use of common benefit and delivery systems for both work- and nonwork-related health problems (Himmelstein and Rest 1996).

**Viatical Settlements**

In 1989, the concept of viatical settlements was introduced into the U.S. health services system, stimulated in part by the number of AIDS patients with life insurance policies who had exhausted other assets to pay for their health services. Viatical settlement companies buy the life insurance policies of the terminally ill, paying the insured 50 to 80 percent of the policy's face value. The policyholder thereby acquires cash to pay living and medical expenses. The viatical settlement company continues to pay the policy premiums and collects the policy's face value when the former policyholder dies.

In 1998, more than 50 viatical settlement companies provided their services in the United States. One trade association, the National Viatical Association, notes that some or all of the proceeds of the settlement may be taxable, the settlement could be subject to the claims of creditors, and receipt of a viatical settlement may adversely affect the recipient's eligibility for Medicaid or other government benefits or programs (National Viatical Association 1996). The role of viatical settlement companies may change as new drug therapies appear to increase the life spans of people who are HIV positive.

Despite the extent of private health insurance coverage and the steady growth and expansion of some public health insurance programs, particularly Medicare and vendor payment programs such as Medicaid, an estimated 15 to 20 percent of the U.S. population does not have health insurance for some or all of any given calendar year. Chapter 3 discusses this population and the problems it faces in obtaining health services.

**People Without Private or Public Health Insurance**

## Regulation of Health Insurance

Health insurance, particularly private health insurance, is regulated primarily at the state government level as a result of the 1945 McCarran-Ferguson Act (Kuttner 1997). Prior to a discussion of the scope of state government regulation of health insurance, however, three federal statutes that significantly affect health insurance and preempt state regulation—ERISA, COBRA 1985, and HIPAA—are addressed.

### *ERISA*

The 1974 Employee Retirement Income Security Act (ERISA) provides a federal framework for regulating employer-sponsored pension and welfare plans, including health plans, whether established by employers, employee organizations such as unions, or both. ERISA preemption effectively blocks states from directly regulating most employer-sponsored (self-funded) plans, but it permits states to regulate health insurers (USGAO 1995b). ERISA governs the reporting, disclosure, fiduciary obligation, and claims-filing procedures, whether or not the business is self-funded.

ERISA is important to the state's regulation of health insurance for two major reasons. First, if a state wants to develop and sponsor a statewide program of health insurance, as Hawaii did in 1974, it must obtain a statutory exemption from Congress. Several states—including Minnesota, New York, Oregon, and Washington—proposed, but did not obtain, such exemptions in the mid-1990s.

Second, as a federal statute, ERISA preempts states from regulating health insurance plans that are self-funded by employers. Because an increasing proportion of individuals who have employer-sponsored health insurance are covered by self-funded plans, state proposals to reform health insurance may not affect the majority of those who have employer-sponsored health insurance. In a 1995 report, the National Governors Association identified the following potential state actions that it believed were prohibited, due to judicial interpretations of ERISA (USGAO 1995b):

- establishing minimum guaranteed benefits packages for all employers;
- developing standard data collection systems applicable to all health plans;

- developing uniform administrative processes, including standardized claims forms;
- establishing all-payer rate-setting systems;
- establishing a statewide employer mandate;
- imposing a level playing field through premium taxes on self-funded plans; and
- imposing a level playing field through provider taxes where the tax is interpreted as having an impermissible direct or indirect effect on self-funded plans.

### COBRA 1985

The 1985 COBRA (Consolidated Omnibus Budget Reconciliation Act) established the opportunity for employees with group health insurance coverage who lost their jobs due to work-related (e.g., resignation, layoff, termination) or family-related (e.g., divorce, death) reasons to retain their health insurance coverage for up to 36 months if they pay the premium plus an additional administrative charge. COBRA provisions also apply to the dependents of such employees who lose their coverage due to the death of, separation from, or divorce from an insured.

Under COBRA provisions, firms with 20 or more full-time or part-time employees during 50 percent of the business days in the preceding calendar year must offer continuing coverage after a qualifying event for up to 18 months for work-related events and up to 36 months for family-related events. Employees pay a price not to exceed 102 percent of the total premium. If coverage is lost due to disability, an additional 11 months of coverage are available, and costs to the former employee may be increased in that 11 months to 150 percent of total premiums (Flynn 1994).

A study of COBRA utilization found that 22 percent of COBRA participants were ages 62–64, suggesting that COBRA is a major bridge to Medicare coverage. Most of the qualifying events were work related. Of those who qualified for COBRA coverage due to family events, the most frequently reported reason for loss of coverage was when a dependent child reached age 19, or age 23 in the case of a full-time student, and thus lost coverage under the parent's policy (Flynn 1994).

HIPAA made some changes in COBRA requirements that became effective January 1, 1997. Among these required changes are:

- clarification that disabled beneficiaries of covered employees are eligible for the maximum coverage period of 29 months;
- provision for extended coverage if the former employee becomes disabled during the first 60 days of COBRA coverage;
- provision for termination of COBRA coverage for individuals becoming eligible for new group health plans; and

- extension of the definition of a qualified beneficiary to include a child born to or adopted by the covered employee while covered under COBRA.

Additional provisions of this act are explained in later sections.

### The Health Insurance Portability and Accountability Act of 1996

In 1996, Congress, unable to agree to the sweeping health insurance changes proposed in the 1993 Health Security Act (HSA), agreed to incremental changes set out in the Health Insurance Portability and Accountability Act (HIPAA) of 1996. This act:

- imposed limits on preexisting-condition waiting periods;
- required group health plans to offer special enrollment periods for individuals who originally declined coverage because of other coverage or who exhausted or lost their COBRA benefits under specified circumstances;
- prohibited group health plans from excluding, on a variety of grounds, an otherwise eligible individual from coverage;
- required insurance carriers to guarantee renewal of all group health plans, including those sponsored by small and large employers;
- provided for the portability of insurance from group to individual plans;
- changed aspects of both ERISA and COBRA; and
- provided favorable tax treatments to medical savings accounts (Blue Cross/Blue Shield 1996).

### State Regulation of Health Insurance

The sale of and reporting on all types of insurance is regulated by state governments, often by a state insurance commission or comparable entity. Key insurance regulatory activities include monitoring the insurer's financial solvency, reviewing premium rates, reviewing policies, and investigating consumer complaints and insurer marketing practices (USGAO 1993a).

Even though self-funded health insurance plans, which cover the majority of people with employer-sponsored health insurance in most states, are exempt from state regulations, many states devote considerable resources to regulating health insurance. An important aspect of state regulation is the monitoring of state-mandated benefits, which any health insurer licensed to do business in that state must offer. Table 6.12 shows the types of benefits states typically mandate, including treatments, certain types of service providers, and special populations. Of the more than nine hundred different benefits mandated nationally (Iglehart 1992), the

**Mandated Health Insurance Benefits**

**TABLE 6.12**
Number
of States
with Specific
Mandates
for Health
Insurance
Policies, 2003

**Treatment Mandates (2003)**

| | |
|---|---|
| Mammography screening | 46 |
| Diabetic supplies, education | 43 |
| Off-label drug use | 33 |
| Mental health parity | 30 |
| Formula for phenylketonuria | 27 |
| Well-child care | 27 |
| Alcoholism treatment | 26 |
| Prostate cancer screening | 26 |
| Dental anesthesia | 24 |
| Minimum mastectomy stays | 24 |
| Contraceptives | 20 |
| Drug abuse treatment | 20 |
| Clinical trials | 17 |
| Mental health coverage | 17 |
| Colorectal screen | 15 |

**Provider Mandates (1995)**

| | |
|---|---|
| Psychologists | 40 |
| Chiropractors | 39 |
| Optometrists | 35 |
| Podiatrists | 30 |
| Nurse midwives | 28 |
| Social workers | 21 |
| Nurse practitioners | 17 |
| Psychiatric nurses | 15 |
| Osteopaths | 13 |
| Physical therapists | 10 |
| Nurse anesthetists | 10 |
| Professional counselors | 9 |
| Speech/hearing therapists | 5 |
| Occupational therapists | 6 |
| Acupuncturists | 5 |

**Special-Population Mandates (1995)**

| | |
|---|---|
| Newborns | 48 |
| Handicapped dependents | 35 |
| Continuation dependent coverage | 32 |
| Dependent students | 7 |

SOURCES: USGAO 1995a, 2003.

following are mandated by a majority of states: mammography screening by 46 states, diabetic supplies by 43 states, psychologists' services by 40 states, chiropractic services by 39 states, coverage of newborns by 48 states, and coverage of handicapped dependents by 35 states (USGAO 1995b, 2003).

States regulate the offering of Medisup/Medigap policies to Medicare beneficiaries within their states and may authorize the sale of additional types of Medisup/Medigap policies as long as the minimum benefit package is offered. The Federal Employee Health Benefit Program (FEHBP), which provides health insurance to federal workers is not subject, however, to most state regulation (USGAO 1995b).

State insurance commissions, at the direction of state statutes, have on occasion waived mandated benefit requirements or permitted premium-cutting measures to induce more small businesses to be able to offer health insurance coverage. Such waivers appear to have had only a modest effect on increasing access to health insurance (USGAO 1992a).

## Proposed Changes in the U.S. Health Insurance Industry

Health insurers are critical to the financing of health services in the United States and are also central to discussions about how and why the system should change. Employers are active in supporting reforms, and politicians at all governmental levels are also proposing changes. This section outlines some of the major proposed and effected reforms of recent years.

### Employer Reforms to Health Insurance

As employers have become more aware of how providing employee health insurance affects their balance sheets, they have initiated business groups on health, multiple-employer trusts, purchasing alliances and cooperatives, and benefit redesign in the form of tiered benefits, and have also proposed new HealthMarts.

New insurance products, some of them the result of the consumer (and provider) backlash against managed care, are also being offered. These include consumer-directed health plans, health savings accounts (HSAs), health reimbursement arrangements (HRAs), and flexible spending arrangements (FSAs).

One of the first business groups on health, the Washington Business Group on Health, was established in 1974, initially to defeat national health insurance but later to become involved with a range of medical policy issues, **Business Groups on Health** including cost containment (Starr 1982). Multiple-employer trusts (METs), which are legal trusts established by a plan sponsor to bring together a number of small, unrelated employers for the purpose of providing medical coverage on an insured or self-funded basis (HIAA 2002), began to appear on the U.S. scene in the late 1970s. A current and powerful example of a MET is the Pacific Business Group on Health, established in 1989.

**Health Insurance Purchasing Cooperatives**

For more than two decades, purchasing cooperatives have provided ways to obtain more affordable health insurance coverage. Health insurance purchasing cooperatives (HIPCs) were, in fact, a centerpiece of the 1993 Health Security Act, the Clinton administration's unsuccessful national health insurance initiative. Among the better-known purchasing cooperatives are the California Public Employees Retirement System and Health Insurance Plan of California, a government-sponsored voluntary purchasing pool for 80,000 employees of small businesses (Bowen 1995).

Using pooled buying power, HIPCs obtain insurance coverage for the workers of all employers and make that coverage more affordable by spreading the risk over a larger population (USGAO 1994a). HIPCs may be either public or private and are formed to contract with health plans, enroll individuals in these plans, collect and distribute premiums, and provide comparative information to consumers on health plan quality and price. In addition, they may:

- determine how many plans with which to contract;
- decide what types of health plans to offer;
- develop self-funded plans to ensure coverage in rural areas;
- review and control health plan marketing materials;
- analyze and distribute quality data submitted by plans to improve member services;
- develop risk adjustment methods; and
- negotiate premiums with health plans (USGAO 1994a).

**Association Health Insurance Plans**

Businesses may also establish an association health insurance plan in which members of a trade or professional association form a group for the purpose of obtaining health insurance under one master contract. Chambers of Commerce and the American Public Health Association, for example, are groups that have established association health plans. The GAO (1995d) estimates that 17 percent of small employers that offer insurance do so as a local business association, trade group, employer coalition, or other group of small purchasers.

**Defined Contribution and Premium Support**

Large employers—those who employ ten thousand or more workers—are working to change the environment in which employees make their health coverage decisions. Convinced that the market principles can apply effectively to health services, some large employers are giving employees increasing responsibility for their health services cost decisions. These employers are simultaneously instituting and publicizing measures of quality and efficiency, not only for managed care organizations (MCOs) in their service areas but also for hospitals and clinicians (Galvin and Milstein 2002).

Among the ways under consideration for increasing the employee or beneficiary's cost-consciousness is to move away from the direct provision of health insurance benefits to mechanisms such as defined contributions or premium support. A defined contribution would provide a fixed allowance per employee for the individual purchase of health insurance. With premium support, frequently linked with proposed Medicare reform, the federal government would pay a defined portion of the premium for a standard benefit package, and the beneficiary would pay the balance (Smith and Rosenbaum 1999).

**Tiered Benefit Design**

Employers who sponsor employee health insurance have worked with insurers or insurance consultants to redesign part or all of the benefit packages in an effort to force employees to become more cost-conscious in their decision making. One such redesign began with tiered prescription drug benefits in which an employee could choose: (1) a generic drug with a small or no copay; (2) a brand-name drug for which no generic equivalent is available; or (3) a brand-name drug when a generic is available, requiring the highest copay. This approach has now expanded to choices of hospitals and medical groups and physicians in some instances (Iglehart 2002; Blostin 2003). In tiered health plans, an insurer groups together hospitals based on their costs of care. As is true in tiered prescription drug plans, the enrollee pays more for care in a higher-tiered hospital.

**HealthMarts**

Other forms of group health insurance purchasing arrangements such as HealthMarts are emerging. The purpose of such proposed entities as HealthMarts is to enable the small-group market to function more like a large-group market. HealthMarts seek to permit pooled purchasing and to amend ERISA to preempt mandated state benefits (Hall, Wicks, and Lawlor 2001).

All efforts to increase the insured's responsibility in decision making and cost containment are predicated on informed consumers competent to make the best choice for their circumstances. Spirited debate continues about the appropriateness and likely effectiveness of these proposals and strategies.

**New Insurance Products**

Consumer-directed health care—efforts on the part of the insured to gain greater control over coverage and service delivery—has stimulated the development of new insurance products. One such product is the high-deductible plan, in which an employer offers a plan with an annual deductible of, for example, $1,000, for individual coverage. Persons who do not expect the need for many health services may choose this type of plan over the most costly options available.

Health savings accounts (HSAs) are a type of high-deductible plan. Enrollees have higher cost sharing but broader choices than are typically offered by HMOs. HSAs were authorized by the MMA of 2003. Consumers can own and control their health care spending and save for future health care costs with tax-free interest until retirement. As of 2005, more than one million persons were enrolled in HSAs (Marchetta and Rogal 2005). Maximum lifetime benefits are established for HSAs, differing by whether the plan is individually purchased or purchased by a small or a large employer.

HSAs have both positive and negative effects on the delivery system. On the positive side, they may affect the overuse of discretionary services by promoting greater awareness of costs. HSAs may help to focus attention on the current pay-as-you-go entitlement programs, such as Medicare, and the attendant inequities such programs foster for the workers who pay for them. The individual ownership of HSAs may encourage individual recognition of place and responsibility in supporting a system of care. The potential downsides are that HSAs may foster inappropriate underuse of services, with the responsibility now accruing to the insured person rather than to the provider. HSAs may also continue to affect the distribution of financial responsibility between the healthy and the sick, and they may weaken society's sense of responsibility for its must vulnerable members (Robinson 2005).

Health reimbursement arrangements (HRAs) are spending accounts established by an employer from which an employee can draw to reimburse medical expenses. If the account becomes depleted, the employee must pay out-of-pocket until an established deductible is met, at which time the HRA becomes a traditional major medical plan. At the employer's discretion, HRA funds may be carried over to a subsequent year; they are not portable (Gabel et al. 2004).

Flexible savings arrangements (FSAs) generally allow individuals to elect to receive tax-free funds diverted from wages instead of cash wages to use for qualifying expenses, such as medical care or child care. Employees annually sign up for FSA plans along with their election of other health insurance benefits (Fuchs and James 2005). A cap is set on the maximum amount that may be diverted from wages, the amount must be expended according to the employer's rules, and it may not be carried forward from year to year.

## Political Reforms to Health Insurance

Like employers, the political system also recognizes the importance of the insurance industry in the U.S. delivery system. Enabling initiatives include relaxation of state standards to stimulate the availability of health insurance to smaller businesses.

In an effort to increase the availability of health insurance to the workforce, many states, as well as the unsuccessful Health Security Act of 1993, considered instituting a "play or pay" mandate to employers. This mandate would have required employers either to provide a specified benefits package to their employees (to play) or to contribute (to pay) to a pool of funds that would then purchase health insurance for those who could not obtain it through their workplace. This proposed mandate has not been instituted at any major level.

**Play or Pay**

Medical savings accounts (MSAs) are tax-deferred accounts set up to pay for routine medical expenses and are designed to cover the predicable front-end costs of preventive care and diagnostic services. MSAs are usually established with savings from premium costs when an employer or an individual chooses to forego comprehensive coverage with higher premiums for catastrophic policies with high deductibles and low premiums. The Balanced Budget Act of 1997 (PL 105-33) permits Medicare beneficiaries to enroll in MSAs under certain conditions.

**Medical Savings Accounts**

    An advantage of MSAs is that they lower administrative costs. Disadvantages are that they do not correct flaws in the current health insurance system and are used by some as a tax shelter (ALPHA Center 1994). Medicare beneficiary and other enrollment in MSAs has been low to negligible, with only about 140,000 plans established since their inception (Fuchs and James 2005).

Politicians and others have also expressed interest in vouchers or refundable tax credits as additional ways to increase access to health insurance. Vouchers would require a sponsor to create an environment in which providers have incentives to deliver high-quality, economical care. Voucher payments would require a very large redistribution of existing public subsidies if health insurance were to be made more affordable for low-income people and would likely require substantial tax increases (Kronick 1991).

**Vouchers and Tax Credits**

    Proposed tax credit options in 2002 ranged from modest to sweeping, the latter of which would replace the current tax subsidies for employer-sponsored health insurance with tax credits for the individual purchase of health insurance (Fuchs, Merlis, and James 2002). Congress has not yet acted on the tax credit options for health insurance.

In August 2001, the Bush administration introduced the Health Insurance Flexibility and Accountability Initiative to give states greater flexibility in covering low-income uninsured populations. States may request from the secretary of the Department of Health and Human Services (HHS) a waiver under Section 1115 provisions of the Social Security Act that will allow them to streamline benefit packages, create public-private partnerships, and

**Health Insurance Flexibility and Accountability Initiative**

increase cost sharing for optional and expansion populations covered under Medicaid and SCHIP (Engquist and Burns 2002). The GAO (2003a) has raised concerns about the appropriateness of some SCHIP waivers granted by the HHS.

**Premium Subsidies for Employer-Sponsored Health Insurance**

Because nearly three-quarters of the uninsured live in households with at least one full-time worker, several states are experimenting with ways to cover more of the uninsured by providing premium subsidies for employer-sponsored health insurance. The subsidies may be directed to employees, as is being done in New Jersey, or to the employers, as is being done in Massachusetts. Analysts indicate that these types of subsidies are being explored because: (1) a public-private blend reduces the drain on public coffers; (2) this same blend avoids the stigmatization of enrollment in a public program; and (3) such an approach allows children and their parents to have the same source of coverage (Cornwell and Short 2001).

## Summary

Health insurance, both private and public, has been the principal financing mechanism for U.S. health services since the end of World War II. About 63 percent of the population under age 65 has some type of insurance coverage, and the majority of people age 65 and older are Medicare beneficiaries. Still, an estimated 20 percent of the population does not have health insurance coverage at some point or for the entirety of a calendar year. The majority of people with private health insurance obtain it as a benefit of employment or by being a dependent of someone who is an insured employee. Major public health insurance programs include Medicare and TRICARE. Medicaid, although not technically a health insurance program, is included in this chapter's discussion of public insurance because it pays for health services to about 13 percent of the nation's population.

Costs of providing health insurance have risen steadily. Between 1980 and 1990, annual growth in private health insurance premiums averaged nearly 21 percent. In 1994 and 1995, the growth in premium rates declined but has increased annually since 2001. Costs of providing public health insurance, Medicare in particular, have increased as the number of beneficiaries and the amount spent per beneficiary have grown. Premium increases for Part B of Medicare have risen steadily, but premium revenues fund only one-quarter of Part B costs; three-quarters of Part B expenditures come from federal general revenue funds. Additional increases are certain as a result of the 2003 MMA Medicare outpatient prescription drug coverage, a benefit that was implemented on January 1, 2006. Expansions in Medicaid eligibility and in covered services have driven increases in the costs and the total expenditures for paying for health services for low-income people. Reform in welfare legislation initially appeared to slow Medicaid expenditure growth, but downturns in the economy portend resumed expenditure increases.

Because the provision of employer-sponsored health insurance has become a major business expense as well as a major cost to governments, a range of cost-containment strategies has been introduced in the last quarter-century. Most of these strategies have had disappointing results, primarily because they could affect only one segment of the health services industry. Efforts are now focused on the implementation of new insurance products.

Although public opinion polls continue to show that most people in the United States favor the provision of a basic set of health services benefits to all, efforts to provide these benefits through a program of national health insurance have been proposed—and have failed—as recently as 1993. Incremental changes, both to employer-sponsored and public insurance programs, appear to be the way in which access to coverage by the uninsured is likely to occur.

## Note

1. The Supplement Security Income (SSI) program is a federal cash assistance program for low-income aged and disabled people that has standard eligibility requirements. It was established to replace state-provided cash assistance programs to low-income aged and disabled persons. The AFDC program was replaced by the Temporary Assistance to Needy Families (TANF) program as part of the 1996 Personal Responsibility and Work Opportunity Reconciliation Act (PL 104-193).

## Key Words

actuary

administrative load

administrative services only (ASO)

Aid to Families with Dependent
    Children (AFDC)

American Hospital Association
    (AHA)

baby boomer

black lung program

Blue Cross

Blue Shield

Centers for Medicare and Medicaid
    Services (CMS)

CHAMPUS Reform Initiative

cherry picking

Civilian Health and Medical Program
    of the Uniformed Services
    (CHAMPUS)
claims processing
co-insurance
commercial health insurance
community rating
Consolidated Omnibus Budget
    Reconciliation Act (COBRA)
copayments
cost containment
cost sharing
cream skimming
crossover population
deductible
Deficit Reduction Act (DEFRA)
defined benefit
defined contribution
Dependents Medical Care Program
disability insurance
"dread disease" insurance policies
dually entitled
durational rating
efficiency
Emergency Maternal and Infant Care
    Program (EMIC)
Employee Retirement Income
    Security Act (ERISA)
employer-sponsored health insurance
end-stage renal disease (ESRD)
entitlement programs
equity
expenditures caps
experience rating
Federal Employees' Compensation Act
Federal Employee Health Benefits
    Program (FEHBP)
Federal Employers Liability Act
federal match rate
fee-for-service delivery system
first-dollar coverage
guaranteed issue
guaranteed renewal
Health Insurance Flexibility and
    Accountability Initiative

Health Insurance Portability and
    Accountability Act (HIPAA)
health insurance purchasing
    cooperatives (HIPC)
health maintenance organizations
    (HMOs)
HealthMarts
Health Security Act (HSA)
home health care
hospice care
hospital service contract
indemnity insurance plans
individual health insurance policies
insurance vouchers
Longshoremen and Harbor Workers
    Act
long-term care (LTC) insurance
loss leader
loss ratio
managed care
managed care organizations (MCOs)
mandated health insurance benefits
maximum lifetime benefits
means test
Medicaid
Medicaid optional services
Medical Information Bureau
medically indigent
medically needy
medical savings accounts
medical screening
Medicare
Medicare+Choice
Medicare Hospital Insurance (Part A)
Medicare Prescription Drug
    Improvement and
    Modernization Act (MMA)
Medicare Supplementary Medical
    Insurance (Part B)
Medicare trust funds
Medigap policies
Medisup policies
Military Health Services System
    (MHSS)
multiple-employer trusts (METs)

national health insurance (NHI)
not-for-profit organization
omnibus budget reconciliation act
    (OBRA)
Pacific Business Group on Health
payer of first/last resort
Personal Responsibility and Work
    Opportunity Reconciliation Act
play or pay
point-of-service (POS) plan
portability of health insurance
precertification
preexisting conditions
preferred provider organization
    (PPO)
premium support
prepaid group practices (PGPs)
prior authorization
private health insurance
proprietary health organization
public/social health insurance
purchasing alliances
Qualified Medicare Beneficiaries
    (QMB)
RAND Health Insurance Experiment
    (HIE)
redlining
reinsurance
retention rate
retiree health insurance
risk
risk adjustment

risk assessment
risk pooling
second surgical opinion
selection bias
self-funded/self-insured
State Child Health Insurance Program
    (SCHIP)
state health insurance commissions
state health insurance programs
Supplemental Security Income
    (SSI)
tax credits
Tax Equity and Fiscal Responsibility
    Act (TEFRA)
Temporary Assistance for Needy
    Families (TANF) block grant
third-party administrator (TPA)
tiered benefit design
tier rating
TRICARE
triple option
unbundled services
underwriting
uninsurable
universal coverage
utilization management
vendor payment program
viatical settlements
vouchers
welfare reform
willing-provider laws
workers' compensation insurance

# References

AcademyHealth. 2006. *State of the States: Finding Their Own Way.* Washington, DC: AcademyHealth.

———. 2002. *State of the States.* Washington, DC: AcademyHealth.

ALPHA Center. 1994. "New York Adopts Pure Community Rating—Other States Take Incremental Approach." State Initiatives in Health Care Reform, No. 7. New York: ALPHA Center.

American Hospital Association. 1988. *Promoting Health Insurance in the Workplace: State and Local Initiatives to Increase Private Coverage.* Chicago: American Hospital Association..

Blostin, A. P. 2003. "Tiered Hospital Plans. Compensation and Working Conditions Online." [Online information; retrieved 1/2/06.] www.bls.golv/opub/cwc/print/;cm20030715ar01p1.htm.

Blue Cross/Blue Shield Association. 1996. "Kassenbaum-Kennedy Review." (unpublished). Chicago: Blue Cross/Blue Shield Association.

Bowen, B. 1995. "The Practice of Risk Adjustment." *Inquiry* 32 (1): 33–40.

Brook, R. H. 1991. "Health, Health Insurance, and the Uninsured." *Journal of the American Medical Association* 265 (22): 2998–3002.

Butler, P. 2000. *ERISA Preemption Primer.* Washington, DC: ALPHA Center and National Academy for State Health Policy.

Centers for Medicare and Medicaid Services (CMS). 2005. *Medicare and Medicaid Statistical Supplement, 2003.* Pub. No. 03460. Baltimore, MD: CMS.

———. 2004. "Highlights—National Health Expenditures 2004." [Online information; retrieved 1/12/2006.] http://cms.hhs.gov/statistics/nhe/historical/highlights.asp.

_____. 2000. *Medicare and Medicaid Statistical Supplement 2000.* Pub No. 03424. Baltimore, MD: CMS.

Commerce Clearing House Medicare and Medicaid Guide. 1995. "CBO Memorandum on Managed Care and Medicare." Internal Memorandum, Congressional Budget Office, April 26, Paragraph 43, 208.

Congressional Research Service. 1993. *Medicaid Source Book: Background Data and Analysis (an Update).* Washington, DC: U.S. Government Printing Office.

Cornwell, L. J., and A. C. Short. 2001. "Premium Subsidies for Employer-sponsored Health Coverage: An Emerging State and Local Strategy to Reach the Uninsured." *Issue Brief: Findings from Health Systems Change, No. 47.* Washington, DC: The Center for Studying Health System Change.

Cunningham III, R., and R. M. Cunningham, Jr. 1997. *The Blues: A History of the Blue Cross and Blue Shield System.* Dekalb, IL: Northern Illinois University Press.

Desonia, R. A. 2004. "The Promise and the Reality of Long-Term Care Insurance." NHPF Background Paper. Washington, DC: National Health Policy Forum.

Engquist, G., and P. Burns. 2002. "Health Insurance Flexibility and Accountability Initiative: Opportunities and Issues for States." *State Coverage Initiatives Issue Briefs* 3 (2): 1–6. Washington, DC: AcademyHealth.

Feldman, R., D. Wholey, and J. Christianson. 1989. "Economic and Organizational Determinants of HMO Mergers and Failures." *Inquiry* 33 (2): 118–32

Feldstein, P. J., and T. M. Wickizer. 1995. "Analysis of Private Health Insurance Premium Growth Rates: 1985–1992." *Medical Care* 33 (10): 1035–50.

Flynn, P. 1994. "COBRA Qualifying Events and Elections, 1987–1991." *Inquiry* 31 (2): 215–20.

Fuchs, B., and J. A. James. 2005. "Health Savings Accounts: The Fundamentals." NHPF Background Paper. Washington, DC: National Health Policy Forum.

Fuchs, B., M. Merlis, and J. James. 2002. "Expanding Health Coverage for the Uninsured: Fundamentals of the Tax Credit Option." NHPF Background Paper. Washington, DC: National Health Policy Forum.

Gabel, J. R., H. Whitmore, T. Rice, and A. T. LoSasso. 2004. "Employers' Contradictory Views about Consumer-Driven Health Care: Results from a National Survey." *Health Affairs Web Exclusive* W4-210, April 21, 2004.

Galvin, R., and A. Milstein. 2002. "Large Employers' New Strategies in Health Care." *New England Journal of Medicine* 374 (12): 939–42.

Gates, V. S. 2002. *State of the States: State Coverage Initiatives.* Washington, DC: Academy for Health Services Research and Health Policy.

Gauthier, A. K., J. A. Lamphere, and N. L. Barrand. 1995. "Risk Selection in the Health Care Market: A Workshop Overview." *Inquiry* 32 (1): 14–22.

Ginsburg, P. D., and J. D. Pickreign. 1997. "Tracking Health Care Costs: An Update." *Health Affairs* 16 (4): 151–55.

Glazner, J., W. R. Braithwaite, and S. Hull. 1995. "The Questionable Value of Medical Screening in the Small-Group Health Insurance Market." *Health Affairs* 12 (2): 224–34.

Goff, V. 2004. "Consumer Cost Sharing in Private Health Insurance: On the Threshold of Change." NHPF Issue Brief No. 798. Washington, DC: National Health Policy Forum.

Hall, M. A. 1992. "The Political Economies of Health Insurance Market Reform." *Health Affairs* 11 (2): 108–24.

Hall, M. A., and C. J. Conover. 2003. "The Impact of Blue Cross Conversions on Accessibility, Affordability, and the Public Interest." *The Milbank Quarterly* 81(40): 509-42.

Hall, M. A., E. K. Wicks, and J. S. Lawlor. 2001. "HealthMarts, HIPCs, MEWAs, and AHPs: A Guide for the Perplexed." *Health Affairs* 20 (1): 142–53.

Health Insurance Association of America. 1992. *Source Book of Health Insurance Data.* Washington, DC: HIAA.

———. 2002. *Source Book of Health Insurance Data.* Washington, DC: HIAA.

Himmelstein, J., and K. Rest. 1996. "Working on Reform: How Workers' Comp Medical Care Is Affected by Health Care Reform." *Public Health Reports* 111 (1): 12–24.

Iglehart, J. K. 2002. "Changing Health Insurance Trends." *New England Journal of Medicine* 347 (12): 956–62.

———. 1992. "The American Health Care System: Private Insurance." *New England Journal of Medicine* 326 (25): 1715–20.

Kenney, G., and D. I. Chang. 2004. "The State Children's Health Insurance Program: Successes, Shortcomings, and Challenges." *Health Affairs* 23 (5): 51-62.

Kiplinger's Retirement Report. 2005. "Disappearing Retiree Health Benefits." [Online information; retrieved 1/17/06.] www.kiplinger.com/retirementreport/features/Cover_Dec21005_01.html.

Kronick, R. 1991. "Health Insurance, 1979–1989: The Frayed Connection Between Employment and Insurance." *Inquiry* 28 (4): 318–32.

Kuttner, R. 1997. "The Kassenbaum-Kennedy Bill—the Limits of Incrementalism." *New England Journal of Medicine* 337 (1): 64–67

Lee, T. H., and K. Zapert. 2005. "Do High-Deductible Health Plans Threaten Quality of Care? *New England Journal of Medicine* 353(12): 1202–04.

Levit, K. R., H. C. Lazenby, and L. Sivarajan. 1996. "Health Care Spending in 1994: Slowest in Decades." *Health Affairs* 15 (2): 130–44.

Levit, K. R., G. L. Olin, and S. W. Letsch. 1992. "Americans' Health Insurance Coverage, 1980–1991." *Health Care Financing Review* 14 (1): 31–57.

Light, D. W. 1992. "The Practice and Ethics of Risk-Rated Health Insurance." *Journal of the American Medical Association* 267 (18): 2503–08.

Liska, D. W., N. J. Brennan, and B. K. Bruen. 1998. *State-Level Databook on Health Care Access and Financing,* 3d ed. Washington, DC: Urban Institute.

Litman, T. J. 1997. *Health Politics and Policy,* 3d ed. Albany, NY: Delmar Publishers.

———. 1992. "Appendix." In *Health Politics and Policy,* 2d edition, by T. J. Litman and L. S. Robins. New York: Delmar Publishers.

Litman, T. J., and L. S. Robins. 1991. *Health Politics and Policy,* 2d ed. New York: Delmar Publishers.

Luft, H. S. 1986. "Compensating for Biased Selection in Health Insurance." *The Milbank Quarterly* 64 (4): 566–91.

Lurie N., W. G. Manning, and C. Peterson. 1987. "Preventive Care: Do We Practice What We Preach?" *American Journal of Public Health* 77 (7): 801–04.

Marchetta, M., and D. Rogal. 2005. "Health Savings Accounts as a Tool for Market Change." Changes in Health Care Financing & Organization Issue Brief No. 4. Washington, DC: Academy Health.

McCormack, L. A., J. R. Gabel, N. D. Berkman, H. Whitmore, K. Hutchinson, W. L. Anderson, J. Pickreign, and N. West. 2002a. "Retiree Health Insurance: Recent Trends and Tomorrow's Prospects." *Health Care Financing Review* 23 (3): 17–34.

McCormack, L. A., J. R. Gabel, H. Whitmore, W. L. Anderson, and J. Pickreign. 2002b. "Trends in Retiree Health Benefits." *Health Affairs* 21 (6): 169–76.

Medical Study News. 2005. "Impact of Medicare Drug Law on Retiree Health Benefits." [Online information; retrieved 12/16/05.] www.news-medical.net/print_article.asp?id=15005.

Monheit, A. C., and M. L. Berk. 1992. "The Concentration of Health Expenditures: An Update." *Health Affairs* 11 (4): 145–49.

Monheit, A. C., L. M. Nichols, and T. M. Selden. 1996. "How Are Net Health Insurance Benefits Distributed in the Employment-Related Insurance Market?" *Inquiry* 32 (4): 379–91.

Monheit, A. C., and C. L. Schur. 1989. *National Medical Expenditure Survey: Health Insurance Coverage of Retired Persons.* Washington, DC: National Center for Health Services Research.

National Viatical Association. 1996. *National Viatical Association Information Booklet.* Washington, DC: National Viatical Association.

Neuman, P. 2004. *The State of Retiree Health Benefits: Historical Trends and Future Uncertainties.* Washington, DC: The Kaiser Family Fund Foundation.

Newhouse, J. P. 1993. *Free for All? Lessons from the RAND Health Insurance Experiment.* Cambridge: Harvard University Press.

Norton, E. C., and J. P. Newhouse. 1994. "Policy Changes for Public Long-Term Care Insurance." *Journal of the American Medical Association* 271 (19): 1520–24.

Rasell, M. E. 1995. "Cost-Sharing in Health Insurance: A Reexamination." *New England Journal of Medicine* 332 (17): 1164–68.

Reichard, J. 1997. "Study Says Medigap May Become Unaffordable to Oldest, Sickest." *Medicine and Health* 51 (35): 2.

Reinhardt, U. E. 1993. "Reorganizing the Financial Flows in American Health Care." *Health Affairs* 12 (Supplement): 172–93.

Robert Wood Johnson Foundation. 2004a. "Kaiser/HRET Employer Benefits Survey as Reported in Robert Wood Johnson Foundation." In *About Coverage: Health Insurance in the United States.* Princeton, N.J.: Robert Wood Johnson Foundation.

———. 2004b. *State Coverage Initiatives: About Coverage: Health Insurance in the United States.* Princeton, NJ: Robert Wood Johnson Foundation.

Robinson, J. 2005. "Health Savings Accounts – The Ownership Society in Health Care." *New England Journal of Medicine* 353 (12): 1199-1202.

Rosenblatt, A. 2004. "The Underwriting Cycle: The Rule of Six." *Health Affairs* 23 (6): 103–06.

Shonick, W. 1995. *Government and Health Services.* New York: Oxford University Press.

Smith, B. M., and S. Rosenbaum. 1999. "Potential Effects of the 'Premium Support' Proposal on the Security of Medicare." *New England Journal of Medicine* 282 (10): 1760–63.

Spillman, B. C. 1992. "The Impact of Being Uninsured on Utilization of Basic Health Care Services." *Inquiry* 29 (4): 457–66.

Starr, P. 1982. *The Social Transformation of American Medicine.* New York: Basic Books, Inc.

Stearns, S. C., and T. A. Mroz. 1996. "Premium Increases and Disenrollment from State Risk Pools." *Inquiry* 32 (4): 392–406.

Sullivan, C. B., M. Miller, R. Feldman, and B. Dowd. 1992. "Employer-Sponsored Health Insurance in 1991." *Health Affairs* 11 (4): 172–85.

Swartz, K. 1994. "Dynamics of People Without Health Insurance: Don't Let the Numbers Fool You." *Journal of the American Medical Association* 271 (1): 64–66.

Thorpe, K. E. 1992. "Inside the Black Box of Administrative Costs." *Health Affairs* 11 (2): 41–55.

"Three Years into SCHIP, State Spending Rises." 2001. *New Federalism Policy Research and Resources, Issue 12.* Washington, DC: Urban Institute.

TRICARE. 2002. "Stakeholders' Report, Volume IV." [Online information; retrieved 6/19/02.] www.TRICARE.osd.mil/onestop/index.html.

United Seniors Health Cooperative. 1995. *1995 Medigap Update and Medicare Summary.* Washington, DC: United Seniors Health Cooperative Newsletter.

U.S. Bipartisan Commission on Comprehensive Health Care. 1990. *A Call for Action: The Pepper Commission Final Report.* Washington, DC: U.S. Government Printing Office.

U.S. Department of Health and Human Services. 2006. *Medicare and Medicaid Statistical Supplement.* Pub. No. (PHS) C3-24-07. Baltimore, MD: USDHHS.

———. 2005. *Health, United States, 2005.* Pub. No. (PHS) 05-1232. Hyattsville, MD: USDHHS.

———. 2003. *Medicare and Medicaid Statistical Supplement.* Pub. No. (PHS) 03386. Baltimore, MD: USDHHS.

———. 2001. *Medicare and Medicaid Statistical Supplement.* Baltimore, MD: USDHHS.

———. 2000. *Medicare and Medicaid Statistical Supplement, 2000.* Baltimore, MD: USDHHS.

———. 1995a. *Health, United States, 1995.* Pub. No. (PHS) 96-1232. Hyattsville, MD: USDHHS.

———. 1995b. *Medicare and Medicaid Statistical Supplement, 1995.* Pub. No. (PHS) 03386. Hyattsville, MD: USDHHS.

U.S. Department of Health and Human Services/Health Care Financing Administration. 1990. *Health Care Financing Program Statistics: Medicare and Medicaid Databook, 1990.* HCFA Pub. No. 03314. Baltimore, MD: USDHHS/HCFA.

U.S. Government Accountability Office (formerly the U.S. General Accounting Office). 2005. *Long-Term Care Financing: Growing Demand and Cost of Services Are Straining Federal and State Budgets.* GAO-05-564T. Washington, DC: USGAO.

———. 2003. *Private Health Insurance: Federal and State Requirements Affecting Coverage Offered by Small Businesses.* GAO-03-1133. Washington, DC: USGAO.

———. 2002. *Medigap: Current Policies Contain Coverage Gaps, Undermine Cost Control Incentives.* GAO-02-533T. March. Washington, DC: USGAO.

———. 2001. *Retiree Health Insurance: Gaps in Coverage and Availability.* GAO-02-178T. November. Washington, DC: USGAO.

———. 1997a. *Medicaid: Sustainability of Low 1996 Spending Growth Is Uncertain.* GAO/HEHS-97-128. June. Washington, DC: USGAO.

———. 1997b. *Private Health Insurance: Continued Erosion of Coverage Linked to Cost Pressures.* GAO/HEHS-97-122. July. Washington, DC: USGAO.

———. 1995a. *Defense Health Care: Despite TRICARE Procurement Improvements, Problems Remain.* GAO/HEHS-95-142. August. Washington, DC: USGAO.

———. 1995b. *Employer-Based Health Plans: Issues, Trends, and Challenges Posed by ERISA*. GAO/HEHS-95–167. July. Washington, DC: USGAO.

———. 1995c. *Health Insurance Portability: Reform Could Ensure Continued Coverage for Up to 25 Million Americans*. GAO-HEHS-95-257. September. Washington, DC: USGAO.

———. 1995d. *Testimony on Employer Association Health Plans*. GAO/HEHS-96-59R. December. Washington, DC: USGAO.

———. 1994a. *Access to Health Insurance: Public and Private Employers' Experiences with Purchasing Cooperatives*. GAO/HEHS-94-142. May. Washington, DC: USGAO.

———. 1994b. *Blue Cross and Blue Shield: Experiences of Weak Plans Underscore the Role of Effective State Oversight*. GAO/HEHS-94-71. April. Washington, DC: USGAO.

———. 1994c. *Health Care Reform: Considerations for Risk Adjustment under Community Rating*. GAO-HEHS-94-173. September. Washington, DC: USGAO.

———. 1993a. *Health Insurance: How Health Care Reform May Affect State Regulation*. GAO/T-HRD-94-55. November. Washington, DC: USGAO.

———. 1993b. *Long-Term Care Insurance: High Percentage of Policyholders Drop Policies*. GAO/HRD-93-129. August. Washington, DC: USGAO.

———. 1992a. *Access to Health Insurance: State Efforts to Assist Small Businesses*. GAO/HRD-92-90. May. Washington, DC: USGAO.

———. 1992b. *Employer-Based Health Insurance: High Costs, Wide Variation Threaten System*. GAO/HRD-92-125. September. Washington, DC: USGAO.

———. 1991a. Medicaid Expansions: Coverage Improves but State Fiscal Problems Jeopardize Continued Progress. GAO/HRD-91-78. Washington, DC: USGAO.

———. 1991b. *Private Health Insurance: Problems Caused by a Segmented Market*. GAO/HRD-91-114. July. Washington, DC: USGAO.

Weil, A. 1997. *The New Children's Health Insurance Program: Should States Expand Medicaid? New Federalism Issues and Options for States*. Series A, No. A-13. Washington, DC: The Urban Institute.

Wickizer, T. M., and P. J. Feldstein. 1995. "The Impact of HMO Competition on Private Health Insurance Premiums, 1985–1992." *Inquiry* 32 (3): 241–51.

Wilensky, G. R., P. J. Farley, and A. K. Taylor. 1984. "Variations in Health Insurance Coverage: Benefits vs. Premiums." *The Milbank Quarterly* 62 (1): 53–81.

Young, C. 2001. "Recent Research Findings on Medicare+Choice." The Monitoring Medicare+Choice Project of Mathematica Policy Research, Inc., No. 6., November. Washington, DC: Mathematica Policy Research, Inc.

Zellers, W. K., C. G. McLaughlin, and K. D. Frick. 1992. "Small Business Health Insurance: Only the Healthy Need Apply." *Health Affairs* 11 (1): 174–80.

**APPENDIX 6.1**

Historic
Initiatives
Intended to
Affect Health
Insurance
Coverage
and/or
Establish
National
Health
Insurance

| Year | Event |
|------|-------|
| 1912 | Social insurance, including health insurance, is endorsed in the platform of the Progressive Party and espoused by its candidate, Theodore Roosevelt. |
| 1917 | Congress passes amendment to War Risk Insurance Act to provide medical benefits to veterans with service-connected disabilities. |
| 1917 | American Medical Association (AMA) House of Delegates passes a resolution stating principles to be followed in government health insurance payments. |
| 1920 | AMA declares unequivocal opposition to compulsory health insurance. |
| 1932 | Committee on the Costs of Medical Care reports that the prevailing form of medical practice should be group practice supported by health insurance; there is a division of opinion among committee members as to whether this insurance should be private and voluntary or governmental and compulsory. |
| 1935 | President Franklin D. Roosevelt sends to Congress the Report of the President's Committee on Economic Security, which is to form the basis of the Social Security Act. The report endorses the principle of compulsory national health insurance but makes no specific recommendations. |
| 1935 | The Epstein Bill, sponsored by Senator Capper, is the first bill introduced into Congress to provide for governmental health insurance. |
| 1938 | The National Health Conference calls for the provision of medical insurance at the state level. |
| 1939 | Senator Robert Wagner of New York introduces a congressional bill calling for federally subsidized state medical care compensation. |
| 1941 | Members of the New York County Medical Society form the Physicians Forum to work for the adoption of compulsory health insurance. |
| 1942 | Rhode Island becomes the first state to pass a health insurance law. |
| 1942 | The Social Security Board expresses support for a unified and comprehensive Social Security system to include health benefits. |
| 1943 | The first Wagner Bill calling for a compulsory national health system for people of all ages is introduced in the Senate and House but is not enacted. |
| 1945 | The Wagner Bill, first introduced in 1943, is reintroduced. |
| 1945 | President Harry Truman sends a message to Congress calling for comprehensive, prepaid medical insurance for people of all ages. |
| 1946 | California passes a compulsory health insurance act. |
| 1948 | The administrator of the Federal Security Agency, the predecessor of the Department of Health, Education, and Welfare, calls a National Health Assembly to mobilize support for national health insurance bills. |
| 1949 | President Truman, in his State of the Union message, again calls for compulsory national health insurance. |
| 1952 | Senator Murray and Representatives Dingell and Celler introduce a bill calling for the payment of hospital costs for retirees and their dependents under the Old Age and Survivors Insurance (OASI) program. |
| 1955 | Major U.S. trade unions set health insurance for the aged as a top priority. |

*(continued)*

| | |
|---|---|
| 1955 | The American Hospital Association's (AHA) Board of Trustees passes a resolution recommending federal subsidies to states to begin voluntary health insurance programs for older people. |
| 1956 | The Dependents Medical Care Act (PL 84-5691) sets up the CHAMPUS program of primarily inpatient care for military dependents. |
| 1957 | The Forand Bill is introduced in Congress. It calls for an increase in the OASI payroll tax to provide for up to 120 days of combined hospital and nursing home care as well as necessary surgery for OASI beneficiaries. The bill is killed by a House Ways and Means Committee in 1960. |
| 1960 | The Eisenhower administration introduces its own "Medicare" program to help the needy aged meet the costs of catastrophic care without using compulsory national health insurance. |
| 1960 | Kerr-Mills Act is passed, which provides federal matching funds to states to pay for health services for aged persons. |
| 1961 | King-Anderson Bill to provide health insurance for the elderly through the Social Security system is introduced in both houses of Congress. |
| 1962 | AMA establishes AMPAC, a political action committee to oppose proposals for medical care for the aged. |
| 1964 | President Johnson calls for the passage of a National Health Insurance Act for the Aged. |
| 1965 | Title XVIII (Medicare) and Title XIX (Medicaid) are added to the Social Security Act, increasing access to health services for persons over age 65, the disabled, and low-income children and their adult caregivers. |
| 1971 | President Nixon, in a message to Congress, proposes the use of HMOs as the cornerstone of his administration's proposal for national health insurance. |
| 1973 | The Catastrophic Health Insurance and Medical Assistance Reform Act sponsored by Senators Long and Ribicoff proposes to cover only unforeseen large losses and includes a large deductible to reduce moral hazard. |
| 1973 | Health Care Insurance Act of 1973, the AMA's "Medicredit" proposal, is introduced in both the House and the Senate and provides on a voluntary participation basis for personal income tax credits to offset the premium costs of privately marketed qualified health insurance policies. |
| 1973 | The Health Security Act—the Griffiths-Kennedy bill—proposes compulsory coverage for all eligible U.S. residents with broad benefits and limited cost sharing. |
| 1974 | Comprehensive Health Insurance Act of 1974 proposed by the Nixon administration mandates employers to offer specified minimum-benefit packages to employees, provides insurance for low-income persons and those with medical risks, and provides for expansion of Medicare. |
| 1974 | The Comprehensive National Health Insurance Act, the Kennedy-Mills Bill, provides for compulsory participation and universal coverage of all legal residents. |
| 1977 | President Carter sponsors the National Health Plan Act, which calls for a two-tier health insurance system. The first tier is for the poor and aged, and the second is for the less-poor working population younger than age 65. This bill includes a major role for the private health insurance industry. |

*(continued)*

**APPENDIX 6.1**
Continued

| | |
|---|---|
| 1977 | Kennedy-Waxman Health Care for All Americans Bill is introduced and is a compromise that would continue the use of private health insurance companies as fiscal intermediaries. |
| 1987 | Senator Edward Kennedy introduces legislation that would require employers to provide a minimum benefit package to employees who work at least 17.5 hours per week. |
| 1988 | The Medicare Catastrophic Health Act passes to expand health coverage, including prescription drugs, to Medicare beneficiaries. |
| 1988 | Massachusetts enacts the first law in the nation to mandate competitive universal health insurance coverage of an entire state's population. |
| 1988 | The state of Washington institutes a voluntary program that offers subsidized health insurance to low-income individuals. |
| 1989 | The Medicare Catastrophic Health Act provisions pertaining to expanded benefits coverage for Medicare beneficiaries are repealed. |
| 1993 | President Clinton's Health Security Act is introduced in Congress. It proposes adding Part C to Medicare and considerably expanding access to health insurance coverage to other parts of the population. |
| 1994 | Oregon's Health Plan, which offers a basic set of benefits to Medicaid beneficiaries and other populations that are not Medicaid-eligible, becomes operational under a waiver from the Health Care Financing Administration. |
| 1997 | Balanced Budget Act introduces Medicare+Choice and other Medicare and Medicaid changes and establishes the State Child Health Insurance Program (SCHIP). |
| 1999 | Balanced Budget Retirement Act institutes changes in Medicare payment to correct some of the imbalances created by the 1997 Balanced Budget Act. |
| 2000 | Benefit Improvement and Protection Act (BIPA) of 2000 creates additional requirements to Medicare, Medicaid, and SCHIP programs. |

SOURCES: Shonick 1995; Litman 1992.

**APPENDIX 6.2**

Major Federal Expansions of Medicaid Eligibility and Services (1984–1990)

| Law | Affected Population | Expansion | M+ | O+ + |
|---|---|---|---|---|
| DEFRA 1984 (PL 98-369) | Infants[1] and children | • Requires coverage of all children born after 9/30/83 meeting state AFDC income and resource standards, regardless of family structure | X | |
| | Pregnant women | • Requires coverage from date of medical verification of pregnancy, providing (1) woman would qualify for AFDC once child is born or (2) woman would qualify for AFDC-UP[2] once child is born, regardless of whether state has AFDC-UP mandate | X | |
| | Infants | • Requires automatic coverage for one year after birth if mother already is receiving Medicaid and remains eligible and infant resides with her | X | |
| | AFDC families | • Requires limited extension of Medicaid coverage if AFDC eligibility is lost due to earnings | X | |
| | SSI recipients | • Extends family income disregard from 4 to 12 months | X | |
| | | • Increases qualifying asset limits for applicants for limited time period (1984–1989) | X | |
| COBRA 1985 (PL 99-272) | Pregnant women | • Requires coverage if family income and resources are below state AFDC levels, regardless of family structure | X | |
| | Postpartum women | • Requires 60-day extension of coverage postpartum if eligibility was pregnancy-related | X | |
| | Terminally ill pregnant women | • Allows provision of hospice services | | X |
| | | • Allows provision of enhanced benefits | | X |
| | Infants and children | • Allows extension of DEFRA coverage up to age 5 immediately, instead of requiring phase-in by birth date | | X |
| | Adopted/foster children, special-needs children | • Requires coverage even if adoption/foster agreement was entered into in another state | X | |
| | | • Requires coverage regardless of income/resources of adoptive/foster parents | X | |

(continued)

**APPENDIX 6.2** Continued

| Law | Affected Population | Expansion | M+ | O++ |
|---|---|---|---|---|
| OBRA 1986 | Aged and disabled | • Creates new optional categorically needy group for those with income below 100 percent of (PL 99-509) poverty line under certain resource constraints. Option can be exercised for this group only if exercised also for pregnant women and infants | | X |
| | Aged and disabled | • Allows Medicare buy-in[3] up to 100 percent of poverty line for qualified Medicare beneficiaries under certain resource constraints | | X |
| | Pregnant women and infants | • Creates new optional categorically needy group for those with income below 100 percent of poverty line; women receive pregnancy-related services only | | X |
| | Pregnant women | • Allows assets test to be dropped for this newly defined category of applicants | | X |
| | | • Allows presumptive eligibility for up to 45 days to be determined by qualified provider | | X |
| | | • Allows guarantee of continuous eligibility through postpartum period | | X |
| | Children | • Allows coverage up to age 5 if income is below 100 percent of poverty line (phased in) | | X |
| | Infants and children | • Requires continuation of eligibility (for those who otherwise would become ineligible) if they are hospital inpatients when age limit is reached | X | |
| | Severely impaired | • Establishes new mandatory categorically needy coverage group for qualified individuals under age 65 | X | |
| | Ventilator-dependent | • Allows coverage of at-home respiratory care services | | X |
| | Aliens | • Requires provision of emergency services if otherwise eligible (financially and categorically) | X | |
| | SSI recipients | • Makes permanent the previous temporary provision requiring coverage of some former disabled SSI recipients who have returned to work | X | |
| Employment Opportunities for Disabled Americans Act (PL 99-643) | Disabled | • Makes permanent a previous demonstration program for individuals able to engage in substantial gainful activity despite severe medical impairments | X | |

*(continued)*

| Legislation | Group | Provision | |
|---|---|---|---|
| Immigration Reform and Control Act of 1986 (PL 99-603) | Newly legalized aliens | • Requires provision of emergency and pregnancy-related services if otherwise eligible; also requires full coverage for eligibles under 18 | X |
| Anti-Drug Abuse Act 1986 (PL 99-570) | Homeless | • Requires state to provide proof of eligibility for individuals otherwise eligible but having no permanent address | X |
| OBRA 1987 (PL 100-203) | Pregnant women and infants | • Allows coverage if income level below 185 percent of poverty line | X |
| | | • Allows immediate extension of OBRA 1986 up to 100 percent of poverty line up to age 5 | X |
| | Children | • Clarifies that states may provide in-home services for qualified disabled children | X |
| | | • Allows coverage for children ages 5–7, up to state AFDC level (phased in by age) | X |
| | | • Allows coverage for children below age 9, up to 100 percent of poverty line (phased in by age) | X |
| | Elderly | • Allows provision of home and community-based services to those who otherwise would need nursing home care[4] | X |
| | Nursing home applicants | • Requires states to establish preadmission screening programs for mentally ill and retarded | X |
| Medicare Catastrophic Care Coverage Act (PL 100-360) | Pregnant women and infants | • Makes mandatory the OBRA 1986 option of coverage up to 100 percent of poverty level (phased in by percentage of poverty line) | X |
| | | • Makes mandatory the OBRA 1986 option of Medicare buy-in up to 100 percent of poverty level (phased in by percentage of poverty line) | X |
| Family Support Act of 1988 (PL 100-485) | AFDC families | • Increases required period of Medicaid coverage if AFDC cash assistance is lost due to earnings | X |
| | AFDC families with unemployed parent | • Requires coverage if otherwise qualified | X |

*(continued)*

**APPENDIX 6.2** Continued

| Law | Affected Population | Expansion | M+ | O++ |
|---|---|---|---|---|
| OBRA 1987 (PL 100-203) | Nursing home residents | • Requires preadmission screening and annual resident review for mentally ill or retarded residents | X | |
| OBRA 1989 (PL 101-239) | Pregnant women and infants | • Requires coverage if income is below 133 percent of poverty line | X | |
| | Children | • Requires coverage up to age 6, if income below 133 percent of poverty line | X | |
| | | • Requires provision of Medicaid-allowed treatment to correct problems identified during EPSDT screenings even if treatment is not covered otherwise under a state's Medicaid plan | X | |
| | | • Requires interperiodic screenings under EPSDT when medical problems are suspected[5] | X | |
| OBRA 1990 (PL 101-508) | Children | • Requires coverage up to age 18 if income is below 100 percent of poverty line (phased in by age) | X | |
| | Pregnant women | • Makes mandatory the OBRA 1986 option of continuous eligibility through postpartum period | X | |
| | Pregnant women and children | • Extends period of presumptive eligibility before written application must be submitted | X | |
| | | • Requires state to receive and process applications at convenient outreach sites | X | |
| | Infants | • Requires continuous eligibility if (1) born to Medicaid-eligible mother who would remain eligible if pregnant and (2) remaining in mother's household | X | |
| | Elderly and disabled | • Extends the MCCA QMB provision of 120 percent of poverty line (phased in by percentage of poverty line) | X | |
| | | • Allows limited program permitting states to provide home and community-based services to functionally disabled, and community-supported living arrangements to mentally retarded/developmentally disabled | | X |

SOURCE: USGAO 1991.

NOTES: EPDST = early periodic screening, detection, and treatment; M = mandated; O = optional; QMB = qualified Medicare beneficiaries.

[1] Infants are children up to age 1

[2] AFDC-UP allows coverage in two-parent families if the principal wage-earner is unemployed

[3] Medicaid covers Medicare cost-sharing charges: premiums, deductibles, co-insurance

[4] This is not automatic. HCFA must grant a waiver to any state wishing to provide these services.

[5] States establish a screening schedule. "Interperiodic" visits are added to the standard schedule if a problem is suspected.

# FINANCING THE U.S. HEALTH SERVICES SYSTEM

## Introduction

The financing of health services in the United States is unique among industrialized countries. Both public (i.e., governmental) and private sources finance care, which is the case in other countries. However, U.S. employers and insurers, frequently called third-party payers, are more involved than their counterparts in other countries. Per capita expenditures for health services in the United States are the highest in the world, yet as much as 20 percent of the population may not have assured financial access to health services at some point during any given year.

This chapter describes the U.S. health services financing system, explores expenditures and expenditure trends in health services, outlines recent efforts to contain health services expenditures, and discusses provider payment mechanisms and their influence on expenditures. The chapter concludes with a discussion of the policy implications of growing health services expenditures.

## How Health Services Are Financed

Although health services were available to some segments of the U.S. population as early as 1798 through the U.S. Marine Hospital Service (see Chapter 4), a system of health services to cover more of the population did not really begin to develop until after World War II. This war is a significant marker in the development of the system for several reasons. First, World War II introduced military forces and their family members to regular, systematic care. Active-duty members needed to maintain good health to accomplish their military missions, and a system of clinics and hospitals was expanded for this purpose. A program for military dependents—the Emergency Maternal and Infant Child Care Program (EMIC)—was established in 1943 (Shonick 1995).

Second, for those in the workforce at home, health services benefits were introduced as a way to compensate for wages and salaries that had been frozen to control the wartime economy. At the end of the war,

**TABLE 7.1**
Major Events
in Financing
U.S. Health
Services

| Year | Event |
|------|-------|
| 1798 | U.S. Marine Hospital Services is established. |
| 1918 | First federal grants to states provide public health services. |
| 1921 | Maternity and Infancy (Sheppard-Towner) Act is passed. |
| 1924 | World War Veterans Act is passed. |
| 1929 | First Blue Cross plan is established at Baylor University, Texas. |
| 1933 | Federal Emergency Relief Act provides federal financing of medical care for aged. |
| 1935 | Social Security Act, which includes funds for maternal and child health, crippled children, aged, blind, and disabled, is passed. |
| 1939 | Blue Shield is established in California and Michigan by state medical societies. |
| 1942 | Rhode Island becomes first state to pass a health insurance law. |
| 1948 | Every state has a Workers' Compensation law. |
| 1956 | Dependents Medical Care Act sets up CHAMPUS program. |
| 1959 | Blue Cross negotiates contract with Civil Service Commission to provide health insurance coverage for federal employees under Federal Employees Health Benefit Act (PL 86-352). |
| 1960 | Title XVI of the Social Security Act creates Medical Assistance for Aged program. |
| 1962 | Health Services for Agricultural Migrant Workers Act is passed. |
| 1965 | Titles XVIII (Medicare) and XIX (Medicaid) are added to Social Security Act. |
| 1974 | Employee Retirement and Income Security Act (ERISA) exempts self-insured companies from state-mandated health insurance benefits. |

*(continued)*

an on-site and returning workforce held expectations of health services as a benefit of employment. Between 1945 and 1960, the number of people with hospital insurance jumped from 32 million to 122 million, and the number with insurance for physician services soared from fewer than 5 million to more than 83 million (Health Insurance Association of America [HIAA] 1985).

Table 7.1 outlines the major events in the evolution of financing today's health services system. The early events emanated from the public sector. Until the 1930s and the development of the Blue Cross system, the private-sector's role was principally one of individual relationships between providers and patients.

Today, the private sector strongly influences how the system is financed. To provide a better understanding of health services financing, this chapter first focuses on the revenue sources that pay for care and then turns to how these sources are expended. Information about financing U.S. health services—financial data on all public and private health services ren-

| Year | Event | TABLE 7.1 |
|------|-------|-----------|
| | | Continued |

| Year | Event |
|------|-------|
| 1975 | Rhode Island enacts first state catastrophic health insurance program. |
| 1983 | Medicare's prospective payment system (PPS) for hospitals is established. |
| 1988 | Medicare Catastrophic Health Act (PL 100-360) is enacted. |
| 1988 | Massachusetts enacts nation's first law to mandate competitive universal health insurance coverage of entire state. |
| 1989 | Parts of Medicare Catastrophic Health Act are repealed. |
| 1989 | Congress mandates Medicare physician payment reform. |
| 1992 | Medicare physician payment reform is implemented. |
| 1997 | Title XXI (Medicare) State Children's Health Insurance Program is added to Social Security Act. |
| 2000 | Benefits Improvement and Protection Act (BIPA) increases the disproportionate share hospital (DSH) allotments for 2001 and 2002 and makes other changes to DSH provisions that result in increased costs to the Medicaid program. |
| 2002 | Medical Device User Fee and Modernization Act (MDUFMA) provides the FDA with additional resources to ensure prompt approval or clearance of applications for marketing medical devices and licensing biological products. |
| 2003 | Medicare Prescription Drug Improvement and Modernization Act (MMA) has many provisions, but chief among them is coverage of outpatient prescription drugs for Medicare beneficiaries, beginning January 1, 2006. |

SOURCE: Adapted from Litman 1997. Reproduced by permission.

dered and sources of funding—comes from the National Health Accounts and is maintained by the Office of Health Statistics in the Centers for Medicare and Medicaid Services (CMS) Office of the Actuary. The CMS, formerly the Health Care Financing Administration (HCFA), publishes data for each year on its web site and in an issue of the *Health Care Financing Review* journal as well as an annual issue of *Health Affairs*.

## Revenue Sources for U.S. Health Services

Figure 7.1 shows the sources of funds for U.S. health services expenditures in 2004. Private insurance, estimated to cover about 63 percent of the nonelderly population (see Chapters 3 and 6), is the source of one-third of the funds expended for health services. The federal government, through its support of Medicare, the Department of Veterans Affairs (VA) health system, military health services, the Indian Health Service (IHS), and other federal health programs, is the funding source of another 30 percent of health services expenditures. Medicaid and SCHIP, jointly funded by federal and state governments, account for 16 percent of health expenditures.

**FIGURE 7.1**
Sources
of Funds
(Revenue)
That Finance
U.S. Health
Services (2004)

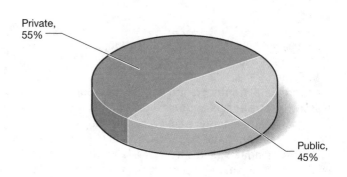

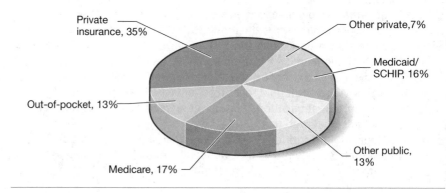

SOURCE: CMS 2005.

Out-of-pocket payments by individuals are the source for 13 percent of health expenditures. These payments include private health insurance premiums, copayments, deductibles, and cash payments for services in lieu of insurance coverage, either because the service is not covered by insurance (e.g., most over-the-counter drugs) or because the individual is not covered by health insurance.[1]

The private sector still accounts for 55 percent of the revenue sources, including private health insurance premiums, out-of-pocket payments, and charitable donations and other funding sources. The public sector provides 45 percent of the sources of funds, with a federal-to-state ratio of 2.4 to 1.

The balance between public- and private-sector sources of financing for the U.S. system has changed dramatically in the last several decades. Until the passage of the Medicare and Medicaid amendments to the Social Security Act (SSA) in 1965, the public sector contributed only modestly to financing health care. As Figure 7.2 shows, however, the public-sector's contributions have increased significantly since 1965. Projections for future spending on health services, discussed later in this chapter, suggest that this trend will continue.

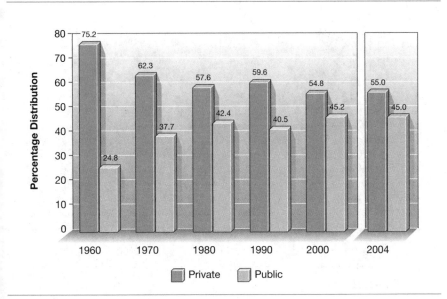

SOURCE: CMS 2005.

**FIGURE 7.2**

Percentage of Public- and Private-Sector Sources of Financing, U.S. Health Services, (Select Years, 1960–2004)

## *Expenditures for U.S. Health Services*

It is important for this discussion to define such key financing terms as *cost, cost containment, expenditures,* and *price.* Cost is the amount spent to produce a good or service. Cost containment strategies are regulatory or other interventions, usually made by employers or payers, to control health services costs; the term is sometimes applied more broadly to mean the containment or control of expenditures. Expenditures are the amounts spent for health services goods or services. Price is the amount charged for a health services good or service.

In 2004, the United States spent $1.9 trillion on health services, an average of $4,094 per person. Figure 7.3 shows the growth in health services expenditures between 1960 (before the passage of Medicare and Medicaid) and 2004. Expenditures grew nearly 70-fold in this 44-year period. Expenditures for health services constitute the second largest category of governmental expenditures, exceeded only by interest payments on the national debt (Ross, Ratner, and Fein 1991).

**Growth in Health Expenditures**

Figure 7.4 identifies the major categories of health services expenditures for 2004: personal health services, including hospitals, physician services, drugs, nursing home care, and other personal services; and program administration, including the net cost of private health insurance (the difference

**Major Categories of Health Expenditures**

**FIGURE 7.3**
Expenditures
for U.S.
Health Services
(Select Years,
1960–2004)

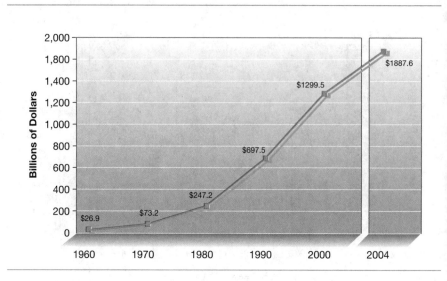

SOURCE: CMS 2005.

**FIGURE 7.4**
Categories
of Expenditures
for U.S. Health
Services (2004)

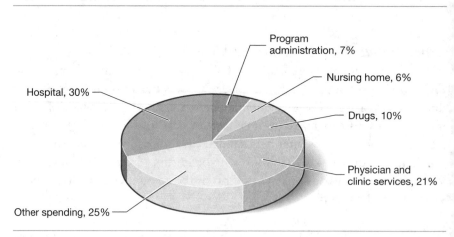

SOURCE: CMS 2005.

NOTE: The category "drugs" now includes only prescription drugs.

between premiums collected and benefits paid out). Payment for hospital care constitutes the largest category of personal health services expenditures (30 percent), followed by payment for physician and clinic services at 21 percent. The nonpersonal health services expenditure categories together constitute about 17 percent of all expenditures: public health (2.9 percent), program administration and net cost of private health insurance (7 percent), and research and construction (6.6 percent).

| Expenditure Category | 1960 | 1970 | 1980 | 1990 | 2000 | 2004 |
|---|---|---|---|---|---|---|
| Hospital | 34.6 | 38.3 | 41.5 | 36.7 | 31.7 | 30.4 |
| Physician services | 19.7 | 18.6 | 18.3 | 21.0 | 22.0 | 21.3 |
| Home health care | <.01 | <.01 | <.01 | 1.9 | 2.3 | 2.3 |
| Drugs and nondurable medical equipment | 15.6 | 12.0 | 8.7 | 8.6 | 9.4* | 10.0* |
| Nursing home | 2.9 | 5.7 | 7.1 | 7.3 | 7.0 | 6.1 |
| Other personal care | 14.9 | 12.7 | 12.2 | 12.7 | 8.5 | 10.0 |
| Public health | 1.5 | 1.8 | 2.7 | 2.8 | 3.4 | 3.0 |
| Program administration and net cost of private health insurance | 4.5 | 3.7 | 4.8 | 5.5 | 6.2 | 7.3 |
| Research and construction | 6.3 | 7.2 | 4.7 | 3.5 | 3.4 | 6.7 |
| Other medical products | N/A | N/A | N/A | N/A | 3.8 | 2.9 |
| *Total Expenditures* | $26.9 billion | $73.2 billion | $247.2 billion | $697.5 billion | $1.3 trillion | 1.9 tril lion |

**TABLE 7.2**
Distribution of Expenditures for Health Services (Select Years, 1960–2004) and Percentage of Total Expenditures

SOURCE: CMS 2005.

*This category includes ONLY prescription drugs for 2000 and 2004.

Changes in the distribution of health expenditures over time are shown in Table 7.2. From 1960 to 2004, the share of expenditures directed to hospital care remained relatively stable, from 34.6 percent in 1960 to 30.4 percent in 2004. Expenditures for physician and clinic services also remained relatively stable (1960 = 19.7 percent; 2004 = 21.3 percent). Home health care represented less than one-tenth of 1 percent of expenditures through 1980, but with Medicare and Medicaid coverage of this service approved in 1974 and 1965, respectively, the home health care share of expenditures

**Changes in Distribution of All Health Expenditures**

has grown to 2.3 percent in 2004. Although this is a small proportion of overall expenditures, it has been, until recently, the fastest growing Medicare expenditure category. Nursing homes' share of expenditures has more than doubled, from 2.9 percent in 1960 to 6.1 percent in 2004. In this interval, Medicare added very limited coverage for skilled nursing home services, and Medicaid added coverage for both skilled and intermediate care, including care for people with developmental disabilities. The proportion of expenditures directed to drugs and other nondurable medical equipment in 2004 is two-thirds of what it was in 1960. It is important to note, however, that the types of expenditures that the National Health Accounts include in this category are subject to change over time.

Expenditures for one category of nonpersonal health services program—administration and net cost of private health insurance—increased from 4.5 percent in 1960 to 7.3 percent in 2004. Two other categories also show change: Public health expenditures increased, from 1.5 percent of total expenditures in 1960 to 3.0 percent in 2004, and expenditures for research and construction increased from 6.3 percent of total 1960 expenditures to 6.7 percent in 2004.

**Changes in Distribution for Personal Health Services Expenditures**

Personal health services expenditures (exclusive of public health, program administration, and research and construction expenditures) for 2004 are shown in Figure 7.5, with changes in the distribution for 1960 to 2004 shown in Table 7.3. Expenditures for hospital care continue to constitute the largest proportion of personal health services expenditures, reflective of the intensity of care provided, even though the total number of admis-

**FIGURE 7.5**
Expenditures for Personal Health Services (2004)

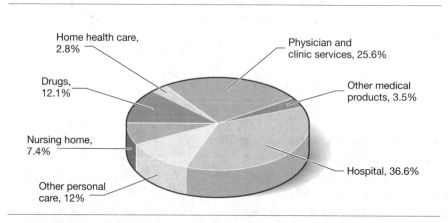

SOURCE: CMS 2005.

NOTE: The "drugs" category includes only prescription drugs. The "other personal care" category includes dental, vision, and other.

| Expenditure Category | 1960 | 1970 | 1980 | 1990 | 2000 | 2004 |
|---|---|---|---|---|---|---|
| Hospital | 39.4 | 41.0 | 47.3 | 41.7 | 36.5 | 36.6 |
| Physician services | 22.5 | 19.9 | 20.8 | 23.8 | 25.3 | 25.6 |
| Home health care | <.01 | <.01 | 1.1 | 2.1 | 2.9 | 2.8 |
| Drugs and nondurable medical equipment | 17.8 | 12.9 | 10.0 | 9.7 | 10.8* | 12.1* |
| Nursing home | 3.3 | 6.1 | 8.1 | 8.3 | 8.2 | 7.4 |
| Other personal care | 17.0 | 21.0 | 12.7 | 14.7 | 12.0 | 12.0 |
| *Total Personal Care Expenditures ($ billions)* | $23.6 | $68.3 | $217.0 | $614.7 | $1,130.4 | $1,560.2 |

**TABLE 7.3** Distribution of Expenditures for Personal Health Services (Select Years, 1960–2004) and Percentage of Total Expenditures

SOURCE: CMS 2005.

*This category includes ONLY prescription drugs for 2000 and 2004.

sions, the number of inpatient days, and the length of stay have declined in recent years.

Examining the proportion of total expenditures, by type of service, covered by various sources of funds, provides additional insight into how the U.S. health services system is financed. Figure 7.6 charts the funding sources for various components of personal health services, including hospital care, physician services, home health services, drugs and other nondurable medical equipment, and nursing home care.

    In 2004, the federal government was the payer for 45.3 percent of all hospital care, 28.5 percent of all physician services, 56 percent of home health care, 17.5 percent of drugs and nondurable medical equipment, and 42 percent of nursing home care. Private insurance is the source of funds for 35.6 percent of hospital expenditures, 48.5 percent of physician services, 12 percent of home health care, 47.5 percent of drug and nondurable

**Sources of Funds for Select Personal Health Expenditures**

FIGURE 7.6
Sources
of Funds
for Select
Personal
Health Services
(2004)

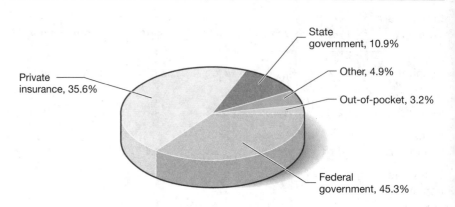

**Hospital Care ($570.8 billion)**

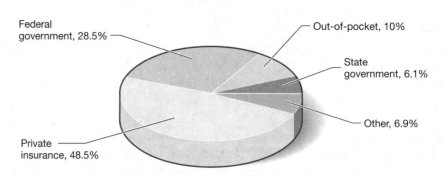

**Physician and Clinical Services ($399.9 billion)**

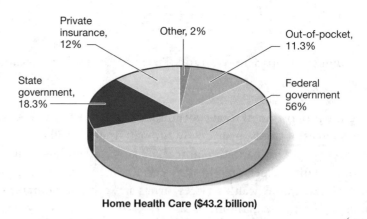

**Home Health Care ($43.2 billion)**

*(continued)*

medical equipment, and 7.8 percent of nursing home care. Out-of-pocket payments fund 3.2 percent of hospital care, 10 percent of expenditures for physician services, 11.3 percent of home health care, nearly 25 percent of prescription drug expenditures, and 27.7 percent of nursing home care.

**FIGURE 7.6**
Continued

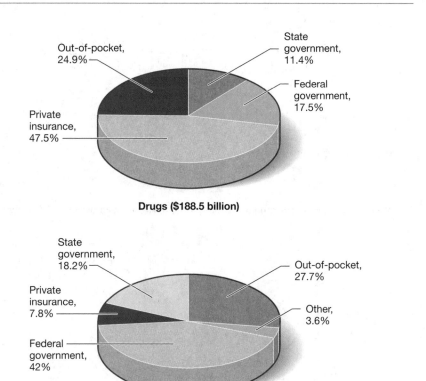

**Drugs ($188.5 billion)**

Out-of-pocket, 24.9%
State government, 11.4%
Federal government, 17.5%
Private insurance, 47.5%

**Nursing Homes ($115.2 billion)**

State government, 18.2%
Out-of-pocket, 27.7%
Private insurance, 7.8%
Other, 3.6%
Federal government, 42%

SOURCE: CMS 2005.

Note that these proportions differ from those in Figure 7.1, which are based on *total* health expenditures.

Sources of funds for program administration and the net cost of private health insurance and public health are shown in Figure 7.7. Private (other) funds are the largest funding sources for program administration and the net cost of private health insurance. Public funds are the sole funding source for public health.

Yet another way to assess the financing of the U.S. health services system is to analyze expenditures by subpopulation groups. Berk and Monheit (1992) used the National Medical Expenditure Survey and other data to examine the concentration of health services expenditures. They reported that for 1987, the top 1 percent of spenders accounted for 30 percent of expenditures and the top 5 percent for 58 percent of expenditures. The bottom half of the population, the low spenders, accounted for only 3 percent

**Expenditures by User Groups**

**FIGURE 7.7**
Sources of
Funds for
Program
Administration
, Net Cost of
Private Health
Insurance, and
Public Health
(2004)

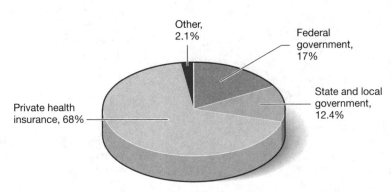

**Program Administration and Net Cost of Private Health Insurance ($136.7 billion)**

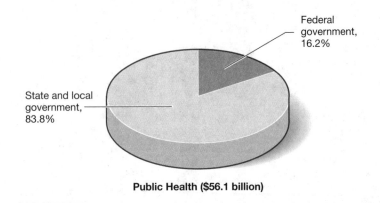

**Public Health ($56.1 billion)**

SOURCE: CMS 2005.

of total expenditures (see Table 7.4). Additional analyses have shown that of the top 1 percent of 1987 spenders, 48 percent were elderly and 16 percent were black, indicating disproportionately poorer health status for these groups than for their younger counterparts from other racial and ethnic groups (Agency for Health Care Policy and Research [AHCPR] 1994).

## Reasons for Growth in Health Services Expenditures

U.S. health services expenditures have experienced nearly uninterrupted growth in the last four decades. Figure 7.8 shows the increase in per capita expenditures for health for select years, from 1960 through 2004. Does this growth reflect a growing and aging population, or are other factors influencing the increases?

| Percentage of U.S. Population Ranked by Expenditures | 1928 | 1963 | 1970 | 1977 | 1980 | 1987 |
|---|---|---|---|---|---|---|
| Top 1 percent | — | 17% | 26% | 27% | 29% | 30% |
| Top 2 percent | — | — | 35% | 38% | 39% | 41% |
| Top 5 percent | 52% | 43% | 50% | 55% | 55% | 58% |
| Top 10 percent | — | 59% | 66% | 70% | 70% | 72% |
| Top 30 percent | 90% | — | 88% | 90% | 90% | 91% |
| Top 50 percent | — | 95% | 96% | 97% | 96% | 97% |
| Bottom 50 percent | — | 5% | 4% | 3% | 4% | 3% |

**TABLE 7.4**
Distribution of Health Expenditures for the U.S. Population by Magnitude of Expenditures (Select Years, 1928–1987)

SOURCE: Berk and Monheit 1992. Copyrighted and published by Project HOPE/*Health Affairs*. The published article is archived and available online at www.healthaffairs.org.

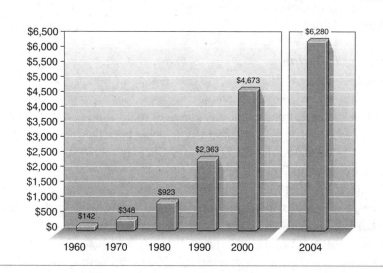

**FIGURE 7.8**
Per Capita Expenditures for U.S. Health Services (Select Years, 1960–2004)

SOURCE: CMS 2005.

    With the exception of 1972—following the Nixon administration's Economic Stabilization Program (ESP), which froze hospital prices—and the full implementation of Medicare's prospective payment system (PPS) for inpatient hospital care in 1984, U.S. health services expenditures have increased each year, and excess medical inflation (inflation above and beyond economy-wide inflation) has generally grown at a rate faster than general inflation. Many reasons are posited for this growth, including:

- general inflation;
- medical price inflation;

- the availability of health insurance and the resulting loss of individual accountability;
- population growth;
- the increased number of elderly in the population, who require more health services;
- technology and the increased intensity of services provided per capita;
- growth in national and personal incomes that permits individuals to spend more on health services;
- the increased complexity of administering a multipayer system;
- fraud and abuse;
- defensive medicine (which may include potenially ineffective care);
- malpractice;
- the growth of government health programs;
- the system's emphasis on curative rather than preventive health services;
- fee-for-service payment systems; and
- market failure.

## Effects of Inflation

Inflation—both general and medical care—is, according to many experts, the major driving force behind expenditure increases, with some researchers attributing about 70 percent of expenditure increases to inflation (Levit, Lazenby, and Sivarajan 1996). Ross, Ratner, and Fein (1991) note that medical care prices increased 44 percent faster than consumer prices in the 1970s and 1980s, due to higher wages and slower increases in productivity in the health sector. From the 1980s to the early 1990s, the rate of medical care inflation averaged 7.5 percent per year, nearly twice the general inflation rate (U.S. General Accounting Office [now known as the U.S. Government Accountability Office— USGAO] 1992a). From 1994 through 1997, health services spending per capita grew at record low levels (Strunk, Ginsburg, and Gabel 2001). This growth slowed even more with the strong economy in the late 1990s but has resumed for the reported health services expenditures for 2004 (CMS 2005).

Although in recent years technology (included in the category of "intensity" when expenditure growth is examined) has been reported to have had the greatest influence on health expenditure growth, the percentage of health expenditure growth attributed to intensity has exceeded either economy-wide inflation or medical inflation in only eight years between 1970 and 2003 (see Chapter 10).

## Role of Health Insurance

The "protective" role of health insurance, whereby the insured are insulated from the true costs of their care, is a major factor in increasing health services expenditures (Peden and Freeland 1995; Fuchs 1990; Congressional Budget Office [CBO] 1992b). About half of the growth in real per capita medical spending between 1960 and 1993 and two-thirds of the growth between 1983 and 1993 resulted either from the health insurance level or expenditure growth, with the level contributing chiefly to expenditure growth (Peden and Freeland 1995).

A study and projection of national health expenditures by the Congressional Budget Office (CBO 1992b) attributes the disproportionate growth of health expenditures to health insurance, designating it a market failure that prevents the forces of competition from working. Health insurance benefits, which are total personal health services expenditures for each payer, exclusive of administrative costs and the insured's deductibles and copayments, increased between 1969 and 1993. For Medicare, the growth averaged 13.7 percent per year, and for private insurance, 13.4 percent per year. In 1994, however, spending for benefits by both insurers declined from prior years: Medicare's 1994 increase in benefit spending was 11.8 percent, and that of private insurance was only 4 percent (Levit, Lazenby, and Sivarajan 1996). Health expenditures in 1998, however, showed that private health insurers increased premiums to restore deteriorating margins and reserves (Cowan et al. 1999). This increase appears to have continued for 1999 and 2000 health expenditures as well. Growth in private health insurance premiums for 2002 was 11.5 percent, for 2003 was 10.4 percent, and for 2004 was 8.4 percent (CMS 2005).

## Other Factors Affecting Health Services Expenditures

**Demographic Effects**
The U.S. population continues to grow, and the proportion of people in older age categories is increasing as the post–World War II baby boomers (people born between 1946 and 1964) age (see Chapter 2). Health status deteriorates and health services utilization increases with age, accounting for an estimated 10 percent of the expenditure growth (Levit, Lazenby, and Sivarajan 1996).

**Technological Effects**
Because the United States has one of the most technologically advanced health services systems in the world, technology also has played a role in increased health expenditures, accounting for an estimated 20 percent of expenditures in the mid-1990s (Levit, Lazenby, and Sivarajan 1996). Schactman et al. (2003) have identified technology as the most important variable driving health care costs, particularly as technology is used in a hospital setting, but also because of technological advances in pharmaceuticals.

**Proportion of the GDP Directed to Health Services**
As national income grows, a country can choose to direct more of its national or domestic product into providing health services for its people. One way to assess a country's commitment to the provision of health services is to examine the proportion of the gross domestic product (GDP) directed to health services expenditures. The GDP measures the value of output produced within the geographic boundaries of that country by the country and

**FIGURE 7.9**
Percentage of
U.S. GDP
Directed to
Health Services
(Select Years,
1960–2004)

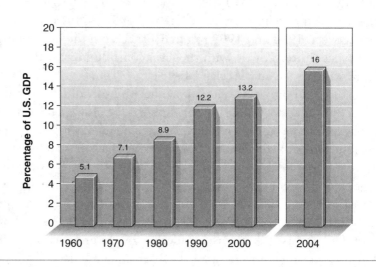

SOURCE: CMS 2005.

NOTE: GDP = gross domestic product.

by foreign citizens and companies. (The gross national product, or GNP, measures the output of the country's citizens and companies, regardless of where the production occurs.) Figure 7.9 shows the proportion of U.S. GDP directed toward health services, which increased from 5.1 percent in 1960 to 16 percent in 2004.

**Expanding Health Services to New Groups**

In the last four decades, the United States has placed a priority on providing health services to certain segments of the population, principally elderly and disabled people and low-income children and their caretakers. Because several health services programs, chiefly Medicare and Medicaid, were established as entitlements, the United States has become locked into the continued allocation of a significant proportion of its resources to health services. As personal incomes grow, individuals have more disposable income to direct toward their health services if they so choose. Of equal potential is the enrichment of a health insurance benefit package in lieu of an increase in wages, which also may increase health expenditures.

**Administrative Costs**

The complexity of administering a multipayer or pluralistic health services system has been identified by some—including the proponents of the unsuccessful 1993 Health Security Act (HSA)—as yet another factor in increased U.S. health services expenditures. Woolhandler and Himmelstein (1991) compared the administrative costs for hospital, physician, and nursing home services in Canada, a single-payer system, with those of the United States and concluded that on a per capita basis, the United States spent significantly more in 1987 on administrative costs ($400 to $497) than did Canada ($117 to $156). Critics claim that this study systematically overstated both the extent of administrative spending and the potential savings that might be achieved. Schwartz and Mendelson (1994) examined waste and inefficiency in hospitals, physician offices, and retail pharmacies and concluded that the potential savings from each source could slow the rate of increase in health services costs from 6.5 to 5 percent annually, but this would not result in dramatic savings.

Fraud and abuse of the U.S. health services system are often touted as major culprits in increasing health services expenditures. In 1992, the GAO (1992b) reported that health industry officials estimated that fraud and abuse contribute some 10 percent ($70 billion out of $700 billion in expenditures for that year) to U.S. health services spending.

**Fraud and Abuse**

The practice of defensive medicine (i.e., providing excessive care in an effort to avert potential legal action) is often cited as a cost- and expenditure-increasing practice whose elimination could result in major health services savings (Fuchs 1990; CBO 1992b). Some would include the provision of potentially ineffective care, formerly labeled futile care, in this category, by which they mean care that can produce no ameliorative or palliative benefits for an intractable condition.

The escalating costs of malpractice premiums that providers pay to protect themselves against litigation are also cited as a driving force behind health services expenditures (CBO 1992a). Schwartz and Mendelson (1994) report that aggressive malpractice reform could result in savings of $8 billion annually, less than 1 percent of total expenditures.

The growth of government health programs, particularly Medicare and Medicaid, has resulted in major increases in health services expenditures (Levit, Lazenby, and Sivarajan 1996; Ross, Ratner, and Fein 1991; Fuchs 1990; Levit and Cowan 1991; Jaggar 1995; Center for Health Economics Research 1994; CBO 1992a, 1992b). Increasing access to services by populations that have been unserved or underserved unquestionably increases utilization and expenditures. As the populations eligible for these programs have grown, either by reaching Medicare's eligibility age or through the expansion of other eligibility criteria, expenditures have also grown. Medicare and Medicaid expenditures in 1970 accounted for only about 5 percent of federal outlays. By 1990, these expenditures were 12 percent and were projected by the CBO (1992a) to be 25 percent of the total budget by 2002.

**Growth of Government Programs**

Medicare, which is financed by employer and employee contributions as well as general revenue funds, consumed 61 cents of every federal health dollar in 1990. The Medicare Hospital Trust Fund, set up as a pay-as-you-go fund, was projected to go bankrupt by the year 2006 (Ross, Ratner, and Fein 1991), but revised estimates suggested that bankruptcy could occur as early as 2001 (Wilensky 1996). Current analyses suggest that this disaster may be forestalled until sometime in the mid-2020s (Wilensky 2001). This moving target is one indicator of the difficulty in making accurate long-range forecasts.

The CMS analysis of national health expenditures for 2004 notes that for the 1987 to 1997 decade, general revenue funding for Medicare increased to a then-record share of federal spending at 33 percent. Although the 1997 to 2000 years showed the slowest overall growth in Medicare spending (2.3 percent), by 2004, the share of federal revenues dedicated to Medicare reached 35 percent.

About 30 percent of all Medicare expenditures are devoted to the 6 percent of beneficiaries in their last year of life, in which utilization of high-technology services is likely to increase (Fuchs 1990). Of the lifetime costs of medical care, 18 percent ($40,000 out of $225,000 in total expenditures) may be incurred in the last year of life. More than 29 percent of Medicare and Medicaid payments for people age 65 and older are for people in the last year of life (Fries, Koop, and Beadle 1993).

Eligibility for federal and state-funded Medicaid began expanding in 1984. The resulting increases in utilization contributed significantly to increases in government spending for health services (Levit and Cowen 1991). Figure 7.10 shows that federal aid to state and local governments for Medicaid increased 2.5 times between 1975 and 2000, from 13.7 percent of all federal aid to states to 41 percent. State budgets to provide the matching Medicaid funds increased as well. Table 7.5 shows CBO estimates of how state budgets are affected if Medicaid expenditures rise above their 1991 share of states' budgets, which they continue to do.

Medicaid, with no dedicated tax to fund it, places a heavy financing burden on the federal government; at times, more than half of all federal spending is on health care. Medicaid spending by the federal government has increased 9 percent annually between 2001 and 2004. The 2001 recession also caused significant problems for states in funding their proportion of Medicaid costs. Medicaid is the second largest item in most state budgets, second only to education (CMS 2005; National Association of State Budget Officers 2004).

**Focus on Acute Rather Than Preventive Care**

The focus in the U.S. health services system on curative and therapeutic interventions, rather than on health promotion and disease prevention, is another cause of increasing health services expenditures (Fries, Koop, and Beadle 1993). Less than 3 percent of expenditures for personal health services are typically spent on health promotion and disease prevention. Pre-

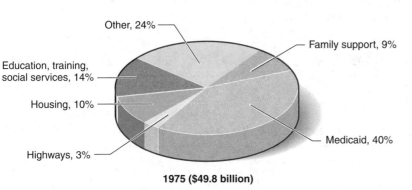

Other, 24%

Family support, 9%

Education, training,
social services, 14%

Housing, 10%

Highways, 3%

Medicaid, 40%

**1975 ($49.8 billion)**

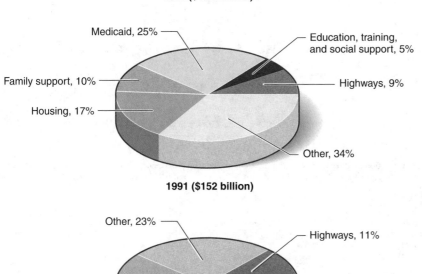

Medicaid, 25%

Education, training,
and social support, 5%

Family support, 10%

Highways, 9%

Housing, 17%

Other, 34%

**1991 ($152 billion)**

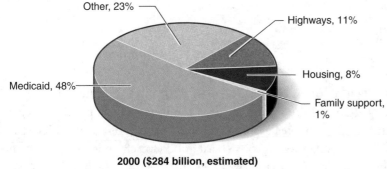

Other, 23%

Highways, 11%

Medicaid, 48%

Housing, 8%

Family support,
1%

**2000 ($284 billion, estimated)**

<br>

**FIGURE 7.10**
Federal Aid to
State and Local
Governments,
by Types of
Aid (1975,
1991, 2000)

SOURCES: U.S. Department of Commerce 1992, 2000.

ventable diseases make up about 70 percent of the burden of illness and associated costs, according to *Healthy People 2000 Objectives* (U.S. Department of Health and Human Services [USDHHS] 1991). Preventable causes of death, many related to personal and lifestyle choices, account for eight of the nine leading death causes (Fries, Koop, and Beadle 1993).

**TABLE 7.5** How State Budgets Are Affected If Medicaid Costs Rise above
Their 1991 Share of GDP: An Illustrative Calculation

|  | 1992 | 1993 | 1994 | 1995 | 1996 | 1997 | 1998 | 1999 | 2000 |
|---|---|---|---|---|---|---|---|---|---|
| **Increase in State Medicaid Costs ($ billions)*** | $9 | $14 | $19 | $25 | $31 | $38 | $47 | $58 | $69 |
| **Increase in State Medicaid Costs** *As a Percentage of State Revenues*†‡ | 2.5 | 3.7 | 4.5 | 5.7 | 6.8 | 7.9 | 9.4 | 11.0 | 12.4 |
| *As a Percentage of State Non-Medicaid Spending*†‡ | 3.2 | 4.9 | 6.0 | 7.7 | 9.2 | 10.8 | 12.9 | 15.3 | 17.6 |

SOURCE: CBO 1992a.

*The difference between the CBO projection for Medicaid costs and the amount that would be spent if state Medicaid expenditures were held to their 1991 share of GDP. In 1991, state spending on Medicaid absorbed an estimated 0.75 percent of GDP. CBO projected that by 2000 it would absorb 1.5 percent.

†Less federal grants-in-aid.

‡CBO does not forecast state revenues and expenditures. In this table, state revenues are assumed to be a fixed share of total state and local revenues, which CBO does project. The shares are based on the 1987 census of government. Similarly, state non-Medicaid expenditures are assumed to be a fixed share of state and local spending.

**Market Failure**    Market failure, often cited as the reason for increasing health expenditures (CBO 1992a, 1992b), reintroduces the long-standing debate regarding whether health services are an economic good (an entity subject to competition and market forces) or a social good (which limits the effects of competitive and market forces) (Gray 1986). A middle ground suggests that health services markets are inefficient for the following reasons (CBO 1992a):

- Consumers lack information.
- Patients delegate authority and responsibility for decision making to physicians.
- Providers often lack needed information.
- Price competition among sellers of care is ineffective.
- Third-party payers are prevalent.
- Governments subsidize much of the market.

The effects of provider payment or reimbursement mechanisms on health services expenditures are discussed later in this chapter.

## Projections of U.S. Health Services Expenditures

Although the 7.9 percent growth in health services expenditures for 2004 is a lower annual increase than the 9.1 percent growth in 2002 and the 8.3 percent growth in 2003, concerns remain that expenditures are out of control and are jeopardizing the use of resources for other societal needs. A review of future expenditures follows, along with a discussion of the implications of increasing health expenditures.

Annual health expenditures reached 1.9 trillion dollars in 2000. The CBO (1992a) projected that spending on health services between 1990 and 2000 would be equivalent to the increase that occurred from 1965 to 1991. The CBO (1992a) also projected that expenditures by the year 2000 would be $1.7 trillion annually and absorb 18 percent of GDP. The CBO projections might have been considered conservative at the time they were reported, inasmuch as their projections of $808 billion in expenditures for 1992 were $25.6 billion lower than the actual expenditures of $833.6 billion. The CMS (then HCFA) analysts projected in 1991 that the proportion of GDP dedicated to health expenditures would be 16.4 percent by 2000 (Levit and Cowan 1991), a figure not quite reached for 2004. Actual health expenditures for 2004 absorbed 16 percent of GDP. Health insurance premiums increased each year between 1999 and 2004; other indicators also suggest a continued increase in annual health expenditures.

Warshawsky (1994) used both a macroeconomic and an actuarial simulation to project health expenditures as a share of GDP. Both approaches projected a continued increase in the relation of health expenditures to the GDP. Warshawsky found that under the most conservative assumptions, the health services sector will consume more than one-quarter of GNP by 2065.

## Efforts to Contain Health Services Costs and Expenditures

The growing consensus is that the increasing costs of and expenditures for health services in the United States must be at least contained, if not reduced. How and by whom this control should be exerted remains a matter of debate. Proponents of a market economy hold that competition, if allowed to freely operate, can stimulate efficiency in the system and ultimately contain costs and expenditures , while proponents of regulation hold that market failures can only be effectively addressed through regulation (Meyer 1985). The result of this debate is a curious patchwork of operative competitive forces and highly regulated segments of the health services sector.

Efforts to contain health services costs and expenditures have been initiated since at least the early 1970s, when the financial effects of the

Medicare and Medicaid programs first became apparent. Cost containment efforts have been targeted at providers, health facility capital development, costs of services and supplies, changing the delivery system, increasing patients' share of costs, controlling utilization, and reducing health insurance costs (see Table 7.6). Initiatives aimed at providers include the 1972 Economic Stabilization Program (ESP) that froze hospital charges, the Medicare prospective payment system (PPS) that established a diagnosis-specific payment system for hospital inpatient care in 1983, and periodic freezes on physician payment by Medicare and Medicaid.

### Containing Health Facility Capital Expenditures

The costs of health facility capital development became part of charges for patient care, and facility development, expansion, modernization, or sales were uncontrolled. As a result, efforts to regulate facility capital development were initiated in the early 1970s: the Section 1122 (of the Social Security Act) capital expenditure review program aimed principally at hospitals and nursing homes in 1972, and the certificate of need (CON) program aimed at these and other providers in 1974. Although the CON program was repealed as federal statute in 1986 and the Section 1122 program was eliminated the following year, several states have elected to maintain a modified CON program as one way to manage their Medicaid expenditures.

Many of the initiatives listed in Table 7.6 were purportedly introduced to resolve issues of access to and quality of care, but the cost and expenditure control remained an important dimension of these programs.

Most of these initiatives failed to contain costs and expenditures for the long term. A common contributor to their failure is the lack of system-wide effect: The majority of these initiatives aim at only one part of the system and cannot address system reactions to avoid these controls. For example, PPS may have contained some expenditures for hospital inpatient care but could not address the resulting shift of care from inpatient to outpatient settings. Analysts hold that many of these initiatives have had only limited and often one-time effects in containing health services costs and expenditures. Schwartz and Mendelson (1994) note that Medicare's PPS and the spread of managed care resulted in a one-time reduction of 30 percent in the use of inpatient hospital days in the 1980s; however, by 1988, the increases in outpatient costs exceeded the savings that resulted from reduced inpatient days.

Provisions of the 1997 Balanced Budget Act slowed overall growth in Medicare expenditures for three years, but expansionary legislation between 2000 and 2002, particularly in the provisions of Part B, have fueled a resumption in increases through 2004 (CMS 2005).

**TABLE 7.6** Initiatives to Contain U.S. Health Services Expenditures

| | |
|---|---|
| Containing Provider Payment | • Economic Stabilization Program (ESP), 1971, to control hospital costs<br>• Voluntary hospital cost containment program, 1974<br>• Medicare's prospective payment system (PPS) for hospitals, 1983<br>• Medicare's resource-based relative value scale physician payment reform, implemented 1992<br>• Selective contracting by payers, including MediCal (California's Medicaid program)<br>• Periodic freezes on provider reimbursement by Medicare and Medicaid |
| Health Facility Capital Development | • Section 1122, Social Security Act, requiring preauthorization for capital development, 1972<br>• Certificate of need (CON) requires state preauthorization of all health facility capital development and equipment expenditures above a certain financial threshold, 1974 |
| Costs of Supplies and Services | • Medicaid drug rebates authorized by Omnibus Budget Reconciliation Act, 1990<br>• Medicaid competitive bidding for services initiated by various Medicaid programs |
| Changing the Delivery System | • Health Maintenance Organizations (HMO) Act, 1973<br>• Managed care demonstrations for Medicare and Medicaid, 1982<br>• Medicare+Choice, a managed care option for Medicare beneficiaries established by the 1997 Balanced Budget Act<br>• Medicare Advantage, the managed care option created by the 2003 Medicare Modernization and Prescription Drug Act |
| Increasing Patient's Share of Costs | • Use of cost sharing for premium, deductibles, copayments, and co-insurance<br>• Limits on services (reimbursement for only a set number of prescriptions per month)<br>• Limits on expenditures for certain services or a lifetime cap on benefits or expenditures<br>• Reductions or caps on employer's contribution to health insurance premium for employees<br>• Elimination of dependent coverage or increased premium for this coverage |
| Utilization Control | • Medicare's professional standards review organizations (PSRO), 1972<br>• Medicare's peer review organizations (PROs), 1982<br>• Payers' preauthorization, precertification, second surgical opinion programs<br>• Quality improvement organizations (QIOs) replaced PROs to focus on improving quality of care in specific disease categories |
| Reducing Costs of Health Insurance | • Employer ability to self-insure following Employee Retirement Income Security Act (ERISA) of 1974<br>• Business-industry coalitions |

## Provider Payment Mechanisms

The ways in which health services providers are paid for their services is important to understanding the financing of a health services system. Payment mechanisms directly affect expenditures as well. Four major payment mechanisms have typically been used in the U.S. health services system—fee-for-service, flat fee per medical case, flat fee per patient per month or year, and global budgeting—and are discussed in the sections that follow. Table 7.7 summarizes the types of payment systems used for various services—hospital inpatient and outpatient, physicians, and nursing homes—by major types of payers. The extent of financial risk to providers is also noted. The section begins with a discussion of a proposed modification in provider payment: pay-for-performance (P4P).

### Pay-for-Performance

In the interest of tying provider compensation more closely to performance, Medicare and other groups (including the National Quality Forum [NQF], the Joint Commission on Accreditation of Healthcare Organizations [JCAHO], the National Committee for Quality Assurance [NCQA], the Agency for Healthcare Research and Quality [AHRQ], and the American Medical Association [AMA]) collaborated in 2004 to establish payment standards for hospital and physician services. This collaboration was grounded in provisions of the 2003 Medicare Modernization Act and proposed that providers be paid on a fee-for-service basis but that payments be augmented through the receipt of bonuses for meeting performance standards. The performance standards or goal measures are linked to a condition or diagnosis and take into account the patient's severity of illness.

A CMS demonstration on pay-for-performance, conducted in both the public and the private sectors, was initiated in 2003. Early results are just beginning to be reported. The Rewarding Results program reported in November 2005 that P4P programs can improve patients' quality of care (*Medicine and Health* 2006). Another report on an early experience with P4P (Rosenthal et al. 2005) concludes that paying clinicians to reach a common, fixed performance target may produce little gain in quality for the money spent and will largely reward those with higher performance at baseline. This study measured changes in performance among clinicians in West Coast locations who were evaluating performance in cervical cancer screening, mammography, and hemoglobin A1C tests.

Forward movement on the P4P program appears to have been stalled by the inability to achieve a federal budget for fiscal year 2006 on schedule. This delay has affected other provider reimbursement changes proposed by the CMS.

**TABLE 7.7** Provider Payment Mechanisms

| | Provider | | | | |
|---|---|---|---|---|---|
| Payer | Hospital Inpatient | Hospital Outpatient | Physician | Nursing Home | Provider Risk |
| *Commercial Private Insurance* | | | | | |
| Indemnity FFS | Per diem and procedure Global budgeting | Encounter/ visit | Usual, customary, and reasonable (UCR) | If covered: per diem | Little risk to provider |
| HMO | Depends on whether HMO owns hospital | Capitation | Capitation | Usually not covered | Provider likely to bear some risk |
| PPO | Discount | Discount | Discounted FFS | If covered: per diem | Provider likely to bear some risk |
| *Social Insurance Programs* | | | | | |
| Medicare Part A | DRG | NA | | Per diem, SNF only | Provider likely to bear some risk |
| Medicare Part B | NA | RBRVS | RBRVS | NA | Provider likely to bear some risk |
| Medicare Part C Medicare+Choice | DRG | Capitation | Capitation | NA | Provider likely to bear significant risk |
| Medicaid FFS | Per diem and procedure | Encounter/ visit | Fee schedule | Per diem | Payment usually below private-sector level |
| Medicaid prepaid | Depends on provider contract | Capitation | Capitation | If covered: discounted per diem | Provider likely to bear some risk |
| Medicaid prospective payment | Modified DRG | NA | NA | NA | Provider likely to bear some risk |

NOTES: DRG = diagnosis-related group; FFS = fee for service; NA = not applicable; RBRVS = resource-based relative value scale; SNF = skilled nursing facilities.

## Fee-for-Service Payment

The spread of indemnity health insurance after World War II, followed by the establishment in the mid-1960s of two major social programs—Medicare and Medicaid—instituted formal payment or reimbursement systems for health services providers. The primary payment basis for hospitals was per day or per stay, and billing included the hospital's operational and capital costs. The primary payment mechanism for physicians was fee-for-service, wherein the patient was charged a fee for each service or set of services provided. If the patient had health insurance, his or her insurer paid this charge or some insurance-policy–specified portion of it. Charges varied by geographic area, specialty of provider, and other variables, which led some payers, including Medicare, to institute a uniform payment schedule based on usual, customary, and reasonable (UCR) charges for a given area.

Medicare also introduced a payment strategy—provider assignment—to reduce the beneficiary's out-of-pocket payments for physician care. A physician who accepts Medicare assignment agrees to accept Medicare's payment as payment in full and cannot bill the beneficiary for the difference between physician charges and Medicare's payment. A physician who does not accept assignment may bill the patient for the portion of the bill that Medicare does not pay. This is known as extra billing. In 1989, Medicare set limits on the amount of extra billing a physician could charge a beneficiary (USDHHS 1995).

Per-day or per-service payment mechanisms embody the incentive for adding unneeded days of care or "interesting-to-know-about-but-perhaps-nonessential" tests and other services. In this payment system, the payer bears the risk; the services provider bears no financial risk. Such payment mechanisms can drive up health services expenditures, especially when the patient is outside the loop of fiscal accountability because his or her insurance handles all the financial transactions. Among several studies that cite the inflationary effects of these payment mechanisms on increasing health services expenditures is that of economist Uwe Reinhardt (1994). The policy spotlight on increasing health services expenditures helped stimulate alternative payment mechanisms.

## Medicare-Specific Payment Mechanisms

**Medicare's Prospective Payment System**

Medicare led the drive to change how hospitals were paid for inpatient care with the institution of its prospective payment system (PPS) in 1983. Hospital payments had become an ever-larger share of Medicare expenditures, and hospital billing practices enabled hospitals to recover some uncompensated billings by shifting these costs to Medicare and other payers. To deter this practice of cost shifting, Medicare developed an initial list of 467 diagnosis-related groups (DRGs) and established a payment schedule for each code. The payment schedule included geographic (i.e., urban and rural) and teaching hospital adjustments. Hospitals could also seek additional compensation for outlier cases, those whose stay or need for intensity of services significantly exceeded the norm. Four major classes of specialty hospitals (children's, psychiatric, rehabilitation, and long-term care) and two major types of distinct-part units of short-stay hospitals (psychiatric and rehabilitation) are excluded from participating in Medicare's PPS (USD-HHS 1995).

Other payers, including Medicaid, began to follow Medicare's lead. By 1991, 22 Medicaid programs used a modified DRG system as their basis of payment for hospital services (Congressional Research Service 1993). The CMS, the federal administrative agency for Medicare and Medicaid, has supported research into the development of DRGs for outpatient and ambulatory care and for psychiatric and rehabilitative services, and these reimbursement changes are in pilot testing or early implementation phases.

Medicare is also leading the way in changing physician payment mechanisms. In 1992, Medicare began to implement its resource-based relative value scale (RBRVS), a system created to better rationalize payments across specialties and to better reimburse the less technical but critically important aspects of care, such as history taking, physical examination, and counseling. A national Medicare fee schedule, a volume performance standard (VPS) to restrain the annual rate of increase in Medicare physician payments, and a limit on the amount that nonparticipating physicians can charge Medicare beneficiaries on unassigned claims are features of the Medicare Physician Payment Reform Program of 1989 (USDHHS 1995).

**Medicare's Relative-Based Resource Value Scale**

### *Flat Fee Per Patient Per Month or Year*

An entirely different payment system, based on a flat advance payment per patient per month or per year, is a feature of some types of health maintenance organizations (HMOs) and other managed care hybrids. This payment mechanism is commonly referred to as *capitation,* and at least some of the risk for providing the appropriate level of care is borne by the provider.

Capitation was introduced as a way to increase the efficiency of the system, permitting individuals to get as much as, but no more than, the amount of care needed. It introduces conflicting provider incentives: to keep patients well and to avert costly care that stems from delayed medical intervention, but also to potentially underserve patients to retain as much capitation as possible as profit.

Is capitation a more efficient payment mechanism than fee-for-service? Results from earlier studies (Luft 1981; Manning et al. 1984) indicate that capitation-reimbursed care in many HMOs was less costly than fee-for-service care, principally because HMOs were able to reduce the number of inpatient hospitalizations. Schwartz and Mendelson (1994) report that for 1950 to 1980, patients enrolled in HMOs used 30 percent fewer inpatient hospital days than patients in fee-for-service systems. This may be the one-time, limited effect of an intervention because only an additional 1.8 percent of hospital days were eliminated between 1988 and 1991. Before a definitive answer can be offered, the case-mix of populations whose care was reimbursed by each mechanism needs to be compared.

**Capitation's Effect on Health Expenditures**

Staines (1993) explored the potential for capitation systems to reduce health services expenditures. He estimated the potential effects of managed care on national health spending and concluded that if all acute health services spending were delivered through staff or group model HMOs, national health spending would be about 10 percent lower. If the delivery of all acute services not already provided by HMOs were subject to utilization review arrangements incorporating precertification and concurrent review of inpatient care, spending might be 1 percent lower. The effectiveness of capitation payment mechanisms in reducing health services expenditures will continue to be examined as the delivery of health services moves increasingly toward managed care models.

Analysts describe a backlash against managed care (Blendon et al. 1998), beginning in the late 1990s; pure capitation payment methods appear to be decreasing in prominence. Zuvekas and Hill (2004) and Bazzoli et al. (2000) have reported studies that question whether capitation can help control costs.

**Use of Capitation in Medicare and Medicaid Programs**

Medicare and Medicaid have, to varying degrees, introduced capitation payment systems for their eligible populations. In 1982, Medicare initiated a series of risk-based demonstrations with providers for the care of Medicare beneficiaries and opened this option to all interested providers in 1985. Provider payment is based on an adjusted average per capita cost (AAPCC); the AAPCC is calculated as 95 percent of a geographic area's historic expenditures per Medicare beneficiary, adjusted for age and gender.

Whether Medicare has been able to contain its expenditures for beneficiaries in capitated systems remains open to debate. Studies show that the Medicare beneficiaries who enroll in capitated programs are typically younger and healthier than other beneficiaries (USGAO 1994), a phenomenon known as selection bias. Other studies suggest that the AAPCC payment rate is excessive, paying providers more, on average, than they would have earned under the fee-for-service system.

The 1997 Balanced Budget Act created a new form of Medicare managed care—the Medicare+Choice plans. The intent was to attract a greater proportion of Medicare beneficiaries into managed care plans, which the federal government believed would help project and control expenditures. At the time of the act's passage, the Medicare market seemed to be an attractive line of business, particularly because Medicare beneficiaries who typically enrolled in managed care plans were frequently the younger and healthier beneficiaries, and enrollments began to grow. By 2000 and 2001, however, the growth momentum had stalled, and soon Medicare+Choice plans were closing their enrollments of Medicare beneficiaries and in some cases closing their doors because of financial reversals. Grossman, Strunk, and Hurley (2002) attribute this roller-coaster effect to rising health services cost trends, the effects of the commercial insurance underwriting cycle (see Chapter 6), and the plans' inabilities to negotiate provider discounts.

The Medicare Prescription Drug Improvement and Modernization Act (MMA) of 2003 replaced the Medicare+Choice program with the Medicare Advantage plan. Major types of Medicare Advantage plans may reimburse providers on a capitation or modified capitation basis or may be private unrestricted fee-for-service plans (CMS 2005).

In 1982, the Medicaid program initiated a similar series of demonstration studies of capitated care. An assessment of 25 Medicaid managed care programs concluded that the evidence available did not indicate that risk-based (capitation) methods of payment had a material effect on cost and utilization of services, with the exception of physician visits where the number of visits was not changed or was lower than the number in the fee-for-service system (Hurley, Freund, and Paul 1993).

### Global Budgeting

A fourth provider payment mechanism, used typically with hospitals, is the global budget. Widely used in Canada for hospital care, global budgeting involves provinces providing a prospectively determined fixed amount to facilities for their full operational expenses. Depreciation and capital development expenses may be included in this amount or may be separately funded.

# Implications of Increasing Health Services Expenditures

What are the implications for governments, businesses, and individuals of a society's choice to direct a significant proportion of its GDP toward supporting health services? This question continues to arise as policymakers consider the prospects of growing health services expenditures. Pauly (1993) argues that high medical services costs are not a problem per se but become a problem when they are worth less than the forgone consumption; that is, one must consider the opportunity costs of health services.

Even with the 2004 lower rate of increase in expenditures compared to many prior years, health spending still grew faster than the GDP (CMS 2000). Figure 7.9 shows the proportion of GDP directed to health services for select years from 1960 to 2004. The health services share of GDP has increased threefold in this 44-year period. The implications of increasing health services expenditures for government, employers and businesses, and the individual are now considered.

### Implications for Government

Since 1980, health spending has been the second fastest growing component of the federal budget, surpassed only by the interest payments on the national debt (Ross, Ratner, and Fein 1991). By 1990, federal government outlays for health services were more than double those for national defense (CBO 1992a). During the 1980s, federal spending on health increased 50 percent in constant (adjusted for inflation) dollars, while spending on science and education fell 22 percent (Center for Health Economic Research 1994). Medicaid support is frequently the largest or second largest component of state government budgets, sometimes exceeding state support for education. Spending for health services, therefore, has the potential to squeeze out or eliminate government support for other services.

**Tax Expenditures**    Another implication for the federal government of increased health services expenditures is the way they are treated in the U.S. tax code. Because employer health premiums are not taxed and other health-related expenses are tax deductible, federal and state governments lose billions in tax revenue each year. This loss is referred to as tax expenditure and is considered by many policymakers to be a substantial tax loophole.

The most significant loophole is the exclusion from employee-taxable income of employer-paid premiums. In 1998, this amounted to an estimated tax expenditure of $75.2 billion (Sheils and Hogan 1999), which had grown to $188.5 billion by 2004 (Sheils and Haught 2004). Untaxed employer health premiums are the third largest source of lost federal revenues, behind pensions and mortgage interest, and surpass deductions for state and local taxes (Center for Health Economic Research 1994). Since 2003, qualifying individuals have had the option of obtaining a health coverage tax credit (HCTC) to help them reduce the cost of their health coverage. A recent GAO report indicates that in 2003, more than 19,000 individuals received about $37 million in benefits from the IRS for the HCTC for themselves and their dependents (USGAO 2004).

### Implications for Employers and Businesses

The implications of health services expenditures for employers and businesses are increasingly evident in business financial reports. U.S. corporations spend a significant amount on employee health services. From 1980 to 1990, the cost of employer-sponsored health services increased about threefold and consumed 3.9 percent of the GDP. In 1990, health services spending by businesses was equivalent to 61.1 percent of corporate profits before taxes and was 107.9 percent more than the amount of corporate profits after taxes. Business health services spending as a share of total labor compensation was 10.2 percent for state and local government and 6.8 percent for private industry in 2001 (USDHHS 2005), up from 2 percent in 1965 (Levit and Cowan 1991).

Increasing health services expenditures also affect businesses' ability to adequately fund retiree health programs that current and former employees believed were a benefit of their employment. Generous benefit packages often were established long before the consequences of increasing health services expenditures were fully understood. To protect the receipt of an earned benefit, federal law (Financial Accounting Standards Board Release 106) now requires that businesses report and show how they will fund the future costs of retiree health benefits (Ross, Ratner, and Fein 1991). Nonetheless, the number of firms offering health benefits to persons who retire before they reach the age of Medicare eligibility or who are fully retired continues to decline (see Chapter 6).

**Effects on Retiree Health Benefit Programs**

Allocation of resources to maintain a healthy workforce is generally considered a good business investment, but when the proportion of such resources precludes other potential investments without proportionately improving employee health, businesses may begin to reassess these commitments.

**Effects on Employee Cost Sharing**

One result of this reassessment is that more companies are increasing the cost-sharing requirements for their employees. Between 1980 and 1988, the share of employees holding policies requiring deductibles of $100 or more rose more than fivefold (Ross, Ratner, and Fein 1991). Other business strategies for containing health services expenditures include refusing to offer insurance, self-insuring, seeking exemption from state-mandated benefits (applicable to small businesses), and increasing employees' share of co-insurance (Levit and Cowan 1991).

Since 2000, the employer share of employer-sponsored health insurance has declined more than 3 percentage points, from 74.7 percent to 71.3 percent. A favorable labor market has allowed businesses to pass on more of the annual increases in health care costs to their employees (CMS 2005).

## Implications for the Individual

The implications of increasing health services expenditures on individuals are mixed. For individuals in the workforce, the fear of losing all their assets to a catastrophic medical event may be mitigated by the availability of employer-sponsored health insurance. Insured employees may find, however, that their share of costs is increasing, lifetime coverage of expenditures may be limited or capped, and benefits may be reduced for both the employee and his or her dependents as employers address their costs of providing health insurance. Salaries and wages may remain static or even decrease in real dollars as a consequence of employers providing ever-more-costly health insurance benefits.

Economist Uwe Reinhardt (1993) points out that real cash wages have hardly grown in the last two decades because of the increasing costs that employers pay for health insurance. For individuals who do not have employer-sponsored health insurance, either because it is not a benefit of their employment or they are not in the workforce, rising costs of providing health services do not increase their likelihood of obtaining health services. Many such individuals or families may be in lower-income categories and, if they obtain health services at all, may spend proportionately more of their incomes on health services than do higher-income families (Center for Health Economic Research 1994).

## Summary

Health services in the United States are financed by a combination of private- and public-sector sources. The public sector finances about 45 percent of all expenditures, nearly double the 1960 public share of 24.5 percent. Per capita expenditures for health services—$6,280 in 2004—are the highest in the world, but nearly 20 percent of the U.S. population does not have assured access to regular care.

Expenditures for health services have been driven by inflation, demographic changes, the use of technology, and other reasons—chief among them the growth of public programs such as Medicare and Medicaid. The dedication of an ever-increasing proportion of GDP to health services (16 percent in 2004) raises questions about resource allocations to meet a range of needs.

Numerous initiatives to control expenditures have been largely unsuccessful in the long term, primarily because each has targeted only one part of the health services system. Barring major system changes, health services expenditures are projected to continue to increase. The amount of the GDP that health expenditures absorb will depend on the strength of the economy. In a strong economy, the percentage of GDP could remain relatively constant or show an increase, whereas in a weaker economy, the proportion will depend on whether health expenditures match a slowdown or decrease in overall economic growth.

## Note

1. Although individuals frequently pay a share of the premiums for their health insurance, often as a payroll deduction, this expenditure is included in the appropriate health insurance expenditure category, rather than in the out-of-pocket category in the National Health Accounts.

## Key Words

adjusted average per capita cost (AAPCC)

administrative costs

Agency for Healthcare Research and Quality (AHRQ)

American Medical Association (AMA)

Balanced Budget Act of 1997

capital expenditure review

capitation

case-mix

Centers for Medicare and Medicaid Services (CMS)

certificate of need (CON) program

co-insurance

competition

concurrent review

cost

cost containment

cost sharing

defensive medicine

Department of Veterans Affairs (VA)

developmental disabilities

diagnosis-related groups (DRGs)

Economic Stabilization Program (ESP)

Emergency Maternal and Infant Child Care Program (EMIC)

entitlement programs

expenditures

extra billing

fee-for-service payment

Financial Accounting Standards Board Release 106

flat fee per medical case

flat fee per patient

fraud and abuse

general inflation

global budgeting

gross domestic product (GDP)

gross national product (GNP)

group model HMO

Health Care Financing Administration (HCFA)

health maintenance organization (HMO)

Health Security Act (HSA)

indemnity health insurance

Indian Health Service (IHS)

Joint Commission on Accreditation of Healthcare Organizations (JCAHO)

malpractice

managed care

Marine Hospital Service

Medicaid

medical inflation

Medicare

Medicare+Choice

Medicare Hospital Trust Fund

Medicare Physician Payment Reform Program

Medicare Prescription Drug
   Improvement and
     Modernization Act (MMA)
Medicare's prospective payment
   system (PPS)
National Committee for Quality
   Assurance (NCQA)
National Medical Expenditure Survey
National Quality Forum (NQF)
net cost of private health insurance
nondurable medical equipment
nursing home
opportunity costs
out-of-pocket payments
pay for performance (P4P)
personal health care expenditures
pluralistic health system

precertification
price
private sector
provider assignment
public sector
regulation
retiree health benefits
resource-based relative value scale
   (RBRVS)
selection bias
Social Security Act (SSA)
staff model HMO
tax expenditures
usual, customary, reasonable
   charge (UCR)
utilization review
volume performance standard (VPS)

## References

Agency for Health Care Policy and Research. 1994. Growth in Health Care Expenditures for Children and Adults. Bethesda, MD: Intramural Research Highlights: NMES, No. 37, AHCPR Pub. No. 94-0136.

Bazzoli G., L. Dynan, D. R. Burns, and R. Lindroom. 2000. "Is Provider Capitation Working? Effects on Physician-Hospital Integration of Costs of Care." *Medical Care* 38 (3): 311–324.

Berk, M. L., and A. C. Monheit. 1992. "The Concentration of Health Expenditures: An Update." *Health Affairs* 11 (4): 145–49.

Blendon, R. J., M. Brodie, J. M. Benson, D. E. Altman, L. Levitt, T. Hoff, and L. Huzick. 1998. "Understanding the Managed Care Backlash." *Health Affairs* 17 (4): 80–94.

Center for Health Economic Research. 1994. *The Nation's Health Care: Who Bears the Burden?* Waltham, MA: Center for Health Economic Research.

Centers for Medicare and Medicaid Services (CMS). 2005. "Highlights, National Health Expenditures, 2004." [Online information; retrieved 1/12/06.] http://cms.hhs.gov/statistics/nhe/historical/highlights.asp.

———. 2000. "Highlights, National Health Expenditures, 2000." [Online information; retrieved 2/17/03.] http://cms.hhs.gov/statistics/nhe/historical/highlights.asp.

Congressional Budget Office. 1992a. *Economic Implications of Rising Health Care Costs.* Washington, DC: CBO.

———. 1992b. *Projections of National Health Expenditures.* Washington, DC: CBO.

Congressional Research Service. 1993. *Medicaid Source Book: Background Data and Analysis (an Update)*. Washington, DC: U.S. Government Printing Office.

Cowan C. A., H. C. Lazenby, A. B. Martin, P. A. McDonnell, A. L. Sensenig, J. M. Stiller, L. S. Whittle, K. A. Kotova, M. A. Zezza, C. S. Donham, A. M. Long, and M. W. Stewart. 1999. "National Health Expenditures, 1998." *Health Care Financing Review* 21 (2): 165–210.

Fries, J. F., C. E. Koop, and C. E Beadle. 1993. "Reducing Health Care Costs by Reducing the Need and Demand for Medical Services." *New England Journal of Medicine* 329 (5): 321–25.

Fuchs, V. R. 1990. "The Health Sector's Share of the Gross National Product." *Science* 247 (4942): 534–38.

Gray, B. H. 1986. *For-Profit Enterprise in Health Care*. Washington, DC: National Academy Press.

Grossman, J. M., B. C. Strunk, and R. E. Hurley. 2002. "Reversal of Fortune: Medicare+Choice Collides with Market Forces." Issue Brief No. 52. Washington, DC: Center for Studying Health System Change.

Health Insurance Association of America. 1985. *Source Book of Health Insurance Data*. Washington, DC: HIAA.

Hurley, R. E., D. A. Freund, and J. E. Paul. 1993. *Managed Care in Medicaid: Lessons for Policy and Program Design*. Chicago: Health Administration Press.

Jaggar, S. F. 1995. *Medicare and Medicaid: Opportunities to Save Program Dollars by Reducing Fraud and Abuse*. GAO/T-HEHS-95-110. Washington, DC: USGAO.

Levit, K. R., and C. A. Cowan. 1991. "Businesses, Households, and Governments: Health Care Costs, 1990." *Health Care Financing Review* 12 (2): 83–93.

Levit, K. R., H. C. Lazenby, and L. Sivarajan. 1996. "Health Care Spending in 1994: Slowest in Decades." *Health Affairs* 15 (2): 130–44.

Litman, T. J. 1997. *Health Politics and Policy*, 3d ed. New York: Delmar.

Luft, H. S. 1981. *Health Maintenance Organizations: Dimensions of Performance*. New York: John Wiley.

Manning, W., A. Leibowitz, G. A. Goldberg, W. H. Rogers, and J. P. Newhouse. 1984. "A Controlled Trial of the Effect of a Prepaid Group Practice on the Use of Services." *New England Journal of Medicine* 310 (23): 1505–10.

Medicine and Health. 2006. "Pay for Performance Not Reaching Small Physician Practices." *Medicine and Health* 60 (2): 1,4. Washington, DC: Health Care Information Center.

Meyer, J. A. 1985. *Incentives vs. Controls in Health Policy*. Washington, DC: American Enterprise Institute for Public Policy Research.

National Association of State Budget Officers. 2004. "The Fiscal Survey of States: April 2004." [Online article or information; retrieved 12/28/05.] www.nasbo.org/publications/fiscsurvey/2004/fsapril2004.pdf.

Pauly, M. V. 1993. "U.S. Health Care Costs: The Untold True Story." *Health Affairs* 12 (3): 152–29.

Peden, E. A., and M. S. Freeland. 1995. "A Historical Analysis of Medical Spending Growth, 1960–1993." *Health Affairs* 14 (2): 235–47.

Reinhardt, U. E. 1994. "Planning the Nation's Workforce: Let the Market In." *Inquiry* 31 (3): 250–63.

———. 1993. "Reorganizing the Financial Flows in American Health Care." *Health Affairs* 12 (Supplement): 172–93.

Rosenthal, M. B., R. G. Frank, L. Zhonghi, and A. M. Epstein. 2005. "Early Experience with Pay for Performance: From Concept to Practice." *Journal of the American Medical Association* 294 (14): 1788–93.

Ross, J., J. Ratner, and H. Fein. 1991. *U.S. Health Care Spending: Trends, Contributing Factors, and Proposals for Reform.* GAO/HRD 91–102. Washington, DC: USGAO.

Schactman, D., S. H. Altman, E. Eilat, K. E. Thorpe, and M. Doonan. 2003. "The Outlook for Hospital Spending." *Health Affairs* 22 (6): 12–26.

Schwartz, W. B., and D. M. Mendelson. 1994. "Eliminating Waste and Inefficiency Can Do Little to Contain Costs." *Health Affairs* 13 (1): 224–38.

Sheils, J., and R. Haught. 2004. "The Cost of Tax-Exempt Health Benefits in 2004." *Health Affairs Web Exclusive*, W4-106-112, February 25, 2004.

Sheils, J., and P. Hogan. 1999. "Cost of Tax-Exempt Health Benefits in 1998. *Health Affairs* 18 (2): 176–81.

Shonick, W. 1995. *Government and Health Services.* New York: Oxford University Press.

Staines, V. S. 1993. "Potential Impact of Managed Care on National Health Spending." *Health Affairs* 12 (Supplement): 248–57.

Strunk, B. C., P. B. Ginsburg, and J. R. Gabel. 2001. "Tracking Health Care Costs." *Health Affairs Web Exclusive*, September 26.

U.S. Department of Commerce. 2000. *Statistical Abstract of the United States.* Washington, DC: U.S. Government Printing Office.

———. 1992. *Statistical Abstract of the United States.* Washington, DC: U.S. Government Printing Office.

U.S. Department of Health and Human Services. 2005. *Health, United States, 2005.* Pub. No. (PHS) 2005-1232. Hyattsville, MD: USDHHS.

———. 1995. *Medicare and Medicaid Statistical Supplement, 1995.* Pub. No. (PHS) 03386. Baltimore, MD: USDHHS.

———. 1991. *Healthy People 2000: National Health Promotion and Disease Prevention Objectives.* Washington, DC: U.S. Government Printing Office.

U.S. Government Accountability Office (formerly the U.S. General Accounting Office). 2004. *Health Coverage Tax Credit: Simplified and More Timely Enrollment Process Could Increase Participation.* GAO-04-1029. September. Washington, DC: USGAO.

———. 1994. *Health Care Reform: Considerations for Risk Adjustment under Community Rating.* GAO/HEHS-94-173. Washington, DC: USGAO.

———. 1992a. *Employer-Based Health Insurance: High Costs, Wide Variation Threaten System.* USGAO/HRD-92-125. September. Washington, DC: USGAO.

———. 1992b. *Health Insurance: Vulnerable Payers Lose Billions to Fraud and Abuse*. USGAO/HRD-92-69. Washington, DC: USGAO.

Warshawsky, M. J. 1994. "Projections of Health Care Expenditures as a Share of the GDP: Actuarial and Macroeconomic Approaches." *Health Services Research* 29 (3): 293–313.

Wilensky, G. 2001. "Medicare Reform: Now Is the Time." *New England Journal of Medicine* 345 (6): 458–62.

———. 1996. "Presentation to Kaiser Founder's Day Dinner." Unpublished presentation, Denver, CO. November.

Woolhandler, S., and D. Himmelstein. 1991. "The Deteriorating Administrative Efficiency of the U.S. Health Care System." *New England Journal of Medicine* 324 (18): 1253–38.

Zuvekas, S. H., and S. C. Hill. 2004. "Does Capitation Matter? Impacts on Access, Use, and Quality." *Inquiry* 41 (3): 316–335.

# RESOURCE PRODUCTION

# THE HEALTH SERVICES WORKFORCE

## Introduction

From its beginning as a cottage industry at the turn of the twentieth century to its current position as the nation's largest industry, the U.S. health services system today employs more than 13.9 million workers (U.S. Department of Health and Human Services [USDHHS] 2005) and is projected to grow even more to meet the increasing health services needs of an aging population. Traditionally organized with the physician as leader, today's health services workforce is undergoing major changes in its roles and functions. Questions of supply and distribution occupy much of the workforce discussion.

This chapter focuses on several of the key health services provider professions, including physicians; midlevel practitioners, such as physicians' assistants and advanced practice nurses; nurses; pharmacists; and dentists. Each profession is reviewed in terms of its origin and current role in the delivery of health services, training, supply and distribution, and the issues currently facing the profession, including the effects of managed care. Physicians are addressed first because more than 20 percent of personal health services expenditures are directed to them, and because they control an estimated 75 percent of all health services expenditures through their admission of patients to hospitals and nursing homes, referral of patients to other providers, prescribing of medications, and other physician-directed exchanges (Ginzberg 1992; Tarlov 1995; Mullan, Politzer, and Davis 1995).

Many other types of caregivers are also important, including other allied health professionals, informal caregivers, and lay healers. In recent years, the alternative and complementary health services industry has grown significantly; Cooper and Stoflet (1996) project that the per capita supply of alternative medicine clinicians—chiropractors, naturopaths, and practitioners of oriental medicine—will grow by 88 percent between 1994 and 2010, while physician supply will grow by 16 percent. Among the many other employees in the health services workforce are the more than 900,000 workers in the health insurance industry (Health Insurance Association of America [HIAA] 1996), as well as workers in health services equipment and supply businesses, the pharmaceutical industry, and other health-related businesses.

In addition to physicians, nurses, other care providers, and administrators, the public health workforce also includes specialists in specific public health areas, including sanitarians, environmental health workers, and health facility licensure staff. Administrators and financial and billing experts constitute yet another essential component of the health services workforce. Although this chapter cannot do justice to all of them, their contributions to the provision of health services are important to note.

## Physicians

Economic and other forces are pushing for changes in the physician's role in the U.S. health services system. As a context for proposed changes, this section reviews the development of the medical profession in the United States; medical education and training (including graduate medical education); physician demand, supply, and distribution; and other issues the medical profession currently faces.

### The Role of the Physician in the U.S. Health Services System

The physician is the first point of contact with the traditional health services system for most users, whether that contact is in the physician's office or clinic, or a hospital emergency department. Figure 8.1 shows the practice settings for U.S. physicians. The physician is generally perceived as the leader or director of health services, the entry point for hospital or nursing home admission, and the controller of access to prescription drugs, medical equipment, and other services.

The physician's leadership role in the provision of health services emerged as the system developed in scope and sophistication. Today, that leadership role is being challenged as business owners and payers exert greater influence on the delivery of care in their efforts to constrain expenditures. Once an autonomous provider with nearly complete authority over how care was delivered, today's physician is finding his or her practice increas-

**FIGURE 8.1**

Physician
Practice
Settings (2003)

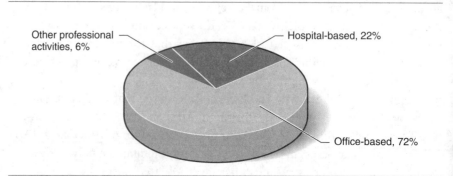

SOURCE: USDHHS 2005.

ingly circumscribed. Prior to a discussion of the range of issues that portend continued change in the physician's role, the profession's origin in the United States is reviewed, followed by material on the evolution of medical education, the resulting supply of physicians, and their distribution.

## The Development of the Medical Profession in the United States

The U.S. medical profession was adapted from the British system of physicians, surgeons, and apothecaries that colonials brought to this country. Physicians in the colonial era were trained principally through apprenticeships and later in nonstandardized programs that often had no university affiliation (Starr 1982).

Medicine as a profession began to emerge by the mid-nineteenth century. The American Medical Association (AMA) was established in 1846, states began to assume responsibility for licensing physicians, and the reform of medical education began. Shortly after 1900, a broad consensus about the desirability to improve medical education, establish and maintain more rigorous educational standards, introduce the scientific foundations of medicine, and emphasize the necessity of independent research began to emerge in the medical profession. In 1906, the AMA Council on Medical Education conducted an independent site visit of U.S. schools and identified findings similar to those of the subsequent Flexner Report (Ludmerer 1985). Educators committed to reform pointed to the scholarship traditions of German and other European universities.

A key element of reform was the 1910 Bulletin Number Four prepared by Abraham Flexner for the Carnegie Foundation for the Advancement of Teaching. Flexner, along with a representative of the AMA, visited the 131 U.S. medical colleges, as well as the Canadian medical schools. He detailed the wide variability in facilities, faculties, admission practices, and educational requirements, and recommended that the number of U.S. medical schools be reduced to 31. Flexner also recommended that remaining schools be modeled after the Johns Hopkins Medical School, which in the 1870s had established a rigorous curriculum, set stringent admissions standards (including the prerequisite of a baccalaureate degree), and emphasized high academic standards for participating faculty members (Starr 1982).

## Medical Education and Training

Flexner did not succeed in reducing the number of medical schools to 31. By 1915, the number had been reduced to 95, and by 1965, the number was 88. However, by 1980, the number had increased to 126 (Starr 1982) and in 2005 was 125. Additionally, 19 schools of osteopathy produce about 5 percent of the physician workforce, and several additional schools of osteopathy are currently proposed for development (Schroeder 1994; Cooper 1995; American Osteopathic Association 2002).

Medical schools today are associated with both private and public universities. The number of applicants generally far exceeds the number of available slots, but the number of graduates has remained relatively constant, at about 17,000 annually from 1980 through 2005 (USDHHS 2005).

The basic training and graduate medical education of physicians—the sole and carefully guarded purview of the private sector until the early 1960s (Ginzberg 1992)—has become increasingly dependent on governmental support. This governmental support stemmed from perceived shortages of physicians at various times and was intended to correct this "market failure." Governmental support has taken many forms: the construction of educational facilities, capitation grants to support new faculty, student scholarships and loans, and research funds that also provide laboratory learning experiences for medical students, interns, and residents.

Medical education is costly. Annual tuition costs for the four years of basic medical education vary widely, but tuition generates less than 5 percent of medical school revenues. Nearly half of medical school revenues are derived from the provision of medical services by teaching faculty, medical students, interns, and residents (Reinhardt 1994). Other sources of revenue for basic medical education include allocations from state governments, clinical earnings from teaching faculty practices, revenues from inpatient care, research monies, and grants and contributions from foundations and other sources.

### Graduate Medical Education (GME)

Graduate medical education (GME), the specialty training beyond medical school that ranges from three to seven or more years, is also costly. GME is provided in residencies of various lengths, depending on the degree of subspecialization sought. Residents receive an annual stipend in exchange for the care they provide to patients as part of their training. The costs of GME to the federal government, averaging $70,000 per year per resident (Wennberg et al. 1993; Rivo, Mays, and Katzoff 1995; National Health Policy Forum [NHPF] 2002), are of particular interest to policymakers because the Medicare program is a major payer for GME. In 1995, Medicare support of GME amounted to about $7 billion per year (NHPF 2002). By contrast, managed care organizations are relatively uninvolved in the provision of GME. Only an estimated 10 percent of managed care organizations have limited involvement in GME (Eisenberg 1994).

Medicaid is the second largest explicit payer of GME, with all but five states paying for the clinical training of physicians. In 1998, the total paid by 45 states was $2.4 billion (Henderson 2000). Whether this level of support will change depends in part on the extent to which Medicaid programs direct their enrollees into managed care plans; as of 2000, only 16 state Medicaid programs carved out the Medicaid GME payments from capitated rates to be redirected to clinical teaching programs (Henderson 2000).

In 2000, Minnesota instituted a unique use of tobacco settlement funds, allocating them to finance a new Medical Education and Research Cost (MERC) fund to finance GME (Blewett and Weslowski 2000). The MERC fund will finance about 6 percent of GME costs in the state and will be used to defray educational expenses among the state's academic health centers.

The costs of GME, particularly to Medicare, are of interest because of their volume and because the number of residencies and residents is not centrally controlled. Rather, the number is determined by the individual institutions wishing to offer such programs and thus requires open-ended support from the various payers. As a result, the number of residency positions exceeds the number of annual U.S. medical school graduates (USMGs) by about 40 percent (Eisenberg 1994; Tarlov 1995). International medical graduates (IMGs), formerly referred to as foreign medical graduates (FMGs), generally fill these excess positions. About 10 percent of these IMGs are native U.S. citizens and another 12 percent are naturalized citizens who received their basic medical education outside the United States (Mullan, Politzer, and Davis 1995). The majority of IMGs are residents of other countries and received their basic medical education outside the United States.

IMG participation in the U.S. health services system historically had at least three purposes: (1) to provide advanced training to physicians from other countries, particularly developing countries, so that they could offer the most current care when they returned home; (2) to provide a relatively inexpensive labor supply to teaching hospitals, which is true of USMG residents as well; and (3) to augment the supply of U.S. physicians as needed.

IMGs play an important role in the U.S. health services system. When immigration policies have been relaxed, as was the case in the 1960s and early 1970s (Mullan, Politzer, and Davis 1995), IMGs have swelled the ranks of U.S. physicians in times of perceived shortages. IMGs often accepted positions in mental hospitals, prison dispensaries, and inner-city hospitals, positions that many USMGs found less desirable. The health services systems in some states, such as New Jersey, New York, Florida, and Illinois, are highly dependent on the participation of IMGs, who constitute 44 percent of New Jersey's physician workforce, 39 percent of New York's physician workforce, and about one-third of the physician workforces in Florida and Illinois (AMA 2004).

The appropriateness of providing GME access to IMGs is debated for many reasons. One is the effect of IMGs on the overall supply of physicians in the United States. Although one intent behind IMG participation in GME in the United States is to better prepare IMGs to provide care in their native countries, an estimated 70 to 75 percent of IMGs actually remain in the United States immediately after their training or return to the United States to practice after only a brief period in their native countries.

The approximate five thousand IMGs who join the permanent U.S. workforce every year represent the equivalent of the entire graduating classes of 50 medical schools around the world. The settling out of IMGs in the United States increased through the mid-1990s due to changes in the treatment of immigration visas (Mullan, Politzer, and Davis 1995). Such changes in immigration policy and the lack of a central body to determine the number of needed residency slots make projecting the need for physicians in this country increasingly difficult, and controlling the physician supply impossible. A subsequent section of this chapter ("IMG Participation in GME") discusses other changes in the supply of IMGs related to recent requirements for clinical skill assessments.

### Supply and Distribution of Physicians

In 2003, 871,535 physicians were licensed in the United States, 736,211 of whom were active in the profession. Of the active U.S. physician pool, 94 percent are involved in providing patient care; 22 percent are hospital-based; 6 percent are involved in other professional activities, such as medical teaching, administration, and research; and 3 percent are federal physicians (USDHHS 2005). About one-third of U.S. physicians are generalists or primary care physicians, including general practitioners, family practitioners, general internal medicine physicians, and general pediatricians without advanced subspecialty training. Two-thirds of U.S. physicians are specialists and subspecialists.

How many physicians, and what types of specialties, are needed to provide appropriate levels of care to a population? Determining an acceptable answer to this seemingly straightforward question remains elusive for many reasons:

- With as much as 20 percent of the population uninsured at some point in a year, not all people have ready and regular access to a physician's services.
- A significant proportion of health services provided, as much as 20 to 50 percent, is believed to produce few beneficial results and may, in certain instances, be harmful (Brook 1991; Ginzberg 1992; Schroeder 1992).
- The supply and distribution of physicians has not been amenable to market forces, resulting in high numbers of physicians in some areas and none in others.
- The varying lengths of physician training complicate the ability to project production of physician supply.
- Pressures are mounting to shift the focus of medical care from treatment of illness and disease to an increased emphasis on health promotion and disease prevention, thus altering the physician's role in health services.

**Determining the Demand for Physicians**

Because determining the demand for physicians is difficult, analysts have focused instead on evaluating proxies for demand, including determining physician utilization and projecting it to the full population; determining physician utilization in managed care settings, which exert more control over utilization, and projecting it to the full population; determining need based on the actual incidence of illness in the population and the ideal level of care to meet these needs; and using an adjusted needs model, which recognizes that not all events require a physician's care (Schroeder 1994; Weiner 1994).

Using current utilization of physician services to determine demand presents a major problem in a system where access to health services is inequitable. Such a calculation measures actual utilization rather than the complete utilization of services that would occur if all who needed care could regularly access it.

Determining demand by assessing actual utilization in managed care settings and then projecting such utilization to the full population may come closer to targeting the number and types of physicians needed. The projections for physician demand that have been made using this methodology (Weiner 1994; Cooper 1995) have, however, assumed universal access to care, which is not yet a reality.

This methodology has also assumed a high level of participation in managed care, which is occurring in more populous areas but lagging in less populous ones; a wide geographic variation in managed care enrollment still exists (Rivo, Mays, and Katzoff 1995). Both approaches and the two based on estimated needs for medical care emphasize a focus on illness and disease rather than on health and do not fully address the importance of the physician's role in health promotion and disease prevention.

**Calculating Physician Supply**

Calculating physician supply is easier than calculating demand because the supply can be influenced in only two ways: the number of slots available in U.S. medical schools for basic medical education and the number of GME slots available based on immigration and IMG policies (Tarlov 1995). The supply of physicians is most frequently reported as a ratio of the number of physicians to a population of 100,000 people. What is important to know is which physicians are included—are all licensed physicians, all active physicians, all nongovernment physicians, or other physician groups included?

Table 8.1 shows the physician-to-population ratios at various intervals, beginning in 1950 and projected to the year 2020. The calculation of physician-to-population ratios and the projection of future ratios clearly show that the supply of physicians is increasing. The current physician-to-population ratio is 235 physicians per 100,000 population (USDHHS 2005). From the mid-1970s through the mid-1990s, the supply of physicians grew 1.5 times as fast as the overall population (Lohr, Vanselow, and Detmer 1996).

Does this physician-to-population ratio indicate a physician surplus, as is currently being debated? The word *surplus* may be misleading inasmuch as it suggests that surplus physicians may be unemployed

**TABLE 8.1**
Physician-to-
Population
Ratios
1950–1990
(Actual) and
2000–2020
(Projected)

| | Number of Physicians per 100,000 Population |
|---|---|
| 1950 | 146 |
| 1960 | 146 |
| 1970 | 156.9 |
| 1980 | 197.8 |
| 1990 | 233 |
| 2000 | 270.6 |
| 2010 | 292.2 and 247 |
| 2020 | 297.5 and 237 |

SOURCES: Alliance for Human Reform 1994; Cooper 1995.

(Tarlov 1995)—a situation that some analysts anticipate but that is not yet realized. As early as 1974, the potential for an oversupply of physicians was recognized (Ginzberg 1992). A physician oversupply presents more problems than it solves in a health services system (Lohr, Vanselow, and Detmer 1996), particularly if the oversupply is of specialists. Such an oversupply contributes to very high rates of expensive, invasive procedures that often result in only marginal improvements in health, potential inadequate access to the services of generalists, and excessive medical care expenditures (Schroeder 1992; Ginzberg 1992).

Physician-to-population ratios reveal nothing about the balance between primary caregivers (or generalists) and specialists. Most countries' health services systems are organized around the primary caregiver, or generalist, who is the first medical contact, provides care that is both longitudinal and comprehensive (Grumbach, Becker, and Osborn 1995), and refers a patient to a specialist as needed. In most countries, the number of generalists is at least equal to and usually significantly higher than the number of specialists.

Managed care in the United States is predicated on this same principle: a patient first sees a primary care physician and then may be referred to a specialist.[1] In the United States, however, the ratio of specialists to generalists is nearly 2 to 1, with less than 30 percent of the physician workforce classified as generalists (Schroeder 1992; Grumbach, Becker, and Osborn 1995). Patients in the United States who are not in managed care may self-refer to a generalist or specialist. The growing influence of managed care, however, has implications for the ability of patients to self-refer to specialists and for the number of specialists needed to participate in managed care.

Physician-to-population ratios also reveal nothing about the distribution of physicians. The economic principles of supply and demand suggest that the distribution of physicians among a population would be somewhat uniform—that physicians would establish practices where they could expect a competitive edge. Such is not the case in the U.S. system, where physicians are concentrated in more populous areas and entirely absent from some less populous areas. Twenty-eight percent of all practicing U.S. physicians are located in the Boston–Washington, DC corridor—a populous but geographically small area. By contrast, Alaska, Idaho, Montana, and Wyoming encompass 25 percent of the U.S. landmass but have only 1 percent of the population and far less than 1 percent of all practicing physicians (Cooper 1995). Thus, regardless of what physician-to-population ratio is deemed the appropriate level of supply, some areas will likely always be underserved in the current health services system.

Under traditional fee-for-service practice, the addition of physicians to a medically saturated area does not drive down prices or incomes. Rather, incomes remain constant or even increase. This contrary-to-market expectation is attributed, in part, to the physician's ability to induce demand for medical services (Wennberg et al. 1993; Schwartz and Mendelson 1990; Eisenberg 1994; Starr 1982, Reinhardt 1994). Even in times of physician surplus, a fee-for-service reimbursement system permits physicians to remain self-employed entrepreneurs and to control their income through volume of services provided. Under capitation or other managed care payment systems, the physician's role may convert from employer to employee.

The difficulty in measuring physician demand has in no way inhibited the government and the medical profession from attempting to affect physician supply. Table 8.2 summarizes various initiatives, beginning as early as 1959, to either increase physician supply or address a perceived oversupply. Nearly four decades of tinkering demonstrate the difficulty of defining and achieving a satisfactory physician supply. Significant changes in the available supply of physicians take a very long time, even when drastic changes are made in the supply pipeline (Wennberg et al. 1993). **Efforts to Affect the Physician Supply**

One reason why change takes so long is physicians' high level of specialization—they cannot easily assume different roles (e.g., a pediatric oncologist and a family physician could not successfully reverse roles or job share). Added to the challenge of effecting immediate supply changes is the fact that a physician's work career generally spans 35 to 40 years after the completion of medical training (Schroeder 1992; Schwartz, Ginzburg, and LeRoy 1993).

To summarize the current status of physicians:

- No consensus has been reached on how to measure demand for physicians.
- The supply of physicians has grown steadily since 1970 and faster than the population growth in the 1980s and 1990s.
- Specialists outnumber generalists by nearly 2 to 1.

**TABLE 8.2**
Initiatives
Intended to
Affect the
Supply of U.S.
Physicians

**Initiatives to Increase Physician Supply**

| | |
|---|---|
| 1959 | Bane Report, U.S. Surgeon General |
| 1963 | Health Professions Educational Assistance Act |
| 1965 | Coggeshall Report, Association of American Medical Colleges |
| 1966 | Citizens Committee on Graduate Medical Education |
| 1967 | National Advisory Committee on Health Manpower |
| 1968 | Health Manpower Act |
| 1970 | Carnegie Committee on Health Education |
| 1970 | Emergency Health Personnel Act |
| 1972 | Creation of Uniformed Services University of the Health Sciences and the Armed Forces Professional Scholarship Program |
| 1972 | Veterans Administration authorized to help establish eight new medical schools |
| 1972 | Establishment of National Health Services Corps |

**Initiatives to Address Oversupply**

| | |
|---|---|
| 1981 | Omnibus Budget Reconciliation Act eliminates capitation grants for training physicians |
| 1981 | Report by Graduate Medical Education National Advisory Committee on physician oversupply |
| 1986 | Council on Graduate Medical Education (COGME) established |
| 1993 | Report by Physicians Payment Reform Commission on oversupply |
| 1994 | COGME report on oversupply |
| 1995 | COGME report on oversupply |
| 1996 | Institute of Medicine report on oversupply |

SOURCES: Tarlov 1995; Litman 1997, reproduced by permission; Ginzberg 1992.

- Managed care and other changes in the financing and delivery of health services are changing the role of the physician and will likely affect the physician supply and future employment.

## Issues Facing the U.S. Medical Profession

A series of interrelated issues have significant implications for how medicine will be practiced in the United States in coming years. These issues include:

- how GME should be supported;
- whether the number of GME training slots should be reduced;
- whether the number of IMGs participating in GME should be reduced;

- the effects of recent changes in the number of hours that residents may work;
- whether the ratio of specialists to generalists should be changed, and if so, how;
- whether physician reimbursement for outpatient care through Medicare is achieving its desired ends;
- the effects of reduced Medicare reimbursement on access to care for Medicare beneficiaries, as well as the effects on physician incomes; and
- the effects of managed care on the physician workforce.

## Support for GME

Given the increasing volume of Medicare expenditures and concerns about the projected bankruptcy of its hospital trust fund within the second decade of the century, the appropriateness of the considerable Medicare investment in GME will continue to be debated. The role of academic medical centers, teaching hospitals, and ambulatory care settings in providing GME must be a part of this discussion.

GME positions are concentrated in academic medical centers and major teaching hospitals, but the shift away from specialist to generalist medical training that began in the mid-1990s assumed that ambulatory care sites might also require support (Eisenberg 1994). The 1997 Balanced Budget Act (PL 105-33) provided GME support to train "qualified non-hospital providers" in approved medical residency training programs located in federally qualified health centers, rural health clinics, and other sites determined by the secretary of the U.S. Department of Health and Human Services (HHS) as appropriate training sites.

## The Number of GME Slots

The number of residencies and available slots for residents has traditionally been determined by the teaching institutions that train them. This structure created incentives for specialist training over generalist training, and for institutions to at least maintain—if not expand—the number of GME slots, regardless of the need for those specialists.

Recent studies of physician supply by the Institute of Medicine, the Council on Graduate Medical Education (COGME), the Physician Payment Reform Commission, and others suggest that a national body, perhaps modeled on the Defense Base Closure and Realignment Commission, be established to set a cap on the number of GME slots and determine how these slots are to be allocated across training programs.

The 1997 Balanced Budget Act places limits on the number of residents for which Medicare will reimburse hospitals. The total number of resident full-time equivalents (FTEs) in allopathic and osteopathic medicine may not exceed the total number of FTEs in the hospital during its most recent cost-reporting period ending on or before December 31, 1996. The limit does not apply to dentistry or podiatry residents.

## IMG Participation in GME

The participation of IMGs in GME has had a significant effect on physician supply and the generalist-to-specialist ratio. Between 1988 and 1993, the number of IMGs nearly doubled, and the number of IMG residents increased by more than 80 percent. IMGs constitute a substantial share of the total physician workforce, up from 10 percent in 1963 to 24 percent in 2004. IMGs specialize disproportionately when compared to USMGs and through the mid-1990s filled more than half of all nephrology slots and about 30 percent of all cardiology slots (Mullan, Politzer, and Davis 1995). By 2004, 30 percent of IMGs named anesthesiology as their specialty, and another 30 percent identified psychiatry as their primary care specialty. Because only about 25 percent of all IMGs return to their countries of origin, their numbers continued to swell the U.S. workforce until 1998 requirements that IMGs must pass a clinical skills assessment reduced the number of IMG applicants. The extent to which Medicare and other payers should continue to support the training and eventual practice of non-U.S. physicians who are not native or naturalized U.S. citizens, when many believe that the United States already has a physician oversupply, will continue to be debated.

Congressional concern about the extent to which Medicare subsidized GME led to a provision in the Balanced Budget Act that essentially caps Medicare's support of GME at 1997 levels. Academic health centers and other clinical settings that provide graduate (specialist) training to physicians may create and fill more training slots than Medicare's funds support, but they will need to find other funding sources to do so.

Changes in the supply of IMGs will directly affect U.S. physician supply. In 1998, the Educational Commission for Foreign Medical Graduates (ECFMG), the U.S. body that certifies IMGs for entrance into U.S. GME programs, instituted a requirement that IMGs must pass a clinical skills assessment (CSA) to achieve ECFMG certification. This requirement was imposed because of concerns that IMGs might be deficient in some clinical skill areas, such as history taking, physical exams, and communicating with patients in spoken English. Whelen et al. (2002) studied IMGs seeking certification from 1995 through 2001 and found that the number of IMGs taking the Step 1 exam decreased by 46 percent and the number of IMGs registered to take the Step 2 exam decreased by 38 percent. The number of ECFMG certificates issued annually dropped from a range of 9,000 to 12,000 for the years 1995 through 1998 to 6,000 for the years 1999 through 2001.

In the few years since their implementation, the CSA requirements appear to have influenced a decrease in the number of IMGs seeking certification to enter practice in the United States. At the same time, however, the number of U.S.-born IMGs has grown. Salsberg and Forte (2002) note that while the U.S. allopathic schools responded to public policy concerns about producing too many physicians, the growth in osteopathic medical school graduates and in IMGs was a counterforce to efforts made to limit the number of physicians produced in this country.

## Changes in Number of Hours Residents Can Work

Until 2003, the number of hours that a resident could be expected to be attending or on call was largely unregulated. The national spotlight on inpatient medical errors, some of which could be attributed to long hours of sleep-deprived service by residents, brought about work-hour restrictions mandated by the Accreditation Council for Graduate Medical Education (ACGME) in July 2003.

These changes were expected to result in quality-of-life improvements for the residents and quality-of-care improvements for the patients the residents serve. Fletcher et al. (2005) systematically reviewed the effects of the work-hour reduction on residents' lives but were challenged in interpreting the 54 chosen studies, largely because of suboptimal study design and the use of nonvalidated instruments. This topic merits more study and analysis.

## Specialists versus Generalists

Even those who are not persuaded of an oversupply of physicians generally agree that an imbalance exists between the number of specialists and generalists, or in physician distribution (Schwartz and Mendelson 1990; Cooper 1995). This imbalance contributes to rising health services expenditures. Even if health insurance coverage were universal, this imbalance would not, in the short term, likely aid in addressing equity-of-access issues. Even when medical schools alter their basic curricula to place greater emphasis on generalist training, appropriate generalist training in tertiary referral hospitals is not easily available, and the available GME slots do not reflect a growing emphasis on generalist training. Additionally, the best ways to utilize a valuable resource—highly trained subspecialists who may be in oversupply—in meeting the needs for more generalists has not yet been resolved.

## Physician Reimbursement

Outpatient care provided by specialists has typically been reimbursed at higher rates than care provided by primary care physicians. The resource-based relative value scale (RBRVS) implemented by Medicare in 1992 attempted to address these inequities and to better reimburse physician interviewing, physical examination, and counseling. Because of the way physician office overhead was calculated, however, the extent of intended adjustment may not occur (Ginzberg 1992; Schroeder and Sandy 1993).

Primary care physicians are likely to continue to push for greater fee equity for their Medicare patients who are not in capitated managed care systems.

Of immediate concern to physicians are the reduced Medicare payments specified on a phase-in basis by the 1997 Balanced Budget Act. How this payment reduction, the most recent of which was to be implemented in 2003, affects patient access is not yet fully known. Anecdotally, at least, Medicare patients in certain geographic areas report difficulty in accessing a physician. Speculation abounds that physicians may reduce the number of Medicare patients they treat and/or refuse to accept new Medicare patients.

### Effects of Managed Care on the Physician Workforce

Managed care, which in 2000 covered as much as 91 percent of the U.S. population that has employer-sponsored health insurance, 60 percent of Medicaid enrollees, and 17 percent of Medicare beneficiaries (see Chapter 19), has a number of implications for the physician workforce. Most types of managed care depend on primary care physicians as their first line of medical contact for subscribers and the control point for the use of specialists. Many types of managed care may also make substantial use of advanced nurse practitioners and physician assistants, thus potentially reducing their reliance on physicians. Managed care subscribers may have financial sanctions that discourage self-referral to specialists.

One potential consequence of these changes in the ways in which health services are being financed and delivered is the potential for some physicians, especially subspecialists, to have difficulty in maintaining the size of practice to which they are accustomed (Mullan, Politzer, and Davis 1995).

Weiner (1994) forecast the effects of health reform, including the growth of managed care, on physician workforce requirements and reported that the supply of specialists could outstrip their requirements by as much as 60 percent by the beginning of the twenty-first century. Other studies echo the view that the growth in managed care will result in a large and growing oversupply of specialists and subspecialists and will have major effects on medical education systems and teaching institutions that may result in decreasing financial support for medical education (Rivo, Mays, and Katzoff 1995).

The effect of managed care on the production of primary care (generalist) physicians over specialists appears to have been only modest and short-lived. Resident exit surveys conducted in New York, where 68 percent of practicing physicians are nonprimary care, and in California, which has a high level of managed care penetration, indicate that the marketplace demand for nonprimary care physicians exceeds the demand for primary care physicians (Salsberg and Forte 2002).

The spread of managed care magnifies the imbalances in the physician workforce, but it also presents opportunities (Rivo, Mays, and Katzoff 1995). One potential opportunity is the evolution of a new kind of specialist—the hospitalist—who focuses on the care of inpatients so that the primary care physician can focus on all other aspects of patient care (Wachter and Goldman 1996).

The hospitalist provides inpatient care in place of primary care physicians or academic attendings. Wachter and Goldman (2002) report that by 1999, 65 percent of internists had hospitalists in their community, and 28 percent reported using them for patient care. In certain geographic areas, such as California, the usage of hospitalists by community physicians is more than 60 percent. Pham et al. (2004) report eight thousand hospitalists nationally in 2004. In their review of the literature on hospitalists, Wachter and Goldman (2002) found that empirical research supports the premise that hospitalists improve inpatient efficiency without harmful effects on quality of patient satisfaction.

Hospitalists have grown as a profession for several reasons: (1) financial pressures from reimbursement rates that did not keep pace with rising costs helped spur physician support; (2) accelerating growth in health care costs prompted increasing interest in hospitalist use; (3) hospitalists may improve patient throughput in hospitals experiencing capacity constraints; (4) hospitalists have been attractive as a way for physicians to avoid inpatient care and emergency department calls and thus reduce exposure to malpractice; and (5) hospitalists have been used to assist in patient safety improvement (Pham et al. 2004).

This relatively new profession also faces some challenges, identified by Pham et al. (2004). First, education, training, and professional identity are a challenge due to the diversity of the sponsors, employers, and roles. Second, some organizations promoting quality and patient safety improvement did not explicitly anticipate the use of hospitalists as substitutes for board-certified intensivists. Third, the growing use of hospitalists could influence physician-hospital relationships.

## Physician Workforce Recommendations

The role of physicians, governmental support for medical education, and physician supply and distribution continue to be scrutinized as the U.S. health services system experiences change. A number of recommendations regarding the physician workforce are currently under consideration by the profession, payers, educators, and others. Table 8.3 summarizes recommendations that address physician education, generalist versus specialist training, supply, distribution, funding of hospital care for indigents, and new roles for physicians.

**TABLE 8.3**
Recommenda-
tions Regarding
Physicians in
the Workforce

### Physician Education

— Change the structure of medical education.
— Establish an all-payer pool to finance residencies.
— Sever the connection between care and residency training that exists in the current GME.
— Consider a system of vouchers where medical students can choose their residency sites.
— Increase minority representation in medicine.
— Train more physicians in ambulatory and managed care settings.
— Shift the amount and length of GME support currently provided by Medicare; rechannel it from teaching hospitals to academic medical centers.

### Generalist vs. Specialist Training

— Restructure the economic incentives under which physicians practice.
— Place a congressional limit on the total number of funded residencies.
— Establish a federal body to distribute GME slots by specialty.
— Use an accrediting body to select residency slots to be funded based on the quality of the educational program.
— To increase the number of generalists, create a way to pay for office-based teaching through the use of special billing codes or other mechanisms.
— Decrease the number of specialists trained.
— Modestly increase the number of generalists trained and improve the quality of primary care teaching.

### Supply

— Develop an early retirement program for physicians.
— Do not open any new medical schools and do not increase medical school class sizes.
— Change the funding of GME and reduce the number of slots to closer approximate the number of USMGs.

### Distribution

— Reallocate physicians to underserved regions of the country and the world.
— Expand the National Health Service Corps to alleviate the problems of student debt and medically underserved areas.

### Funding of Hospital Care for Indigents

— Provide transitional funding to teaching hospitals that have become dependent on Medicare GME funding.
— Assist state and local governments in developing mechanisms to replace funding for IMG-dependent hospitals that provide substantial amounts of care to the poor and disadvantaged.

### New Roles for Physicians

— Develop and promote new opportunities in medical outcomes research and quality management.
— Develop new programs of lifelong learning and retraining.

SOURCES: Council on Graduate Medical Education 1995; Eisenberg 1994; Ginzberg 1992; Lohr, Vanselow, and Detmer (eds.) 1996; Wennberg et al. 1993. Copyright © 1993. The People-to-People Health Foundation, Inc. All Rights Reserved. Adapted with permission.

## Other Types of Health Services Providers

Midlevel practitioners (such as physician assistants and nurse practitioners), nurses, pharmacists, and dentists are among other major health services providers. Categorized as nonphysician providers (NPPs) or nonphysician clinicians (NPCs) by some (Weiner 1994; Cooper 1995), each profession has a different relationship with organized medicine. The sections that follow describe these professions in terms of their origin and role in modern health services, the education and training required, provider supply and distribution, and current issues.

Complementary and alternative medicine (CAM) providers have become more visible and more accepted in the U.S. delivery system. A section on CAM providers follows the discussion of the more traditional health services professions.

Public health workers are also an important part of the health services workforce. An estimated 448,000 workers were in salaried public health positions in 2001, and 11 percent of those were public health nurses. Some public health workers—public health nurses in particular—provide direct services to clients. Many others are involved in maintaining a safe environment (e.g., clean water and air) and in administering a broad range of public health programs, including those related to bioterrorism. A major concern about the public health workforce is the lack of specific training in public health by a majority of those fulfilling public health functions (Gebbie and Merrill 2001).

Although a full review of additional health services providers is not possible, many of them fit under the umbrella term of "allied health" (USDHHS 1990):

- clinical laboratory personnel;
- physical and occupational therapists;
- radiologic technicians;
- workers in dietetics;
- medical records administrators;
- speech and language pathologists and audiologists;
- respiratory therapists;
- clinical psychologists; and
- medical social workers.

## Midlevel Practitioners

Two categories of health services providers—physician assistants and advanced practice nurses, which includes nurse practitioners and nurse midwives—are called midlevel practitioners, indicating that their functions and responsibilities are higher than those of entry-level caregivers but below those of physicians. Table 8.4 summarizes the required education, number of schools offering training, number of annual graduates, licensure and certification requirements, practice settings, and current supply of different health professions. Figure 8.2 shows the ratio of these professionals per 100,000 population.

### Physician Assistants

Physician assistants (PAs) emerged as a profession at the close of the Vietnam War, when members of the medical corps sought a way to use their training in the peacetime economy. Duke University is credited with establishing the first PA training program in the early 1960s. In 2004, 135 programs graduated PAs to work in hospitals, clinics, and physician practices (see Table 8.4).

**Physician Assistant Education and Training**

The majority of PA training programs are university-affiliated and require 20 to 36 months of didactic and clinical training. Most PA programs are affiliated with medical schools; the medical model of care, as opposed to the nursing or the social models, is therefore emphasized. PAs receive a certificate of program completion, and some may also receive baccalaureate or master's degrees if their programs are structured to offer them.

PAs function according to each state's Medical Practice Act. Each act specifies the degree of independence of practice permitted, including whether the PA must function in a side-by-side, over-the-shoulder, or at-a-distance relationship with the supervising physician. Forty-seven states and the District of Columbia permit limited prescribing powers for their PAs (Hocker and Berlin 2002). Payers vary in their recognition of PA independence. PAs are certified by a national board—the National Commission on Certification of Physician Assistants. Federal support of PA training comes through Title VII of the Public Health Service Act, which since 1972 has provided $135 million to educate PAs. The education funds are earmarked to prepare PAs for roles in primary care settings and utilization in medically underserved areas.

**Supply and Distribution of Physician Assistants**

As of 2003, 52,200 PAs were in practice in both urban and rural health services settings (Hocker and Berlin 2002). An estimated 33 percent practice in rural communities. Figure 8.3 shows the range of PA practice settings. Although white males dominated the profession in its early years, 54 percent of all PAs today are women (Hocker and Berlin 2002).

The PA role and function may evolve as a result of other changes occurring in the health services workforce. Managed care, with its emphasis on primary and generalist care, often makes greater use of PAs to enhance efficiency and cost-effectiveness. At least one study (Cooper 1995) projects the need for 50,000 additional PAs by the year 2010.

**TABLE 8.4** Health Professions Education, Supply, and Current Issues

| Category | Education Level | Number of Schools | Number of Annual Graduates | Licensure/ Certification | Practice Setting | Current Supply |
|---|---|---|---|---|---|---|
| *Physician* | 4 years medical school, 3–7 years residency | 125 allopathic 23 osteopathic | 17,736 (2005) | State licensure, 24 specialty boards for certification | 71% office-based, 20% hospital-based, 9% other | 736,211 active (2004), 23.7% female, 24% IMGs |
| *Physician assistant* | 20–36 months; May receive BA or BS or master's degree | 135 programs | 4,100 (2000) | National certification | 28% hospital-based, 26% group practice, 11% solo MD, 17% clinic, 16% other | 52,700 active (2005) |
| *Nurse* (2004), | Certified nursing assistant (CNA), LPN/LVN (12 months), RN | 1,484 programs | 76,618 RNs (2003) | State licensure | 67% hospital-based, 33% other | 2.3 million active including 58,500 nurse practitioners (2001) |
| *Dentist* | 3 years post-baccalaureate plus specialty | 58 schools | 4,443 (2003) | State licensure | 66% private or group practice | 196,000 (2003) |
| *Pharmacist* | 4–5 years post-baccalaureate plus post-baccalaureate training | 89 schools | 8,158 (2003–04) | State licensure | 66% commercial pharmacy, 20% hospital pharmacy, 14% other | 170,000 (2003) |

SOURCE: USDHHS 2005.

FIGURE 8.2
Active Health
Services
Personnel
per 100,000
Population
(2003)

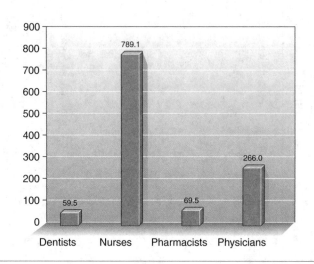

SOURCE: USDHHS 2005.

FIGURE 8.3
Physician
Assistant
Practice
Settings
(2000)

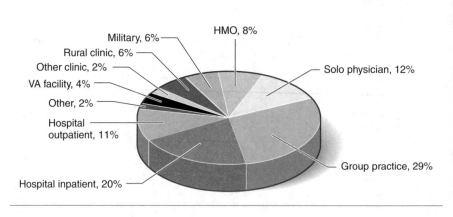

SOURCE: USDHHS 2002.

Much of the early stimulus for the development of PA programs was to create a type of health services provider who could fill the gap left by too few primary care physicians. Although 45 percent of PAs practice in generalist areas, 55 percent are associated with specialist practices (USDHHS/ HRSA 1994; Hocker and Berlin 2002). Even though studies indicate that PAs can effectively handle about 80 percent of the patient problems in an ambulatory care setting, the PA profession is structured to work in close association with a physician (Jones and Cawley 1994; U.S. General Accounting Office [now known as U.S. Government Accountability Office—

USGAO] 1994). The PA profession thus faces issues of professional terri-
torialism, including licensure restrictions.

## Advanced Practice Nurses

Two types of advanced practice nurses (APNs)—nurse midwives and nurse
practitioners (NPs)—have been health services providers since the early
1970s. In states that permit them to practice, nurse midwives provide prenatal care, labor and delivery services, and postpartum care for the mother
and infant. Nurse midwife training programs are usually based in nursing
schools. An estimated five thousand nurse midwives were in active practice
in hospitals, clinics, and other health services settings as of 2002 (Brigham
and Women's Hospital 2002)

The nurse practitioner profession developed not only to address the
perceived shortages of primary care physicians but also in recognition that
nurses could function clinically well above their customary levels. With additional training, nurses could handle an estimated 50 to 90 percent of the patient
encounters in an ambulatory care setting (Schroeder 1994; USGAO 1994).

Some of the early programs trained pediatric nurse practitioners. Programs were also developed to train family nurse practitioners, geriatric health
practitioners, and nurse practitioners that specialize in women's health services. APNs function according to each state's Nurse Practice Act, which
specifies the degree of independence of practice permitted. Medicare does
not directly reimburse APNs, and other payers vary in their recognition of
APN practice independence.

**Education and Training of Nurse Practitioners**

Nurse practitioners are registered nurses who receive advanced training,
usually in schools of nursing affiliated with universities. Their training thus
emphasizes the nursing model of care. NPs may receive a baccalaureate or
master's degree as part of their training program. NPs function under the
auspices of a state's Nurse Practice Act, but they work under the supervision of a physician rather than another nurse. Like PAs, NPs may have a
relationship with a physician that is side-by-side, over-the-shoulder, or at-
a-distance.

**Supply and Distribution of Advanced Practice Nurses**

More than 58,500 NPs were practicing in the United States in 2001 (Hocker
and Berlin 2002). Cooper (1995) projected that the number of APNs would
increase to 102,000 by the year 2010. Just as the majority of nurses are
female, so are the majority (96 percent) of NPs.

Several key issues relate to the future role and function of APNs.
Aiken and Salmon (1994) note the need for national standards for APNs.
Such standards would permit greater uniformity of function, perhaps over-
coming the vagaries of individual state Nurse Practice Acts. How APNs

would interface with a hoped-for increase in the number of generalist physicians and a potential increase in the number of PAs also must be considered. The issue of direct reimbursement to APNs, long a contentious one, will continue to be raised until it is resolved.

## Nurses

Nurses constitute the largest group of health services providers, with more than 2.3 million active nurses in the workforce in 2004. Modern nursing traces its origins to Florence Nightingale, whose emphasis on hygiene is credited with reducing the death rate in British hospitals from 40 to 2 percent during the Crimean War of 1853 to 1856 (Starr 1982). Nurse training schools were established in New York City, New Haven, and Boston in 1873, fostered by upper-class women who were committed to improving institutions such as public hospitals and almshouses (Starr 1982). Although nurses have a degree of professional independence, as evidenced by visiting nurses' associations, they usually function as members of a team under the direction of a physician or an APN.

Two-thirds of nurses are hospital employees, but the market for nurses in outpatient settings is growing rapidly (see Figure 8.4). Between 1988 and 1992, employment of nurses in hospital outpatient settings increased 68 percent, and employment in public health and community settings increased 62 percent, whereas nurse employment in hospital inpatient settings grew less than 6 percent (Aiken and Gwyther 1995).

Alternate work settings, such as home health care, school-based health, and workplace health centers, continue to attract nurses away from the intensity of inpatient hospital and nursing-home work, where the acuity of the patient load continues to increase.

**FIGURE 8.4**
Nurse Practice
Settings (2000)

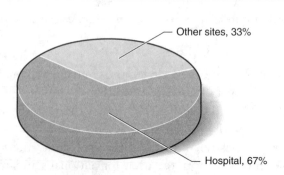

Other sites, 33%

Hospital, 67%

SOURCE: USDHHS 2002.

## Nurse Education and Training

Five levels of nursing preparation exist, although hierarchical progression through them is not a customary career path. In addition, nurses may obtain advanced degrees, including Ph.D.s in nursing and Doctor of Nursing (ND).

The entry level is the certified nurse assistant (CNA), whose training may consist of institution-specific, on-the-job training. No licensure is associated with this level of nursing, though a certificate of completion may be awarded. The licensed practical nurse (LPN) or licensed vocational nurse (LVN) is the next level of nursing and requires an average 12 months of formalized training, often in a community college technical or vocational program. State licensure is required for the LPN/LVN. The third level of nursing preparation, and what is generally considered the first level of professional training, is that of the registered nurse (RN). RNs may achieve their education and training in one of three ways:

1. hospital diploma programs, the original method of training, which requires an average of three years of training (145 hospital diploma programs exist in the United States, training about 8 percent of the nursing workforce [Aiken and Salmon 1994; Aiken and Gwyther 1995]);
2. associate degree programs (AA or AS) offered by community colleges, the source of 65 percent of RNs (Aiken and Salmon 1994); and
3. college and university baccalaureate programs.

RNs must be licensed by the state to practice.

The fourth level of practice is the advanced practice nurse (a nurse midwife or a nurse practitioner), described earlier. The fifth level of nursing is the clinical specialist, whose preparation requires a master's degree.

Federal support for nursing education began in 1964 with passage of the Nurse Training Act, which was renewed in subsequent congressional sessions until 1981, when capitation grants for nursing and other health professions were eliminated by the Omnibus Budget Reconciliation Act (OBRA) of 1981. Preprofessional nursing education support from the federal government is available through Medicare direct GME funds, 15 percent of which is targeted for hospitals to use to train nurses and other paramedical personnel. Two-thirds of Medicare funds earmarked for nursing education have gone to the 145 hospitals operating diploma programs. The only types of graduate nursing education that receive Medicare funds are the 86 nurse anesthetist programs (Council on Accreditation of Nurse Anesthesia Programs 2003).

## Supply and Distribution of Nurses

The total active workforce of nurses numbered more than 2.3 million, or 82 percent of the licensed profession, in 2004 (U.S. Department of

Labor 2004). About 50,000 nurses were trained in each year between 1980 and 1990 (Aiken and Gwyther 1995) in 1,484 programs. Despite the high number of nurses and the nurse-to-population ratio of 789 to 100,000, nurse shortages are experienced periodically.

In many parts of the United States, a nursing shortage is evident. Hospitals may have to hire contract nurses, often at salaries twice that of their regular nurses, in order to staff units and keep them open. This strategy can create discontinuities in care and also elevate the stresses and tensions inherent in the work situation, which may be exacerbated by salary differentials. The duration of the current nursing shortage is not known. Analyses of the nursing workforce and of the declines in enrollment in nursing programs, however, do not promise prompt solutions. Buerhaus and Staiger (2000) report on the implications of an aging registered nurse workforce, noting that the average age of RNs is forecast to be 45.5 years within the next 10 years, with more than 40 percent of the workforce expected to be older than 50 years. In March 2004, the average age of the working registered nurse was 43.3 years (American Association of Colleges of Nursing [AACN] 2004). By 2020, the RN workforce is projected to be about the same size as it was in 2000, which will be nearly 20 percent below the projected RN workforce requirements. Bednash (2000) points out that enrollments in nursing programs decreased for the five-year period 1995 through 1999 and calls for nursing education reform, restructuring work environments, and developing systems of care that allow RNs to fully use their professional skills. According to the National Council of the State Boards of Nursing, the number of first-time, U.S.-educated nursing school graduates who sat for the NCLEX-RN, the national licensure exam for registered nurses, decreased by 20 percent from 1995 to 2003 (AACN 2004). The percentage of registered nurses who are not working in nursing rose from 17.3 percent in 1992 to 18.3 percent in 2000 (Sochalski 2002).

Prior to 2002, the two most recent nursing shortages occurred in 1979 and from 1986 to 1988. Both shortages were due less to a truly limited supply than to the flattening of nursing wages, due in part to an influx of nurses into the labor pool (Newschaffer and Schoenman 1990). Delayed market responses seem largely responsible for recent nursing shortages, and the market corrects itself when nursing salaries increase (Newschaffer and Schoenman 1990; Reinhardt 1994). In contrast to the potential for salary growth in other health professions, over the span of a professional career, a nurse could anticipate a salary increase of only 36 percent through the 1980s (Delevan and Koff 1990). Since 1992, according to a recent study, nursing wages on average have done no better than keep pace with inflation in the general economy (Sochalski 2002).

Many analysts believe that the emphasis of nurse education and training should be redirected (Ward and Berkowitz 2002; Aiken and Gwyther 1995; USDHHS 1990). Sixty percent of all nurses are prepared at less than a baccalaureate level (USDHHS/Bureau of Health Professions 1996), but ongoing changes in the health services system continue to require nurses with a minimum preparation of a baccalaureate degree.

One way that the United States has periodically dealt with its nurse shortages is to import them from other countries, often from developing countries such as the Philippines, India, or some African nations. Although this importation may benefit the individual nurse and the U.S. delivery system, it often leaves the country of origin with a nursing deficit. The United Kingdom has also used the importation solution, but agreed in 2001 to stop directly recruiting nurses from countries with nursing shortages (Chaguturu and Vallabhaneni 2005). Such promises to desist from these recruitments do not apply to large private institutions, and the health systems in developing countries are beginning to speak out about the negative effects to their systems from these recruitments.

## *Issues Facing the Nursing Profession*

As the largest group of health services providers, nurses have many issues facing their profession. Maintaining the appropriate supply of nurses will continue to be a challenge, and nursing salaries may fluctuate with their supply. The downsizing of hospitals, as well as continuous changes in the delivery system, will affect nursing supply, although the full range of effects is not yet known.

Functioning to the limit of their licensure is another challenge for nurses. Studies have shown that medical residents perform many functions that do not require their level of training and skill (Schroeder 1994); studies have also noted that nearly 75 percent of the functions that registered nurses routinely perform do not require actual nursing skills and training (Aiken and Salmon 1994).

An effective career ladder that creates a logical progression from CNA to clinical specialist has long been sought in nursing but is not universally available.

Future roles for nurses are currently unclear. New functions or possible areas of focus include the potential for nurses to contribute to the restructuring of the hospital, enhance the viability of the academic medical center, provide more care to the underserved, and identify new roles for public health nursing (Aiken and Salmon 1994).

# Pharmacists

In its developmental stages, pharmacy was closely allied with medicine. Early pharmacies, especially in small frontier towns, were frequently owned and operated by the town's physician; conversely, nonphysician druggists often acquired medical practice as a part of their role. Distinction between the two fields began emerging in the late nineteenth century, aided in part by differing views on the efficacy of some medications, particularly some proprietary drugs popularly known as patent medicines.

Organized medicine stimulated broad-scale informational campaigns against many nostrums, focusing on their opium and alcohol content as well as on specious claims of cure. The AMA established a Council on Pharmacy and Chemistry in 1905 to set standards for drugs and drug evaluation, and physicians began controlling access to drugs for their patients through the practice of prescribing. As a consequence, drug companies began to seek earlier physician involvement in the development of new products (Starr 1982).

### Pharmacist Education and Training

Eighty-nine schools of pharmacy, all affiliated with an institution of higher learning, provide two entry-level pharmacy degrees—the five-year baccalaureate degree or the six-year Doctor of Pharmacy (PharmD) degree—either of which qualifies the individual to take the licensure examination (USDHHS 1990). Individuals with baccalaureate degrees in pharmacy may earn a PharmD as a graduate-level degree. Accrediting bodies appear to be emphasizing the PharmD over the baccalaureate degree.

Early federal health services workforce legislation, such as the 1960 Health Manpower Act and the 1971 Comprehensive Health Manpower Training Act, included funds for institutional grants to schools of pharmacy. These funds provided for scholarships, loans, construction, and faculty resources to increase the supply of pharmacists.

### Supply and Distribution of Pharmacists

In 2003, 196,000 pharmacists were in active practice in the United States (USDHHS 2005), and 46 percent of them were women (Cooksey et al. 2002). Enrollments in pharmacy schools peaked in 1974 to 1975, sharply declined in the early 1980s, and currently remain below the mid-1970s high. About eight thousand students graduate from pharmacy schools each year.

Although the growing population of elders, who use a higher number of prescription drugs than other age groups (and have the potential for greater outpatient prescription drug coverage as a result of the 2003 Medicare Prescription Drug Improvement and Modernization Act [MMA]), could indicate a need for more pharmacists, one workforce commission recommended a reduction of 20 to 30 percent in the number of pharmacists (Pew Memorial Trust 1995). The role of the pharmacist is also changing with the use of new information, communication, and robotics technologies (USDHHS 1990).

Pharmacists are geographically disbursed but are dependent on the availability of physicians to generate the prescriptions they fill. Figure 8.5

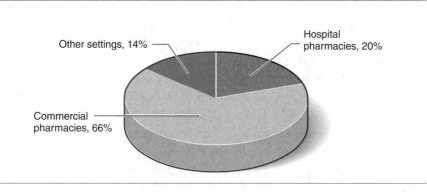

**FIGURE 8.5**

Pharmacist Practice Settings (2000)

SOURCE: USDHHS 2002.

shows the practice settings of pharmacists, with two-thirds employed in independent or chain pharmacies.

## Issues Facing the Pharmacy Profession

New communication, information, and other technologies have the potential for decreasing the demand for pharmacists. Another force that may affect the demand for pharmacists is the growing market share of mail-order pharmacies. Maintenance drugs for conditions such as ulcers or high cholesterol are particularly well suited to mail ordering, which generally specifies a 14-day turnaround time, although the turnaround may be much shorter. Mail-order pharmacies compete by making volume purchases of drugs, sometimes at deep discounts, and by issuing longer-term supplies of the prescription, which results in fewer dispensing fees. Additionally, mail-order pharmacies aggressively pursue the rewriting of prescriptions, seeking the physician's permission to substitute a drug that is less expensive than the one prescribed or, as critics point out, a drug that is more readily available to the mail-order pharmacy (Barton, Bondy, and Glazner 1993).

An increasing number of people in the United States are obtaining prescription drugs from Internet pharmacies, which began online service early in 1999. By July 1999, an estimated two hundred to four hundred businesses were selling prescription drugs online. In that first year, ten million Americans used the Internet to shop for health products, spending an estimated $160 million on prescription drugs. A GAO study (2000) reported that in 1999, 111 online pharmacies required a physician's prescription, 54 would provide a prescription if the consumer completed an online questionnaire, and 25 did not require a prescription. Purchase of prescription drugs over the Internet avoids the regulation of the pharmacy profession and the dispensing of drugs that traditionally occurs at the state level of government.

The GAO updated its study of Internet pharmacies in 2004 (USGAO 2004). Three types of Internet pharmacies sell prescription drugs directly to consumers. The first type operates much like a traditional drugstore, selling a wide range of drugs and requiring consumers to submit a prescription from their physician before their orders are filled. A second type of Internet pharmacy specializes in certain lifestyle medications, such as those that treat weight control or sexual dysfunction. The third type of Internet pharmacy dispenses drugs without a prescription.

The authors of the GAO study targeted 13 drugs, including drugs with safety restrictions or handling requirements; drugs that had, in the past, been counterfeited; and narcotics. They attempted to purchase these drugs from U.S., Canadian, and other international Internet pharmacies without a physician's prescription, and they produced their own prescriptions to enable their purchases. They were able to obtain the majority of the prescription drugs they targeted from a wide variety of domestic and foreign pharmacies without providing a physician's prescription. The GAO identified several problems with the handling, FDA-approval status, and authenticity of the 21 drug samples received from other foreign Internet pharmacies but fewer problems from samples provided by U.S. and Canadian pharmacies. This study pointed not only to issues of consumer safety but also suggests the potential changing role of pharmacists if more consumers seek their prescriptions from Internet providers.

New roles for pharmacists include their increased management of complex drug therapies and an expanded function in patient education about drugs and potential drug interactions.

## Dentists

Dentistry emerged as a profession as technological advances permitted the retention of diseased teeth, the prevention of dental decay, and the ability to correct dental malformations. Unlike the previously discussed categories of health services providers, dentistry has never had a dependent relationship with medicine, and dentists do not function under the authority of a physician. Figure 8.6 shows the practice settings of dentists, with most in solo or group private practice.

### Dental Education and Training

About 170,000 dentists are active in the U.S. health services workforce today (USDHHS 2005). About 8 percent of all dentists are female, and 3 percent are African American. Fifty-five dental schools, most in affiliation with a college or university, graduate about 4,400 dentists each year. Basic dental training generally requires four years of study, but about 16 percent

FIGURE 8.6
Dentist Practice
Settings (2000)

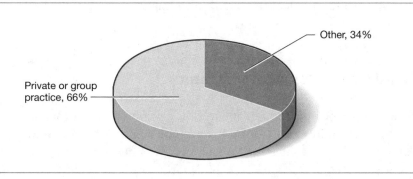

Other, 34%

Private or group
practice, 66%

SOURCE: USDHHS 2002.

of dentists specialize in one of the following recognized specialties: ortho-
dontics, oral and maxillofacial surgery, periodontics, pedodontics, endodon-
tics, and prosthodontics (USDHHS 2002).

Dentists also benefited from federal support of their education through
the 1960 Health Professions Education Assistance Act and its subsequent
amendments and the 1971 Comprehensive Health Manpower Training Act,
which provided funds for scholarships, loans, construction, and faculty support to increase the supply of dentists.

### Supply and Distribution of Dentists

Dentists have so effectively dealt with dental health problems that dental
decay in insured children has dropped dramatically, affecting the demand
for this type of dental care. Given the changes in dental disease patterns,
the increased requirements for dental infection control as a result of the
acquired immune deficiency syndrome (AIDS), and technologic advances
that permit the individual to retain teeth for a lifetime, the role of the dentist is shifting to meet these new needs (USDHHS 1990). Dental implants
are also aiding the retention of teeth. Without an expansion of dental insurance coverage for a greater proportion of the population, the need for additional dentists remains unclear.

Because dentists function autonomously, their distribution is less constrained than that of health services providers who are dependent on associations with physicians. Dentists are, however, dependent on the availability
of hygienists and technicians to support an effective practice.

### Issues Facing the Dental Profession

A major issue facing the dental profession is its role in managed care. Ensuring that basic and comprehensive dental care is part of the benefits package for both indemnity insurance and various managed care programs is

essential in allowing dentists to remain an important part of the health services team.

## Health Services Administrators

Maintaining the operation of an increasingly complex health services delivery system requires an administrative complement to the provision of care.
Administration was once the domain of a provider, whose principal training was as a clinician; today's administrators must be highly trained busi-
nesspeople and managers.

### Education and Training

Executives in the U.S. health services system generally have graduate-level
training that they earn in one of three ways: by earning a master's degree
in a field such as hospital administration, by entering administration from
a clinical profession such as medicine or nursing, or by assuming administrative responsibilities after completing education programs in general business, law, accounting, or a related field. Administrators are responsible for
a range of functions, including:

- strategic planning and marketing;
- accounting and financial management;
- clinical and management information;
- human resources (recruiting, training, benefits, and compensation); and
- maintaining the physical plant.

### Supply and Distribution of Health Services Administrators

Determining the supply of health services administrators depends on the
organizational levels included in the count. One source (Griffith 1995)
estimates the total executive pool to be about 60,000. The leading professional organization, the American College of Healthcare Executives
(ACHE), has a current membership of about 30,300 (ACHE 2003). Growth
areas in the field include mergers and acquisitions, contracting, rate setting, and marketing.

### Issues Facing Health Services Administrators

The volatility of the U.S. health services delivery system requires an executive workforce that demonstrates leadership and flexibility. Administrators
must be prepared to address the prospect of new owners or employers as a
result of mergers and acquisitions. Reengineering and downsizing of facilities, the reconfiguration of facilities into new systems, and new links with
other providers require the commitment of significant administrative

resources. Maintaining currency with new technologies, including procedures and drugs, is essential to the provision of cutting-edge care. Retaining and expanding market share—major administrative functions—are crucial to an institution's survival.

## Complementary and Alternative Medicine (CAM) Providers

Complementary and alternative medicine (CAM) providers in actuality represent some of the earliest practitioners of the healing arts. Included under this CAM umbrella are acupuncturists, chiropractors, homeopaths, naturopaths, and those who practice traditional Chinese medicine, relaxation, biofeedback, hypnotherapy, prayer and spiritual applications, and other therapies. "Complementary" means in addition to, and "alternative" means in place of Western medicine. A recent topic of discussion and debate is the extent to which CAM and Western medicine may become integrated.

CAM practitioners have always been a part of the U.S. health services delivery system, but until the last decade or so, they were frequently not only unacknowledged but often nearly an underground element of the system. Demand for CAM services has made their roles more visible. One result was official CAM recognition by the establishment in 1992 within the National Institutes of Health (NIH) of the Office of Alternative Medicine, which became the National Center for Complementary and Alternative Medicine in 1999.

Data on CAM are still somewhat sparse. Giordano et al. (2002) identify some of the barriers to CAM research, including lack of funding, lack of research skills, lack of an academic infrastructure, insufficient patient numbers (or, more likely, lack of insurance claims data to reveal such numbers), difficulty in undertaking and interpreting systematic reviews, and even lack of motivation because these health-promoting therapies cannot be patented and, therefore, are not commercially profitable.

Periodic surveys of CAM providers by the National Center for Health Statistics (NCHS) (within the Centers for Disease Control and Prevention [CDC]) offer some insight into CAM utilization. A 2002 survey, reported in 2004, indicates that CAM usage is associated with gender (more women use CAM), education levels (those with higher levels of education are more frequent CAM users), and place of residence (those who live along the West Coast are greater utilizers than those who live in the eastern United States (Barnes et al. 2004). The most recent year for which expenditure data are available is 1997; in that year, U.S. citizens spent between $36 and $47 billion on CAM providers, of which between $12.2 and $19.6 billion was paid out-of-pocket. Table 8.5 provides other highlights about CAM from the 2002 survey.

TABLE 8.5
Frequencies and Age-Adjusted Percentages of Adults Age 18 and Older Who Used Complementary and Alternative Medicine (CAM) Providers, by Type of Therapy, United States (2002)

| | Ever Used (in Thousands) | Used in Past 12 Months (in Thousands) |
|---|---|---|
| *Any CAM Use* | 149,271 | 123,606 |
| *Alternative Medical Systems* | | |
| Acupuncture | 8,188 | 2,136 |
| Homeopathic treatment | 7,379 | 3,433 |
| Naturopathy | 1,795 | 498 |
| *Biologically Based Therapies* | | |
| Chelation therapy | 270 | 66 |
| Folk medicine | 1,393 | 233 |
| Diet-based therapies | 13,799 | 7,099 |
| *Manipulative and Body-Based Therapies* | | |
| Chiropractic care | 40,242 | 15,226 |
| Massage | 18,899 | 10,052 |
| *Mind-Body Therapies* | | |
| Biofeedback | 1,986 | 278 |
| Meditation | 20,698 | 15,336 |
| Deep-breathing exercises | 29,658 | 23,457 |
| Yoga | 15,232 | 10,386 |
| Prayer for health reasons | 110,012 | 89,624 |

SOURCE: Barnes et al. 2004.

## Summary

The provision of the standard of health services expected by most people in the United States is labor intensive. Health services providers constitute about 70 percent of the operational expense of any major provider organization (O'Neil and Riley 1996). Changes in the organization and financing of health services are directly affecting the roles and functions of various health services providers. Roles are changing as business leaders and payers exert greater influence on the system. Decisions about referrals, medications, or therapies that once were the sole purview of the physician are now being influenced in subtle—and not so subtle—ways by others in the system. Providers are being pushed to function to the highest level of licensure (O'Neil and Riley 1996). For nurses, for example, this means reconsidering responsibilities and possibly eliminating more than half of their current tasks, which studies have shown could be performed by others with less training (Aiken and Salmon 1994).

## Changes in Roles and Functions

Changes in roles and functions stimulate a reconsideration of professional turf, practice acts, licensure requirements, and the role of oversight boards. Changes of these magnitudes raise tensions about job security and job satisfaction, contributing to a general sense of uncertainty about where the health services system is heading.

## Changes in Provider Demographics

The demographics of health services providers are changing, too. More women physicians in the workforce, who work fewer hours than their male counterparts during childbearing years, are stimulating new discussions about the quality of a physician's life. More women are becoming PAs. The dominant gender in nursing is female, with many entering the profession at later ages, contributing to an older workforce. In all health services provider professions, members of racial and ethnic minority groups are still seriously underrepresented, although their presence in the workforce is slowly increasing.

## Supply and Distribution

One of the most pervasive and controversial issues surrounding the ongoing changes in the organization and financing of the U.S. health services system is the supply and distribution of the health services workforce. During the 1970s and 1980s, growth in the medical, nursing, pharmacy, and dental fields outpaced population growth (USDHHS 1990). Several decades of efforts by the government, educators, and others to influence the supply and distribution of the workforce in response to perceived shortages or surpluses provide evidence of how difficult this issue is to resolve.

A number of variables affect health services provider supply, including population demographics, technologic advances, decisions about total health services expenditures, the proportion of the population without regular access to care, provider income expectations, constraints on the autonomy of practice, and the influence of managed care.

Governmental efforts to correct the market by offering scholarships, loan forgiveness, or other incentives to providers who will practice in medically underserved areas (MUAs) or in health professional shortage areas (HPSAs), or who will train for disciplines deemed in short supply, have met with mixed success, at best.

## Governmental Involvement in Health Professions Training

The extent of governmental involvement in the preparation of the health services workforce is indeed open to question (Reinhardt 1994). Since the early 1960s, the federal government has supported the training of physicians, general dentists, physician assistants, and allied health providers under Title VII of the Public Health Service Act, and of nurses, nurse practitioners, and nurse midwives under Title VIII of the act (USGAO 1994). Challenges to the appropriateness of this support resulted in termination of capitated educational grants in the early 1980s. Health professionals still continue, however, to receive more federal support than do most other professionals.

## Note

1. Specialists may be self-declared or may be certified by a board of specialty practice. Of all practicing physicians who have completed residency training, 79 percent are board certified (Grumbach, Becker, and Osborn 1995).

## Key Words

advanced practice nurse (APN)

allied health provider

allopathic physician

American Medical Association (AMA)

Balanced Budget Act of 1997

board certification

capitation grants

complementary and alternative
    medicine (CAM) provider

Council on Graduate Medical
    Education (COGME)

Educational Commission for Foreign
    Medical Graduate (ECFMG)

Flexner Report

foreign medical graduate (FMG)

graduate medical education (GME)

health professional shortage area
    (HPSA)

hospital diploma nursing program

hospitalist

international medical graduate (IMG)

Internet pharmacy

mail-order pharmacy

medically underserved area (MUA)

Medical Practice Act

midlevel practitioner

National Health Interview Survey
    (NHIS)

National Health Service Corps (NHSC)

nonphysician clinician (NPC)

nonphysician provider (NPP)

nurse midwife

Nurse Practice Act

nurse practitioner

omnibus budget reconciliation act
    (OBRA)

osteopathic physician

patent medications

physician assistant (PA)

physician-induced demand

professional certification

resource-based relative value scale
    (RBRVS)

U.S. medical graduate (USMG)

# References

Aiken, L. H., and M. E. Gwyther. 1995. "Medicare Funding of Education." *Journal of the American Medical Association* 273 (19): 1528–32.

Aiken, L. H., and M. E. Salmon. 1994. "Health Care Workforce Priorities: What Nursing Should Do Now." *Inquiry* 31 (3): 318–29.

Alliance for Human Reform. 1994. *The Doctor Track*. Washington, DC: AHR.

American Association of Colleges of Nursing. 2004. "Nursing Shortage Fact Sheet." [Online information; retrieved 1/3/2006.] www.aacn.nche.edu/Media/Backgrounders/shortagefacts.htm.

American College of Healthcare Executives. 2003. "February Fact Sheet." Chicago: ACHE.

American Medical Association. 2004. "International Medical Graduates: IMGS in the U.S." [Online information; retrieved 1/3/06.] www.ama-assn.org/ama/pub/category/211.html.

American Osteopathic Association. 2002. "College of Osteopathic Medicine." [Online information; retrieved 8/26/02.] www.aoa-net.org/students/colleges.htm.

Barnes, P. M., E. Powell-Griner, K. McFann, and R. L. Nahin. 2004. "Complementary and Alternative Medicine Use among Adults, United States, 2002." *Advance Data from Vital and Health Statistics, No. 343*. Hyattsville, MD: Centers for Disease Control and Prevention (National Center for Health Statistics).

Barton, P. L., J. Bondy, and J. Glazner. 1993. *Colorado Medicaid Reform Study*. Denver: University of Colorado Health Sciences Center.

Bednash, G. 2000. "The Decreasing Supply of Registered Nurses: Inevitable Future or Call to Action?" *Journal of American Medical Association* 283 (22): 2985–87.

Blewett, L. A., and V. Weslowski. 2000. "New Roles for States in Financing Graduate Medical Education: Minnesota's Trust Fund." *Health Affairs* 19 (1): 248–52.

Brigham and Women's Hospital. 2002. "Facts about Nurse Midwives." [Online information; retrieved 1/3/2006.] http://brighamandwomens.org/midwifery/Patient/facts.asp.

Brook, R. H. 1991. "Health, Health Insurance, and the Uninsured." *Journal of the American Medical Association* 265 (22): 2998–3002.

Buerhaus, P. I., and D. O. Staiger. 2000. "Implications of an Aging Registered Nurse Workforce." *Journal of the American Medical Association* 283 (22): 2948–54.

Chaguturu, S., and S. Vallabhaneni. 2005. "Aiding and Abetting—Nursing Crises at Home and Abroad." *New England Journal of Medicine* 353 (17): 1761–63.

Cooksey, J. A., K. K. Knapp, S. M. Walton, and J. M. Cultice. 2002. "Challenges to the Pharmacist Profession from Escalating Pharmaceutical Demand." *Health Affairs* 21 (5): 182–88.

Cooper, R. A. 1995. "Perspectives on the Physician Workforce to the Year 2020." *Journal of the American Medical Association* 274 (19): 1534–43.

Cooper, R. A., and S. J. Stoflet. 1996. "Trends in the Education and Practice of Alternative Medicine Clinicians." *Health Affairs* 15 (3): 226–38.

Council on Accreditation of Nurse Anesthesia Programs. 2003. "Accredited Nurse Anesthesia Programs." [Online information; retrieved 3/27/03.] www.aana.com/coa/accreditedprograms.asp.

Council on Graduate Medical Education. 1995. *7th Report-COGME 1995 Physician Workforce Funding Recommendations for DHHS Programs.* Rockville, MD: COGME.

Delevan, S. M., and S. Z. Koff. 1990. "The Nursing Shortage and Provider Attitudes: A Political Perspective." *Journal of Health Politics, Policy and Law* 11 (1): 62–80.

Eisenberg, J. M. 1994. "If Trickle-Down Physician Workforce Policy Fails, Is the Choice Now Between the Market and Government Regulation?" *Inquiry* 31 (3): 241–49.

Fletcher, K. E., W. Underwood, S. Q. Davis, R. S. Mangrulkar, L. F. McMahon, and S. Saint. 2005. "Effects of Work Hour Reduction on Residents' Lives: A Systematic Review." *Journal of the American Medical Association* 294 (9): 1088–1100.

Gebbie, K. M., and R. Merrill. 2001. "Enumerations of the Public Health Workforce: Developing a System." *Journal of Public Health Management and Practice* 9 (60): 440–42.

Ginzberg, E. 1992. "Physician Supply Policies and Health Reform." *Journal of the American Medical Association* 268 (21): 3115–18.

Giordano, J., D. Boatwright, S. Stapelton, and L. Huff. 2002. "Blending the Boundaries: Steps Toward an Integration of Complementary and Alternative Medicine into Mainstream Practice. *Journal of Alternative and Complementary Medicine* 8 (6): 897–906.

Ginzberg, E. 1992. "Physician Supply Policies and Health Reform." *Journal of the American Medical Association* 268 (21): 3115–18.

Griffith, J. R. 1995. *The Well-Managed Health Care Organization.* Chicago: Health Administration Press.

Grumbach, K., S. H. Becker, and E. H. S. Osborn. 1995. "The Challenge of Defining and Counting Generalist Physicians: An Analysis of Physician Masterfile Data." *American Journal of Public Health* 85 (10): 1402–07.

Health Insurance Association of America. 1996. *Source Book of Health Insurance Data.* Washington, DC: HIAA.

Henderson, T. M. 2000. Medicaid's Role in Financing Graduate Medical Education. *Health Affairs* 19 (1): 221–29.

Hocker, R. S., and L. E. Berlin. 2002. "Trends in the Supply of Physician Assistants and Nurse Practitioners in the United States." *Health Affairs* 21 (5): 174–81.

Jones, P. E., and J. F. Cawley. 1994. "Physician's Assistants and Health System Reform." *Journal of the American Medical Association* 271 (16): 1266–72.

Litman, T. J. 1997. *Health Politics and Policy,* 3d ed. New York: Delmar.

Lohr, K. N., N. A. Vanselow, and D. E. Detmer (eds.). 1996. *The Nation's Physician Workforce: Options for Balancing Supply and Requirements. Summary.* Washington, DC: National Academy Press.

Ludmerer, K. M. 1985. *Learning to Heal—the Development of American Medical Education.* New York: Basic Books

Mullan, F., R. M. Politzer, and C. H. Davis. 1995. "Medical Migration and the Physician Workforce: International Medical Graduates and American Medicine." *Journal of the American Medical Association* 273 (19): 1521–27.

National Health Policy Forum (NHPF). 2002. "Too Few? Too Many? The Right Kind? Physician Supply in an Aging and Multicultural Society." Washington, DC: NHPF meeting announcement. September 10.

Newschaffer, C. J., and J. A. Schoenman. 1990. "Registered Nurse Shortages: The Road to Appropriate Public Policy." *Health Affairs* 9 (1): 98–106.

O'Neil, E., and T. Riley. 1996. "Health Workforce and Education Issues During System Transition." *Health Affairs* 15 (1): 105–12.

Pew Memorial Trust. 1995. *Critical Challenges: Revitalizing the Health Professions for the 21st Century. Third Report.* Philadelphia: Pew Memorial Trust.

Pham, H. H., K. J. Devers, S. Kus, R. Berenson. 2004. "Health Care Market Trends and the Evaluation of Hospitalists and Roles." *Journal of General Internal Medicine* 20: 101–07.

Reinhardt, U. E. 1994. "Planning the Nation's Workforce: Let the Market In." *Inquiry* 31 (3): 250–63.

Rivo, M. L., H. L. Mays, and J. Katzoff. 1995. "Managed Health Care: Implications for the Physician Workforce and Medical Education." *Journal of the American Medical Association* 274 (9): 712–15.

Salsberg, E. S., and G. J. Forte. 2002. "Trends in the Physician Workforce, 1980–2000." *Health Affairs* 21 (5): 165–81.

Schroeder, S. A. 1994. "Managing the U.S. Health Care Workforce: Creating Policy Amidst Uncertainty." *Inquiry* 31 (3): 266–75.

———. 1992. "Physician Supply and the U.S. Medical Marketplace." *Health Affairs* 11 (1): 235–43.

Schroeder, S. A., and L. G. Sandy. 1993. "Specialty Distribution of U.S. Physicians—The Invisible Driver of Health Care Costs." *New England Journal of Medicine* 328 (13): 961–63.

Schwartz, A., P. B. Ginzburg, and L. B. LeRoy. 1993. "Reforming Graduate Medical Education: Summary Report of the Physicians Payment Review Commission." *Journal of the American Medical Association* 270 (9): 1079–82.

Schwartz, W. B., and D. M. Mendelson. 1990. "No Evidence of an Emerging Physician Surplus." *Journal of the American Medical Association* 263 (14): 557–60.

Sochalski, J. 2002. "Nursing Shortage Redux: Turning the Corner on an Enduring Problem." *Health Affairs* 21 (5): 157–73.

Starr, P. 1982. *The Social Transformation of American Medicine.* New York: Basic Books.

Tarlov, A. R. 1995. "Estimating Physician Workforce Requirements: The Devil Is in the Assumptions." *Journal of the American Medical Association* 274 (19): 1558–60.

U.S. Department of Health and Human Services. 2005. *Health, United States, 2005.* Pub. No. 05-1232. Hyattsville, MD: USDHHS. [Online information accessed in 2005 and 2006.] www.aacn.nche.edu/Media/Backgrounders/shortagefacts.htm.; www.ama-assn.org/ama/pub/category/1550.html.; www.aoa-net.org/students/college.htm.; http://brighamandwomens.org/midwifery/Patient/facts.asp.; www.aana.com/coa/accreditedprograms.asp.

———. 2002. *Health, United States 2002.* Hyattsville, MD: USDHHS.

———. 1990. *Seventh Report to the President and Congress on the Status of Health Personnel in the United States.* Pub. No. HRS-P-OD-90-3. Washington, DC: USDHHS.

U.S. Department of Health and Human Services/Bureau of Health Professions. 1996. "Health Workforce." *Newslink* 2 (1): 1–12.

U.S. Department of Health and Human Services/Health Resources and Services Administration. 1994. *Physician's Assistants in the Health Workforce.* Washington, DC: USDHHS.

U.S. Department of Labor. 2004. "Occupation and Employment." [Online information; retrieved 1/3/2006.] http://stats.bls.gov/oes/2004/may/oes291111.htm.

U.S. Government Accountability Office (formerly the U.S. General Accounting Office). 2004. *Internet Pharmacies: Some Pose Safety Risks for Consumers.* GAO-04-820. Washington, DC: USGAO.

———. 1994. *Health Professions Education: Role of Title VII/VIII Programs in Improving Access to Care Is Unclear.* HEHS-94–164. Washington, DC: USGAO.

Wachter, R. M., and L. Goldman. 2002. "The Hospitalist Movement 5 Years Later." *Journal of the American Medical Association* 287 (4): 487–94.

———. 1996. "The Emerging Role of 'Hospitalists' in the American Health Care System." *New England Journal of Medicine* 335 (7): 514–17.

Ward, D., and B. Berkowitz. 2002. "Arching the Flood: How to Bridge the Gap Between Nursing Schools and Hospitals." *Health Affairs* 21 (5): 42–52.

Weiner, J. P. 1994. "Forecasting the Effects of Health Reform on U.S. Physician Workforce Requirements: Evidence from HMO Staffing Patterns." *Journal of the American Medical Association* 272 (3): 222–40.

Wennberg, J. E., D. C. Goodman, R. F. Nease, and R. B. Keller. 1993. "Finding Equilibrium in U.S. Physician Supply." *Health Affairs* 12 (2): 89–103.

Whelen, G. P., N. E. Gary, J. Kostes, J. R. Boulet, and J. A. Hallock. 2002. "The Changing Pool of International Medical Graduates Seeking Certification Training in U.S. GME Programs." *Journal of the American Medical Association* 288 (9): 1079–84.

# HOSPITALS

## Introduction

Changes in the U.S. hospital industry dramatize the transformations occurring throughout the entire health services system and illustrate the ongoing tensions between conflicting views of health services as a social good to which all should have basic access or a commodity responsive to market forces. Hospitals' central role in the evolution of the U.S. acute care system is eroding as a result of changes occurring in the ways in which health services are delivered and financed.

Following a brief review of the development of the U.S. hospital industry, this chapter addresses the current status of hospitals and then turns to the many organizational, financing, and health services delivery issues hospitals face today.

## Development of the Hospital in the U.S. System

U.S. hospitals had their origins in almshouses established as early as the seventeenth century as domiciliaries for the destitute and sick. The provision of medical care, rudimentary at best at that time, was secondary to the provision of the more basic needs of food and shelter. Hospitals that provided care for the very poor were the next evolutionary phase of today's institution. Stimulated by physicians' interests in establishing their own workshops to provide care to a broader social class, both private hospitals and the predecessors of community hospitals began to emerge.

Paul Starr (1982), in his book *The Social Transformation of American Medicine*, identifies three phases of hospital development that shape the current institution. Phase I, lasting from approximately 1751 to the mid-1800s, featured the development of voluntary and public hospitals. Voluntary hospitals were so designated because voluntary donations rather than taxes supported them. Public hospitals were in large part tax-supported.

In Phase II, from the mid-1800s to 1890, "particularistic" hospitals to treat special populations such as children or specific diseases such as tuberculosis emerged. Near the end of Phase II, 172 hospitals existed in the United States.

In Phase III, from 1890 to about 1920, profit-making (proprietary) hospitals appeared on the U.S. health services scene. By the end of this phase, more than four thousand hospitals of all types were available, and an additional 521 mental illness hospitals had been established.

Throughout these phases, the hospital was being reconstituted from an institution of social welfare to one of medical science, from being organized as a charity to being organized as a business, and from an orientation toward the poor and their patrons to a focus on health services professionals and their patients. As part of this reconstitution, the hospital moved from the periphery to the center or hub of medical education and medical practice and developed three separate lines of authority: medical/clinical, administrative, and governing.

## The Hospital in Today's Health Services System

Table 9.1 shows the variety of ways the hospital is categorized, ranging from geographic location to bed size to ownership. These categorizations are not mutually exclusive; a hospital may fit multiple classifications. Several of these classifications, such as geographic, organizational configuration, and teaching status, factor in to the way that payers, particularly Medicare, reimburse hospitals for the care of their subscribers.

As of 2003, 5,625 general short-stay, nonfederal hospitals provided a range of medical and surgical services to those requiring inpatient hospitalization. As shown in Figure 9.1, the number of hospitals peaked at 6,774 in 1975; the hospital count for 2003 is about the same as it was in 1960 (5,768). The number of total hospital beds has followed a similar pattern, with 1,333,882 nonfederal beds available in 1985, but only 965,256 beds available in 2003. The three intervening decades between 1960 and the early 1990s included spurts of growth often followed by retrenchments and repositioning.

Figure 9.2 shows the distribution of short-stay hospitals by government status and type of ownership. Only about 4 percent of all hospitals are federal, and more than 70 percent of all hospitals are not-for-profit institutions. Figure 9.3 shows hospital distribution by bed size, with 48 percent of all hospitals having fewer than one hundred beds and only 5 percent having five hundred or more beds.

In addition to general short-stay hospitals, other classes of hospitals include federal, long-term, and specialty hospitals, such as rehabilitation hospitals, children's hospitals, substance abuse treatment hospitals, and hospitals that treat only burn patients, cancer patients, or those with other specific diseases or conditions.

TABLE 9.1
Types of
Hospital
Classifications

| Category | Example |
|---|---|
| Geographic | • Rural<br>• Urban |
| Organizational configuration | • Sole community hospital<br>• Freestanding hospital<br>• Member of multihospital system<br>• Critical access hospitals |
| Bed size | • 0–99 beds<br>• 100–199 beds<br>• 200–299 beds<br>• 300–499 beds<br>• 500+ beds |
| Level of care | • Secondary hospital<br>• Tertiary hospital<br>• Teaching hospital |
| Ownership | • Investor-owned or proprietary<br>• Public<br>• Not-for-profit |
| Government status | • Federal government facility<br>• State or local government facility<br>• Nongovernmental facility |
| Teaching status | • Teaching hospital<br>• Academic health center hospital<br>• Nonteaching hospital |
| Duration of care | • Short-stay hospital<br>• Long-term care hospital |
| Specialty status | • General acute care<br>• Children's hospital<br>• Substance abuse treatment hospital<br>• Psychiatric hospital<br>• Rehabilitation hospital |
| Other designators | • Community hospital<br>• Voluntary hospital |

## Hospital Supply and Distribution

In addition to the financial resources to establish and maintain the physical plant, hospitals require two other kinds of resources: a complement of medical and allied health professionals to provide inpatient care and a large enough population base to utilize the available services. Although hospitals can be found in locales with limited professional and consumer populations, hospital long-term viability and high-quality care depend on adequate levels of these resources.

**FIGURE 9.1**
Number of
U.S. Short-
Stay
Nonfederal
Hospitals
(Select Years,
1975–2003)

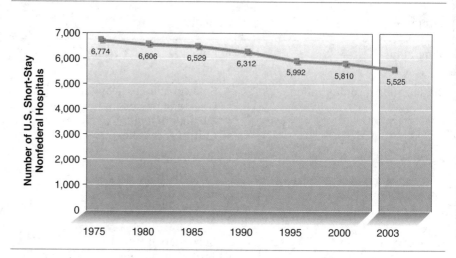

SOURCE: U.S. Department of Health and Human Services (USDHHS) 2005.

**FIGURE 9.2**
U.S. Short-
Stay Hospitals
by
Governmental
Status and
Type of
Ownership
(2003)

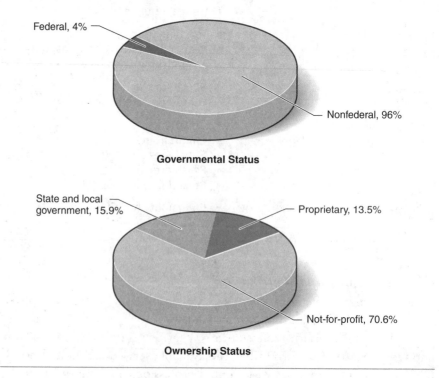

SOURCE: USDHHS 2005.

**FIGURE 9.3**
U.S. Short-
Stay Hospitals
by Bed Size
(2003)

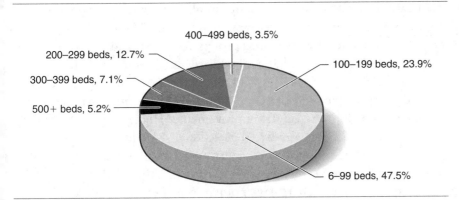

400–499 beds, 3.5%

200–299 beds, 12.7%

300–399 beds, 7.1%

500+ beds, 5.2%

100–199 beds, 23.9%

6–99 beds, 47.5%

SOURCE: USDHHS 2005.

**Supply: The Hill-Burton Program to Build Hospitals**

As the nation turned to rebuilding and strengthening its industrial base following World War II, a shortage of hospitals and health services providers was declared. To remedy the hospital shortage, the Hospital Survey and Construction Act of 1946, also referred to as the Hill-Burton Act, initially provided funds for hospital construction in rural areas. Subsequent amendments to the act expanded the program's scope, making funds available for replacement facilities in more metropolitan areas as well as for ambulatory care centers, nursing homes, rehabilitation facilities, and chronic disease facilities. In its later years, the Hill-Burton program expanded its focus to the modernization of existing hospitals, particularly those involved in the education of physicians (Rohrer 1987). States were required to provide matching funds and to establish a Hill-Burton planning council to determine priorities for construction, replacement, renovation, or modernization. Later provisions of the act also required participating hospitals to provide specific levels of care to patients unable to pay for that care.

Under the auspices of the Hill-Burton program, hospitals were established in rural areas that did not necessarily have either a complement of health professionals or a sizable consumer population, which ultimately jeopardized their long-term financial viability. Nonetheless, these facilities provided access to care in the short term to some populations that had never before experienced such access.

**Supply: Hospital Capital Expenditure Review Programs**

The Hill-Burton program influenced the distribution of hospitals by creating financial incentives to place them in rural and other underserved areas where they might not otherwise have been established. Two other federal initiatives, both focused on the prior review and authorization of capital expenditures, had a limited effect on hospital distribution. These initiatives—the 1122 program of the Social Security Act and the certificate of need (CON) program established by the National Health Planning and Resources Development Act of 1974—required governmental bodies aided by consumer groups to review and approve or disapprove health facility capital expenditures, including those for new or replacement plants, renovations, and modernizations. Rather than expand access to hospital services, these initiatives tried to control health services expenditures by limiting capital improvements. Highly unpopular among providers, the 1122 program was repealed in 1987 and the national CON program in 1986, though some states opted to retain their CON programs (see Chapter 5). As a move toward hospital growth appears to be underway, some researchers have pointed out the need to determine the extent to which states have retained any planning and regulatory controls on hospital growth and development (Bazzoli et al. 2003).

**Distribution: Sole Community Hospitals and Critical Access Hospitals**

Although the effects of the market are increasingly evident in the hospital industry, hospital distribution has traditionally not been entirely responsive to market forces. Hospitals may be situated in areas that have limited populations and provider resources simply because no other facility is within a reasonable distance. Sole community hospitals (SCHs) are a hospital class identified under the 1982 Tax Equity and Fiscal Responsibility Act (TEFRA) for special treatment by the Centers for Medicare and Medicaid Services (CMS) under Medicare's prospective payment system (PPS).

In general, an SCH constitutes the primary and often the only source of inpatient services for the residents of a market area. The CMS designates SCHs based on the distance of the hospital from neighboring facilities, the proportion of patients in the service area receiving treatment at other hospitals, and a requirement that the hospital be located in a rural, nonmetropolitan statistical area (nonMSA) (Farley 1985). SCH designation provides some exemptions to service volume, intensity, and other requirements that the CMS enforces for the Medicare and Medicaid programs it administers. For example, SCHs may be licensed for swing beds, beds that may function either for acute or long-term care, depending on the patient's need. This exception is important to the hospital's reimbursement by Medicare.

Equitable payment to rural hospitals has always posed a challenge to Medicare and other payers. The use of diagnosis-related groups (DRGs) and prospective payment may not meet the operational needs of small facilities with low censuses. Most persons, especially community members, agree that these often small and isolated facilities need to be retained to provide at least a first line of inpatient care to rural residents, many of whom may be Medicare beneficiaries. Such facilities may also provide essential psychiatric and rehabilitative services to their communities.

Cost-based reimbursement for rural hospitals, designated by Medicare as critical access hospitals (CAHs), has proven to be a better way to maintain the viability of these facilities. The CAH designation was established by the 1997 Balanced Budget Act to replace the previous payment classification system of the essential access community hospital (EACH) and the rural primary care hospital (RPCH). CAHs can be no larger than 25 (swing or acute) beds, and the average length of stay (ALOS) for acute-care patients can be no longer than 96 hours. CAHs are also limited to a census of 15 patients per day (currently an absolute number and not an annual average), and they are not to have distinct part units (DPUs), such as psychiatry or rehabilitation. By the end of 2002, 681 rural hospitals had received CAH designation (U.S. General Accounting Office [now known as the U.S. Government Accountability Office—USGAO] 2003). A GAO study of CAHs, mandated by the 1997 Balanced Budget Act, suggests that other rural hospitals are potential candidates for this designation but have not sought it, in part because the prohibition of DPUs as well as the census requirements pose obstacles to their delivery of care.

**Distribution: Centers of Excellence**

At the other end of the distribution spectrum, certain medical or surgical functions, because of the costs to maintain adequately trained professionals and provide the necessary equipment or operatories, may be regionalized into centers of excellence. Aware that a certain volume of procedures is necessary to maintain high-quality outcomes, payers may designate certain hospitals as centers of excellence for particular services, paying for such care to their subscribers only if the care is obtained in a designated center. The Medicare program, for example, has designated centers of excellence for heart transplants and reimburses Medicare beneficiaries for them only in these centers. The CMS has several demonstration centers of excellence programs for select cardiovascular procedures, total joint replacements, coronary artery bypass grafts (CABGs), and outpatient cataract surgery. The CABG program saved Medicare nearly $40 million in ten thousand cases at seven sites, and the cataract demonstration saved more than $500,000 in seven thousand cases at four sites (Faulkner & Gray 1996a).

## Hospital Organization

Three dimensions of hospital organization are important to an understanding of the health services system: (1) how an individual hospital is organized to perform its functions, (2) how hospitals may be linked into systems, and (3) the hospital's relationship to other health services functions and facilities in its community. The discussion begins with the internal organization of a generic hospital.

Most hospitals have traditionally been organized along three related but separate lines of authority: the medical staff, hospital administration, and the governing body. The balance of power among this trinity continues to shift as hospitals respond to accelerating changes in the health services system.

**Hospital Medical Staff**

Until recent changes in the U.S. health services system (addressed later in this chapter in "The Hospital in Transition" section), most physicians on the hospital's medical staff generally were not hospital employees. Some types of physician specialists, such as pathologists and radiologists, may be direct employees of the hospital, providing a support service to all admitted patients. Similarly, emergency care physicians may also be hospital employees. In the past, however, most other physicians who met membership conditions established by the governing body served on the medical staff and were given the privilege of admitting their patients to that hospital but were not salaried by the hospital.

The marked exceptions are physicians who participate in a staff model health maintenance organization (HMO) that owns or operates its own hospital, physicians who are salaried employees of state or local governments who staff public hospitals, and physicians paid directly by governmental programs for military veterans, active-duty military personnel, and others, such as indigenous populations, for whom the government is obligated to provide health services.

**Hospital Administration**

Hospital administration has been a recognized profession in the United States since the early 1900s and allows experts in facility organization and finance to professionally operate the hospital, leaving physicians free to concentrate on patient care. As the financing of health services has increased in complexity, as health services expenditures have escalated and commensurate efforts been made to contain them, and as competitive forces have mushroomed, hospital administrators have become subject to increasing demands and skill requirements.

During the growth and expansion of the hospital industry, which has only recently slowed, administrators focused much of their attention on ensuring that the needs and demands of their medical staffs were met and that their physical plants and equipment were as comprehensive and up-to-date as possible. To survive in today's competitive environment, the administrator is much more likely to be focusing on market share, developing new organizational structures with physicians and other providers, and concentrating on strategically positioning the hospital to respond to continuous change. Since the terrorist attacks of September 2001, hospitals have also had to determine how they would handle a range of potential bioterrorist events and have had to file plans with their state health departments that indicate how they would provide services under unusual emergency situations.

**Hospital Governance**

The type of governing body serving a hospital depends on the hospital's tax status. Even though the for-profit (proprietary) hospital industry has grown significantly in recent years, the majority of nonfederal short-stay hospitals are organized as not-for-profit hospitals (see Figure 9.2). Not-for-profit hospitals have traditionally been governed by boards of trustees, made up of influential business and community leaders who can assist the hospital in fundraising and other activities to maintain its viability. In recent years, the fundraising role of trustees has diminished as not-for-profit hospitals have turned to debt financing of their capital development (Potter and Longest 1994). For-profit hospitals are governed by boards of directors, most of whom are likely to have a shareholder interest in the hospital.

In addition to the internal organization of a generic hospital, two other aspects of hospital organization bear examination: (1) whether the hospital is a discrete entity or is affiliated with a system of hospitals, and (2) the hospital's relationship to other health services functions and facilities in its community.

**Freestanding Hospitals**

Freestanding hospitals—discrete organizational entities unaffiliated with other hospitals in a multihospital system—are an increasingly rare species in the hospital world. Few hospitals have the luxury of depending on their communities for the full range of support required to remain viable. The increasingly competitive forces generated by managed care and other dynamics are forcing hospitals to align themselves with one another and with other health services providers in ways that would not have been anticipated in the 1980s. The remaining freestanding hospitals are likely to be located in rural, more isolated areas, where affiliations and alliances are impractical because there are few partners with whom to ally.

**Hospital Systems**

The majority of nonfederal short-stay hospitals, both proprietary and not-for-profit, are either allied with other hospitals in their markets through cooperative agreements, joint ventures, or other organizational linkages, and/or they are members of a multihospital organization. Early collaborative efforts included shared services agreements, group purchasing consortia to reduce the costs of equipment and supplies to participating members, and negotiations to avoid replicating expensive services, such as emergency departments and neonatal intensive care units.

Public hospitals may also have alliances with other hospitals but are less likely to be part of large multihospital organizations because of the challenge, and often limited benefits, of linking the various governmental sponsors of public hospitals. Although they remain the source of inpatient care for the uninsured and other populations, earning them the label "safety-net" hospitals, many public hospitals, facing competition for their Medicaid and other insured patients from area hospitals, are devising new organizational structures to retain and enhance their market share. One such strategy is the creation of an independent hospital authority, which allows the public hospital to disengage from the often-cumbersome personnel, inefficient purchasing, and other local governmental services in favor of establishing their own more effective systems.

Many multihospital organizations represent only their specific market areas; others are national in scope. Both not-for-profit and for-profit hospitals are organized into hospital systems. Religious sponsors, such as the Sisters of Mercy and Sisters of Providence, created some of the early multihospital organizations. Much of today's focus on the hospital industry centers on the recent growth, through acquisition and merger, of proprietary hospital groups such as HCA—The Healthcare Company. By 2001, 52.6 percent of U.S. community hospitals were affiliated with systems, up from 30.8 percent in 1979 (Bazzoli 2004).

**Hospital Antitrust Issues**

In effecting collaborative arrangements, partnerships, and other complex system agreements, hospitals must be careful to avoid violating antitrust stipulations. Three major federal antitrust statutes regulate hospitals and other aspects of the health services system: the 1890 Sherman Act regarding restraint of trade, the 1914 Clayton Act pertaining to potential monopoly power, and the 1914 Federal Trade Commission Act addressing unfair competition (USGAO 1994a). A 1996 U.S. District Court ruling, which found that not-for-profit hospitals are fundamentally different from other businesses and behave differently, with less self interest, in highly concentrated markets than do for-profit hospitals, may ease the way for more hospital mergers (Faulkner & Gray 1996d).

**Hospital Integration with Other Health Services Providers**

The second level of external hospital organization of interest is the hospital's relationship to other health services providers and facilities. In the early days of modern hospital development—the 1950s and 1960s, for example—hospitals concentrated on providing medical and surgical services for acutely ill patients in need of inpatient care. Some hospitals, particularly in smaller, more rural communities, may have had a long-term care unit, but most focused on traditional hospital inpatient services. A number of external forces, however, have stimulated hospitals to broaden their spectrum of care.

Among these external forces are advancing technologies that permit more procedures and therapies to occur on an outpatient basis and incentives from payers to shift the provision of such services to settings less expensive than hospital inpatient care. These forces and the need to maintain and expand market share have prompted hospitals to expand their missions and their operations. Hospitals have used several strategies to effect expansion, including horizontal and vertical integration. Each of these forms of integration extends the reach of hospitals to a wider population of potential inpatients.

*Horizontal Integration*

Horizontal hospital integration focuses on the development of a continuum of care, from health promotion to disease prevention to inpatient acute care to long-term and palliative care. As such, it is the opposite of out-sourcing, which is obtaining key services through subcontracts or other arrangements with external providers.

*Vertical Integration*

Vertical integration is when a hospital extends its reach to capture and control more services that lead to inpatient hospitalization. Vertical integration may include the acquisition of pre- and post-hospital services, such as outpatient clinics, trauma or urgent care centers, rehabilitation units, or nursing homes. It may be forward integration, moving toward the consumer, or backward integration, moving toward the supplier. In the 1990s, vertical integration strategies were expanded to incorporate physicians and medical groups.

*Provider-Sponsored Organizations and Specialty Hospitals*

Vertical integration set the stage for hospitals to sponsor or participate in other new organizational forms, such as provider-sponsored organizations (PSOs), management services organizations (MSOs), and integrated health services networks. Larger, urban teaching hospitals with more than 15 percent of their revenues from managed care are most likely to participate in new organizational forms (Morrisey, Alexander, and Burns 1996).

PSOs take many forms. One of the earliest, the physician-hospital organization (PHO), is a joint venture between a hospital and its medical staff to contract with HMOs or self-insuring employers to provide services to an enrolled population. PHOs typically assume risk for the services they provide under a capitation arrangement. In 1994, two-thirds of hospital top executives reported in a Deloitte & Touche survey that PHOs were "absolutely necessary" to the future success of their facilities and 87 percent had or planned to establish a PHO. The ardor for this type of organization seems to have since cooled on both sides. In mid-1996, only 28 percent of hospitals had PHOs, and 37 percent said they saw no need to create one (Faulkner & Gray 1996c).

Although the development of PHOs has slowed, the development of PSOs was expected to take on new life with the passage of the 1997 Balanced Budget Act. This act defines a PSO as a public or private entity that:

- is established or organized and operated by a health care provider, or group of affiliated health care providers;
- provides a substantial proportion of the health care items and services under its contract through the provider or affiliated group of providers;
- shares directly or indirectly substantial financial risk with the providers, with respect to the provision of such items and services; and
- has at least a majority financial interest in the entity.

The act envisioned that PSOs, licensed in their respective states, would enroll Medicare beneficiaries into these managed care organizations. Medicare beneficiary enrollment in PSOs has been much slower than anticipated, and the expected growth of this form of delivery system has not materialized.

Specialty hospitals, particularly cardiac, surgical, and orthopedic hospitals, have eclipsed the development of PSOs. About one hundred specialty hospitals were operating in June 2003, and two-thirds of those had opened since 1990 (USGAO 2005). Approximately 70 percent of them were owned, in part or in whole, by physicians (USGAO 2005).

Debate about specialty hospitals' effect on other types of hospitals, as well as about the potential conflict of interest posed by physician ownership, resulted in an 18-month moratorium (through June 2005) on Medicare's reimbursement for services its beneficiaries received in specialty hospitals. Some have called for an extension of the moratorium to allow more time to evaluate this new type of hospital.

A study by the Medicare Payment Advisory Commission (MEDPac) found that: (1) in comparison to general hospitals, specialty hospitals were financially rewarded due to favorable Medicare payments for certain types of patients that specialty hospitals were more likely to treat; (2) specialty hospitals tended to treat patients in the more profitable DRGs or had a higher share of less severely ill patients within each DRG than general hospitals; or (3) both conditions. Proponents of specialty hospitals hold that these hospitals foster innovation and drive down costs (Dummit 2005). The jury is still out on this debate.

*Management*
*Services*
*Organizations*

MSOs buy the physical assets of their participating physicians, provide administrative services, and negotiate with managed care firms. Integrated health services organizations may take many forms: formal organizational entities distinct from both physicians and hospitals, contractual or practice ownership linkages between physicians and hospitals, or other organizational configurations that involve risk sharing to varying degrees.

The extensive changes occurring in the health services system ensure that the new organizational forms in which the hospital plays some, although not necessarily the central, role will continue to emerge. They are discussed more extensively in Chapter 19.

## *Hospital Revenue Sources and Financing*

A full appreciation of the challenges facing today's hospitals requires an understanding of hospital revenue sources and how hospitals finance their operations and capital development. Revenue streams are common to all types of hospitals, but one aspect of hospital revenue—uncompensated care—is less likely to be an issue in investor-owned facilities. Some financing issues are common to all types of hospitals. Other financing issues are specifically related to the hospital's tax status—whether it is a public hospital, a not-for-profit hospital, or a for-profit hospital.

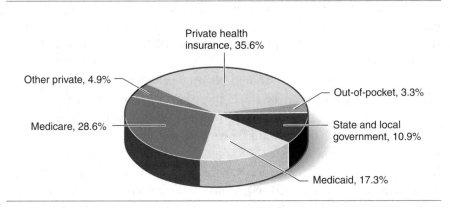

SOURCE: CMS 2005.

**FIGURE 9.4**

Hospital Revenue Sources (2004)

**Hospital Revenue Sources**

Figure 9.4 shows the major sources of patient care revenues to hospitals, with private health insurance providing 35.6 percent of all hospital inpatient revenues, seconded by Medicare, which provides 28.6 percent. Medicare's significance as a payer of both inpatient and outpatient hospital care gives it increasing leverage to shape hospital payment policies.

**Uncompensated Hospital Care**

What about the patient who is uninsured and has no means to pay for inpatient hospital care? A patient who presents at a hospital emergency department in need of care must receive treatment if that hospital participates in the Medicare program (Potter and Longest 1994), and nearly all general short-stay hospitals participate in Medicare. Voluntary and proprietary hospitals are not required to treat such patients for all conditions; however, they must stabilize the patients and then may transfer them to a public hospital (Siegel 1996), which must render care.

The financial implications to any hospital that renders care to patients unable to pay are substantial, particularly to public hospitals that receive a disproportionate share of such patients. Such unreimbursed care is variously classified as uncompensated care, bad debt, or charity care. Traditionally, the cost of uncompensated care has been the sum of charity and bad debt deductions from gross patient revenues or charges (Lewin, Eckels, and Miller 1988).

The uninsured accounted for almost 5 percent of all hospital inpatient discharges in 2000 (McLaughlin and Mortensen 2003), meaning that these individuals did not generally pay the hospitals for services rendered. The American Hospital Association (AHA) reported that hospitals spent about $25 billion on uncompensated care in 2004 (Weissman 2005). Classes of hospitals are disproportionately affected by uncompensated care. Urban public hospitals account for one-third of the uncompensated care in the

United States; this is double their share of the hospital market. Major teaching hospitals provide three times the amount of uncompensated care, relative to their share of the overall hospital market (Mann, Melnick, and Bamezai 1997).

The debate about who should be responsible for uncompensated care continues. Some hold that the tax-exempt status of not-for-profit hospitals holds them to a higher standard of providing uncompensated care and other community services than would be expected of investor-owned facilities. The Internal Revenue Service (IRS), in fact, has not required not-for-profit hospitals to provide uncompensated care as a condition of their tax-exempt status since 1969 (USGAO 2005). Even so, not-for-profit hospitals are wary about the lack of IRS specification about community service (such as sponsoring community health screenings and participating in professional education and training) or uncompensated care as conditions of retaining their tax-exempt status.

Both Medicare and Medicaid provide additional disproportionate share hospital (DSH) payments to hospitals, in recognition of the burden that unpaid treatments can place on hospital operations. Additional one-time funding increases have also occurred: the 1997 Balanced Budget Act made $100 million available in 12 states for fiscal years 1998 through 2001 for emergency services provided to undocumented aliens. The Medicare Prescription Drug Improvement and Modernization Act of 2003 also authorizes $1 billion over fiscal years 2005 through 2008 for emergency services provided to undocumented and certain other aliens (USGAO 2004). It is unlikely, however, that these incremental approaches will solve the problem of uncompensated care.

## Financing of Not-for-Profit Hospitals, Including Public Hospitals

This review of hospital financing begins with issues that are specific to a hospital's tax structure. Not-for-profit hospitals are organized under Section 501(c)(3) of the IRS tax code, and as such, are exempt from federal and state taxes and generally from local property and other taxes. Not-for-profit hospitals also have access to tax-exempt bond financing and have tax-deductible status for gifts and contributions (USGAO 1993).

Public hospitals are also likely to be organized as not-for-profit hospitals, but their financing streams differ from those of other not-for-profit hospitals. Public hospitals are largely dependent on tax-based support from their government sponsors and from patient revenues for their operating funds. Public hospitals may have a greater proportion of patient revenues from Medicaid (an average of 38 percent and as much as 50 percent) than do other types of hospitals (which average about 14 percent) because public hospitals frequently provide care to less affluent populations (Siegel 1996). Public hospitals are likely to have the highest proportion of uncompensated care of any category of hospital because as publicly supported institutions, they are obligated to serve all who seek their services. On average, about one-third of all public hospital billings remain unpaid (Kassirer 1995). For capital expenditures, public hospitals may compete with other governmental units for a share of the capital budget. Governmental sponsors may also place capital bond initiatives on the ballot for public decision. Obtaining capital funds for public facilities is difficult, and many public hospitals struggle to provide care in outdated and inadequate physical plants.

*Not-for-Profit Hospitals*

For operating expenses, not-for-profit hospitals depend to varying extents on their sponsor, whether it is a religious or fraternal order, or a charitable, community-based, or other type of organization. Revenues for patient care also provide a major source of operational support. Capital development for not-for-profit hospitals, once the purview of boards of trustees, now occurs principally through debt financing. Both not-for-profit and for-profit hospitals gained an expanded capacity to carry debt when the Medicare and Medicaid programs adopted cost reimbursement principles and treated depreciation and interest as reimbursable costs (Potter and Longest 1994).

*Tax Basis for Hospital Not-for-Profit Status*

Not-for-profit hospitals must generate revenue to cover expenses and to keep their physical plant, their medical and allied health staff, and their complement of services competitive. Net-of-expenses revenues are reinvested in the facility's improvement and growth, whereas in for-profit hospitals, some of those revenues may be returned to shareholders as dividends on their investments.

The not-for-profit status of hospitals has come under fire from several sources; the primary criticism is that not-for-profits receive more from their communities in tax exemptions than they return to their communities in services. Critics add that it is difficult to distinguish some not-for-profits from proprietaries because not-for-profits have diversified, developing for-profit ventures, such as diagnostic imaging centers, outpatient surgeries, and primary care clinics, under their not-for-profit umbrellas. The contention centers around whether not-for-profits should be expected to return at least the equivalent dollar value of the tax exemptions they receive in the form of care for the indigent, the provision of community programs such as immunization drives, the training of physicians and other health services workers, or the availability of generally expensive and unprofitable services, such as burn units, trauma services, or substance abuse treatment.

Prior to 1969, the IRS, which determines tax status, required that a hospital would be recognized as a corporation organized for charitable purposes only if it were "operated to the extent of its financial ability for those not able to pay for services rendered and not exclusively for those who are able and expected to pay." A 1969 revenue ruling revised this policy to emphasize that the promotion of health is itself a charitable purpose. The ruling stated that a hospital that "ordinarily limits admissions to those who can pay the cost of their hospitalizations, either themselves or through private health insurance, or with the aid of public programs such as Medicare" can still qualify for 501(c)(3) status. By 1974, it was clear that federal policy did not require the provision of free care to the poor as a condition for income tax exemption for not-for-profit hospitals (Potter and Longest 1994).

The current position of the IRS seems to be that not-for-profit hospitals provide a benefit to the community (USGAO 1993). In addition to the previous list of community service benefits, types of social benefits provided by not-for-profit hospitals include the public trusteeship of assets, including the use of surplus earnings, for the benefit of the community; a disincentive for private gain offsetting the information disparity between the provider and the patient that distorts the market economy; and relief of the governmental burden of providing services not available from or adequately supplied by private enterprise (Potter and Longest 1994). The IRS has not yet specifically mandated a dollar-for-dollar tradeoff.

Some state courts have tested this issue with varying results. The Utah Supreme Court established specific criteria in 1985 for the annual determination of the charitable status of hospitals, with emphasis placed on the amount of free care provided to a local population. A 1989 Vermont Supreme Court affirmed the broader view of a charitable hospital, holding that the main determinant was the availability rather than the amount of free care (O'Donnell and Taylor 1990).

Pennsylvania has also denied exemptions for hospital property that had never before been taxed, and a Texas attorney general initiated an investigation to determine whether not-for-profit hospitals were fulfilling their charitable obligations (Potter and Longest 1994). Other states, such as Colorado, have attempted ballot initiatives to require that all not-for-profit organizations, including hospitals, be subject to property taxes; to date, such initiatives have failed.

## Financing of For-Profit (Proprietary) Hospitals

Since the early development of for-profit hospitals from 1890 to 1910, their presence has fluctuated in the U.S. health services sector. A favorable economic climate for growth and access to equity capital stimulated a wave of for-profit hospital growth and development in the 1970s and early 1980s. The growth and performance of for-profit hospitals, particularly those in hospital systems, have been attributed to their economies of scale, establishment of strong management structures and control systems, tighter controls on the use of nursing and other support personnel, and ability to respond more quickly and more effectively to patient demands.

By the mid-1980s, hurt by their inability to attract key medical and business leaders, the growth of for-profit hospitals appeared to be on the wane, with one respected analyst suggesting that ". . . there is little basis for believing that their [for-profit hospital chains] share of the total health care market will grow" (Ginzberg 1988). Within a decade, however, for-profit hospitals, once dominant in only a handful of states, achieved a resurgence with far-reaching effects. Issues regarding specialty hospitals, most of which are organized as for-profit hospitals, typify the debate issues about for-profit hospitals in general.

Rather than building new facilities to increase their holdings, proprietary hospitals rebounded in the mid-1990s through the conversion of not-for-profit hospitals to investor-owned hospitals. In 1994, 34 not-for-profit hospitals were converted to investor-owned hospitals, and in 1995, 58 additional hospitals were converted, with as many as 447 community hospitals in takeover negotiations in 1995 (Kuttner 1996).

**Resurgence of For-Profit Hospitals**

The scope of this conversion may be more tangible if one considers changes in the number of hospital beds. Between the first quarter of 1994 and the third quarter of 1995, not-for-profits lost 16,827 beds and for-profits gained 21,840 beds (Fabini 1996). These kinds of conversions require that the charitable assets of the not-for-profit hospital be converted to a community use, often through the establishment of a foundation for health-related research and development.

One reason for the resurgence of for-profit hospitals in the mid-1990s may have been the enactment of "safe harbor" regulations that provide greater flexibility for physicians to refer patients to facilities in which they have a financial interest. Under the safe harbor regulations, a clinical lab to which a physician-owner cannot legally refer patients in ordinary business circumstances becomes a legal referral facility if it is part of a large, integrated entity in which the physician holds stock (Kuttner 1996).

Proprietary hospitals remain a modest proportion (13 percent) of the overall hospital industry, and the growth spurts of the mid-1990s were not sustained in subsequent years. The modest exception is the relatively recent development and potential growth of specialty hospitals.

For-profit hospitals serve as a focal point for the debate about whether health services are a social or a market good and, therefore, whether competition or regulation should manage development of the hospital industry. In the 1970s, a surge of for-profit hospital growth and development stimulated still unresolved discussions about the propriety of shareholders profiting from an industry servicing the sick. Although proprietary operations occur in many parts of the health services sector—in the development and sale of pharmaceuticals, and in nursing homes, independent laboratories, urgent care centers, home health care, and most recently, health maintenance organizations—the proprietary hospital has come to symbolize what is right, or wrong, about the application of market principles to the health services industry.

**Competition versus Regulation in the Hospital Industry**

**TABLE 9.2**
Regulatory
Programs for
Hospitals

| Focus of Control | Regulatory Program |
|---|---|
| *Quality of Care* | • Hospital licensure by state government<br>• Medicare and Medicaid certification<br>• Joint Commission on Accreditation of Healthcare Organizations voluntary accreditation |
| *Utilization* | • Quality improvement organization review of Medicare inpatient hospitalizations<br>• Preauthorization, precertification, second surgical opinion requirements by payers |
| *Capital Development* | • 1122 capital development review program*<br>• Certificate of need program* |
| *Costs/Provider Payment* | • Economic Stabilization Program, 1971*<br>• Medicare's prospective payment system, 1983<br>• Hospital selective contracting<br>• Periodic freezes on provider payment by Medicare and Medicaid<br>• Statewide hospital all-payer systems such as that in the state of Maryland<br>• Statewide hospital cost containment boards such as that in the state of Florida |

*No longer in effect.

The regulation versus competition debate is likely to remain unsettled in the short term. Table 9.2 outlines some of the major regulatory actions of the last several decades pertaining to quality of care, utilization, capital development, cost containment, and provider payment that have variously affected hospital development and operation. Each endeavor has or had a limited focus, which narrows its ability to fully regulate the industry. Yet any regulation prevents the industry from being fully competitive.

Some economists and analysts note that some markets, such as hospital markets, are not truly competitive (Fein 1990) and that not-for-profit hospitals have goals outside the market (Kuttner 1996). Anderson, Heyssel, and Dickler (1993), in comparing the effects of competition and regulation on hospitals, note that regulation has had a greater effect on hospital production processes, primarily by controlling expenditures per discharge, whereas the effects of competition have been greater on utilization by decreasing the number of discharges per capita.

The rights or wrongs of for-profit hospitals cannot be resolved here. What can be said is that some for-profit hospitals may be more efficient than some not-for-profit hospitals, which have goals outside the market

(Kuttner 1996). A not-for-profit status may help to assure appropriate, high-quality care, research, and professional education, but these may occur at the cost of efficiency (Potter and Longest 1994).

For-profit hospitals are more likely to avoid offering services that are unprofitable and less likely to have large amounts of uncompensated care than are not-for-profit hospitals (Lewin, Eckels, and Miller 1988). For-profit hospitals may have higher administrative overhead costs but may also be more profitable. They may have fewer employees per occupied bed but pay their employees higher wages. For-profit hospitals may fund more capital development through debt financing and have significantly higher capital costs in proportion to their operational costs than do not-for-profit hospitals (Watt, Derzon, and Renn 1986).

**Financing Issues Common to All Hospitals**

To varying extents, all hospitals have two other revenue streams: Medicare teaching adjustment funds and Medicare and Medicaid disproportionate share funds.

*Medicare Teaching Adjustment Funds*

The Medicare legislation passed as Title XVIII of the Social Security Act in 1965 included authority to compensate hospitals for Medicare's "share of the costs associated with medical education [graduate medical education (GME)]," which is the specialty training that occurs beyond basic medical education.

The GME provision was in response to a perceived shortage of physicians and includes reimbursement to teaching hospitals for both direct and indirect medical education costs. Direct GME (DGME) costs include salaries and benefits for residents and teaching physicians, costs of conference and classroom space, costs of additional equipment and supplies, and allocated overhead costs.

Indirect medical education (IME) costs are intended to compensate teaching hospitals for the proportion of their higher costs due to increased diagnostic testing, larger number of procedures performed, higher staffing ratios, and additional record keeping (USGAO 1994b). Payment formulas incorporating fixed-base costs, the number of full-time equivalent (FTE) residents, and the proportion of Medicare days of care are used for both direct and indirect medical education costs.

The 1997 Balanced Budget Act changed in several ways the methods by which rates are calculated for the Medicare teaching adjustment. First, DGME and IME payments currently embedded in the managed care rates that Medicare pays to health plans were carved out over five years. Second, the IME payments to teaching hospitals were decreased by reducing the multiplier in the IME formula between 1998 and 2002. Third, the number of full-time equivalent (FTE) residents for which a hospital may receive DGME and IME payments is now limited. Fourth, incentive payments are provided, under specific conditions, to hospitals that undertake a voluntary residency reduction plan to reduce the number of residency slots for which they receive DGME and IME payments (Association of American Medical Colleges [AAMC] 1997).

*Medicare and Medicaid Disproportionate Share Funds*

Medicare's prospective payment system (PPS) contains a mechanism, established in 1986, to provide additional reimbursement to hospitals that care for a disproportionate share of low-income patients. The payment formula is complex; different groups of hospitals need different percentages of low-income patients to qualify for the increase, and they receive different levels of increases when they do qualify. The sum of two percentages is used to determine eligibility: the percentage of Medicare patient days accounted for by people who receive Supplemental Security Income (SSI) payments made to low-income elderly and disabled people and the percentage of patient days, including Medicare, accounted for by people eligible for Medicaid. Large hospitals, particularly those in inner-city settings, are most likely to be recipients of disproportionate share funding (Russell 1989).

The Medicaid program has also had a disproportionate share hospital (DSH) payment mechanism, authorized by the 1980 and 1981 Omnibus Budget Reconciliation Acts (OBRAs), to compensate hospitals that treat a disproportionate share of Medicaid patients. The DSH payments were in recognition that hospitals were at financial risk if the care provided to a significant proportion of their patients was reimbursed at low rates or unreimbursed. State Medicaid programs soon found ways to increase their share of federal Medicaid matching funds through creative provider taxes or provider "donation" programs, some of which were subsequently disallowed by the federal government. The 1997 Balanced Budget Act scheduled a $10 billion reduction in Medicaid DSH payments through the year 2002 as one way to reduce federal expenditures for Medicaid. Medicaid DSH payments are the largest source of financial assistance for uncompensated care and are funded jointly by the states and the federal government (USGAO 2005).

## The Hospital in Transition

Hospitals are now shifting away from their longtime role of being the hub of the health services system to becoming service organizations in the health services system (Shortell, Gillies, and Anderson 1996). This section explores the reasons for and implications of this major change.

### The Hospital: Major Focus of Health Services Expenditures
Even before the passage of Medicare and Medicaid authorization in 1965, which increased access to inpatient hospital and other health services, hospitals accounted for the majority of health services expenditures—nearly

**FIGURE 9.5**
Hospital
Expenditures
as a Percentage
of Personal
Health Care
Expenditures
(PHCE)
(Select Years,
1960–2004)

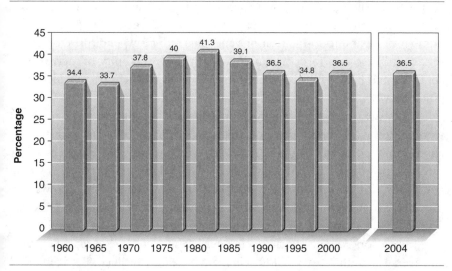

SOURCE: USDHHS 2005.

39 percent in 1960. In 2004, hospitals accounted for 36.5 percent of all *personal* health services expenditures (Figure 9.5). Hospitals, therefore, are the most obvious targets as concerns about health services costs and expenditures continue to rise.

### Changes in Hospital Reimbursement Lead to Changes in Care Delivery

Hospitals account for such a significant proportion of total health services expenditures not only because of the volume and intensity of the high technology services they provide but also, until recent changes in the Medicare program, because of the ways in which hospital services were reimbursed. Until Medicare's PPS was established in 1983, hospitals based their charges on their costs, both capital and operating, plus a profit margin. Costs were essentially distributed across payers so that some of the costs of providing care to uninsured and other nonpaying patients were shifted to paying patients.

Because the majority of Medicare expenditures was directed to inpatient hospital care and Medicare outlays for this care were growing at a rapid rate, Medicare imposed a payment system based on the patient's specific diagnosis. Two major effects resulted: hospitals could not shift non-Medicare costs to Medicare, and hospitals now had incentives to provide as many services as possible on an outpatient basis, since payment for outpatient services was not initially regulated by the PPS.

Medicare's PPS affected other payers as well, none of whom wished to cross-subsidize the care for nonsubscribers. Simultaneous with efforts to curtail hospital cost shifting was a growing interest among employers who sponsored health insurance in the potential of managed care to reduce the number of inpatient hospitalizations and thus reduce expenditures for health services. These two forces, combined with the availability of increasingly sophisticated health services technologies, changed the ways in which hospitals provide care.

Instead of a patient being admitted in advance for diagnostic tests and workup, tests can be performed on an outpatient basis, prior authorization by an insurance company might be required before admission for nonemergent care, and postoperative inpatient recovery time might be shortened. A whole new industry of services, formerly provided on an inpatient basis, is now being provided on an outpatient basis: birthing centers, urgent care centers, trauma centers, freestanding surgery centers, and centers for diagnostic imaging.

As a consequence of these changes in inpatient care, occupancy rates and average lengths of stay (ALOS) in many hospitals declined. Between 1980 and 1995, total inpatient admissions per one thousand people and ALOS each declined about 20 percent, and inpatient days per one thousand people declined about 40 percent (Reinhardt 1996). Such declines directly and negatively affected hospital revenues and the hospital's full financial picture, resulting in fewer patients over whom to spread capital and operating costs.

### Hospital Acquisitions, Mergers, and Closures

Hospital acquisitions, mergers, and closures have changed the configuration of hospitals in the U.S. delivery system. Hospital capacity has been reduced through downsizing and reengineering. Each of these changes is described in the sections that follow.

**Hospital Leveraged Buyouts**

Industry-wide changes have occurred in hospitals as well. Hospital acquisitions, mergers, and closures became hallmarks of the industry in the 1980s and early 1990s. In the 1980s, hospitals were as susceptible to the leveraged buyout (LBO) frenzy as any other major business. Under an LBO, control of one corporation is purchased by another, with substantial amounts of debt financing and the elimination of publicly held equity. Whether such buyouts improve revenue, expense, or profitability performances of the affected organizations is debatable. One study of LBOs by major proprietary chains reported that operating expenses grew more than for other hospitals in their areas, the total number of employees did not really change, and capital investment did not decline following the LBOs (Clement and McCue 1996).

**Hospital Mergers**

Hospital mergers also occurred with increasing regularity during this period. Between 1990 and 1997, 176 full-asset mergers resulted in consolidated ownership (Bazzoli 2004). The number of mergers peaked at 152 in 1996, but by 2000, the total had dropped to 18. The number of mergers and acquisitions combined peaked at 310 in 1997 and remained high at 132 in 2000 (Cuellar and Gertler 2003). A trade-off between efficiency and market share occurs with the consolidation of hospital markets through mergers and acquisitions. The advantages of such ventures are that hospitals can increase efficiency by reducing excess capacity and eliminating duplication of services, as well as give themselves increased bargaining power with managed care plans. Among the disadvantages is the potential for hospitals to negate the advantages of competitive markets if they acquire too much market power and raise prices or avoid lowering costs (Schactman and Altman 1995).

Some mergers, particularly those between not-for-profit hospitals in which the combined entity has the market power to raise prices above competitive levels, have come under scrutiny from the Federal Trade Commission (FTC). A key issue in such mergers is whether not-for-profits with market power will behave anticompetitively in concentrated markets (Faulkner & Gray 1996b).

**Hospital Downsizing and Reengineering**

The number of hospitals continues to decline, although some of the reduction in numbers may be due to mergers and consolidations. Particularly in the mid- to late-1990s, hospitals downsized by way of reengineering and, in some instances, closing. Between 1983 and 1993, the number of community hospitals declined by 9 percent and the number of staffed beds by 10 percent (Robinson 1996). Between 1980 and 1993, 949 hospitals closed (Shortell, Gillies, and Devers 1995). Downsizing and closures may result from excess capacity and may occur as the result of hospital market consolidation through mergers and acquisitions. Closures, especially rural hospital closures, have given rise to concerns about access. Between 1980 and 1988, 200 rural hospitals closed, representing about half of all community hospital closures for this period (USGAO 1991). Closed rural hospitals shared many common characteristics:

- They had suffered substantial and increasing losses in the three years prior to closure.
- Their losses were due primarily to a high cost per case compared to other hospitals.
- Losses on Medicare patients due to the PPS were not a major factor in their closures except for the smallest hospitals with fewer than 50 beds.
- A rural location did not increase the risk of closure.
- Risk factors for closure included low occupancy, small size, for-profit ownership, a weak economy, competition from other health services providers, and their provision of less complex levels of care (USGAO 1990, 1991).

### The Effects of Managed Care on the Hospital Industry

Managed care, which in its broadest definition means that the type and scope of an individual's health services is overseen by someone with a fiduciary interest in that care, has influenced the evolving role of the hospital. Managed care programs often include fiscal incentives for reducing the level and amount of care provided in the most costly setting—the hospital. To survive in markets that are highly saturated by managed care, hospitals have had to negotiate discounts, consider new types of insurance products, and adjust their traditional operational styles in other ways as well.

The effects of managed care on hospitals as well as on other sectors of the health services industry are of widespread interest, and research results are beginning to be reported. A study of California hospitals between 1983 and 1993 found that hospital expenditures grew 44 percent less rapidly in markets with a high HMO penetration. This decline was due to reductions in volume and mix of services (28 percent), reductions in bed capacity (6 percent), and changes in the intensity of services provided (10 percent). The substitution of outpatient for inpatient surgery, the shift from acute to subacute inpatient days, and the reductions in psychiatric hospitalizations were accelerated by the presence of an HMO (Robinson 1996). What remains unknown is the effect of these changes on overall hospital operation and performance.

The backlash against managed care suggests that hospital growth is resuming as part of a retreat from highly managed care. For the period 1994 through 1998, hospital spending actually declined year to year by as much as 5.3 percent, but it increased at a rate of 2.8 percent in 2000, a 1.2 percentage point increase over 1999 (Strunk, Ginsburg, and Gabel 2001). Growth in hospital outpatient spending also increased in 2000, so that the 2000 increases represent the largest since 1992. Growth in spending for both inpatient and outpatient hospital services also accelerated in 2001 (Strunk, Ginsburg, and Gabel 2001). Hospital spending increased 8.6 percent in 2004. The growth in hospital spending for this year accounted for 33 percent of the overall increase in health spending, greater than its 30 percent share of aggregate spending for total national health expenditures (Centers for Medicare and Medicaid Services [CMS] 2005).

### The Changing Role of the Hospital

The role of the hospital is clearly changing. Some see this role becoming more narrow and specialized; others see a transition from an institution providing primarily acute inpatient care to a health system offering a continuum of care. Table 9.3 shows the dimensions of ongoing change evaluated by Shortell and colleagues (1995).

Whether a hospital's role ultimately expands or contracts, its most immediate concern is survival. To survive, analysts suggest that a hospital

| Hospital | Health Services System | |
|---|---|---|
| Acute inpatient care | → | Continuum of care |
| Treating illness | → | Maintaining, promoting wellness |
| Care for individual patients defined | → | Accountable for the health status of populations |
| Commodity product | → | Value-added services, with emphasis on primary care, health-promotion, ongoing management of chronic illness |
| Market share of admissions | → | Covered lives |
| Fill beds | → | Care provided at appropriate level |
| Manage an institution | → | Manage a network of services |
| Manage a department | → | Manage a market |
| Coordinate services | → | Actively manage and improve quality |

**TABLE 9.3**
Transition from Hospital to Health Services System

SOURCE: Shortell, Gillies, and Devers 1995. Used with permission.

must reduce its costs; develop a pricing strategy that loads more of the over-head costs in the early stages of the stay and makes the incremental costs of additional days more competitive; assume a utilization review role based on the use of clinical epidemiology, computers, and continuous quality improvement (CQI); and seek other partners in downsizing (Brennan 1996; Reinhardt 1996).

## Summary

The role of the hospital, once the hub of the acute care system, is evolving in response to changes in health services financing and delivery. The number of hospitals and the number of staffed beds, as well as the patient's average length of stay, have declined in recent years as emphasis on outpatient care increases. Although the industry overall has downsized, the for-profit sector increased its market share in the mid-1990s; however, that growth has since leveled off.

Many analysts expect that the growth of managed care will continue to have implications for the hospital industry, particularly for further reductions in excess capacity. Some express concern that the "obsessive quest to gut the hospital" may not significantly reduce hospital expenditures and may even add to total health spending if the cuts are too severe (Reinhardt 1996). An analogy may exist between changes in the hospital industry and the dismantling of inpatient mental health care in favor of deinstitutionalization. Deinstitutionalization was intended to improve the care and quality of life for the person with mental illness and certainly did so for some, but not all, of this population. Further, it was accomplished at increased cost, both monetary and social, inasmuch as the community infrastructure had to be developed but the overhead and operational costs for the inpatient facilities still had to be covered.

## Key Words

antitrust

average length of stay (ALOS)

backlash against managed care

backward integration

bad debt care

Balanced Budget Act of 1997

birthing centers

capital expenditure review

capitation

centers of excellence

Centers for Medicare and Medicaid
    Services (CMS)

certificate of need (CON) programs

charity care

Clayton Act

community hospital

competition

continuous quality improvement
    (CQI)

cost shifting

critical access hospital (CAH)

cross-subsidization

debt financing

deinstitutionalization

direct graduate medical education
    (GME) costs

disproportionate share hospital
    (DSH) payments

downsizing

excess capacity

Federal Trade Commission Act

for-profit hospitals

forward integration

freestanding hospital

freestanding surgery centers

graduate medical education (GME)

group purchasing consortia

health maintenance organizations
    (HMOs)

Hill-Burton program

horizontal integration

hospital authority

hospital joint ventures

hospital mergers

Hospital Survey and Construction
    Act of 1946

hospital system

indirect medical education (IME)
    payments

integrated health care networks

investor-owned hospitals

leveraged buyout

managed care

management services organization
    (MSO)

multi-institutional systems

not-for-profit hospitals

outsourcing

physician-hospital organization

proprietary hospital

provider-sponsored organization
    (PSO)

public hospital

reengineering

regulation

safe harbor regulations

"safety-net" hospital

shared services

Sherman Act

sole community hospital

staff model HMO

Supplemental Security
    Income (SSI)

swing bed

<table>
<tr><td>Tax Equity and Fiscal Responsibility Act (TEFRA) of 1982</td><td>urgent care centers</td></tr>
</table>

Tax Equity and Fiscal Responsibility
   Act (TEFRA) of 1982
teaching hospital
uncompensated care

urgent care centers
utilization review
vertical integration
voluntary hospital

# References

Anderson, G., R. Heyssel, and R. Dickler. 1993. "Competition vs. Regulation: Its Effect on Hospitals." *Health Affairs* 12 (1): 70–80.

Association of American Medical Colleges. 1997. *Legislative and Regulatory Update.* Washington, DC: AAMC Office of Governmental Regulations.

Bazzoli, G. J. 2004. "The Corporatization of American Hospitals." *Journal of Health Politics, Policy and Law* 29 (4-5): 885–905.

Bazzoli, G. J., L. R. Brewster, G. Liu, and S. Kuo. 2003. "Does U.S. Hospital Capacity Need to Be Expanded?" *Health Affairs* 22 (6): 40–54.

Brennan, T. A. 1996. "What Role for Hospitals in the Health Care Endgame?" *Inquiry* 32 (2): 106–09.

Centers for Medicare and Medicaid Services (CMS). 2005. "Highlights—National Health Expenditures 2004." [Online information; retrieved 1/12/2006.] http://cms.hhs.gov/statistics/nhe/historical/highlights.asp.

Clement, J. P., and M. J. McCue. 1996. "The Performance of Hospital Corporation of America and Healthtrust Hospitals after Leveraged Buyouts." *Medical Care* 34 (7): 672–85.

Cuellar, A. E., and P. J. Gertler. 2003. "Trends in Hospital Consolidation: The Formation of Local Systems." *Health Affairs* 22 (6): 77–87.

Dummit, L. A. 2005. "Specialty Hospitals: Can General Hospitals Compete?" *Issue Brief No. 804.* Washington, DC: National Health Policy Forum.

Fabini, S. 1996. "Not-for-Profits vs. For-Profits: Reading the Tea Leaves." *Healthcare Trends Reporter* 10 (4): 1–2.

Farley, D. 1985. *Sole Community Hospitals: Are They Different?* Pub. No. 85-3348. Washington, DC: USDHHS/NCHSR.

Faulkner & Gray. 1996a. "'Excellence' Centers' Bargains Sought." *Medicine and Health* 50 (16): 3.

———. 1996b. "FTC Won't Ease Up on Mergers Creating Dominant Nonprofits." *Medicine and Health* 50 (46): 1.

———. 1996c. "Interest in PHOs Wanes, Survey Says." *Medicine and Health* 50 (28): 3.

———. 1996d. "More Nonprofit Hospital Mergers Predicted in Wake of FTC Defeat." *Medicine and Health* 50 (41): 3.

Fein, R. 1990. "For Profits: A Look at the Bottom Line." *Journal of Public Health Policy* 11 (1): 49–61.

Ginzberg, E. 1988. "For Profit Medicine: A Reassessment." *New England Journal of Medicine* 319 (12): 757–61.

Kassirer, J. P. 1995. "Our Ailing Public Hospitals: Cure Them or Close Them?" *New England Journal of Medicine* 333 (20): 1348–49.

Kuttner, R. 1996. "Columbia/HCA and the Resurgence of the For-Profit Hospital Business (1st part)." *New England Journal of Medicine* 335 (5): 362–76.

Lewin, L. S., T. J. Eckels, and L. B. Miller. 1988. "Setting the Record Straight: The Provision of Uncompensated Care by Not-for-Profit Hospitals." *New England Journal of Medicine* 318 (18): 1212–15.

McLaughlin, C. G., and K. Mortensen. 2003. "Who Walks Through the Door: The Effect of the Uninsured on Hospital Use." *Health Affairs* 22 (6): 143–55.

Mann, J. M., G. A. Melnick, and A. Bamezai. 1997. "A Profile of Uncompensated Hospital Care, 1983–1995." *Health Affairs* 16 (4): 223–32.

Morrissey, M. A., J. Alexander, and L. R. Burns. 1996. "Managed Care and Physician/Hospital Integration." *Health Affairs* 15 (4): 62–73.

O'Donnell, J. W., and J. H. Taylor. 1990. "The Bounds of Charity: The Current Status of the Hospital Property-Tax Exemption." *New England Journal of Medicine* 322 (1): 65–68.

Potter, M. A., and B. B. Longest, Jr. 1994. "The Divergence of Federal and State Policies on the Charitable Tax Exemption of Nonprofit Hospitals." *Journal of Health Politics, Policy, and Law* 19 (2): 393–419.

Reinhardt, U. E. 1996. "Perspective: Our Obsessive Quest to Gut the Hospital." *Health Affairs* 15 (2): 145–54.

Robinson, J. C. 1996. "Decline in Hospital Utilization and Cost Inflation under Managed Care in California." *Journal of the American Medical Association* 276 (13): 1060–64.

Rohrer, J. E. 1987. "The Political Development of the Hill-Burton Program: A Case Study in Distributive Policy." *Journal of Health Politics, Policy, and Law* 12 (1): 137–75.

Russell, L. B. 1989. *Medicare's New Hospital Payment System: Is It Working?* Washington, DC: The Brookings Institute.

Schactman, D., and S. Altman. 1995. *Market Consolidation, Antitrust, and Public Policy in the Health Care Industry.* Princeton, NJ: The Robert Wood Johnson Foundation.

Shortell, S. M., R. R. Gillies, and K. J. Devers. 1995. "Reinventing the American Hospital." *The Milbank Quarterly* 73 (2): 131–60.

Shortell, S. M., R. R. Gillies, and D. A. Anderson. 1996. *Remaking Health Care in America: Building Organized Delivery Systems.* San Francisco: Jossey-Bass, Inc.

Siegel, B. 1996. *Public Hospitals—A Prescription for Survival.* New York: Commonwealth Fund.

Starr, P. 1982. *The Social Transformation of American Medicine.* New York: Basic Books, Inc.

Strunk, B. C., P. B. Ginsburg, and J. R. Gabel. 2001. "Tracking Health Care Costs." *Health Affairs Web Exclusives,* September 26.

U.S. Department of Health and Human Services. 2005. *Health, United States, 2005.* Publication No. (PHS) 2005–1232. Hyattsville, MD: USDHHS.

U.S. Government Accountability Office (formerly the U.S. General Accounting Office). 2005. *Nonprofit, For-Profit, and Government Hospitals: Uncompensated Care and Other Community Benefits.* USGAO-05-743T. May. Washington, DC: USGAO.

———. 2004. *Undocumented Aliens: Questions Persist about Their Impact on Hospitals' Uncompensated Care Costs.* USGAO-04-472. May. Washington, DC: USGAO.

———. 2003. *Medicare: Modest Eligibility Expansion for Critical Access Hospital Program Should Be Considered.* USGAO-03-948. September. Washington, DC: USGAO.

———. 1994a. *Health Care: Federal and State Antitrust Actions Concerning the Health Care Industry.* USGAO/HEHS 94-220. August. Washington, DC: USGAO.

———. 1994b. *Medicare: Graduate Medical Education Payment Policy Needs to Be Examined.* USGAO/HEHS-94-33. May. Washington, DC: USGAO.

———. 1993. *Nonprofit Hospitals: For-Profit Ventures Pose Access and Capacity Problems.* USGAO/HRD 93-124. July. Washington, DC: USGAO.

———. 1991. *Rural Hospitals: Federal Efforts Should Target Areas Where Closures Would Threaten Access to Care.* USGAO/HRD 91-41. Washington, DC: USGAO.

———. 1990. *Rural Hospitals: Factors That Affect Risk of Closure.* USGAO/HRD-90-134. June. Washington, DC: USGAO.

Watt, J. M., R. A. Derzon, and S. C. Renn. 1986. "The Comparative Economic Performance of Investor-Owned Chains and Not-for-Profit Hospitals." *New England Journal of Medicine* 314 (2): 89–96.

Weissman, J. 2005. "The Trouble with Uncompensated Hospital Care." *New England Journal of Medicine* 352 (12): 1171.

# BIOMEDICAL RESEARCH, HEALTH SERVICES TECHNOLOGY, AND TECHNOLOGY ASSESSMENT

## Introduction

Results from biomedical research and developments in health services technology—which include drugs, devices, medical and surgical procedures used in medical care, and the organizational and supportive systems with which such care is rendered—provide the underpinnings of a progressive health services system. The U.S. health services system enjoys an international reputation as a leader in biomedical research and in the development and application of new health services technologies. This chapter begins with a review of the biomedical research role in the U.S. system. The development, dissemination, and application of health services technologies, such as drugs, medical devices, and medical and surgical procedures, are then addressed. The final section of the chapter explores the use of technology assessment, which aims to rationalize the use of technology and the resulting expenditures for it.

## Biomedical Research

Interest in and support for biomedical research to improve patient care have distinguished the U.S. health services system since the mid-twentieth century. The federal government's role can be traced to a science adviser of President Franklin D. Roosevelt, who in 1945 recommended that the government provide $5 million to support biomedical research (Ginzberg 1990). In the intervening 50 years, that amount steadily increased; nearly $94.3 billion was spent on biomedical research in the United States in 2003 (Moses et al. 2005).

Table 10.1 shows national health expenditures on biomedical research through 2004. The data in this table are exclusive of research and development expenditures of drug companies and other manufacturers and providers of medical equipment and supplies. These expenditures reflect principally public sources of funding. Table 10.2 shows that all funding sources for biomedical research, including drugs, equipment, and supplies, was $94.3 billion in 2003, the most recent year for which data are reported[1]

**TABLE 10.1**

National Health Expenditures (NHE) on Biomedical Research (Select Years, 1960–2004)

| Year | Expenditures (in Billions of Dollars) | Percentage of NHE |
|------|---------------------------------------|-------------------|
| 1960 | $0.7  | 2.6 |
| 1970 | 2.0   | 2.7 |
| 1980 | 5.5   | 2.2 |
| 1990 | 12.2  | 1.8 |
| 2000 | 25.6  | 1.9 |
| 2004 | 39.0  | 2.1 |

SOURCES: Levit, Lazenby, and Sivarajan 1996; 2000 and 2004 data are from CMS 2004.

NOTE: Research and development expenditures of drug companies and other manufacturers and providers of medical equipment and supplies are excluded from "research" expenditures but are included in the expenditure class in which the product falls.

**TABLE 10.2**

National Funding for Health Research and Development (Millions of Dollars Through 1999; Billions of Dollars for 2003)

| Year | All Funding | Federal | State/Local | Industry* | Nonprofits |
|------|-------------|---------|-------------|-----------|------------|
| 1960 | $ 886    | $ 448  | $ 46  | $ 253  | $ 139 |
| 1965 | 1,890    | 1,174  | 90    | 450    | 176   |
| 1970 | 2,847    | 1,667  | 170   | 795    | 215   |
| 1975 | 4,701    | 2,832  | 286   | 1,319  | 264   |
| 1980 | 7,967    | 4,723  | 480   | 2,459  | 305   |
| 1985 | 13,567   | 6,791  | 878   | 5,360  | 538   |
| 1990 | 23,095   | 9,791  | 1,625 | 10,719 | 960   |
| 1995 | 35,816   | 13,423 | 2,423 | 18,645 | 1,325 |
| 1999 | NA       | 17,244 | NA    | NA     | NA    |
| 2003 | $94.3 B  | 33.3 B | 4.3 B | 54.1 B | 2.5 B |

SOURCES: USDHHS 2002; Moses et al. 2005.

NOTE: B = billion; NA = not available.

*Includes expenditures for drug research. These expenditures are included in the "drugs and sundries" component of the national health expenditures, not under "research."

(U.S. Department of Health and Human Services [USDHHS] 2002 and Moses et al. 2005). Figure 10.1, which does not include expenditures for drug, equipment, and supply research, shows that the federal government is the funding source for more than one-third of all other kinds of biomedical research.

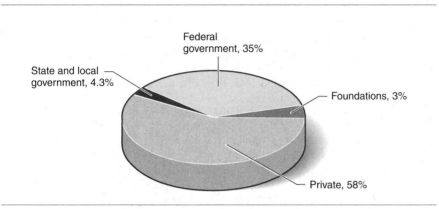

**FIGURE 10.1**
Funding for Health Research and Development, Source of Funds (2004)

SOURCE: Levit, Lazenby, and Sivarajan 1996.

## *The Federal Role in Biomedical Research*

Because drug and medical device research is addressed in subsequent sections of this chapter, the focus here is on basic and applied biomedical research. The major source of support for this type of research is the federal government, and much of the research funding flows through the National Institutes of Health (NIH).

The NIH was established in 1930 to serve as the administrative unit for the medical research of the Public Health Service (PHS), and the NIH remains a unit of the PHS. The first categorical institute—the National Cancer Institute (NCI)—was established in 1937. Today, the NIH houses 19 institutes that focus on specific diseases or conditions or on body systems and the abnormalities that occur within them, the National Library of Medicine, and seven other specialty centers (see Table 10.3).

The advances in health sciences in the last half of the twentieth century, many of them assisted with NIH funds, are impressive. As a result, life spans are lengthening and major causes of death have shifted from infectious agents to malignancies and diseases of the cardiovascular and cerebrovascular systems. Research endeavors now focus on ameliorating the effects of chronic conditions and unraveling the genetic indicators of certain conditions or diseases in human genome research.

In 1995, former NIH director Harold Varmus identified a number of recent advances in health outcomes through the use of new technologies, including new surgical treatments, organ transplantation, implantation of pacemakers and artificial joints, effective therapies for certain leukemias and other cancers, drugs effective against certain mental diseases, and genetic testing for many inherited diseases (Varmus 1995).

TABLE 10.3
National
Institutes
of Health

| | |
|---|---|
| **Institutes** | National Cancer Institute (1937) |
| | National Heart, Lung, and Blood Institute (1948) |
| | National Institute of Diabetes and Digestive and Kidney Diseases (1948) |
| | National Institute of Allergy and Infectious Diseases (1948) |
| | National Institute of Child Health and Human Development (1962) |
| | National Institute on Deafness and Other Communication Disorders (1988) |
| | National Institute of Dental and Craniofacial Research (1948) |
| | National Institute of Neurological Disorders and Stroke (1950) |
| | National Eye Institute (1968) |
| | National Institute on Aging (1974) |
| | National Institute of Arthritis and Musculoskeletal and Skin Diseases (1986) |
| | National Institute on Drug Abuse (1973) |
| | National Institute of Mental Health (1949) |
| | National Human Genome Research Institute (1989) |
| | National Institute on Alcohol Abuse and Alcoholism (1970) |
| | National Institute of Environmental Health Sciences (1969) |
| | National Institute of General Medical Sciences (1986) |
| | National Institute of Nursing Research (1986) |
| | National Institute of Biomedical Imaging and Bioengineering (2000) |
| **Libraries** | National Library of Medicine (1956) |
| **Centers** | NIH Clinical Center (1953) |
| | John E. Fogarty International Center (1968) |
| | Center for Information Technology (1964) |
| | National Center for Research Resources (1990) |
| | Center for Scientific Review (1946) |
| | National Center for Complementary and Alternative Medicine (1992) |
| | National Center on Minority Health and Health Disparities (1993) |

SOURCE: National Institutes of Health 2006.

Federal support of biomedical research, constituting less than 4 percent of total health services expenditures, has grown steadily in the last 35 years. Figure 10.2 shows the growth in congressional appropriations for the NIH, from $1.1 billion in 1970 to $28 billion in 2004. Although the appetite for continued growth in biomedical research is not sated, and even though congressional appropriations have remained relatively immune from regular proposals to trim federal expenditures, the amount of discretionary dollars is an evermore-constrained resource within the federal budget cycle.

Senator Frist (2002) suggests that congressional initiatives to double the NIH budget between 1998 and 2003 have succeeded (see Figure 10.2). He notes that the NIH budget grew 108 percent between 1995 and 2002, more than twice as fast as the overall federal budget. What remains to be seen is how a weaker economy, initiatives in the war on terrorism, and the financial effects of further armed conflict and the continued growth of entitlement programs will affect NIH growth.

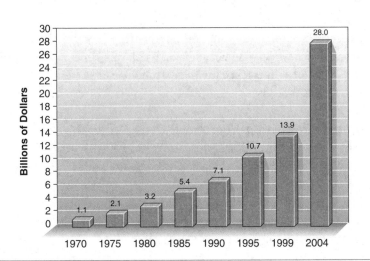

**FIGURE 10.2**
Congressional Appropriations for the NIH (Select Years, 1970–2004)

SOURCES: USDHHS 2002; Varmus 1995; Zerhouni 2005.

NOTE: Data intervals are irregular.

# Health Services Technology

The development, dissemination, and application of health services technologies such as drugs, devices, and medical and surgical procedures are
hallmarks of the U.S. health services system. This technological imperative
has produced one of the most advanced systems of care in the world. Three
major sources stimulate the development of health services technology: general advances in science and technology outside the field of medicine that
are filtered into clinical use, innovation from medical research and development, and innovation from medical practice itself (Rettig 1994).

## Steps in the Development of a New Technology

The development or innovation of a new technology occurs in several stages
that may not always reflect a studied progression or a necessarily sequential
order. McKinley (1981) provides one model for considering the development
of a new technology, noting the following usual stages of an innovation:

1. promising report;
2. professional and organizational acceptance;
3. public acceptance and state and third-party payer endorsements;
4. standard procedure, observational reports, and descriptive accounts;
5. randomized clinical trials;
6. professional denunciation; and
7. erosion and discreditation.

Not all stages are reached with every innovation, but an example of a technology that approximates McKinley's order is the Jarvik artificial heart. A more recent example—the implantable heart, which is currently still an experimental procedure—may be analyzed using this same approach. McKinley's model is helpful in tracing the development and current status of some health services technologies.

## Technology's Effects on Health Services Expenditures

The price for having one of the most advanced health services systems in the world is the regular and substantial growth in expenditures to maintain it—16 percent of the gross domestic product (GDP) in 2004.

Periodic reports of the National Health Accounts (NHA) indicate the growth in personal health services expenditures, per capita, that can be linked to: (1) economy-wide inflation; (2) "excess" medical inflation that is above and beyond economy-wide inflation; and (3) a residual, which includes the use of new technology. In most years since the National Health Accounts have been reported, beginning in 1960, either economy-wide inflation or medical inflation has surpassed the category of "intensity," which is defined as "the residual percent of growth which cannot be attributed to price increases or population growth [and] represents changes in use of kinds of services and supplies." Medical technology development is subsumed under the intensity category. From 1970 to 2003, the percentage of health expenditure growth due to intensity has exceeded either economy-wide or medical inflation in only eight years. Figure 10.3 shows the factors that contributed to growth in personal health care expenditures for 2002–03. The NHA do not purport to estimate expenditure growth pertaining to the overuse of existing technology.

Innovations in the treatment of clinical conditions, major hospital services, or physician specialties affect the costs of and expenditures for health services. Rettig (1994) provides the following examples of such innovations:

**FIGURE 10.3**
Percentage Growth in Personal Health Expenditures, by Cause (2002–03)

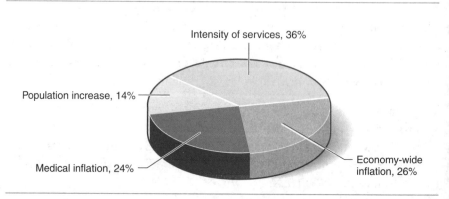

Intensity of services, 36%

Population increase, 14%

Medical inflation, 24%

Economy-wide inflation, 26%

SOURCE: USDHHS 2005.

- Major advances may create a clinical ability to treat previously untreatable terminal conditions, such as end-stage renal disease (ESRD), diabetes, or AIDS, by some long-term maintenance therapy, where unit cost, patient volume, and changing epidemiology drive costs.
- Within the framework of chronic treatment of previously untreatable terminal diseases are two additional effects: secondary diseases within the disease are discovered, and the indications for treatment tend to expand over time.
- Major advances may create a clinical ability to treat previously untreatable acute conditions, such as coronary artery bypass grafts.
- Existing capabilities improve incrementally, such as laparoscopic surgery for gall bladder removal; these improvements are often quality-enhancing and cost-decreasing, but may also be cost-increasing and are strongly influenced by coverage decisions.
- Clinical progress may extend medicine's scope to conditions once regarded as beyond its boundaries, such as mental illness, psychiatric disorders, and substance abuse.

The sections that follow examine drugs as an example of health services technology, and then medical devices, supplies, and new medical and surgical procedures.

### Drugs

The development and use of new drugs is an important part of the U.S. health services system, though per capita drug utilization and the proportion of national health expenditures spent on drugs historically played a smaller role in this culture than in others, such as France and Germany (U.S. General Accounting Office [now known as the U.S. Government Accountability Office—USGAO] 1994b). Following the days of patent medicines and nostrums, drug development became increasingly sophisticated with the use of more complex—and often more toxic—compounds. The increasingly complex drugs being developed ultimately led to increased regulation of the industry (Table 10.4).

The first major act to regulate the pharmaceutical industry—the Biologics Act of 1902—required premarket batch testing and licensing of all biologic drugs. The Food and Drug Act of 1906 standardized drug strength and purity and prohibited drug adulteration and misbranding. A national move to expand drug regulation followed a wave of deaths in 1937 attributed to the new drug elixir sulfanilamide. The drug contained diethylene glycol, a chemical normally used in antifreeze, and had not been tested for safety in human use. The resulting legislation—the Food, Drug, and

**Drug Regulation**

**TABLE 10.4**

Regulation of Food, Drugs, Cosmetics, and Devices

| Year | Legislation or Regulation |
|---|---|
| 1906 | Food and Drug Act required that drugs meet official standards of strength and purity and not be adulterated or misbranded. |
| 1938 | Food, Drug, and Cosmetic Act required manufacturer to provide evidence about new drugs before marketing. |
| 1951 | Durham-Humphrey Amendment established a category of mandatory prescription drugs. |
| 1962 | Kefauver-Harris Drug Amendments required manufacturer to provide evidence of effectiveness of drug in addition to safety before marketing. |
| 1983 | Orphan Drug Act provided tax breaks to manufacturers of drugs that affect conditions among populations of 200,000 or fewer persons. |
| 1984 | Drug Price Competition and Patent Term Restoration Act expanded the number of drugs suitable for the abbreviated new drug application, which makes it easier for a generic drug to reach the market after a patent expires. Pioneer drugs were granted patent extensions up to five years. |
| 1987 | Prescription Drug Marketing Act prohibited the reimportation of exported drugs and initiated major changes in the use of drug samples. |
| 1992 | Prescription Drug User Fee Act allowed FDA to collect fees with each new drug application (NDA) to support the hiring of the additional reviewers required to handle the increased volume of work. |
| 2002 | Medical Device User Fee and Modernization Act provides the FDA with additional resources to ensure prompt approval or clearance of applications for marketing medical devices and licensing biological products. |

SOURCES: Grady 1992; Moore 1996; USGAO 2005.

Cosmetic Act (FDCA) of 1938—was one of the early pieces of consumer protection legislation.

The FDCA required manufacturers to submit to the Food and Drug Administration (FDA)—the federal agency founded in 1906 to regulate the production and dissemination of drugs and medical devices—a notification with data on the safety of a drug before the drug could be marketed. The FDCA was further amended in 1962, as the result of the thalidomide tragedy in Europe. The high incidence of birth defects noted among children born to women who had taken thalidomide during pregnancy led to discontinued use of this drug for pregnant women. The FDA must now approve the safety and efficacy of a new drug, as well as its method of manufacturing and labeling, before the drug can be marketed (Moore 1996). It is interesting to note that thalidomide has experienced a resurgence in its use, though not for its original use as a sedative, but rather for the treatment of such conditions as malignant melanoma (Kudva, Collins, and Dunphy 2001).

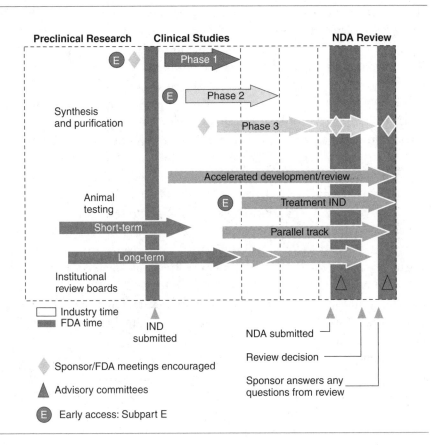

**FIGURE 10.4**
FDA Approval
Process for
New Drugs

SOURCE: FDA 2006.

NOTES: IND = investigational new drug; NDA = new drug application.

The FDA controls the approval and marketing of both prescription and over-the-counter (OTC) drugs. Figure 10.4 charts the progress for the approval of a new drug. Manufacturers who develop a new drug and believe they are ready to test it on humans must submit an investigational new drug (IND) application to the FDA. If the FDA approves this application, the manufacturer begins clinical trials to test the drug's safety and efficacy, and establishes the appropriate production and marketing strategies.

If the trials are successful, the manufacturer submits to the FDA a new drug application (NDA); the FDA can accept the NDA or refuse to file it if the NDA does not meet its standards. If the FDA accepts the NDA, it takes one of three actions: issues an approved letter, clearing the drug to be marketed; issues an approval letter, indicating that the drug can be approved if the sponsor resolves certain issues; or issues a nonapproval letter that specifies the reasons for withholding approval (USGAO 1996).

**Criticism of FDA Drug Review Process**

The FDA review and approval process regularly comes under fire, with manufacturers and anxious consumers lobbying for a shorter, less-rigorous process and consumer protection advocates demanding that the public continue to be protected from unsafe and ineffective products. The rapid spread of AIDS in the mid-1980s brought particular pressure to the FDA. People living with AIDS or those who were HIV-positive, aware that there was no cure for this disease, clamored for access to experimental and in some cases untested therapies, arguing that the unknown risks of such therapies were no greater than the certain death they faced from the disease. The drug review processes in other countries, such as the United Kingdom, were proposed as models for U.S. adaptation.

In response to congressional queries about FDA processes, the GAO was asked to analyze the review and approval times for NDAs submitted between 1987 and 1994 (USGAO 1996). Contrary to manufacturer and consumer claims, the GAO found that the approval time had shortened for NDAs submitted in 1992 to 19 months, compared to the 33-month period for NDAs submitted in 1987. Two factors that affected lengths of NDA approval times were the priority score initially assigned by the FDA and the sponsor's prior experience.

Higher priority scores are assigned to drugs with expected therapeutic benefits beyond drugs already on the market, and they proceed through the FDA's review process, on average, about 10 months faster than drugs not expected to offer additional therapeutic benefits. Only about 17 percent of NDAs achieve this priority status. NDAs submitted by sponsors who have had prior experience with the FDA process proceed, on average, through the process four months faster than NDAs submitted by first-time applicants. Applications from experienced sponsors are three times more likely to be approved than those from less-experienced sponsors. The GAO study also found that approval times for the drug review process in the United Kingdom were no shorter than those in the United States (USGAO 1996). A study by the Tufts Center for the Study of Drug Development (2002), reported in March 2000, indicates that the European Union's Medicines Evaluation Agency (EMEA) rate of approval for biotechnology products takes 417 days, compared to 452 within the United States for the same products.

FDA approval times have decreased since 1980. In 1992, the Prescription Drug User Fee Act (PDUFA) was passed, which allows the FDA to augment its budget (and thus add staff) by charging user fees to drug developers. Olson (2004) found that the availability of PDUFA led to a substantial decrease in drug review times. New drug approval times for new molecular entities dropped from a median of 22 months in 1992 to less than 12 months in 1999 (FDA 2006).

The development of a new drug takes time—an average of 12 years—and is expensive. Not all promising substances result in the issuance of a new drug. The costs for developing a new drug vary widely. Keyhani, Diener-West, and Powe (2005) cite estimates from $57 million to $802 million per drug and note that the variance is due in part to different assumptions and methods used in developmental research. A study of drugs approved from 1994 through 1998 found that only one in five compounds that entered preclinical testing made it to human testing, and only one of those five was approved for sale (Spilker 2002). Some drug products, even though they are effective in treating the condition for which they were developed, are not lucrative enough to warrant production. The reason for this may be either because the condition affects such a small proportion of the population that the manufacturing costs cannot be recouped or because the provision of the drug increases the manufacturer's legal liability. Two national drug-related acts protect the availability of such products: the Orphan Drug Act of 1983 and National Childhood Vaccine Injury Act.

**New Drug Development**

The Orphan Drug Act of 1983 ensures that essential but low-demand drugs remain available to the population in need. Orphan drugs are those for conditions affecting fewer than 200,000 people. The act permits manufacturers to take tax deductions for about 75 percent of the cost of the clinical studies required as part of the IND/NDA process and gives the manufacturer exclusive marketing rights for seven years for the approved drug (Moore 1996).

*Orphan Drug Act*

The National Childhood Vaccine Injury Act was enacted in 1986 as a result of lawsuits directed against manufacturers of whole-cell pertussis and other vaccines, to which some patients reported adverse reactions. The act provided for an independent review of available scientific evidence on adverse events attributed to vaccinations and established the Vaccine Adverse Event Report System (VAERS), jointly operated by the FDA and the Centers for Disease Control and Prevention (CDC). The act also established the National Vaccine Injury Compensation Program to limit the legal actions that may be brought against a vaccine manufacturer.

*National Childhood Vaccine Injury Act*

In 2004, only 10 percent of total personal health services expenditures were directed to the purchase of drugs—about half of the proportion of personal health services expenditures spent on drugs in 1960 (see Table 10.5). Of drug expenditures, 60 percent are for prescription drugs, and 40 percent are for OTC drugs. A number of drugs that were formerly available only through a physician or dentist's prescription, such as Advil, Nuprin, Sudafed, Benadryl, and Claritin, are now available as OTC drugs (Moore 1996). The

**Drug Expenditures as a Proportion of National Health Expenditures**

**TABLE 10.5**
National
Health
Expenditures
(NHE) for
Prescription
Drugs
(Select Years,
1960–2004)

| Year | Expenditures (in Billions of Dollars) | Percentage of NHE |
|---|---|---|
| 1960* | 4.2 | 15.6 |
| 1970* | 8.8 | 12.0 |
| 1980 | 12.0 | 5.0 |
| 1990 | 40.3 | 5.8 |
| 2000 | 121.8 | 9.4 |
| 2004 | 188.5 | 10.0 |

SOURCES: Levit, Lazenby, and Sivarajan 1996; USDHHS 2002; CMS 2004.

*Data for 1960 and 1970 also include expenditures for other medical nondurables.

Congressional Budget Office (1992) projected in 1992 that spending on drugs would increase 7.5 percent per year between 1991 and 2000, with increases attributed to both price and quantity. The annual increases for select years between 1993 and 2004 ranged from 8.2 percent to 18.2 percent, and averaged 12.7 percent (CMS 2005).

Despite increasing insurance coverage for drugs, nearly 25 percent of drug expenditures are out-of-pocket payments. One major reason for this high proportion of out-of-pocket payments is that Medicare beneficiaries, who because of their age and/or conditions of disability use more drugs per capita than other population subgroups, did not receive Medicare coverage for outpatient prescription drugs until January 1, 2006, after any of these data were reported.

**Drug Prices**    Drug prices periodically come under fire from consumers and from such payers as the federal government. The federal-state Medicaid program, for example, provides optional coverage for prescription drugs; this optional coverage absorbed 11.5 percent of all Medicaid expenditures for 2001 (CMS 2005). Concern about the amount of federal funds being spent on drugs prompted Congress to require, as part of the 1990 Omnibus Budget Reconciliation Act (OBRA), that manufacturers pay rebates to states to have their prescription drugs covered by state Medicaid programs. The 1992 Veteran's Health Care Act extended this rebate to health services programs operated by the Department of Veteran's Affairs (VA), the Public Health Service (PHS), and the Department of Defense (DOD) (Moore 1996).The Bureau of Labor Statistics prepares a Producer Price Index for Prescription Drugs, called PPI-DRUGS, that reports drug price statistics. PPI-DRUGS reported that the price of prescription drugs increased an average of three times the increase in economy-wide inflation between 1980 and 1990. However, subsequent analyses by the GAO (1995d) suggest that this index overstated drug prices substantially because of the way it sampled drugs to measure and other calculation errors. The GAO noted that price indexes measure price changes rather than price levels. The indexes can thus be used to determine whether prices rise rapidly, but not whether the prices are excessive.

## Medical Devices

A medical device is any item promoted for a medical purpose that does not rely on a chemical action to achieve its desired effect. Types of medical devices range from the simple tongue depressor to complex imaging equipment. Medical devices are most generally used by a health services provider, rather than the patient. Assistive technology devices, such as powered mobility devices to aid a person with physical or other limitations, are addressed in the discussion of durable medical equipment and supplies later in the chapter.

*FDA Review of Medical Devices*

As of 1976, the FDA must review medical devices to ensure their safety and effectiveness. The FDA categorizes medical devices into three classes and assesses three tiers of risk or hazard. Class I devices are the least regulated; about 40 percent of the 1,700 types of devices reviewed by the FDA are categorized in Class I. About 12 percent of the devices reviewed by the FDA are categorized as Class III, the most regulated devices (USGAO 1995b; Kessler, Pape, and Sundwall 1987).

*FDA Premarket Notification*

About 90 percent of all device applications reach the market through the FDA premarket notification process, also called the 510k process because its authority resides in Section 510k of the FDCA. In the premarket notification process, manufacturers notify the FDA of their plans to market a product that is similar to one already approved by the agency and thus not likely to pose a significant risk to public safety. If the FDA agrees that the proposed device is substantially equivalent to the predicate device, it may approve the product's development and distribution (USGAO 1995b; Kessler, Pape, and Sundwall 1987; Zimmerman 1994).

New types of devices require a more stringent level of FDA review, which is called the premarket approval (PMA) process. The FDA makes its determination on the device's safety and effectiveness from clinical trial data submitted by the sponsor (USGAO 1995b). The data may be derived from well-controlled clinical trials, partially controlled studies, studies and objective trials without controls, well-documented case histories, or significant human experience with a marketed device (Grady 1992). The FDA assigns all new devices and transitional devices, which are devices that were regulated as drugs prior to 1976, to Class III for the most rigorous level of assessment.

FDA
Investigational
Device
Exemption

The FDA also regulates research conducted to determine the safety and effectiveness of unapproved devices and must approve those deemed to hold significant risk in their use. Such research is conducted under the auspices of an investigational device exemption (IDE) granted by the FDA to exempt the device from the FDA's regulatory requirements while the research is being conducted (USGAO 1995b).

FDA Regulation
of Biologics

The FDA also regulates certain biologics. Two types of applications cover biologics: priority biologics license applications (BLAs) are for products that, if approved, involve a significant improvement in the safety or effectiveness of the treatment, diagnosis, or prevention of a serious or life-threatening disease. Nonpriority BLAs are considered standard BLAs (USGAO 2005).

Criticism of FDA
Device Review
Process

Manufacturers, prospective consumers, and others sometimes fault the FDA for the length of time it takes to review and act on device applications. Critics have proposed that review processes used in other industrialized countries be considered as substitutions for the FDA process. Some point out that less-rigorous review may be appropriate for certain devices, such as those that affect only a very low volume of patients. For such devices, the costs required for the clinical studies to proceed through the approval process may far exceed the financial return from sales (Zimmerman 1994), a situation similar to the orphan drug dilemma.

The GAO evaluated FDA reviews of medical devices that were submitted between 1989 and mid-1995 (USGAO 1995b). Table 10.6 shows the FDA-permitted time limits and the median and mean times for FDA reviews of both premarket notification and PMA devices. The review times include periods during which the manufacturer is responding to FDA queries for additional information or clarification; 20 to 25 percent of the review time has been estimated to be non-FDA review time. The number of premarket notification devices was relatively constant during this period, whereas the number of PMA devices under review declined. The GAO found that the review time for devices varied widely over the study period. The review time for premarket devices was relatively stable from 1989 to 1991, rose sharply in 1992 and 1993, and then dropped in 1994. The review time for PMAs was less clear, in part because a large proportion of applications were not completed at the time of the review.

Suggestions for reducing the FDA review time for medical devices include the establishment of more specific performance standards for the various device classes (Kessler, Pape, and Sundwall 1987), clearer definitions of what constitutes significant versus nonsignificant risk of devices (Sherertz and Streed 1994), and an increased use of external contract research organizations (CROs) to test new drugs and devices (Zimmerman 1994). The European Union (EU) uses private organizations to review some devices, but the EU's approach to regulating devices has not had enough working

**TABLE 10.6**
FDA Review Times for Medical Devices (1988–1994)

### Premarket Notification Devices

| Date of Application Submission | Average Number of Applications under Review | FDA Allowable Time (Days) | Median Review Time (Days) | Mean Review Time (Days) |
|---|---|---|---|---|
| 1989–1991 | 4,801 | 90 | 80–90 | 124 |
| 1993 | 4,654 | 90 | 230 | 263 |
| 1994 | 4,342 | 90 | 152 | 166 |

### Premarket Approval Devices

| Date of Application Submission | Average Number of Applications under Review | FDA Allowable Time (Days) | Median Review Time (Days) | Mean Review Time (Days) |
|---|---|---|---|---|
| 1989 | 84 | 180 | 414 | NA |
| 1992 | 66 | 180 | 984 | 336 |

SOURCE: USGAO 1995b.

NOTE: NA = data not available.

experience to serve as a model for device review in the United States (USGAO 1996).

The 1997 FDA Modernization and Accountability Act permits the FDA to regulate medical devices for uses not named on their labels if "there is a reasonable likelihood that the device will be used for an intended use not identified in the proposed labeling" that could cause harm (Reichard 1997).

In 2002, Congress passed the Medical Device User Fee and Modernization Act (MDUFMA), a counterpart to the PDUFA described earlier. The MDUFMA provides the FDA with additional resources to ensure prompt approval or clearance of applications for marketing medical devices and licensing biological products[2] (USGAO 2005). FDA must set and meet certain performance goals in return for the additional fees received. The GAO is required to annually report on the FDA's achievement of these performance goals. A mid-2005 GAO analysis indicated that the FDA would likely meet a proportion of the 20 performance goals set for that year, but perhaps be unable to meet all 20. A final determination, of course, could not be made until complete data are available for the full year (USGAO 2005).

## Durable Medical Equipment and Supplies

Durable medical equipment (DME) such as wheelchairs and supplies such as surgical dressings, prostheses, and orthoses are aspects of health services technology that are sometimes overlooked. Expenditures for DME, vision products, and other supplies constitute less than 2 percent of total expenditures for personal health care. However, the proportion of the population that requires such aids and supplies due to chronic or disabling conditions is growing as the population ages and as technologic advances salvage more lives and increase life spans.

Both the Medicare and Medicaid programs, which pay for care for elderly and disabled people, have begun to institute controls on expenditures for equipment and supplies. In 2004, Medicare spent $6.5 billion out of $299.6 billion, or 2.2 percent of total expenditures for personal health care, on DME and $1.9 billion (<1 percent of expenditures) on nondurable medical products (CMS 2005). Medicare and Medicaid billings for equipment and supplies have become so vulnerable to fraud that the Centers for Medicare and Medicaid Services (CMS), their administrative agency, has initiated controls to reduce the excessive payments known to have been made for equipment and supplies (USGAO 1995a, 1995c). Medicare and Medicaid practices of leasing rather than purchasing certain kinds of equipment, such as nebulizers, has also occasioned concern about these kinds of expenditures. The long-term costs of such leases may far exceed the equipment's purchase price, but the more economically efficient route of purchase usually runs afoul of governmental regulations on equipment purchases.

A separate but important category of medical equipment is that of assistive technology devices such as mobility aids, microcomputers, and powered mobility devices that an estimated 5 percent of people in the United States require to increase their ability to communicate and to accommodate their physical impairments (LePlante, Hendershot, and Moss 1992). Private or public insurance coverage varies significantly for assistive technology devices.

### Medical and Surgical Procedures

Three types of medical and surgical procedures contribute significantly to health services technology: therapeutic advances, such as heart-lung transplantation; diagnostic advances, both invasive and noninvasive; and preventive advances that avoid the onset or ameliorate the effects of disease (Grady 1992). This section focuses on how medical and surgical advances move from investigative or experimental stages to accepted practice.

Physicians and other scientists continuously seek new ways to treat illness and disease, to improve quality of life, and to prolong life. Search strategies include applying current procedures or drugs in new situations, often called off-label uses, as well as developing new procedures. The point at which a new procedure is safe and effective enough for general application in a population is not easily determined and may be affected by whether the patient's condition is deemed to be terminal or nonterminal (Grady 1992). The controversy over the use of autologous bone marrow transplant

(ABMT) for women with end-stage breast cancer is a case in point. The effectiveness of this costly procedure is not fully known, but it is one of the few therapies available and thus is a sought-after treatment, even though some insurers still consider it experimental. This is one of a number of instances where the decision about a procedure's effectiveness may be made in the legal rather than in the medical system.

When new drugs are developed, their initial use—in animals and eventually in humans—is experimental. As experience with a drug is gained and its principal side effects become known, a drug that produces the desired outcomes moves along a continuum of acceptance from experimental to standard practice. In an effort to clarify the movement of a new procedure along the experimental-accepted practice continuum, the American Medical Association's Diagnosis and Therapeutic Technology Assessment Program includes the following in its definition of "investigational" (Grady 1992):

**Investigational/ Experimental vs. Therapeutic, State-of-the-Art Technologies**

- off-label use of drugs and devices;
- National Cancer Institute Group C cancer drugs and FDA investigational new drugs;
- medical services for which outcomes are not yet known;
- medical services not yet evaluated by well-designed, well-controlled clinical trials;
- medical services whose beneficial effects have not been shown to be attainable outside an investigational setting;
- medical services for which supportive evidence does not exist in the medical community regarding their safety or effectiveness;
- medical services for which beneficial effects are outweighed by harmful ones; and
- alternative medical therapies not widely recognized by the medical community.

In the absence of an assessment of the technology, insurers have several ways to control their coverage for the technology (Newcomer, 1990). They may:

- develop a list of coverage exclusions, which must be kept current;
- establish criteria for what constitutes experimental therapy, including requirements for a minimal number of treated patients whose cases have been reported, a threshold rate of cure and improvement in quality of life, and results of a randomized clinical trial (RCT) that establishes the benefit of a new therapy over the conventional one;
- allow coverage if a patient is enrolled in a RCT; or
- make decisions on a case-by-case basis.

### Halfway Technologies

Along the continuum of investigative to standard practice procedures are technologies sometimes called halfway technologies, meaning that they are an interim procedure that can be used effectively until scientific advances provide a more complete solution. Renal dialysis was considered by some to be a halfway technology, maintaining life for ESRD patients until kidney transplantation was fully developed enough to replace it for suitable patients. The multidrug "cocktails"—the antiviral protease inhibitors that are currently being used to delay the full onset of AIDS or ameliorate its effects—may prove to be a halfway technology, but at this stage in their usage, the long-term effects of this intervention have yet to be fully evaluated.

## Technology Assessment

Assessing the readiness of a new procedure for general application is a relatively recent field of scientific endeavor called technology assessment (TA). TA is any process of examining and reporting properties of medical technology used in health services, such as safety, efficacy, feasibility, indications for use, cost, cost-effectiveness, and the social, economic, and ethical consequences, whether intended or unintended (Rettig 1994). Table 10.7 outlines dimensions that can be considered in performing TAs.

### Randomized Clinical Trials

The gold standard for TA is the randomized clinical (controlled) trial (RCT), in which a carefully designed and controlled research study compares an intervention in treatment and control populations. RCTs do not occur with every innovation for a variety of reasons, including the time and expense required and the difficulty of establishing a control group

**TABLE 10.7**
Dimensions of Health Services Technology Assessment

- Technical performance
- Clinical efficacy
- Safety
- Cost and efficiency
- Acceptability and attractiveness
- Research value
- Effects on medical care system
- Potential need for procedure
- Relevant constraints on available technology
- Benefit-cost and cost effectiveness assessed for economic and social costs, including lives saved
- Quality of life
- Patient preferences

when withholding a treatment, even an experimental one, is deemed unethical. RCTs often may not be conducted or completed until after the intervention has become well established, making it difficult to eradicate ineffective technologies.

## Who Is Responsible for TA?

The question of whether TA is the responsibility of the public sector, the private sector, or both remains unresolved. Governmental initiatives such as the NIH Consensus Development conferences remain in effect, but other governmental programs, such as the congressional Office of Technology Assessment (OTA), have been repealed. The role of the private section remains in flux as well.

Like the health services system from which it emanates, TA is not a centralized or uniform activity. Several major governmental units are responsible for discrete aspects of TA (e.g., the FDA for drugs and devices), but a centralized and authoritative governmental body for TA does not exist.

**Government Role in TA**

One of the earliest federal government efforts at TA was the National Center for Health Care Technology, which existed from 1978 to 1982. In 1983, the Office of Health Technology Assessment (OHTA) was established at the National Center for Health Services Research (NCHSR), which subsequently became the Agency for Health Care Policy and Research (AHCPR), and in 1997, became the Agency for Healthcare Research and Quality (AHRQ). AHRQ has had limited funds to conduct TAs, including some for the Medicare program. The OTA, established in the early 1970s, responded to congressional requests for TAs in many fields, including health services, but was abolished in fiscal year 1996.

Other governmental agencies, such as the U.S. Government Accountability Office (GAO; formerly known as the U.S. General Accounting Office) and the Congressional Budget Office (CBO), do limited TAs in response to congressional requests. The two agencies responsible for making recommendations on Medicare provider payment—the Prospective Payment Assessment Commission (PROPAC) and the Physician Payment Reform Commission (PhysPRC or PPRC; both acronyms have been used)—consider the effects of technologies on Medicare reimbursement rates but do not actively conduct TAs (Rettig 1994). The 1997 Balanced Budget Act consolidated these two separate agencies into the Medicare Payment Advisory Commission (MedPAC).

One TA process to determine the readiness for adoption of a new procedure into general practice is the NIH Consensus Development Conference, which was established in 1976 as a way to help both practitioners and payers determine the clinical status of a new procedure. The NIH convenes a panel of

**NIH Consensus Development Conferences**

experts on the topic, provides the most currently available data and studies, including those that support and oppose the procedure, and requires the expert group to issue a statement of consensus about the procedure. Consensus conference reports issued by the NIH cover a wide range of medical and surgical procedures, including the morbidity and mortality of dialysis (USDHHS 1993), optimum calcium intake (NIH 1994), physical activity and cardiovascular health (NIH 1995), cochlear implants for adults and children (AMA 1996), management of hepatitis C (NIH 1997), and diagnosis and treatment of attention deficit hyperactivity disorder (ADHD) (NIH 1998).

**TA for the Medicare Program**

Medicare is often considered the bellwether for other payers in determining the technologies for which it will reimburse. The AHRQ Office of Health Technology Assessment (OHTA) assesses between one and nine technologies per year for Medicare to determine the appropriateness of Medicare reimbursement (USGAO 1994a). Medicare's administrative body—the CMS—conducts between 20 and 30 national coverage decisions for various technologies each year. The considerations that the CMS takes into account when assessing the coverage potential for a new technology include the likely expense to Medicare, the potential for widespread use in medical practice, the level of disagreement regarding the technology's safety and effectiveness, and the variation among coverage decisions by the 28 Medicare fiscal intermediaries (CMS 2005; USGAO 1994a; Glenn 1989).

**TA in the Private Sector**

The private sector also has had an episodic role in TA. At the national level, the Institute of Medicine (IOM), a unit of the National Academy of Sciences, sponsored a Council on Health Care Technology from 1986 to 1990 (Rettig 1994). Third-party payers are increasingly supporting the assessment of technologies. Individual Blue Cross/Blue Shield plans have long been involved in the support of and requirement for TA as a basis for insurance coverage decisions. Other insurers and health maintenance organizations (HMOs) may assess outcomes to evaluate the use of technologies, whereas hospitals are inclined to use financial analyses as the bases for their technology decisions (Luce and Brown 1995).

Because TA is decentralized, timely assessment of all technologies is not assured. The technologies most likely to be assessed are those with the highest unit cost, such as solid-organ transplantation or the latest generation of imaging equipment. Technologies with lower unit costs, such as some laboratory tests, may actually account for greater expenditures because of their volume but may be less frequently assessed, a phenomenon that some call "big-ticket" versus "little-ticket" technology (Moloney and Rogers 1979).

## Technology Reassessment

Even if a technology is assessed, a one-time assessment may not be sufficient (Banta and Thacker 1990). Health services technology has a life cycle, and periodic reassessment is important to take into account other changes in health services delivery and to assess the technology's effectiveness over a longer time period.

One factor important to the reassessment process is the variability of physician practice, which may vary by age cohort (Ginzberg 1990), geographic region (Wennberg, Bunker, and Barnes 1980), physician specialty, the training focus of the physician's medical school and residency programs, and other factors. The study of variations in physician practice constitutes a growing field of scientific inquiry to better understand the outcomes that derive from the care rendered.

## Eradicating an Ineffective Technology

If a technology is found to be ineffective upon initial assessment or reassessment, that finding alone is not always sufficient to eradicate the practice or usage. Technologies may diffuse widely and quickly, even in advance of an assessment, and their widespread use and often long-standing acceptance may create resistance to their discontinuation, even when solid evidence shows them to be ineffective.

The use of intermittent positive pressure breathing (IPPB) to treat chronic obstructive pulmonary disease (COPD) and other lung conditions exemplifies the difficulty of phasing out an outmoded technology (Duffy and Farley 1993). Results from a 1983 NIH clinical trial concluded that IPPB was no better than the less costly and less dangerous nebulizer for treating stable COPD patients in an outpatient setting. A subsequent assessment by the AHCPR OHTA in 1991 also concluded that IPPB, although useful in certain rare circumstances, is not generally helpful in treating COPD. Although the use of IPPB declined, it has not ceased entirely, despite clear indications of its ineffectiveness for COPD.

Ineffective technologies linger for several reasons, including physician practice habits, the lack of an effective alternative, or because third-party payers still reimburse their use (Duffy and Farley 1993).

# The Role of Health Technology in a Changing Health Services System

Pressures to contain or reduce the U.S. health services system are being exerted by employers who provide health insurance to their employees, by third-party payers such as Medicare and Medicaid, and by others concerned about this industry's growth rates. The development and application of health services technology has had a significant role in the growth of health services expenditures.

How likely is it that this culture can be weaned of its enthusiastic support for and dependence on health services technologies? Rettig (1994) argues that this culture has two competing goals for its health services system: to moderate the growth of medical expenditures and to maintain its world-class capacity to innovate in medicine. The commitment to innovation is perhaps greater and more deeply rooted than is the commitment to moderate medical expenditures. Evidence for this commitment can be seen in the funding for biomedical research, the powerful lobbies for specific diseases, the accelerated rate of FDA approvals of new drugs that may combat life-threatening diseases, orphan drug legislation, and the restoration and expansion of patent terms for drugs.

### Effects of Managed Care on Technology Assessment

Whether technological innovation can continue unabated is not clear. The influences of managed care in changing the delivery system and other efforts to control health services expenditures can be seen on health services technology. The emphasis on technologic innovation is shifting from breakthrough technologies to cost-saving ones, and a parallel shift from inpatient to outpatient technologies is evident (Kessler, Pape, and Sundwall 1987).

The pharmaceutical industry, a major force in health services technology, is feeling the effects of managed care. Extensive restructuring, or reengineering, is occurring in this highly competitive industry. Managed care is also stimulating the increased use of formularies, which limit the types of drugs a provider may prescribe and often emphasize the use of generics over brand-name drugs (Moore 1996).

### Ethical Concerns about Uses of Health Services Technology

What constitutes an ethical use of technology will continue to be debated as the U.S. health services system undergoes change. Scientific advances have in many instances outpaced abilities to reasonably, much less ethically, apply them. The debate about the technological ability to extend lives versus quality of life remains unresolved (Ginzberg 1990; Angell 1990). Potentially ineffective care—care rendered when there is little or no prospect of patient benefit—and its effects on growing health services expenditures is emerging as a topic of consideration. The potential for affecting genetic makeup raises the debate to a higher pitch, but resolutions remain elusive.

### Proposed Controls on the Use of Health Services Technology

Suggestions for controlling the use of health services technologies abound. Melski (1992) recommended that the misapplication or overuse of technology be examined. Must harmless seborrheic keratoses and benign moles be removed? Should an MRI be done for every chronic headache? Are thallium stress tests appropriate for chest pain in low-risk patients? Should endoscopies be done for minor gastrointestinal complaints?

Moloney and Rogers (1979), early spokespeople on health technology issues, identified five strategies for the use of health technologies:

1. Limit the development of certain technologies while they are still in the pipeline.
2. Use benefit-cost studies to set priorities for the development and distribution of technologies.
3. Limit distribution of big and expensive technologies within regions according to population and epidemiologic characteristics.
4. Eliminate the use of technologies that have no clinical value.
5. Provide reimbursement for technologies only when they are used according to protocols.

Luce and Brown (1995) recommend that TA be expanded and strengthened by generating good, timely data; fostering collective efforts for TA; having payers grant interim coverage for a technology in exchange for funding support for effective TAs; increasing expertise and training in TAs; and fostering cost-effectiveness studies.

Rettig (1994) offers several policy options for dealing with the conflict between societal goals of moderating health services expenditure growth and maintaining the system's ability to innovate. These options include watchful waiting, tightening the boundary between existing and new technologies, limiting the supply of medical technology, constraining investment in biomedical research and development, and increasing analytic capabilities for assessing technologies.

## Summary

Biomedical research and the range of health technologies, including drugs, medical devices, and medical and surgical procedures, are major contributors to a world-class health services system. World-class systems, however, require world-class financing, setting up the tension between maintaining health services innovations and moderating the growth of health services expenditures. A more extensive use of technology assessment at the earliest possible point in an innovation, coupled with provider and patient education on the results of such findings, offers one way to address this conflict between primary societal goals.

## Notes

1. The amount of federal research support differs in Table 10.2 and Figure 10.2. The number in Table 10.2 is larger because it includes more than NIH funds.
2. The term *approval* is generally used for applications for new devices, while the term *clearance* is used for devices that are substantially equivalent to those legally on the market.

## Key Words

Agency for Health Care Policy and
    Research (AHCPR)
Agency for Healthcare Research and
    Quality (AHRQ)
American Medical Association (AMA)
assistive technology devices
"big-ticket versus "little-ticket"
    technology
biomedical research
breakthrough technologies
Centers for Disease Control and
    Prevention (CDC)
Congressional Budget Office (CBO)
consumer protection
contract review organization (CRO)
cost-saving technologies
Council on Health Care Technology
Department of Defense (DOD)
Department of Veterans Affairs (VA)
drug rebates
durable medical equipment (DME)
European Union (EU)
FDA premarket approval
FDA premarket notification
fiscal intermediaries
Food and Drug Act
Food and Drug Administration (FDA)
Food, Drug, and Cosmetic Act (FDCA)
formularies
generic drugs
gross domestic product (GDP)

halfway technology
health services technology
health maintenance organization
    (HMO)
Institute of Medicine (IOM)
investigational device exemption
investigational/experimental practice
investigational new drug (IND)
managed care
Medical Device User Fee and
    Modernization Act (MDUFMA)
medical devices
Medicare Payment Advisory
    Commission (MedPAC)
National Center for Health Care
    Technology
National Center for Health Services
    Research (NCHSR)
National Institutes of Health (NIH)
new drug application (NDA)
NIH Consensus Development
    Conference
Office of Health Technology
    Assessment (OHTA)
Office of Technology Assessment
    (OTA)
off-label use
omnibus budget reconciliation act
    (OBRA)
orphan drugs
over-the-counter (OTC) drugs

physician practice variations
Physician Reform Payment
    Commission (PhysPRC)
potentially ineffective care
Prescription Drug User Fee Act (PDUFA)
Producer Price Index for Prescription
    Drugs (PPI-DRUGS)
Prospective Payment Assessment
    Commission (PROPAC)

Public Health Service (PHS)
randomized clinical (controlled) trial
    (RCT)
reengineering
technology assessment (TA)
transitional medical devices
watchful waiting

# References

American Medical Association. 1996. "National Institutes of Health Consensus Statement: Cochlear Implants in Adults and Children." *Technology News* 9 (2): 5, 7–8.

Angell, M. 1990. "Prisoners of Technology: The Case of Nancy Cruzan." *New England Journal of Medicine* 322 (17): 1226–28.

Banta, H. D., and S. B. Thacker. 1990. "The Case for Reassessment of Health Care Technology: Once Is Not Enough." *Journal of the American Medical Association* 264 (2): 235–40.

Centers for Medicare and Medicaid Services (CMS). 2005. "Highlights— National Health Expenditures 2004." [Online information; retrieved 1/12/2006.] http://cms.hhs.gov/statistics/nhe/historical/highlights.asp.

Congressional Budget Office. 1992. *Projections of National Health Expenditures.* Washington, DC: CBO.

Duffy, S. Q., and D. E. Farley. 1993. "Intermittent Positive Pressure Breathing: Old Technologies Rarely Die." *Provider Studies Research Note #8.* Bethesda, MD: Agency for Health Care Policy and Research.

Food and Drug Administration. 2006. [Online information; retrieved 1/17/2006.] www.fda.gov/cder/handbook/develop.htm.

Frist, W. H. 2002. "Federal Funding for Biomedical Research." *Journal of the American Medical Association* 287 (13): 1722–24.

Ginzberg, E. 1990. "High Technology Medicine (HTM) and Rising Health Care Costs." *Journal of the American Medical Association* 263 (13): 1820–22.

Glenn, K. J. 1989. "Perspectives. Assessing Medical Technology." *McGraw-Hill's Medicine & Health* 43 (22): supplement 4p.

Grady, M. L. 1992. *Summary Report, New Medical Technology: Experimental or State of the Art.* AHCPR Pub. No. 92-0057. Rockville, MD: Agency for Health Care Policy and Research.

Keyhani, S., M. Diener-West, and N. Powe. 2005. "Do Drug Prices Reflect Development Time and Government Investment?" *Medical Care* 43 (8): 753–62.

Kessler, D. A., S. M. Pape, and D. N. Sundwall. 1987. "The Federal Regulation of Medical Devices." *New England Journal of Medicine* 217 (6): 357–66.

Kudva, G. C., B. T. Collins, and F. R. Dunphy. 2001. "Thalidomide for Malignant Melanoma." *New England Journal of Medicine* 345 (16): 1214–15.

LePlante, M. P., G. E. Hendershot, and A. J. Moss. 1992. "Assistive Technology Devices and Home Accessibility Features: Prevalence, Payment, Need, and Trends." *Advance Data* 217 (September 16): 1–11.

Levit, K. R., H. C. Lazenby, and L. Sivarajan. 1996. "Health Care Spending in 1994: Slowest in Decades." *Health Affairs* 15 (2): 130–44.

Luce, B. R., and R. E. Brown. 1995. "The Use of Technology Assessment by Hospitals, HMOs, and Third Party Payers in the U.S." *International Journal of Technology Assessment in Health Care* 11 (1): 79–92.

McKinley, J. B. 1981. "From 'Promising Report' to 'Standard Procedure': Seven Stages in the Career of a Medical Innovation." *The Milbank Memorial Fund Quarterly* 59 (3): 374–411.

Melski, J. W. 1992. "Price of Technology: A Blind Spot." *Journal of the American Medical Association* 267 (11): 1516–18.

Moloney, T. W., and D. E. Rogers. 1979. "Medical Technology—A Different View of the Contentious Debate over Costs." *New England Journal of Medicine* 301 (26): 1413–19.

Moore, J. 1996. *The Pharmaceutical Industry.* Washington, DC: National Health Policy Forum.

Moses, H., E. R. Dorsey, D. H. M. Matheson, and S. O. Their. 2005. "Financial Anatomy of Biomedical Research." *Journal of the American Medical Association* 294 (11): 1333–42.

National Institutes of Health. 2006. "Institutes, Centers, and Officers." [Online information; retrieved 6/3/06.] www.nih.gov/icd.

———. 1998. "Diagnosis and Treatment of Attention Deficit Hyperactivity Disorder (ADHD)." *NIH Consensus Statement* 16 (2): 1–37.

———. 1997. "Management of Hepatitis C." *NIH Consensus Statement* 15 (3): 1–41.

———. 1995. "Physical Activity and Cardiovascular Health." *NIH Consensus Statement* 13 (3): 1–33.

———. 1994. "Optimum Calcium Intake." *Journal of the American Medical Association* 272 (24): 1942–48.

Newcomer, L. N. 1990. "Defining Experimental Therapy: A Third Party Payer's Dilemma." *New England Journal of Medicine* 323 (24): 1702–04.

Olson, M. K. 2004. "Explaining Reductions in FDA Drug Review Times: PDUFA Matters." *Health Affairs Web Exclusive.* [Online article; posted 1/30/04.] http://content.healthaffairs.org/cgi/content/full/hlthaff.w4.s1v1/DC1.

Reichard, J. (ed.) 1997. "Study Says Medigap May Become Unaffordable to Oldest, Sickest." *Medicine and Health* 51 (35): 2.

Rettig, R. A. 1994. "Medical Innovation Duels Cost Containment." *Health Affairs* 13 (3): 7–27.

Sherertz, R. J., and S. A. Streed. 1994. "Medical Devices: Significant vs. Nonsignificant Risk." *New England Journal of Medicine* 272 (12): 955–56.

Spilker, B. A. 2002. "The Drug Development and Approval Process." [Online information; retrieved 4/1/03.] www.pharma.org/newmedicines/newmedsdb/phases.pdf.

U.S. Department of Health and Human Services. 2005. *Health, United States, 2005.* Pub. No. (PHS) 05-1232. Hyattsville, MD: USDHHS.

———. 2002. *Health, United States, 2002.* Pub. No. (PHS) 02-1232. Hyattsville, MD: USDHHS.

———. 1993. *Morbidity and Mortality of Dialysis: NIH Consensus Statement.* Bethesda, MD: National Institutes of Health.

U.S. Government Accountability Office (formerly the U.S. General Accounting Office). 2005. *FDA: Limited Available Data Indicate That FDA Has Been Meeting Some Goals for Review of Medical Device Applications.* GAO-05-1042. September. Washington, DC: USGAO.

———. 1996. *Medical Device Regulation: Too Early to Assess European System's Value as Model for FDA.* USGAO/HEHS-96-65. March. Washington, DC: USGAO.

———. 1995a. *Durable Medical Equipment: Regional Carriers' Coverage Criteria are Consistent with Medicare Law.* USGAO/HEHS-95-185. September. Washington, DC: USGAO.

———. 1995b. *Medical Devices: FDA Review Time.* GAO/PEMD-96-2. October. Washington, DC: USGAO.

———. 1995c. *Medicare: Excessive Payments for Medical Supplies Continue Despite Improvements.* USGAO/HEHS-95-171. August. Washington, DC: USGAO.

———. 1995d. *Prescription Drug Prices: Official Index Overstates Producer Price Inflation.* USGAO/HEHS-95-90. April. Washington, DC: USGAO.

———. 1994a. *Medicare: Technology Assessment and Medical Coverage Decisions.* USGAO/HEHS-94-195FS. July. Washington, DC: USGAO.

———. 1994b. *Prescription Drugs: Spending Controls in Four European Countries.* USGAO/HEHS-94-30. May. Washington, DC: USGAO.

Varmus, H. 1995. "Shattuck Lecture: Biomedical Research Enters the Steady State." *New England Journal of Medicine* 333 (12): 811–15.

Wennberg, J. E., J. P. Bunker, and B. Barnes. 1980. "The Need for Assessing the Outcome of Common Medical Practices." *Annual Review of Public Health* 1: 277–95.

Zerhouni, E. H. 2005. "U.S. Biomedical Research—Basic, Translational, and Clinical Sciences." *Journal of the American Medical Association* 294 (11): 1352–58.

Zimmerman, D. L. 1994. *Medical Technology and Health Reform: Devising Policy for the Medical Device Market.* Washington, DC: National Health Policy Forum.

# THE DELIVERY SYSTEM

# OVERVIEW OF THE U.S. HEALTH SERVICES DELIVERY SYSTEM

## Introduction

Parts I through V of this book describe the components of a health services system: its organization and management, the economic support it receives and how it finances health services, and the production of resources, such as the workforce, facilities, and technologies.

Part VI builds on this solid foundation, with a focus on how health services are delivered. Four central aspects of the U.S. health services delivery system are addressed:

1. what kinds of care are delivered (i.e., the continuum of care);
2. how health services are delivered, with an emphasis on the evolving role of managed care and the changes it brings to the delivery system;
3. the care of special disorders or populations, using the population with mental illness and developmental disabilities as an illustration of care of special disorders; and
4. maintaining quality of care in the delivery system.

This chapter provides an overview of the U.S. health services delivery system and outlines how the remainder of Part VI is organized.

## The Continuum of Health Services in the U.S. System

A comprehensive health services system includes womb-to-tomb care, beginning with timely and effective prenatal care and ending with palliative care in the last days of life. Figure 11.1 shows the continuum of services one would expect to find in a comprehensive health services delivery system. As earlier chapters have emphasized, this comprehensive continuum exists in the U.S. system, although not all people have access to all parts of the continuum; access may be inhibited by financial, cultural, temporal, geographic, or other barriers. The continuum begins with prenatal care to ensure, to the extent possible, healthy outcomes for mothers and infants.

**FIGURE 11.1**

Continuum of
Health Services

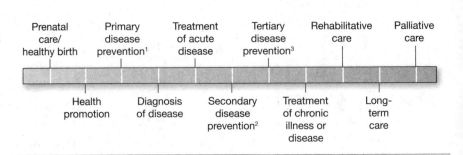

NOTES: 1. Primary disease prevention is preventing agents from causing disease or injury. 2. Secondary disease prevention is early detection and treatment to cure and/or control the cause of disease. 3. Tertiary disease prevention is ameliorating the seriousness of disease by decreasing disability and the dependence resulting from it.

## Prenatal Care

Reproduction to ensure the perpetuation of a species was long assumed to be the most natural of processes, requiring limited involvement of a health services system. Indeed, with only rudimentary knowledge about pregnancy and birth until the advent of modern medicine, few useful interventions were possible. With the increasing sophistication of health services, the importance of prenatal care to healthy outcomes has been widely recognized in industrialized countries with comprehensive delivery systems. Less developed countries may not yet have or employ resources for prenatal care. In recent years, the United States has focused increased attention and resources on improved birth outcomes, but a significant number of pregnant women either do not have access to prenatal care or do not avail themselves of it.

The importance of adequate maternal and child care in the U.S. delivery system was recognized as early as 1921 with the passage of the Shepherd-Towner Act, which provided federal grants to states to establish maternal and child care programs through 1929 (Shonick 1995). Repeated studies have confirmed the importance of adequate prenatal care as early as possible in the gestation. Despite this evidence, nearly 4 percent of all expectant mothers in the United States in 2003 did not receive care until their third trimester or received no care at all (USDHHS 2005). More than twice as many black as white mothers received only third-trimester or no care during this period (see Figure 2.30 in Chapter 2). Advanced technologies have reduced maternal and infant death rates and enabled the survival of even very low-birthweight babies, aiding many of them to lead healthy and productive lives. Many other health problems for the mother and the infant could be averted, however, if all pregnant women received appropriate and timely prenatal care.

## Health Promotion

Promoting good health practices to preserve and enhance health status is the next step on the continuum of services one would expect to find in a comprehensive health services delivery system. Health promotion is a relatively recent focus of the U.S. system, which typically has been oriented to curative care. Advancements in health promotion are due as much to consumer advocates as to health services providers. It has been known for some time that healthy behaviors and lifestyles deter illness and disease, and clinical research results increasingly document how lifestyle and behaviors affect mortality and morbidity (U.S. Department of Health and Human Services [USDHHS] 1991). Health promotion focuses on physical activity and fitness, proper management of body weight, nutrition, eliminating tobacco use, controlling the use of alcohol and other drugs, family planning, support of mental health and mental disorders detection, addressing violent and abusive behavior, and sponsoring educational and community-based health programs.

## Health Protection

Health protection is the preservation of a safe and healthy environment, generally the purview of public health. Public health assumed this role as the transmission of diseases such as cholera that affect the public's health began to be understood. Safe drinking water, clean and uncontaminated air, and appropriate disposal of hazardous and other wastes are essential to the prevention of many communicable and other diseases. A recent focus on health promotion is considering the built environment and the extent to which community design encourages or inhibits healthy behaviors, such as walking, biking, and other outdoor exercise.

## Disease Prevention: Primary, Secondary, and Tertiary

Prevention specialists identify three levels of disease prevention: primary, secondary, and tertiary.

**Primary Disease Prevention**

Primary disease prevention is preventing agents from causing disease or injury to a person or a population. Genetic testing/counseling and health screenings are two ways to recognize and prevent the potential for disease. Each detection method generates both support and opposition.

   Genetic testing and counseling may, for example, assist couples in determining whether a genetically transmitted trait or condition is likely to occur among their offspring. Such testing, as well as human genome research, creates concerns about the ethical applications in a human population, an area that most agree requires much more research and analysis. Screening for potential disease raises at least two issues: First, should screening be done if it can detect the potential for a disease but little or nothing is known about ameliorating the condition? Second, how cost-effective is screening for potential disease? If the incidence rate of the disease is very low, are mass screenings cost-effective? What is the cost of averting one case of the disease? What are the benefits of averting one case of disease?

**Secondary Disease Prevention**

Secondary disease prevention is the early detection and treatment to cure or control the cause of disease. Early detection may occur as the result of routine physical examinations; blood pressure readings; health screenings, including blood tests and cholesterol screens; and regular pap smears and mammograms. The individual, aware of risk factors, may also present to a health services provider with symptoms associated with a disease condition (e.g., a breast lump or a continuous headache) that leads to the early detection of a disease.

Many diseases that are detected at an early stage, including certain kinds of cancers, can be cured. Others, such as hypertension and adult onset diabetes, may be managed and controlled, thereby averting the more serious health consequences associated with these diseases when detected at a later stage.

**Tertiary Disease Prevention**

Tertiary disease prevention is ameliorating the seriousness of disease by decreasing the disability or dependence resulting from it. Tertiary prevention is intended to prevent further deterioration due to a disease and to maintain the individual's physical and functional abilities and independence for as long as possible. Counseling sessions about appropriate diet and awareness of potential foot problems for people with diabetes mellitus are examples of tertiary disease prevention. (See Chapter 12 for information about health promotion and disease prevention.)

### Diagnosis of Disease

A comprehensive health services system depends on the ability of health services providers to diagnose the presence of disease and initiate treatment. Physicians, nurse practitioners, physician assistants, and dentists are the primary diagnosticians of disease. Other health services workers, including nurses and some therapists, are also trained to detect abnormal conditions and refer the patient for medical diagnosis and treatment.

### Primary Care

As per Roemer's model of a health services system discussed in Chapter 1, primary care includes the appropriate treatment of common diseases and injuries, the provision of essential drugs, simple prophylactic and therapeutic dental care, and the identification of potentially serious physical or mental health conditions that require prompt referral for secondary or tertiary care. Primary care generally occurs in the physician's, dentist's, or therapist's office; hospital outpatient clinic; community or neighborhood health center; migrant health center; or other ambulatory care site. Essential drugs may be available through the provider's office or obtained from a pharmacy. (Chapter 13 focuses on the diagnosis of illness and disease and primary care.)

### Secondary Medical Treatment and Long-Term Care

Secondary medical treatment, according to the [Roemer model, is constituted of four types of care: ambulatory care for episodic or chronic conditions and for health maintenance; acute inpatient hospital care; care by nonmedical specialists, including optometrists, podiatrists, and physical therapists; and general long-term care (LTC).]Physicians, nurse practitioners, and physician assistants generally provide the first two types of care, either in their offices or in clinics or hospitals. LTC is often the domain of nurses and various types of therapists, including physical, speech, occupational, and recreational therapists, with periodic physician involvement. (Chapter 14 focuses on secondary medical treatment and Chapter 15 on LTC.)

### Tertiary Medical Care, Including Rehabilitative Care

Tertiary medical care is highly specialized care, usually extremely complex, and usually costly. Tertiary medical care includes, for example, liver and other complex organ transplants, treatment of diseases of the immune system, and treatment of brain and other nervous system disorders. Tertiary medical treatment generally is provided in major teaching hospitals, particularly in the 124 academic health centers (AHCs) that include medical schools and their university teaching hospitals.

Roemer's model also includes rehabilitative care with tertiary medical care. Rehabilitative care has expanded to an increasing number of physical and mental disorders as more is learned about the central nervous system. Rehabilitative care may be provided in a special unit of a tertiary hospital, particularly in a major teaching hospital, or it may be provided in hospitals or facilities that specialize in particular types of rehabilitation, such as spinal cord injuries, closed head traumas, mental illness treatment hospitals, or other centers. (Chapter 16 addresses tertiary medical treatment and rehabilitative care.)

### Palliative Care

Palliative care is end-of-life care provided to ease pain and suffering when no further medical or surgical therapies are available to treat the patient's condition. Palliative care may be provided to patients of any age in a number of settings, including the patient's home, a hospice, or a special hospital or nursing home unit. Cancers are among the principal diagnoses of patients being provided palliative care. (Chapter 17 reviews the palliative care available in the U.S. delivery system.)

## How Health Services Are Delivered

The health services delivery system, traditionally the domain of the health services provider and the individual seeking care, has become increasingly complex. Rather than one universal delivery system, the United States uses multiple modes of delivering care to its diverse populations with their varying levels and types of health insurance or their lack of insurance for care.

The major participants in these delivery systems are sometimes referred to as the "four Ps": the patient, the provider, the payer or insurance company, and the political or governmental unit. Also included as participants are the employer who provides health insurance and the entities that review the quality of care offered and the appropriateness of the utilization of services. The provider and the patient remain the traditional system participants, but some or all of the others may be involved, depending on the patient's type of health services financing.

At the risk of oversimplifying the complexity of the U.S. multisystem, Figures 11.2 through 11.10 model the participants in various delivery system modes. Although these figures cannot capture every variation in delivery system models, they illustrate some of the major models. Ongoing changes in the U.S. health services system will generate changes in the relationships among these participants. Figure 11.2 shows how health services are delivered to individuals with group health insurance employed by either of two types of employers: one that purchases health insurance for its employees and one that is self-insured and serves as both employer and health

**FIGURE 11.2**
Delivery System Participants *(a)* Individual with group health insurance. *(b)* Individual with group insurance employed by a self-insured business.

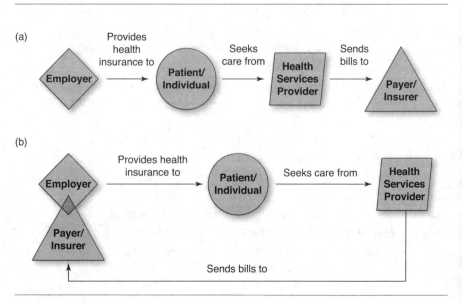

insurer to its employees. Major participants are the employer, the employee/patient, the provider, and the payer.

Figure 11.3 shows the relationships among participants for people who purchase an individual policy because they are ineligible for group health insurance or believe the individual policy is more appropriate for their circumstances. In this instance, the individual may also be self-employed and thus serve as the employer. Major participants in this delivery mode include the patient, the provider, and the payer. Figure 11.3 also shows the delivery system participants for an uninsured individual who pays out-of-pocket for all care. In this instance, the individual serves as the payer; the only other participant is the provider.

Medicare beneficiaries and Medicaid enrollees each have their own delivery system mode. Figure 11.4 portrays the delivery system for Medicare beneficiaries, who, along with their employers, pay into the Medicare trust

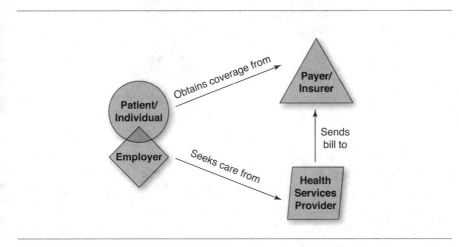

**FIGURE 11.3**
Delivery System Participants, Person with Individual Policy or Self-Pay

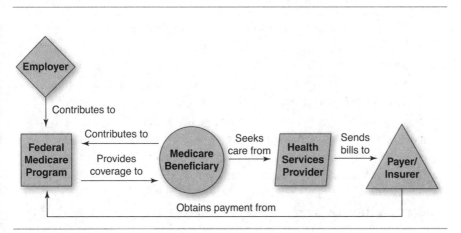

**FIGURE 11.4**
Delivery System Participants, Medicare Program

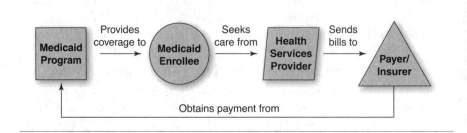

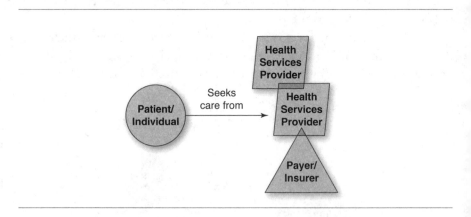

fund during their employment. The delivery system for Medicaid enrollees is shown in Figure 11.5. Medicare beneficiaries and Medicaid enrollees may also receive care in prepaid delivery systems. (In these instances, their delivery systems more closely approximate those in Figures 11.8 and 11.9.) Figure 11.6 shows a delivery system for people whose care is directly provided by governmental programs, such as the Department of Veterans Affairs (VA), the Indian Health Service (IHS), and the Department of Defense (DOD) health services systems.

The person who has neither public nor private insurance and whose funds for out-of-pocket purchases of health services are limited encounters a delivery system like the one shown in Figure 11.7. Such an individual must prevail on providers to make their services available at reduced or no charge.

The models mentioned in the preceding paragraphs apply to care financed by indemnity insurance or fee-for-service payment. They may also apply to certain types of managed care, which in its broadest definition signifies the integration of care financing and delivery. The least integrated forms of managed care, which may still reimburse for care through fee-for-service payment, include preferred provider organizations (PPOs) and independent practice associations (IPAs). The most integrated managed care

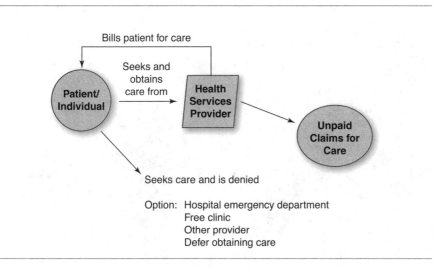

**FIGURE 11.7**
Delivery
System
Participants,
Uninsured
Persons

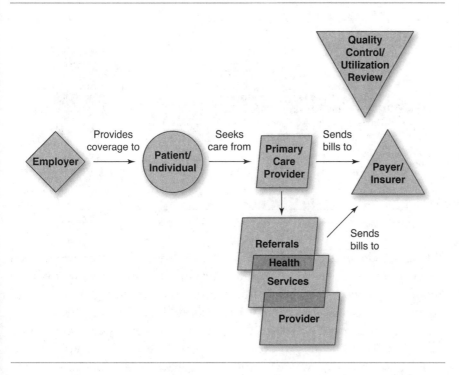

**FIGURE 11.8**
Delivery
System
Participants,
Managed Care,
External
Utilization
Review/
Control

forms include fully capitated staff model health maintenance organizations (HMOs) and integrated health networks.

For people whose health services are provided through a type of managed care, the delivery system includes an entity that reviews the quality of care or the appropriateness of utilization. Figures 11.8 and 11.9 show two

**FIGURE 11.9**
Delivery
System
Participants,
Managed Care,
Internal
Utilization
Review/
Control

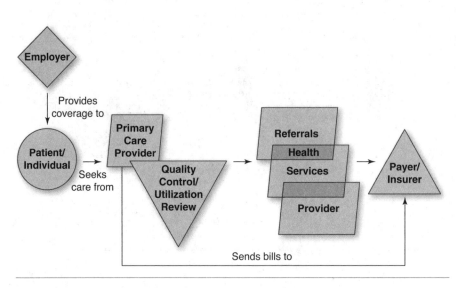

**FIGURE 11.10**
Delivery
System
Participants,
Managed Care,
Self-Insured
Employer

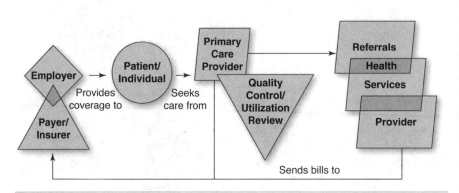

different modes of delivery systems for managed care. The difference between the two modes is where the responsibility for utilization review is vested. People employed by self-insured businesses that use managed care would experience a delivery system similar to that in Figure 11.10.

Managed care, deemed the alternative delivery system as recently as the 1980s, continues to evolve and shape the U.S. delivery system. Managed care does not constitute one standard system but many, inasmuch as a range of managed care models has developed. The relationships among the participants shown in Figures 11.8, 11.9, and 11.10 continue to change as new incentives for financing and delivering care are devised. (The delivery system, with an emphasis on managed care, is the focus of Chapter 19.)

## Care of Special Disorders and Populations

Many health services systems make special provisions for the care of certain disorders or populations that do not readily fit within their existing systems. The U.S. delivery system handles certain disorders (e.g., mental illness) and certain populations (e.g., indigenous peoples, members of the military, veterans) outside the basic health services delivery system and essentially establishes parallel delivery systems. These special provisions may be due to the failure of the traditional delivery system to provide care, as is often true for people with mental illnesses, or to a governmental responsibility for certain populations in return for service to the government, because of treaty obligations, or other reasons.

Examples of exceptions to the standard delivery system in the United States are too numerous for each to be fully addressed in this book. The mental illness treatment system—the focus of Chapter 18—will, therefore, be used as one example of the ways in which special disorders or special populations receive care in the U.S. system.

## Quality of Care

In addition to the components of a traditional health services delivery system, the U.S. system is analyzed in terms of access to care (see Chapter 3), costs of and expenditures for care (see Chapter 7), and quality of care. Quality of care has been of increasing interest to health services providers and researchers as they measure the results or outputs of the current delivery systems and attempt to answer such questions as:

- What constitutes quality health services?
- How should quality be measured?
- Do higher costs and expenditures for care reflect higher quality of care?
- Do lower costs and expenditures indicate lower quality of care?
- Can quality of care be increased without commensurate increases in costs and expenditures?
- Who should be responsible for monitoring quality of care?

The study of quality of care is relatively new and is stimulated by the needs to know about the outcomes of many new interventions and to make optimal use of limited resources. Chapter 20 addresses quality-of-care issues in the U.S. health services system.

## Key Words

| | |
|---|---|
| academic health centers (AHCs) | Medicaid |
| continuum of care | Medicare |
| Department of Defense (DOD) | mental health |
| Department of Veterans | mental illness |
| Affairs (VA) | palliative care |
| developmental disabilities | preferred provider organization |
| genetic testing | (PPO) |
| group health insurance | primary care |
| health maintenance organization | primary disease prevention |
| (HMO) | quality of care |
| health promotion | rehabilitative care |
| hospice | self-insured business |
| human genome research | secondary care |
| independent practice association (IPA) | secondary disease prevention |
| Indian Health Service (IHS) | Shepherd-Towner Act |
| individual health insurance policy | staff model HMO |
| integrated delivery network/system | tertiary care |
| long-term care (LTC) | tertiary disease prevention |
| managed care | uninsured |

## References

Shonick, W. 1995. *Government and Health Services.* New York: Oxford
    University Press.
U.S. Department of Health and Human Services. 2005. *Health, United States,
    2005.* Pub. No. (PHS) 2005-1232. Hyattsville, MD: USDHHS.
———. 1991. *Healthy People 2000: National Health Promotion and Disease
    Prevention Objectives.* Pub. No. (PHS) 91-50212. Washington, DC: U.S.
    Government Printing Office.

# HEALTH PROMOTION
# AND DISEASE PREVENTION

## Introduction

A major goal of a health services system is to protect, maintain, and restore the health of individuals and the population at large. Health promotion, health protection, and disease prevention activities provide three ways to accomplish this goal. This chapter focuses on these, emphasizing the National Health Promotion and Disease Protection Objectives issued by the U.S. Department of Health and Human Services (HHS) in 2000 in the *Healthy People 2010* report. *Healthy People 2010* defines two major goals for the health of the people in the United States: (1) to increase the quality and years of healthy life, and (2) to eliminate health disparities (USDHHS 2000). Periodic assessment of 467 objectives developed for 28 focus areas will monitor progress in achieving the two goals. Table 12.1 lists the 28 focus areas.

First, the areas of health promotion, health protection, and disease prevention are defined, followed by a discussion of those who provide the services and how patients access and utilize them. The chapter concludes with a review of policy issues for each area.

## Health Promotion

Achieving optimal health status is the common goal of health promotion, health protection, and disease prevention activities. Each activity, however, has a separate emphasis to reach this goal. A definition of health promotion and the availability of health promotion services are reviewed in the sections that follow.

### What Is Health Promotion?
Ideally, the promotion of good health practices to preserve and enhance health status is the circumstance under which individuals have their initial contact with a health services system. The U.S. health services system, with its emphasis on curative medicine and crisis intervention, is sometimes faulted for the limited resources it directs to health promotion, health protection, and disease prevention activities, despite the proven cost-effectiveness of

**TABLE 12.1**

*Healthy People 2010* Focus Areas

1. Access to quality health services
2. Arthritis, osteoporosis, and chronic back conditions
3. Cancer
4. Chronic kidney disease
5. Diabetes
6. Disability and secondary conditions
7. Educational and community-based programs
8. Environmental health
9. Family planning
10. Food safety
11. Health communication
12. Heart disease and stroke
13. HIV
14. Immunization and infectious diseases
15. Injury and violence prevention
16. Maternal, infant, and child health
17. Medical product safety
18. Mental health and mental disorders
19. Nutrition and overweight
20. Occupational safety and health
21. Oral health
22. Physical activity and fitness
23. Public health infrastructure
24. Respiratory diseases
25. Sexually transmitted diseases
26. Substance abuse
27. Tobacco use
28. Vision and hearing

SOURCE: USDHHS 2000.

select interventions. Table 12.2 provides information on potential costs savings to the U.S. system if known, effective preventive measures are aggressively implemented. (Costs are calculated on a per patient basis for medical and surgical interventions that could have been avoided had appropriate preventive measures been taken.)

The focus of most health promotion strategies is on individual lifestyle—personal choices made in a social context. These choices affect a person's health status. Several of the *Healthy People 2010* focus areas incorporate measurable objectives in health promotion areas (USDHHS 2000). Some include:

- physical activity and fitness,
- nutrition and overweight,
- tobacco use,

| Condition | Overall Magnitude | Avoidable Intervention* | Cost per Patient† |
|---|---|---|---|
| Heart disease | 7 million with coronary artery disease 500,000 deaths/year 284,000 bypass procedures/year | Coronary bypass surgery | $30,000 |
| Cancer | 1 million new cases/year 510,000 deaths/year | Lung cancer treatment Cervical cancer treatment | $29,000 $28,000 |
| Stroke | 600,000 strokes/year 150,000 deaths/year | Hemiplegia treatment and rehabilitation | $22,000 |
| Injuries | 2.3 million hospitaliza- tions/year 142,500 deaths/year 177,000 persons with spinal-cord injuries | Quadraplegia treatment and rehabilitation Hip fracture treatment and rehabilitation Severe head injury treatment and rehabilitation | $570,000 (lifetime) $40,000 $310,000 |
| HIV infection | 1–1.5 million infected 118,000 AIDS cases (as of January 1990) | AIDS treatment | $75,000 (lifetime) |
| Alcoholism | 18.5 million abuse alcohol 105,000 alcohol-related deaths/year | Liver transplant | $250,000 |
| Drug abuse | Regular users: cocaine: 1.3 million IV drugs: 900,000 heroin: 500,000 Drug-exposed babies: 375,000 | Treatment of drug- affected baby | $63,000 (5 years) |
| Low-birth- weight baby | 260,000 low-birthweight babies born/year 23,000 deaths/year | Neonatal intensive care for low-birth- weight babies | $10,000 |
| Inadequate immunization | Lacking basic immunization series: 20–30% age 2 and younger, 3% age 6 and older | Congenital rubella syndrome treatment | $354,000 (lifetime) |

**TABLE 12.2**

The Economics of Prevention

SOURCE: USDHHS 1991.

*Examples—other interventions may apply.

†Representative first-year costs, except as noted. Not indicated are nonmedical costs, such as lost productivity to society.

- substance abuse,
- family planning,
- mental heath and mental disorders,
- injury and violence prevention, and
- educational and community-based programs.

## Availability and Utilization of Health Promotion Services

Although health promotion activities are important to positive health status, the U.S. health services system is not organized to systematically and comprehensively offer them or to encourage their use. One reason for this gap is the traditional separation of physical health care from behavioral health care. Mental health care, substance abuse treatment, and the recognition and treatment of violent and abusive behaviors are all too frequently segregated from somatic health care, resulting in a fragmented system that may fail to holistically treat an individual's needs.

The availability of health promotional activities, because they center around an individual's lifestyle choices, may depend on an individual's self-awareness and aggressiveness in seeking the activities. Health services providers, including health educators, play important roles in creating awareness of the need for health promotion and in developing strategies with individual patients to increase their participation in health promotion activities. For example, a study by Fleming et al. (1997) shows that a physician who discusses potentially problematic alcohol consumption with a patient can influence that patient to reduce alcohol intake.

The most effective interventions available to clinicians for reducing the incidence and severity of the leading causes of diseases and disabilities in the United States are those that address the personal health practices of patients, according to the U.S. Preventive Services Task Force. The HHS convened the Preventive Services Task Force in the mid-1980s to determine the extent to which providers use preventive services and to assess the effectiveness of a range of available interventions. The resulting first edition of the *Guide to Clinical Preventive Services* assessed the effectiveness of 169 strategies for preventing 60 target conditions (Fisher 1989). The second edition, issued in 1996, reviewed evidence regarding new topics that were added in subsequent years. New topics were added on the basis of the extent to which they satisfied two criteria: (1) the burden of suffering from the target condition and (2) the potential effectiveness of the preventive intervention (diGuiseppi, Atkins, and Woolf 1996).

The area of clinical preventive services deserves additional focus at this point because it denotes a consensus among the provider community about effective preventive services. Recognizing that appropriate preventive services can reduce morbidity and mortality from disease and thus potentially reduce expenditures, the U.S. Preventive Services Task Force analyzed three categories of preventive services: screening, counseling, and immunization/chemoprophylaxis (see Table 12.3). The task force report is important for the guidance it offers providers and for its analytic methodology, which can be used to assess diagnostic, treatment, and preventive interventions.

Providers, however, may not always offer these services or encourage their patients to obtain them elsewhere. The Preventive Services Task Force identified several reasons why physicians fail to provide health promotion and disease prevention services:

- Preventive services are poorly reimbursed or not reimbursed at all.
- A patient care visit is generally limited to resolving the presenting problem, with little time allotted for discussing health-related behaviors or counseling.
- Physicians and other providers may be uncertain about which services should be offered under what circumstances.
- Providers may be skeptical about the effectiveness of some health promotion and disease prevention interventions.

In addition to health services providers, other resources support health promotion. Larger businesses may sponsor on-site fitness centers for their employees or subsidize employee participation in athletic activities and programs. Employee assistance programs (EAPs) may be available to support smoking-cessation programs and to provide confidential access to substance abuse treatment or mental health services. Planned Parenthood organizations and local health departments assist individuals with family planning. Employees insured through managed care programs such as health maintenance organizations (HMOs) may have access to wellness centers that counsel them in areas such as nutrition, assessing body mass index, and developing individualized diet and exercise programs, or that provide substance abuse treatment and smoking-cessation programs.

# Health Protection

Unlike health promotion, which focuses on individual lifestyle issues, health protection emphasizes the health of a population. The following section defines health protection and describes the availability and utilization of health protection services.

## What Is Health Protection?
The major health protection focus areas identified in *Healthy People 2010* include occupational safety and health, environmental health, food safety, and oral health (USDHHS 2000).

**TABLE 12.3**
Effective
Clinical
Preventive
Services

## Screening

*Vascular Diseases*
Asymptomatic coronary artery disease
High blood cholesterol
Hypertension
Peripheral arterial diseases

*Neoplastic Diseases*
Breast cancer
Colorectal cancer
Cervical cancer
Prostate cancer
Lung cancer
Skin cancer
Testicular cancer
Ovarian cancer
Pancreatic cancer
Oral cancer

*Metabolic Diseases*
Diabetes mellitus
Thyroid disease
Obesity
Phenylketonuria

*Hematologic Disorders*
Anemia
Hemoglobinopathies
Lead toxicity

*Ophthalmologic and Ontologic
    Disorders*
Diminished visual acuity
Glaucoma
Hearing impairment

*Infectious Diseases*
Hepatitis B
Tuberculosis
Syphllis
Gonorrhea
Infection with HIV
Chlamydial infection
Genital herpes simplex
Asymptomatic bacteriuria, hematuria
    and proteinuria

*Prenatal Disorders*
Intrauterine growth retardation
Preeclampsia
Rubella
RH compatability
Congenital birth defects
Fetal distress

*Musculoskeletal Disorders*
Postmenopausal osteoporosis
Risk of low back injury

*Mental Disorders/Substance Abuse*
Dementia
Abnormal bereavement
Depression
Suicidal intent
Violent injuries
Alcohol and other drug abuse

## Counseling

Prevention of tobacco abuse
Exercise counseling
Nutritional counseling
Prevention of motor vehicle injuries
Prevention of household and
    environmental injuries
Prevention of HIV infection and other STDs
Prevention of unintended pregnancy
Prevention of dental disease

## Immunization/Chemoprophylaxis

Childhood immunizations
Adult immunizations
Postexposure prophylaxis
Estrogen prophylaxis
Aspirin prophylaxis

SOURCE: Fisher 1989. Copyright Lippincott Williams and Wilkins. Used with permission.

*Availability and Utilization of Health Protection Services*

Primary responsibility for all the health protection objectives resides with the public health sector, although individuals and health services providers also have responsibilities in this area. Federal, state, and local departments of public health, labor, transportation, and others oversee the maintenance of safe living and working environments, including pure water, clean air, safe food and drug products, appropriate waste disposal, elimination of hazardous situations, and reduced risk of automobile accidents. Health educators play the important role of informing the public about how to achieve and maintain safe living and working environments and how to engage in health protective behaviors.

## Disease Prevention: Primary, Secondary, and Tertiary

Three levels of disease prevention—primary, secondary, and tertiary—are identified in a comprehensive health services system.

### What Is Primary Disease Prevention?

Primary disease prevention focuses on preventing agents from causing disease or injury. Primary preventive measures are directed toward individuals who are entirely asymptomatic (i.e., no indication of disease is present). Immunizations are a primary prevention strategy, preventing certain viruses, such as influenza, measles, polio, and chicken pox, from causing diseases.

### What Is Secondary Disease Prevention?

Secondary disease prevention—the early detection and treatment to cure or control the cause of a disease—is also aimed at asymptomatic individuals who have already developed risk factors or preclinical disease but in whom the disease itself has not become clinically apparent (Fisher 1989). Pap smears to detect cervical dysplasia before the development of a cancer are a secondary prevention strategy.

### What Is Tertiary Disease Prevention?

Tertiary disease prevention ameliorates the seriousness of a diagnosed disease by decreasing the resulting disability and dependence. Antibiotic therapy to prevent postoperative wound infection, insulin therapy to prevent the complications of diabetes mellitus, or the use of protease inhibitors to stem the advances of the human immunodeficiency virus (HIV) are examples of tertiary prevention strategies.

*Healthy People 2010* (USDHHS 2000) identifies the following focus areas of preventive services:

* arthritis, osteoporosis, and chronic back conditions;
* cancer;

- chronic kidney disease;
- diabetes;
- disability and secondary conditions;
- heart disease and stroke;
- HIV;
- immunizations and infectious diseases;
- maternal, infant, and child health;
- sexually transmitted diseases; and
- vision and hearing.

### Availability and Utilization of Health Preventive Services

Preventive services are offered by primary care and specialist physicians, nurse practitioners, physician assistants, nurses, and dentists. At least four of these services—maternal, infant, and infant health; HIV; sexually transmitted diseases; and immunization and infectious diseases—are likely to be available through local departments of public health, in community and neighborhood health center clinics, and from other providers of public health services.

## Health Promotion, Health Protection, and Disease Prevention Issues in the U.S. Health Services System

Reorienting the focus from the negative, or disease control, sense of health to a positive focus on health promotion, health protection, and disease prevention remains a challenge in the U.S. system. Issues relating to such a reorientation include applying existing knowledge, the level of responsibility for change, and system issues.

### Applying Existing Knowledge

Although much remains to be learned about how health status relates to individual lifestyle choices and the context in which choices are made, enough solid evidence of the effects of some choices is readily available to warrant prompt and effective action at both the individual and societal level. For example, despite tobacco company protestations to the contrary, evidence about the negative consequences of tobacco use is sufficient to support decisive individual and societal action to curb such use. Evidence about the importance of good nutrition, physical activity, obesity avoidance, and other health-promoting behaviors is also compelling. The issue is not how to obtain additional information, but how to effectively apply existing knowledge to achieve behavioral change.

## Responsibility for Health Promotion, Health Protection, and Disease Prevention

Part of the dilemma in effectively applying existing knowledge regarding health promotion, health protection, and disease prevention is the unclear line of responsibility for these functions (i.e., are they the responsibility of the individual, the health services provider, or society?). The absence of a clear line of responsibility enables each party to easily assume that others are doing what should be done.

Assuming that individuals must be most responsible for their personal health status is easy. However, what about individuals' competency and self-efficacy, and the social context in which they make decisions? Breslow (1990) points out that, for the most part, people use cocaine when it is socially available and when their peers are using it. Asserting that the user has "free choice" may obscure the reality. The argument for individual responsibility, when carried to its extreme, may result in "victim blaming" and in proposals to hold the victim accountable for self-inflicted physical deterioration. Although clearly more easy to prescribe than to implement, a recognition of shared responsibility for health promotion, health protection, and disease prevention, and for the development of effective strategies to improve health status, would markedly improve the U.S. health services system.

## System Issues

In addition to examining and addressing shared responsibility to improve health promotion, health protection, and disease prevention, other changes in the U.S. health services system are influencing the focus on these three areas. These changes include:

- an epidemiologic transition;
- a shift from disease control by specialists to a concentrated focus on health by primary care providers;
- technologic advances;
- the changing influence of managed care;
- the continued debate about whether interventions should be aimed at the individual or at the community; and
- insurance coverage for preventive services.

**Epidemiologic Transition**

Breslow (1990) notes the epidemiologic transition, a concept coined by Omran (1971) and developed by Olshansky and Ault (1986), as part of the recent evolution of health. The epidemiologic transition means that attention on the diagnosis and treatment of disease has transferred from the realm of contagious and communicable diseases—many of which now can be controlled and some of which are close to eradication—to the epidemic diseases (coronary disease, lung cancer, and other noncommunicable diseases) generated by twenty-first century patterns of living.

## Reorientation Toward Primary Care

As one of the most technologically advanced in the world, the U.S. health services system is renowned for its abilities to detect and treat disease. This reputation is reflected in the composition of the physician workforce, where specialists outnumber generalists by a ratio of two to one, and in the reimbursement system, where specialists have traditionally outearned generalists. Results of this emphasis include the provision of high-cost, expenditure-increasing care and potential limitations in accessing primary care.

Several stimuli are effecting a reorientation toward primary care. First, managed care has created a demand for more generalists to serve as patients' first point of contact with their health plan and to control referrals to specialists. This demand has served to decrease the salary differential between the two categories of physicians. Second, some medical schools, sensitive to producing an employable workforce, created or renewed in the mid-1990s a curricular emphasis on primary care. It is not yet clear how many of those changes remain in effect. Third, congressional action on the Medicare program, the predominant support of graduate medical education for both generalist and specialist physicians, is reinforcing this shift through proposals to fund fewer specialty training slots. The 1997 Balanced Budget Act limited the number of residency slots for which the Medicare program would reimburse an academic health center, teaching hospital, or other authorized training site.

## Technologic Advances

Basic scientific research regularly produces results that help to promote and protect health, and in particular, to prevent disease. Unraveling the DNA mysteries, from which is learned the origins and progression of diseases, promises advances on a number of medical fronts. Mapping the human genome and discovering more about the genetic influences on health status are other important advances.

## Managed Care

A major premise of managed care is that health promotion, health protection, and disease prevention, if properly instituted, improve a person's immediate health status and quality of life, and avert more serious—and more costly—health problems later in life. Certain forms of managed care provide financial incentives to keep their subscribers as healthy—and out of the hospital—as possible, which means regular monitoring of individual health status.

Supporting health promotion, health protection, and disease prevention may have immediate payoffs for the individual and the managed care organization; however, the most significant returns for the use of these strategies may not be realized until later in life, when the subscriber may have disenrolled and entered a competitor's health plan. The extent and duration of health promotion, health protection, and preventive services vary greatly by type of managed care plan and are areas in need of additional research and analysis.

Whether intervention to promote and protect health and to prevent disease should be aimed at individuals, their community, or a combination of the two remains unresolved. Breslow (1990) calls attention to a subtle distinction that has occurred over time in defining, and thus attacking, a health problem.

**Level of Intervention**

In earlier times, exposure to hazardous agents, such as contaminated water, constituted the health problem, and the focus of intervention would be at the community level. Access to hazardous agents such as tobacco or alcohol constitutes some of today's health problems, and the focus of intervention would be at the individual and the community levels.

Individual choices about food, exercise, tobacco use, and safe motor vehicle operation suggest that successful interventions for today's health problems should be aimed at the individual. Such choices, however, are made within a social context that often defines access, suggesting that more interventions must involve the community.

Insurers may vary in their coverage of behavioral health and preventive services. Generous health insurance benefit packages may cover weight-loss programs, smoking-cessation assistance, alcohol and substance abuse treatment, and a full range of mental health services. More basic benefit packages, however, may cover few, if any, of these services. Parts of the population most in need of behavioral health and other preventive services may have limited or no access to them, either because they are uninsured or because their benefit package does not adequately cover these services. Even when an insurer covers these services, studies have shown that the availability of services does not ensure their utilization. To enhance patient benefit from preventive services, an organized approach to patient follow-up is essential (Morrissey et al. 1995).

**Insurance Coverage for Preventive Services**

## Summary

Patients, providers, payers, and politicians are turning up the volume on their demands for greater emphasis in the U.S. health services system on health promotion, health protection, and disease prevention. The motivations for these demands include improved quality of life, the desire to positively influence health rather than always intervene in crisis mode, a healthier and more productive workforce, and the need to contain and reduce expenditures for health services. Health promotion, health protection, and disease prevention can be effective in helping to meet these various demands. They cannot, however, eliminate disease and the need for diagnosis, treatment, and rehabilitation in the U.S. health services system.

## Key Words

| | |
|---|---|
| Balanced Budget Act of 1997 | Healthy People 2010 objectives |
| behavioral health | human genome research |
| Guide to Clinical Preventive Services | managed care |
| disease prevention | Planned Parenthood |
| employee assistance programs (EAP) | primary disease prevention |
| epidemiologic transition | secondary disease prevention |
| health maintenance organization | tertiary disease prevention |
| (HMO) | U.S. Preventive Services Task Force |
| health promotion | "victim blaming" |

## References

Breslow, L. 1990. "A Health Promotion Primer for the 1990s." *Health Affairs* 9 (2): 6–21.

diGuiseppi, C., D. Atkins, and S. H. H. Woolf. 1996. *Clinical Preventive Services Report of the U.S. Preventive Services Task Force.* Alexandria, VA: International Medical Publishing.

Fisher, M. 1989. *Guide to Clinical Preventive Services: An Assessment of the Effectiveness of 169 Interventions.* Baltimore, MD: Williams & Wilkins.

Fleming, M. F., K. L. Barry, L. B. Manwell, K. Johnson, and R. London. 1997. "Brief Physician Advice for Problem Alcohol Drinkers: A Randomized Controlled Trial in Community-Based Primary Care Practices." *Journal of the American Medical Association* 277 (13): 1039–45.

Morrissey, J. P., R. P. Harris, J. Kincade-Norburn, C. McLaughlin, J. M. Garrett, A. M. Jackman, J. S. Stein, C. Lannon, R. J. Schwartz, and D. L. Patrick. 1995. "Medicare Reimbursement for Preventive Care: Changes in Performance of Services, Quality of Life, and Health Care Costs." *Medical Care* 33 (4): 315–31.

Olshanksy, S. J., and A. B. Ault. 1986. "The Fourth Stage of Epidemiologic Transition: The Age of Delayed Degenerative Diseases." *The Milbank Memorial Fund Quarterly* 64: 335–91.

Omran, A. R. 1971. "The Epidemiologic Transition." *The Milbank Memorial Fund Quarterly* 49: 509–38.

U.S. Department of Health and Human Services. 2000. *Healthy People 2010.* Washington, DC: U.S. Government Printing Office.

———. 1991. *Healthy People 2000: National Health Promotion and Disease Prevention Objectives.* Pub. No. (PHS) 91-5021. Washington, DC: U.S. Government Printing Office.

# 13

# PRIMARY CARE

## Introduction

Even the most effective system of health promotion, health protection, and disease prevention will not forestall the need for treatment of illness, injury, and disease. A primary care system provides appropriate treatment for common diseases and injuries, essential drugs, and basic dental care, and also identifies potentially serious physical or mental health conditions that require prompt referral for more intensive levels of care.

This chapter defines primary care, discusses who provides it, and addresses how patients access and utilize it. The chapter concludes with a discussion of policy issues related to primary care.

## Defining Primary Care

Primary care is usually the patient's first contact with the treatment system. Roemer's model of a health services system defines primary care as the entry point into the health services system, wherein:

- illness or disease is diagnosed and initial treatment provided;
- episodic care for common, nonchronic illnesses and injuries is rendered;
- prescription drugs to treat common illnesses or injuries are provided;
- routine dental care—examinations, cleaning, repair of dental cavities —occurs; and
- potentially serious physical or mental health conditions that require prompt referral for secondary or tertiary care are diagnosed.

The Institute of Medicine (IOM), which established its first conference on primary care in 1978, convened a Committee on the Future of Primary Care in the early 1990s to re-examine their initial definition. The IOM committee issued the following revised definition of primary care in 1994:

> Primary care is the provision of integrated, accessible health care services by clinicians who are accountable for addressing a large majority of personal health care needs, developing a sustained partnership with patients, and practicing in the context of family and community. (IOM 1995)

Central to this definition are concepts of integrated services, accessibility, provider accountability, provider-patient partnerships, and care oriented to family and community needs.

Although most primary care is provided on an ambulatory basis, some types of secondary care (discussed in Chapter 14) may also be provided on an ambulatory basis. The terms *primary care* and *ambulatory care* therefore overlap but are not synonymous. The data presented in the sections that follow, while inclusive of primary care, are compiled as ambulatory care visits and may include contacts or visits for secondary care. Despite these limitations, the data provide insight into categories of primary care providers and utilization of primary care services.

## Primary Care Providers

The IOM definition of primary care emphasizes the provision of care by clinicians. The first category of clinicians that comes to mind is generally physicians. Figure 13.1 shows the distribution of ambulatory care visits to physicians' offices, by type of physician specialty, for 2003. Nearly 25 percent of ambulatory visits to physicians' offices are made to general practitioners or family practitioners.

Physician assistants (PAs), nurse practitioners (NPs), nurse midwives, nurses, and other categories of providers are also considered clinicians. The

**FIGURE 13.1**

Visits to Primary Care Generalist and Specialist Physicians, by Age Group (2003)

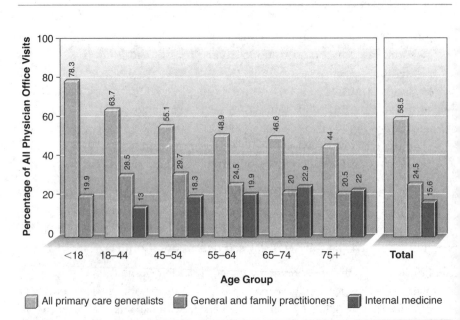

SOURCE: U.S. Department of Health and Human Services (USDHHS) 2005.

definition of primary care provider may be expanded to also include physical and speech therapists, mental health providers, diagnostic and therapeutic laboratory staff, podiatrists, optometrists, home health aides, respiratory therapists, and social workers (Nichols 1996).

## Access to and Utilization of Primary Care

Because primary care is the entry level to diagnosis and treatment of illness, injury, and disease in a comprehensive health services system, it would seem logical that all members of society would have unobstructed access to the system. As was noted in Chapter 3, however, financial and other barriers may limit access to primary and other health services. People with public or private health insurance are more likely to have a connection to one or more primary care providers. People with limited or no health insurance obtain episodic primary and other care from a variety of sources. The Community and Migrant Health Center program, for example, provided comprehensive primary health services to more than seven million people through 1,615 delivery sites in medically underserved areas in 1994 (U.S. General Accounting Office [now known as the U.S. Government Accountability Office—USGAO] 1995).

One measure of access to primary care is the average number of visits to physicians and other primary care providers, including hospital outpatient and emergency departments, per person per year.[1] Figure 13.2 shows that the average number of physician visits per person per year dropped

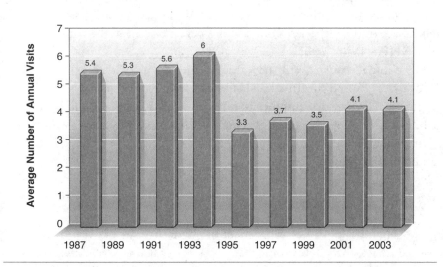

**FIGURE 13.2**
Number of Annual per Person Visits to Primary Care Providers (1987–2003)

SOURCE: USDHHS 2005.

NOTE: Sites of contact include physician offices, hospital outpatient facilities, and emergency departments.

**FIGURE 13.3**
Number of
Annual Visits
to Physicians,
by Age and
Gender (2003)

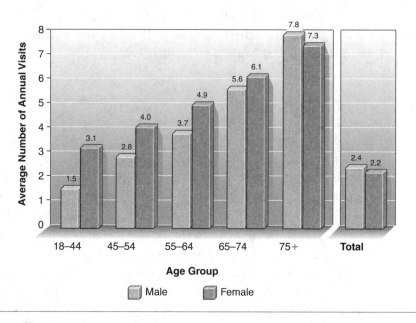

SOURCE: USDHHS 2005.

NOTE: Sites of contact include physician offices, hospital outpatient facilities, and emergency departments.

from a high of 6 visits in 1993 to 3.3 in 1995, and was holding at 4.1 in 2001 and 2003. The increase is likely due to several factors, including increased Medicaid coverage of children and increased utilization of physician services for chronic health problems, some associated with an aging population. Although perhaps the majority of these contacts are for primary care, some are for more intensive care. Of physician contacts, 57 percent take place in the physician's office and 4 percent occur in the patient's home (USDHHS 1995, 2005).

Contacts with a primary care provider are associated with perceived and/or diagnosed health status, age, gender, race/ethnicity, and income. Figure 13.3 shows the number of physician contacts by age and by gender. After reaching age 18, females typically have more physician contacts per year than do males. Some of this difference is related to reproductive health and childbearing.

Figure 13.4 shows the proportion of the population that had a dental visit in 2003. More males than females typically visit a dentist in a year across all age categories.

Figure 13.5 shows the number of physician visits per year by race and by age. Blacks have fewer physician visits per year than do whites in all age categories. The proportion of whites, blacks, Hispanics and other racial and

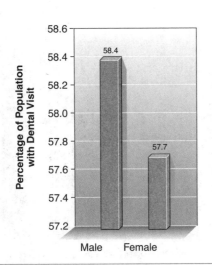

SOURCE: USDHHS 2005.

**FIGURE 13.4**
Dental Visits
in the Past Year,
by Gender
(2003)

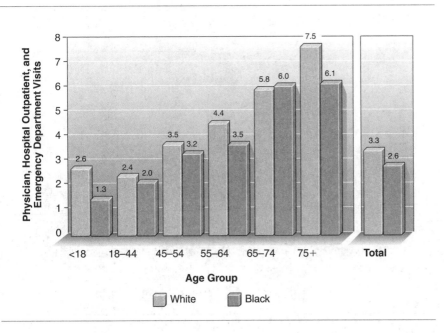

SOURCE: USDHHS 2005.

**FIGURE 13.5**
Annual
Number
of Physician
Visits, by Age
and
Race/Ethnicity
(2003)

**FIGURE 13.6**
Dental Visits
in the Past Year,
by Race/
Ethnicity
(2003)

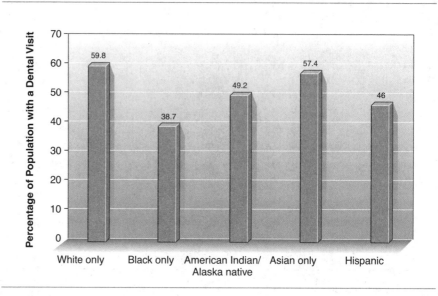

SOURCE: USDHHS 2005.

**FIGURE 13.7**
Percentage
of Population
by Poverty
Status with
Visits to a
Physician's
Office,
Hospital
Outpatient
Facility, or
Emergency
Department
(2003)

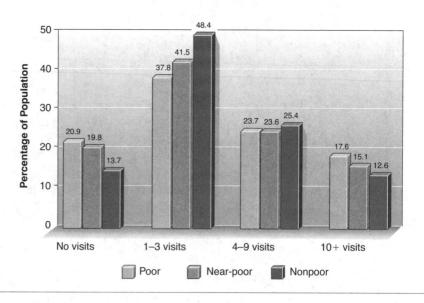

SOURCE: USDHHS 2005.

ethnic groups who saw a dentist in 2003 is shown in Figure 13.6; a higher proportion of whites had a dental visit than all other racial and ethnic groups.

Figure 13.7 shows the relationship between income and the number of primary care provider contacts. A substantially lower proportion of persons in the nonpoor category did not have a primary care visit in 2003.

FIGURE 13.8
Dental Visits
in the Past Year,
by Poverty
Status (2003)

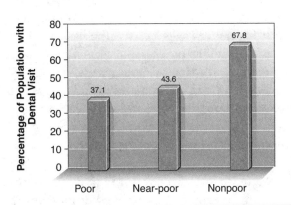

SOURCE: USDHHS 2005.

Nonpoor people had higher proportions of visits in both the 1 to 3 and the 4 to 9 visits per year categories, indicating that they had fewer problems with financial access. A greater proportion of persons in the poor and near-poor categories, however, incurred more than 10 visits per year, suggesting that they may have had poorer health status, including more chronic health problems. A much higher proportion of nonpoor people saw a dentist in 2003 than people considered poor or near-poor (Figure 13.8).

## Primary Care Issues in the U.S. Health Services System

The U.S. health services system faces several major policy issues related to primary care: access to care, the availability of primary care providers, and reimbursement for primary care providers.

### Access to Primary Care

Primary care, as the entry into the treatment system, is important for dealing with routine illnesses and injuries but also for diagnosing and initiating therapy for more severe illnesses and diseases. Unrestricted access to primary care, if appropriately pursued, should result in improved health status for the individual and for a population. When access to primary care is limited or impeded, however, an individual's health status may deteriorate and in turn negatively affect the health of a population. Based on the IOM definition, a comprehensive health services system should assure accessible primary care and other health services.

### Availability of Primary Care Providers

Access to primary care depends, in part, on the type and number of primary care providers available to serve a population. Primary care and other generalist physicians constitute only about one-third of U.S. physicians, an inverse ratio to that of health services systems in other industrialized countries. Efforts are underway (e.g., revising basic medical school training and limiting the number of available slots for specialist training) to increase the number of primary care physicians in the U.S. system. The lengthy pipeline for physician training, however, suggests that the supply and the ratio will not dramatically change in the short term.

### Reimbursement for Primary Care Physicians

The provision of primary care services has traditionally been reimbursed at lower rates than more intensive levels of services, and primary care and generalist physicians have generally had lower incomes than their specialist counterparts. One effect of this differential is an implicit devaluing of primary care providers and a tendency for individuals to self-refer to a range of specialists rather than to access care through a primary provider.

The U.S. health services system's move toward managed care signaled a change in the valuation of primary care providers. Many forms of managed care focus on the primary care provider as the point of entry for other levels of care and services. Primary care physicians and other providers found themselves in demand, and the market forces of supply and demand resulted in increased incomes for primary care providers. How all the managed care forces will play out over time is not yet clear. Recent reports indicate that some managed care entities are reducing or eliminating their gatekeeping functions, which were often filled by primary care physicians (Ferris et al. 2001; Lawrence 2001).

## Summary

Primary care—the first level of diagnosis and treatment of illness, injury, and disease—has transitioned from the edges of the delivery system toward its center. This transition is changing the ways primary care providers are trained, the demand for their services, and the reimbursement for primary care.

## Note

1. Physician and other health care *visits* generally indicate a face-to-face visit between provider and patient. The term *contacts* is often used to include telephone as well as face-to-face communication.

## Key Words

<table>
<tr><td>access to care</td><td>Institute of Medicine (IOM)</td></tr>
<tr><td>ambulatory care</td><td>nurse practitioner (NP)</td></tr>
<tr><td>Community and Migrant Health<br>   Center Program</td><td>physician assistant (PA)<br>primary care</td></tr>
<tr><td>gatekeeping</td><td>utilization of services</td></tr>
</table>

## References

Ferris, T. G., Y. Chang, D. Blumenthal, and S. Pearson. 2001. "Leaving Gatekeeping Behind—Effects of Opening Access to Specialists for Adults in Health Maintenance Organizations." *New England Journal of Medicine* 345 (18): 1312–17.

Institute of Medicine. 1995. *Primary Care: America's Health in a New Era.* Washington, DC: National Academy Press.

Lawrence, D. 2001. "Gatekeeping Reconsidered." *New England Journal of Medicine* 345 (18): 1342–43.

Nichols, L. 1996. *Nonphysician Health Care Providers: Uses of Ambulatory Services, Expenditures, and Sources of Payment.* AHCPR Pub. No. 96-0013. National Medical Expenditure Survey Research Findings, 27. Rockville, MD: Public Health Service/Agency for Health Care Policy and Research.

U.S. Department of Health and Human Services. 2005. *Health, United States, 2005.* Hyattsville, MD: USDHHS.

———. 1995. *Health, United States, 1995.* Pub. No. (PHS) 96-1232. Hyattsville, MD: USDHHS.

U.S. Government Accountability Office (formerly the U.S. General Accounting Office). 1995. *Community Health Centers: Challenges in Transitioning to Prepaid Managed Care.* USGAO/HEHS-95-138. Washington, DC: USGAO.

# 14

# SECONDARY CARE

## Introduction

Secondary care may be rendered on either an ambulatory or an inpatient basis and signals a higher level of intensity, often over a longer period of time, than event-specific primary care. This chapter defines secondary care, provides an overview of secondary care providers, and describes access to and utilization of secondary care services. The chapter concludes with a discussion of policy issues related to the provision of secondary care.

## What Is Secondary Care?

Secondary care includes special ambulatory medical services and commonplace inpatient hospital acute care. Contrasted with primary care, which is also ambulatory care but is centered around episodic, often one-time common illnesses or injuries, secondary care is continuing care for sustained or chronic conditions.

Figure 14.1 shows the percentage of persons with any activity limitation, grouped by age and gender, race/ethnicity, and income level. The prevalence of chronic conditions increases with age, as would be expected. Also as expected, the percentage of the population with activity limitations increases with age; 44 percent of persons in the 75+ age group have some activity limitation due to a chronic disease. Poor persons have a higher proportion of limitations due to chronic disease than do nonpoor persons (23 percent and 9 percent, respectively). The racial or ethnic group with the lowest proportion of limitations due to chronic conditions is the Asian-only group (6.4 percent), whereas the American Indian/Alaska Native group has the highest proportion (21.2 percent). All of these groups are likely to require secondary care as a result of their chronic conditions. Children may also require this level of care.

## Who Provides Secondary Care?

Physicians, singly or as leaders of a health services team, are the predominant care providers. Data on health services providers and users are not typically collected by the level of care provided—primary, secondary, or tertiary—but

**FIGURE 14.1**

Percentage of Persons with Any Activity Limitations (2003)

(*a*) By age group and gender. (*b*) By race/ethnicity. (*c*) By poverty status.

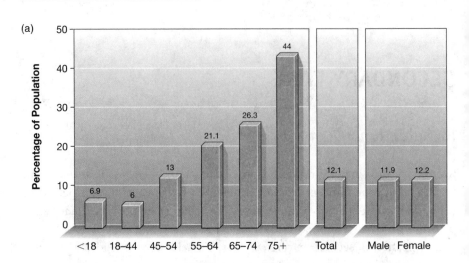

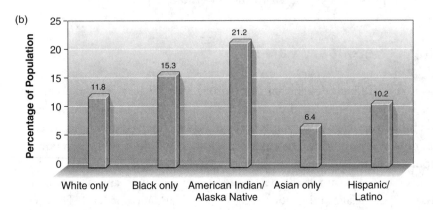

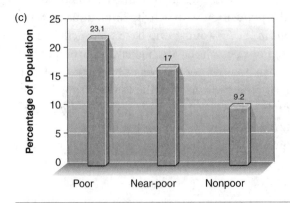

SOURCE: U.S. Department of Health and Human Services (USDHHS) 2005.

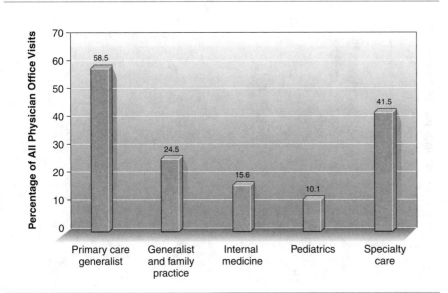

FIGURE 14.2
Visits to
Primary Care
Generalist and
Specialist
Physicians, by
Type of
Physician
(2003)

SOURCE: USDHHS 2005.

NOTE: The data are based on reporting by a sample of office-based physicians. The "primary care generalist" category includes the generalist and family practice, internal medicine, and pediatric categories of physicians, as well as a category of "others," which includes general obstetrics and gynecology. Nearly 59 percent of all visits to physicians' offices are to primary care generalist physicians; the remaining 42 percent of visits are to physicians who identify themselves as specialists.

by provider specialty, diagnosed condition, or patient demographics, for example. Ambulatory care utilization is used to illustrate the use of secondary care, but some of these visits entail primary care.

Figure 14.2 shows the distribution of ambulatory care visits to physicians' offices by type of specialist. All primary care specialists account for 42 percent of visits. Visits to general and family practitioners account for 25 percent of visits, followed by 16 percent to internal medicine, and 10 percent to pediatricians.

Figure 14.3 shows the overall number of ambulatory care visits per one hundred people to physicians' offices, hospital emergency departments, and hospital outpatient departments, and the number of visits per site by age group, gender, and race. In 2003, the majority of visits took place in physicians' offices, and the fewest occurred in hospital outpatient departments. The number of visits increases with age, females have more visits than males (due in part to reproductive health and childbearing), and whites have more visits than blacks.

Secondary care is provided in sites other than those shown in Figure 14.3. Beginning in the late 1970s, groups of physicians, hospitals, and other sponsors established a range of specialty centers, such as ambulatory surgery, radiology, urgent care, childbirthing, and end-stage renal dialysis

FIGURE 14.3

Ambulatory
Care Visits
(2003)
*(a)* By location.
*(b)* By age group
and site.
*(c)* Age-adjusted
by gender
and race.

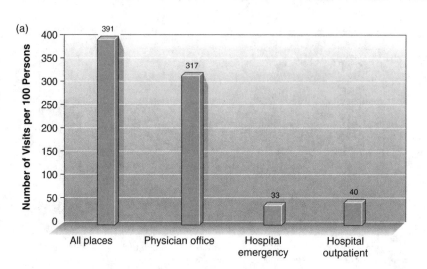

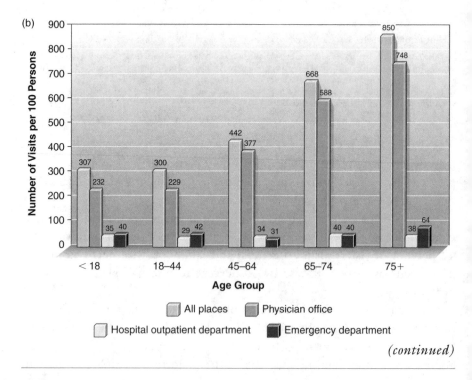

(a) Number of Visits per 100 Persons — All places: 391; Physician office: 317; Hospital emergency: 33; Hospital outpatient: 40

(b) Number of Visits per 100 Persons by Age Group

All places, Physician office, Hospital outpatient department, Emergency department

< 18: 307, 232, 35, 40
18–44: 300, 229, 29, 42
45–64: 442, 377, 34, 31
65–74: 668, 588, 40, 40
75+: 850, 748, 38, 64

*(continued)*

(ESRD). Motivation for developing such centers is high because the centers allow a concentration in one specialty area of medicine or surgery, retain market share, compete for market share, provide care more economically than could be done on a hospital inpatient basis, and attract new user populations.

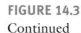

FIGURE 14.3
Continued

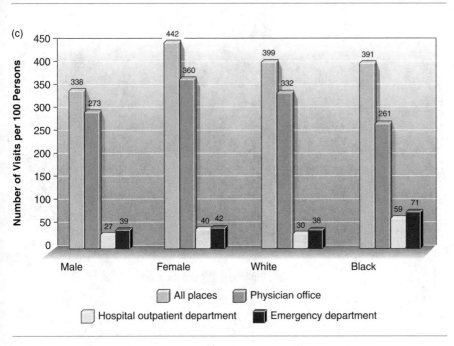

(c)

SOURCE: USDHHS 2005.

## Access to and Utilization of Secondary Care

As discussed in Chapter 3, geographic, cultural, physical, temporal, and financial barriers bind access to secondary care. Financial access may be more crucial in obtaining secondary care than other levels of care because secondary care generally involves sustained or chronic conditions that require frequent treatment. This requirement necessitates regular relationships with—and reimbursement to—health services providers. By contrast, some primary care needs can be met by public health departments or by providers who will accept sliding-scale payments for episodic services. Some tertiary care needs may be met, on an emergency basis, by hospitals that are required to stabilize patients who arrive in need of emergency care.

The provision of chronic care, because it addresses persistent and recurrent health problems, is expensive. The direct costs of care for the 99 million people with chronic conditions in 1995 were estimated at $470 billion (Robert Wood Johnson Foundation 1996). The number of people with chronic conditions is growing due to the increase in chronic conditions as the population ages, the expanding ability to care for and treat

**FIGURE 14.4**
Projected
Number of
Persons with
Chronic
Diseases and
Projected
Expenditures
(Select Years,
1995–2050)

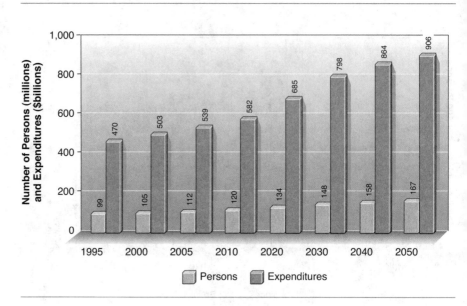

SOURCE: The Robert Wood Johnson Foundation, 1996. Used with permission.

NOTES: Estimates based on the 1987 National Medical Expenditure Survey, University of California–San Francisco—Institute for Health & Aging, 1995. Data intervals are irregular.

chronic conditions and thus prolong life, and other factors. Figure 14.4 shows the projected number of people with chronic diseases and the projected expenditures for their care through the year 2050. The direct medical costs to treat people with chronic conditions will nearly double in that time period.

Although it is true that chronic conditions and disabilities increase with age, recent evidence suggests that some disability rates are declining in older age groups (Wolf, Hunt, and Knickman 2005; Spillman 2004). Some of the declines are in instrumental activities of daily living, as opposed to personal care activities (Spillman 2004). Wolf and colleagues (2005) note three societal trends in areas other than health or functioning that might contribute to declines in disability levels: (1) a reduced supply of informal care (presumably meaning that formal care will be sought), (2) changes in the technology of self-care, and (3) changes in the definitions and perceptions of both "ability" and "disability."

Knowing the number of people with chronic conditions gives an indication of the need for secondary care. However, not all people with chronic conditions or others who need secondary care receive all needed care. Keeping this in mind is important when considering utilization of secondary services; utilization data reflect the population that obtains services, which is almost certainly a smaller number than the population in need of services.

## Utilization of Secondary Services

Figures 14.5 through 14.8 provide utilization information on short-stay, nonfederal hospitals. These data do not distinguish between secondary and tertiary care. They are included in this section because many of the presenting conditions are those that require secondary care.

Figure 14.5 shows the diagnostic and nonsurgical procedures done per 100,000 population for male and female inpatients in 2001–02. For both males and females, the total number of such procedures increases significantly when compared with historic data for the prior 20-year period. Several factors must be considered in analyzing these data: the need for these diagnostic services is growing as the population ages; the ability to provide such services expands as new technologies are implemented; and the number of some services provided on an inpatient basis declined after 1985, when Medicare's prospective payment system (PPS) changed the way in which hospitals were reimbursed for care and created incentives to shift many diagnostic and other services from an inpatient to an outpatient basis.

Figure 14.6 shows discharges, days of care, and average length of stay (ALOS) in short-stay hospitals for 1980, 1990, 2000, and 2003. With the exception of discharges, a steady decline is shown for this 23-year period. Fewer people per thousand are being discharged (with a small blip from 1990 to 2003), they are staying fewer days, and their ALOS is shorter.[1] Both the shift from inpatient to outpatient care and the effects of advanced treatment technologies have influenced these declines. A review of the utilization data for outpatient services would show a commensurate increase as the use of inpatient services declines.

Figure 14.7 shows discharges from short-stay hospitals, by gender, for 1980, 1990, 2000, and 2003. Females have higher utilization than do males, due in part to reproductive health and childbearing admissions. The rate of discharges declines for both genders over this period.

Figure 14.8 shows changes in the ALOS for the same 23-year period, by gender and by age group. The ALOS is known to vary by geographic area, with shorter stays in the West (4.8 days) than in the Northeast (5.3 days), the Midwest (5.8 days), and the South (6.1 days) in 2003 (USD-HHS 2005). This variance is due to physician practice patterns, health status, demographics of the populations of these areas, and other factors. Figure 14.8 shows a general declining trend in ALOS.

FIGURE 14.5
Inpatient
Procedures for
Adults, by
Gender
(2001–02)

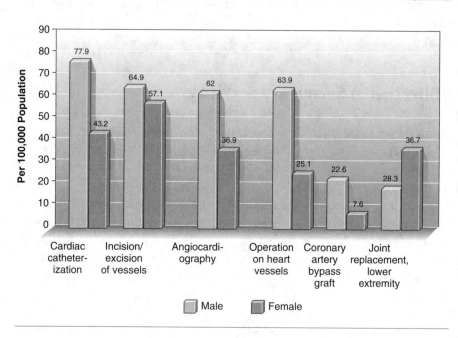

SOURCE: USDHHS 2005.

FIGURE 14.6
Discharges,
Days of Care,
Average Length
of Stay (ALOS),
Short-Stay
Nonfederal
U.S. Hospitals
(Select Years,
1980–2003)

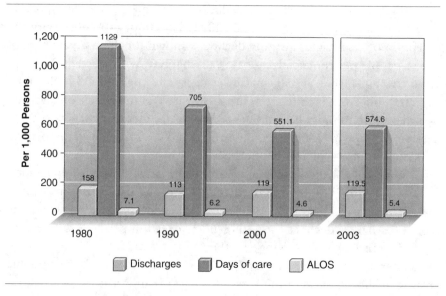

SOURCE: USDHHS 2005.

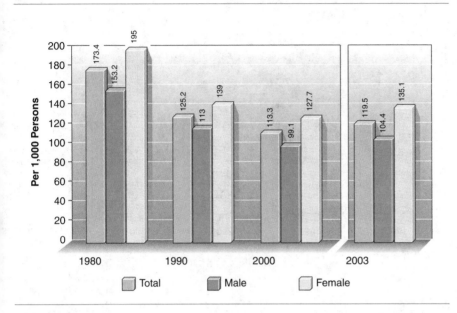

**FIGURE 14.7**
Discharges,
Nonfederal
Short-Stay
U.S. Hospitals,
by Gender
(Select Years,
1980–2003)

SOURCE: USDHHS 2005.

## Policy Issues Related to Secondary Care

Several issues will potentially influence the development of the secondary health services system. First, the various strategies (foremost among which has been a focus on managed care) to reorient the delivery system from a focus on specialty care to primary care has likely affected secondary care, but the nature and the direction(s) of these strategies are not entirely clear. One reason for this lack of clarity is that although primary and specialty care are each distinct and recognizable levels, secondary care constitutes the middle ground and may be provided by either primary or specialty providers.

Second, and related to the shift from specialty to primary care, is the shift in the provision of many secondary services from a hospital inpatient to an outpatient basis. Figure 14.9*a* compares procedures, by gender, for select years, with 1996 being the most recent year for which data are available for the ambulatory procedures, whereas Figure 14.9*b* shows 2001–02 data for the inpatient procedures. The number of procedures done per one thousand persons on an ambulatory basis is increasing, while the number of procedures done per one thousand persons on an inpatient basis is decreasing. The inpatient to outpatient shift has stimulated hospitals to expand their outpatient services and has prompted the development of a prospective payment patient classification system for ambulatory care (Averill et al. 1993). The 1997 Balanced Budget Act created an outpatient prospective payment

**FIGURE 14.8**

Average Length of Stay, Nonfederal Short-Stay U.S. Hospitals (Select Years, 1980–2003)

(*a*) By gender.
(*b*) By age.

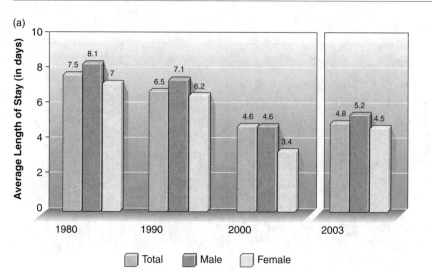

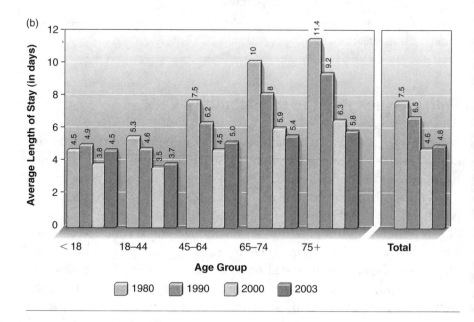

SOURCE: USDHHS 2005.

(a)

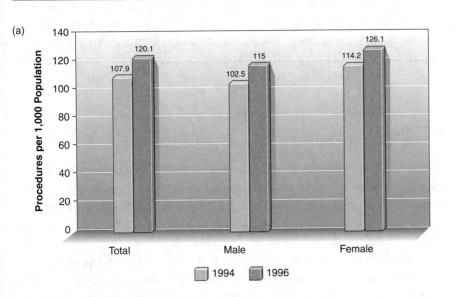

**FIGURE 14.9**
Ambulatory
and Inpatient
Procedures,
by Gender
(Select Years)
*(a)* Ambulatory
procedures, by
gender (1994
and 1996).
*(b)* Inpatient
procedures,
by gender
(select years,
1994–2002).

(b)

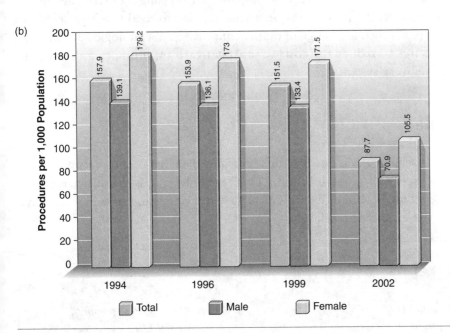

SOURCES: *(a)* USDHHS 2002. *(b)* USDHHS 2005.

NOTE: Data intervals are irregular.

system for services to Medicare beneficiaries (Centers for Medicare and Medicaid Services [CMS] 2005), but this system is not yet in widespread use for non-Medicare beneficiaries. The shift also has implications for greater fragmentation of the delivery system, with market niches for various facets of secondary care, such as ambulatory surgery or outpatient radiology.

## Summary

A significant and growing proportion of the U.S. population needs secondary care for sustained or chronic health problems. Secondary care may be crucial to health maintenance and quality of life. People with comprehensive health insurance coverage are more likely to obtain secondary care than are people with limited or no coverage.

While the need for secondary care grows as the population ages and the number of people with chronic conditions increases, the ways in which some secondary services are being delivered is changing. Many diagnostic and nonsurgical procedures once routinely performed in the hospital are now performed in a range of outpatient settings. Technologic advances and pressures to reduce the costs of inpatient care are prompting this shift in the delivery system.

## Note

1.  Discharge data, rather than admissions data, are often used to describe hospital utilization. One reason for this is that discharge data include both mother and infant, whereas admission data include only the expectant mother.

## Key Words

acute care
ambulatory care
ambulatory surgical centers
    (ASC)
birthing centers
chronic disease care
end-stage renal dialysis (ESRD)
    centers

Medicare prospective payment
    system (PPS)
outpatient care
primary care
secondary care
sliding-scale payments
urgent care centers
utilization of services

# References

Averill, R. F., N. I. Goldfield, M. E. Wynn, T. E. McGuire, R. L. Mullin, L. W. Gregg, and J. A. Bender. 1993. "Design of a Prospective Payment Patient Classification System for Ambulatory Care." *Health Care Financing Review* 15 (1): 71–100.

Centers for Medicare and Medicaid Services. 2005. *Medicare and Medicaid Statistical Supplement 2003*. Pub. No. 03460. Baltimore, MD: CMS.

Robert Wood Johnson Foundation. 1996. *Chronic Care in America: A 21st Century Challenge*. Princeton, NJ: RWJ Foundation.

Spillman, B. C. 2004. "Changes in Elderly Disability Rates and the Implications for Health Care Utilization and Cost." *The Milbank Quarterly* 82 (1): 157–94.

U.S. Department of Health and Human Services. 2005. *Health, United States, 2005*. Pub. No. 05-1232. Hyattsville, MD: USDHHS.

———. 2002. *Health, United States, 2002*. Pub. No. 02-1232. Hyattsville, MD: USDHHS.

Wolf, D. A., K. Hunt, and J. Knickman. 2005. "Perspectives on the Recent Decline in Disability at Older Ages." *The Milbank Quarterly* 83 (3): 365–95.

# 15

# LONG-TERM CARE

## Introduction

As medical technologies continue to save and sustain lives and as the population ages and acquires more chronic health problems, long-term care (LTC) becomes an increasingly important part of the care continuum. Once thought of principally in conjunction with the elderly and identified almost solely with nursing homes, LTC services today are provided to people of all ages in home, community, and institutional settings.

This chapter first provides a definition of long-term care and describes the population requiring LTC services. Formal and informal LTC providers, the utilization of LTC services, and LTC financing are then addressed. The chapter closes with a review of policy issues related to LTC services and programs.

## Defining Long-Term Care

Early definitions of LTC emphasized continuous care over a period of at least 90 days for a range of acute and chronic conditions. Regardless of the length of time (i.e., from weeks to years), LTC is an array of services provided in a range of settings to individuals who have lost some capacity for independence due to an injury, chronic illness, or condition. LTC services assist individuals with basic activities and routines of daily living and may also include skilled and therapeutic care for treatment and management of these conditions (U.S. Bipartisan Commission 1990).

The need for LTC services is often determined by measuring an individual's functional abilities. Two standard measures assess function: activities of daily living (ADLs) and instrumental activities of daily living (IADLs). Table 15.1 identifies the activities included in each category. ADLs are the more basic self-care tasks required for independent functioning, and IADLs are the skills required to perform social tasks and basic household chores to maintain greater self-sufficiency.

How many ADLs and IADLs the individual can demonstrate often determines the person's level of disability. Although these assessment measures are widely used standards to establish an individual's self-care abilities, they do not describe all functional limitations. People with Alzheimer's

| TABLE 15.1 | | |
|---|---|---|
| Activities of Daily Living and Instrumental Activities of Daily Living | | **Generally Include** |
| | **Activities of Daily Living (ADLs)** | • Eating<br>• Bathing<br>• Dressing<br>• Getting to and using bathroom<br>• Getting in or out of bed or chair<br>• Mobility |
| | **Instrumental Activities of Daily Living (IADLs)** | • Going outside the home<br>• Keeping track of money or bills<br>• Preparing meals<br>• Doing light housework<br>• Using the telephone<br>• Taking medicine |

disease or other mental impairments may not have serious ADL limitations but may not be competent to function independently. Other criteria, such as the abilities to attend school or work or to behave in an age-appropriate manner, may be used to further assess functional abilities for people with mental impairments (U.S. General Accounting Office [now known as the U.S. Government Accountability Office—USGAO] 1995).

## Individuals and Populations Requiring LTC Services

More than 12 million people in the United States need LTC services, and nearly 50 percent of this group—an estimated 5 million people—are severely disabled. Figure 15.1 shows the distribution of people, by age group, race and ethnicity, and poverty status, who have limitations of activities caused by chronic conditions. Some of these people need varying levels of LTC. The need for LTC services is often perceived to be linked with an aging population because of the awareness that chronic conditions increase with age. However, a significant proportion of people needing LTC—nearly half—is younger than 65: 40 percent are working-age adults and about 3 percent are children younger than age 18 (USGAO 1995; Feder et al. 2000). Included in these younger age groups are people who require LTC services because of mental impairments or developmental disabilities. Most of the LTC required is not medical in scope, but centers around assistance with the routines of daily living: personal care, meal preparation, housekeeping and chore services, and management of overall care.

FIGURE 15.1

Limitation of
Activity
Caused by
Chronic
Conditions, by
Age Group and
Gender (2000)

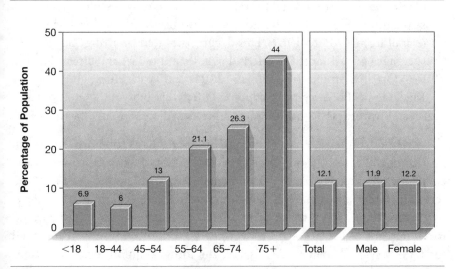

SOURCE: U.S. Department of Health and Human Services (USDHHS) 2005a.

Most analysts believe that the need for LTC services is likely to
increase for at least the next three decades because:

- The population is aging, and the first wave of baby boomers is getting
  close to age 60. People 85 and older—the oldest old—are the fastest-
  growing age group.
- Medical advances enable the saving and sustaining of more lives, but
  those saved may require LTC services—some for relatively short
  periods but others for the duration of their lives. Premature and low-
  birthweight babies who may have had, at best, a limited chance of
  survival 35 years ago are now surviving. Many of them thrive, but
  others require varying periods of LTC during their lives. Accident and
  injury victims whose conditions would once have meant certain death
  are revived and treated, and then resume their lives.
- Medical advances have lengthened the life spans for some congenital
  and disabling conditions. Lung transplants, for example, may provide a
  near-normal life span for people with cystic fibrosis. Prolonging life
  spans affects the demand for LTC services because the need for LTC
  services increases as the population ages and because some remediated
  conditions (e.g., polio) appear to have long-term sequelae that affect
  the individual at a later point in life. Research reported in 1993
  indicates that the extent of chronic and disabling conditions among
  older populations may be lessening. Manton, Corder, and Stallard

(1993) show that the total prevalence of chronically disabled elderly populations in both community and institutional settings declined overall from 1984 to 1989. This decline persisted over three age strata (i.e., ages 65–74; ages 75–84; and age 85 and older) and after adjusting for mortality. Studies by Spillman (2004) and Wolf, Hunt, and Knickman (2005) report changes in elderly disability rates and posit several hypotheses about these changes (see discussion in Chapter 14).

Other studies have attributed disability declines to improvements in nutrition, the care of osteoporosis, and the ability to treat diseases of the circulatory system. Pending developments may also affect the need for LTC services. Potential advances in dementia research may identify ways to deter or prevent the onset of this disease, which currently affects an estimated 5 to 10 percent of the population over age 65 and often results in the need for LTC services. Alzheimer's disease, the most common form of dementia in the United States, affects as many as four million people, and the number of incident cases is expected to be 959,000 in 2050, more than double the number of incident cases (377,000) in 1995 (Hurley and Voliar 2002).

## Long-Term Care Providers

Long-term care providers are categorized as either informal providers (i.e., family members and friends who may render an array of support and assistive services) or formal providers (i.e., trained specialists ranging from physicians to home health aides). Care may be provided in the patient's home or residence, in a community center or other community setting, or in an institution such as a nursing home. Informal LTC providers are discussed first.

### Informal LTC Providers

Of the estimated 12 million people who need LTC, 6.6 million are age 65 or older and are likely to be Medicare beneficiaries and entitled to the LTC coverage that Medicare provides: very limited skilled nursing facility (SNF) care and home health care (see Chapter 6). They may also be part of the 16 percent of the Medicare beneficiaries who are Medicaid-eligible (the dually eligible population), and some may have other health insurance coverage.

The 5.6 million persons under age 65 who need LTC are less likely to have consistent health insurance coverage. Most of this population resides in the community, and about 20 percent are severely impaired, requiring assistance with three or more ADLs (Feder, Komisar, and Niefeld 2000). Of those who receive services, 5 percent receive care from formal providers only, 22 percent receive care from both formal and informal providers, and the majority relies exclusively on unpaid caregivers for their LTC services

(Harrington et al. 1991). More than seven million people in the United States, two million of them in the workforce, provide informal LTC services for a relative or a friend (U.S. Bipartisan Commission on Comprehensive Care 1990; USGAO 1995).

The profile of a typical informal caregiver that follows illustrates why the increasing demand for informal care is worrisome (Harrington et al. 1991; U.S. Bipartisan Commission on Comprehensive Care 1990):

- She is often an older woman herself. More than 75 percent of the providers are women, and more than 35 percent are age 65 or older.
- She is most likely a daughter (24 percent of caregivers), another family member such as a daughter-in-law (26 percent), or a wife (13 percent).
- She may be in poor health as well. More than 33 percent of informal providers are in poor health.
- She generally provides at least four hours of care per day. More than 80 percent of informal caregivers provide this amount of daily care.
- She may have relinquished paid employment to provide care, as do 10 percent of informal caregivers.

For many informal LTC providers, the stress of providing care compromises their personal health status. This fact—along with the geographic dispersion of families, smaller family sizes, the increased number of women working outside the home, the fact that many women are bearing children at older ages, and the longer life spans of cohorts of older people—does not augur well for the expected increased demand for informal LTC services. Adults in midlife who find themselves providing LTC services to older family members while they are still engaged in child-rearing responsibilities may be particularly vulnerable to these stresses. This group is sometimes referred to as the "sandwich generation" because their own needs become sandwiched between those of older parents or other family members and those of children, adolescents, and young adults.

Informal caregivers generally provide LTC services in their own homes or in the homes of the affected family member or friend. Major services may include transportation, assistance with shopping and other household chores, financial management, personal care, and assistance with obtaining medical care and following the regimen, including medications, that the provider prescribes.

### Formal LTC Providers

Formal LTC providers are trained to provide such care and are reimbursed for their services. Although medical and nursing care is included in LTC services, the majority of LTC services provided are nonclinical in nature. Even in a nursing home, a site likely to provide the most intensive level of LTC services, the total amount of nursing-care time a patient receives in a 24-hour period is 1.7 hours. Only about 8 percent of that time is with a registered nurse, and 77 percent of the time is with a nursing assistant (Friedlob 1993).

Usual formal care providers include an array of specialists: home-makers, home health aides, visiting nurses, home health nurses, social workers, mental health services providers, transportation aides, personal care attendants (PCAs), adult day-care providers, meal deliverers, therapists (i.e., speech, physical, occupational, recreational), and others. Usual care sites include the patient's residence, community settings such as senior or community centers, community or neighborhood health centers, adult day-care centers, retirement centers, board and care or shelter homes, assisted living facilities, and nursing homes.

Although 70 percent of all public and private LTC expenditures are for institutional care (USGAO 1995), most people receive LTC services in their residences or in community settings. Figure 15.2 shows that only 16 percent of the population needing LTC resides in institutions; the majority resides in the community.

Several factors influence the site where care is provided. First, the majority of people needing LTC may not require the availability of 24-hour nursing and other care provided in nursing homes; rather, they may need some assistance with one or more ADLs or IADLs.

Second, the supply of nursing home beds is limited. States have been vigilant in controlling nursing home bed supply as a major way of controlling their Medicaid LTC expenditures, and nursing home occupancy is already high, ranging from 74 to 97 percent (Harrington et al. 1992; Cohen and Spector 1996).

Third, few of those who need nursing home care can afford the average annual cost of $46,700 (USDHHS 2002).[1] The annual cost, which

**FIGURE 15.2**
Residence of People Needing LTC, by Age

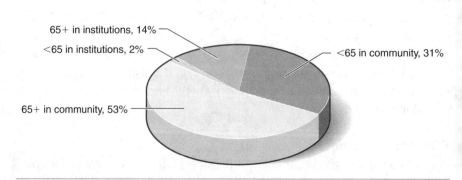

65+ in institutions, 14%
<65 in institutions, 2%
<65 in community, 31%
65+ in community, 53%

SOURCE: U.S. Bipartisan Commission on Comprehensive Health Care 1990.

only 41 percent of nursing home patients are able to bear for the duration of their stay (National Health Policy Forum 1996), is a major reason why Medicaid expenditures have grown so dramatically; Medicaid is the payer for about half of all nursing home expenditures. Nearly 75 percent of total Medicaid expenditures are for acute and LTC services for aged and disabled people; of this expenditure, 90 percent is directed to nursing home or other LTC institutional payments (Coughlin, Holahan, and Ku 1994; Moon 1996).

Fourth, the Medicare program, in an effort to divert beneficiaries from costly nursing home care, expanded its home health care program. In a similar vein, the Medicaid program provides both home health care and, beginning in 1981, initiated reimbursement for a variety of home- and community-based services intended to maintain elderly and/or disabled people in their homes or other settings that are less costly than nursing homes.

## Home Health Care

Home health care services, provided to maintain individuals in their homes and keep them out of more costly institutions, have been available in the U.S. health services system since at least the 1970s. Such services may include blood pressure checks and other monitoring activities, starting intravenous therapies, checking surgical wounds, and administering immunizations or other injections. A limited home health care benefit was included with the passage of Medicare legislation in 1965, and the Medicaid legislation provided for the coverage of personal care services prescribed by a physician. From one of the smallest expenditure categories to one of the fastest growing ones, Medicare home health care expenditures grew from $2.7 billion to $12.7 billion between 1989 and 1994, and were $16.4 billion in 2004. More than 2.4 million Medicare beneficiaries received more than 74 million home health care visits in 2001, averaging 31 visits per person served (Centers for Medicare and Medicaid Services [CMS] 2005b).

The Medicaid home health care program grew at an annual rate of 28.5 percent between 1975 and 1991, the greatest spending increase of any Medicaid service, and represented 5 percent of total Medicaid spending by 1991 (Congressional Research Service 1993). By 2004, Medicaid spent nearly $13.7 billion for home health care, approximately 5 percent of total Medicaid expenditures (CMS 2005a).

Of all home health care services provided, Medicare pays for 38 percent, and Medicaid pays for 32 percent. Private health insurance and out-of-pocket payments account for the remaining 30 percent. Of all of the home health care agencies, Medicare beneficiaries received their services from 6,809 Medicare-certified agencies in 2001. Figure 15.3*a* shows the ownership of these Medicare-certified agencies, with "hospital-based" ownership (29.3 percent of agencies) second to "other" ownership (49.5 percent

**FIGURE 15.3**

Medicare Home Health Agencies by Provider Type and Distribution, Select Years

*(a)* Percentage of home health agency Medicare providers by type (2001).
*(b)* Home health agencies, geographic region, and market share (1999).

(a)

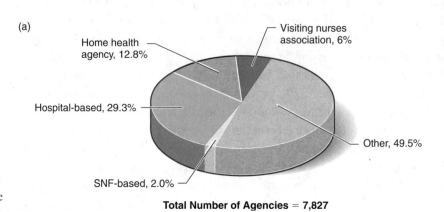

Home health agency, 12.8%
Visiting nurses association, 6%
Hospital-based, 29.3%
Other, 49.5%
SNF-based, 2.0%

**Total Number of Agencies = 7,827**

(b)

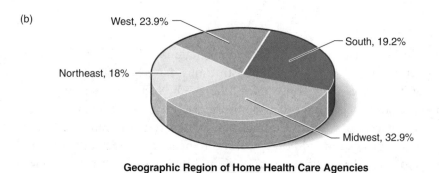

West, 23.9%
South, 19.2%
Northeast, 18%
Midwest, 32.9%

**Geographic Region of Home Health Care Agencies**

SOURCES: *(a)* USDHHS 2005b. *(b)* USDHHS 2005a.
NOTE: SNF = skilled nursing facility.

of agencies) (USDHHS 2005b). Figure 15.3*b* shows the geographic region and market share of Medicare-certified home health agencies.

## Home- and Community-Based Services

The Medicaid provision of LTC services expanded from home health care and nursing home care to home- and community-based services (HCBS) with the passage of the 1981 Omnibus Budget Reconciliation Act (OBRA). This expansion occurred for several reasons:

- State Medicaid programs, because they reimbursed for few HCBS, created perverse incentives for people to use more expensive nursing home care, when it was available.

- Both federal and state governments wanted to reduce their expenditures for nursing home care and restrain expansion of nursing home bed supply.
- Enrollees wanted to obtain services in their homes or communities rather than being institutionalized.

The HCBS provisions of Section 2176 of the 1981 OBRA permitted states to establish waivers authorizing the rendering of community-based LTC services to elderly people, those with developmental disabilities, and other disabled and chronically ill people who would otherwise require nursing home or other forms of institutional care. The Medicaid law (Title XIX of the Social Security Act) authorizes these waivers under its Section 1915(c). Hence, the terms "2176 waiver" and "1915(c) waiver" for HCBS originated from the authorizing legislation.

The 1987 OBRA established a second waiver program to address the special needs of a growing elderly population, sometimes referred to as the "frail elderly," at risk for needing nursing home care. Waivers permit states to cover medical and medically related benefits and to include a range of nonmedical, social, and support services that are essential in allowing people to remain in the community (Congressional Research Service 1993).

Table 15.2 identifies some types of services included in the waiver programs. Additional amendments to the Medicaid waiver authority permit Medicaid to pay for LTC services, including case management, assistance from a home health aide, and respite care, rather than hospital-based services, for chronically ill and disabled children, particularly those who are ventilator-dependent (Model 200 waiver), and for people living with AIDS.

The Medicaid HCBS waivers have unquestionably increased access to LTC services provided in the patient's home or community. As of 2002, Medicaid had approved 263 waiver programs that were operating in 49 states. The fiftieth state, Arizona, operates its entire Medicaid program under an 1115 waiver demonstration program (USGAO 2003).

In 2001, Medicaid expended $20.8 billion for HCBS, about 9.6 percent of its total expenditures (CMS 2005c). The number of Medicaid HCBS enrollees, as of 1999, had grown to 700,000, of whom 55 percent were elderly (USGAO 2003). The GAO, responding to a congressional request to evaluate aspects of Medicaid HCBS, found that the guidance to states offered by the Centers for Medicare and Medicaid Services (CMS) and CMS oversight of HCBS waivers are inadequate to ensure quality of care for waiver enrollees. The GAO also reported that the CMS had not fully complied with statutory and regulatory requirements that base waiver renewals on: (1) the submission by states of annual reports that describe quality assurance approaches and identify deficiencies found through

TABLE 15.2
Examples
of Services
Available
under Medicaid
HCBS Waivers

| | |
|---|---|
| Case management | The development and implementation of a comprehensive care plan for a person with impairments or disabilities |
| Homemaker/home health aide | Assistance in the home with light housekeeping; assistance with medications and other health-related functions |
| Personal care | Assistance with self-care activities such as bathing, dressing, eating |
| Adult day health | Provision of meals and supervision, including recreational therapy, in an out-of-home setting |
| Habilitation | For persons with mental retardation and developmental disabilities, habilitation services are designed to help them acquire, retain, and improve the self-help, socialization, and adaptive skills necessary to reside successfully in community-based settings |
| Respite care | Care provided on a relief basis for a disabled person by special caregivers in order to provide a respite for that person's full-time caregiver |

SOURCE: Congressional Research Service 1993.

monitoring; and (2) the CMS conducting periodic reviews to determine whether states are protecting the health and welfare of waiver enrollees (USGAO 2003).

The CMS is exploring two major questions about Medicaid HCBS waiver programs: (1) Are these programs serving only people at risk of institutionalization? (2) Is the substitution of HCBS for institutionalization resulting in cost savings? Whether all state Medicaid programs are targeting only enrollees at risk of institutionalization is certain to vary by state and by type of waiver program. Weissert, Cready, and Pawalek (1988) found that targeting patients at high risk of institutionalization "has been uneven and best accomplished by a mandatory nursing home preadmission-screening program." Cost savings are difficult to document in HCBS programs, in part because some services provided may not be pure substitutes for institutionalization. The establishment of LTC services in the home and community may generate what some have called the "woodwork" effect: people with needs emerge from the woodwork as soon as services to meet these needs become available (USGAO 1995; Moon 1996).

The chapter focus now turns from LTC services provided in the patient's home or community to LTC services provided in an institutional setting.

## Nursing Home Care

Nursing homes provide nursing care and assistive LTC services on a residential basis for patients of all ages who have a range of disabilities and impairments. In 2003, 1.5 million people, the majority of them elderly, resided in nursing homes in the United States (USDHHS 2005a), and an additional 600,000 lived in other LTC facilities (USGAO 1995). In addition, 2.5 million persons were discharged from nursing homes in 1999, indicating a short stay for recuperation or rehabilitation (CDC 2002).

One challenge in discussing nursing homes is the variety of facilities that may be included under this umbrella term. The Medicare and Medicaid programs, which require that nursing homes that care for their beneficiaries and enrollees be certified as having met certain conditions of participation, distinguished between "skilled" and "intermediate" care until fiscal year 1991, when this distinction was removed and the services were renamed "nursing facility services." Table 15.3 shows Medicare's classification system for skilled nursing facilities (SNFs) based on a resource utilization group (RUG) classification system. Nevertheless, the SNF distinction still appears and is linked to Medicare, which reimburses only for skilled and not for intermediate care. The term *nursing home* is intended to distinguish facilities that provide medical and nursing services from those that provide room, board, and nonmedical care, but some databases combine these different types of facilities.

The most comprehensive data on nursing homes come from the periodic National Long-Term Care Survey, last reported in 1989, and the National Nursing Home Survey of 1999. The lag in the availability of current data, different reporting periods, and different ways in which facilities are defined and categorized limit the ability to draw conclusions about this aspect of the U.S. health services system. A sixth National Nursing Home survey was conducted in 2004, but the data will not be reported until sometime in 2006.

Figure 15.4 shows the distribution of nursing home size, by number of licensed beds, for 1971, 1980, 1986, 1991, 1997, and 1999. Small nursing homes (those with fewer than 25 beds) consistently accounted for 37 percent of all nursing homes until 1991, when the category of smallest nursing homes was reported as fewer than 75 beds. By 1999, 27.5 percent of all nursing homes had more than 200 beds.

Most nursing homes are owned by proprietary organizations, and this proportion remained stable for the 1971 to 1997 period at approximately 70 to 80 percent (see Figure 15.5). By 1999, however, the proportion of proprietary nursing homes had decreased to 40 percent, with a commensurate increase in not-for-profit nursing homes in the same period.

**TABLE 15.3**
Medicare
Skilled Nursing
Facilities,
RUG-III
Classification
System

| Clinical Hierarchy Category (First Level) | | Activities of Daily Living (Second Level) | Problem/ Service Split (Third Level) |
|---|---|---|---|
| Rehabilitation (Special) | Ultra-high intensity | 3 Levels | (not used) (14 groups) |
| | Very high intensity | 3 Levels | |
| | High intensity | 3 Levels | |
| | Medium intensity | 3 Levels | |
| | Low intensity | 2 Levels | |
| Extensive services | | (not used) | Count of services (3 groups) |
| Special care | | 3 Levels | (not used) (3 groups) |
| Clinically complex | | 3 Levels | Signs of depression (6 groups) |
| Impaired cognition | | 2 Levels | Nursing rehabilitation (activity count) (4 groups) |
| Behavior problems | | 2 Levels | Nursing rehabilitation (activity count) (4 groups) |
| Physical functions (reduced) | | 5 Levels | Nursing rehabilitation (activity count) (10 groups) |

SOURCES: Fries 1992; Health Care Financing Administration 2000.

NOTE: RUG-III = Resource Utilization Groups, Version Three.

## Veterans Nursing Homes

Qualified military veterans have access to their own designated nursing homes supported by the Department of Veterans Affairs (VA). The VA provides nursing home care to qualified military veterans in three ways. First, the VA owns nursing home facilities; 40 percent of veterans receiving nursing home care reside in VA-owned facilities. Second, the VA contracts with community nursing homes for beds for veterans; 24 percent of veterans receiving nursing home care reside in community nursing homes. Third, the VA pays a portion of the costs of nursing home care for veterans who reside in state-owned and operated veterans' homes; 36 percent of veterans

**FIGURE 15.4**
Percentage
Distribution
of Nursing
Home Size
(Select Years,
1971–1999)

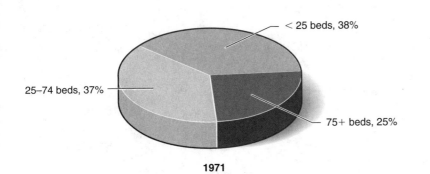

< 25 beds, 38%

25–74 beds, 37%

75+ beds, 25%

**1971**

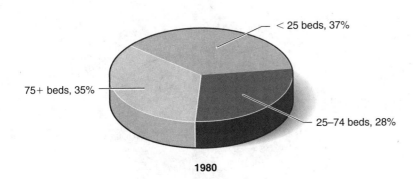

< 25 beds, 37%

75+ beds, 35%

25–74 beds, 28%

**1980**

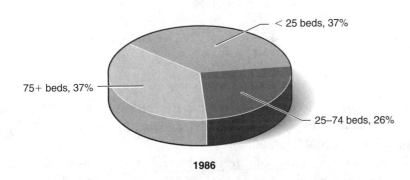

< 25 beds, 37%

75+ beds, 37%

25–74 beds, 26%

**1986**

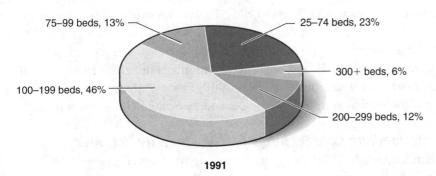

75–99 beds, 13%

25–74 beds, 23%

300+ beds, 6%

100–199 beds, 46%

200–299 beds, 12%

**1991**

*(continued)*

**FIGURE 15.4**
Continued

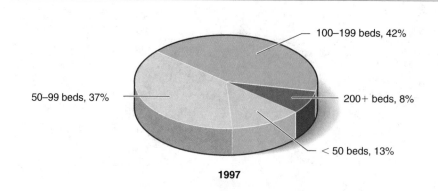

100–199 beds, 42%

50–99 beds, 37%

200+ beds, 8%

< 50 beds, 13%

1997

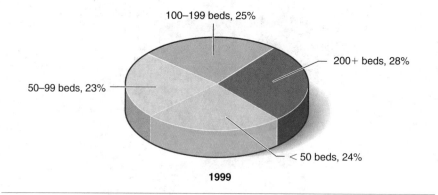

100–199 beds, 25%

50–99 beds, 23%

200+ beds, 28%

< 50 beds, 24%

1999

SOURCES: U.S. Department of Commerce (USDOC) 1995, 2001; USDHHS 2005a.

receiving nursing home care reside in state veterans' homes. More than 93,000 veterans nursing home stays occurred in 2003 at an expenditure of $20.8 billion (USDHHS 2005a).

Despite the number of veterans who received nursing home services, the GAO estimates that only 14 percent of veterans' demand for nursing home care was met (USGAO 1996). Demand is expected to increase as the number of veterans age 65 and older grows from 8.8 million in 1995 to 9.3 million in the year 2000. Much of this demand is expected to come from veterans age 75 and older, whose numbers increased from 2.6 million in 1995 to 4.0 million in the year 2000; this group is at high risk of nursing home admission because of age and associated chronic conditions.

### Intermediate Care Facilities for the Mentally Retarded

Until the early 1970s, the care of people with developmental disabilities, defined as mental retardation and related conditions, was limited to nursing homes, state mental institutions, the individual's family, or private arrangements the family could make. With the passage of PL 92-223 in

**FIGURE 15.5**
Percentage
Distribution of
Nursing Home
Ownership
(Select Years,
1971–1999)

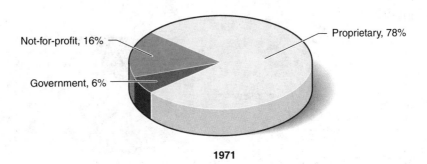

1971

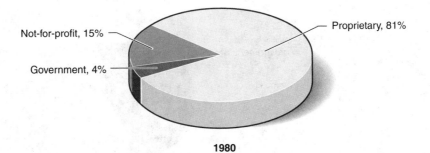

1980

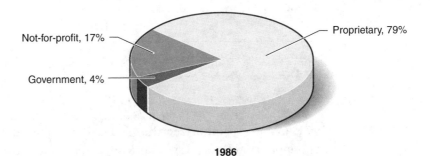

1986

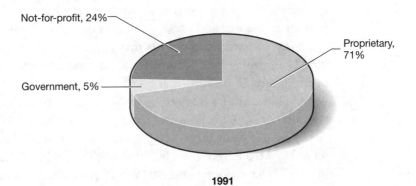

1991

(continued)

**FIGURE 15.5**
Continued

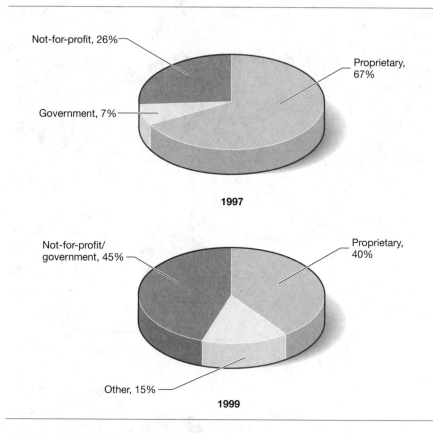

SOURCES: USDOC 1995, 2001; USDHHS 2005a.

1971, Congress authorized the Medicaid program to pay for optional (as opposed to mandated) services provided in facilities that met Medicaid standards for people with developmental disabilities. These facilities are known as Intermediate Care Facilities for the Mentally Retarded (ICFMR). ICFMRs provide residential and social services and arrange for nursing, medical, and therapeutic services their clients may require. The number of ICFMRs grew quickly as existing facilities met Medicaid criteria and new facilities were developed. Figure 15.6 shows that 547 facilities existed in 1977. By 1990, there were 5,404 facilities (Congressional Research Service 1993), and by 2005, the number of ICFMR facilities had grown to about 7,400 (CMS 2005b).

As shown in Figure 15.7a, the number of Medicaid enrollees cared for in ICFMRs ranged from 69,000 in 1975, to 151,000 in 1981, to 117,000 in 2001. The majority of the enrollees are adults over age 21, and only 14 percent are younger than 21 years (USDHHS 2000). ICFMR residents account for only two-tenths of 1 percent of all unduplicated count Medicaid enrollees.

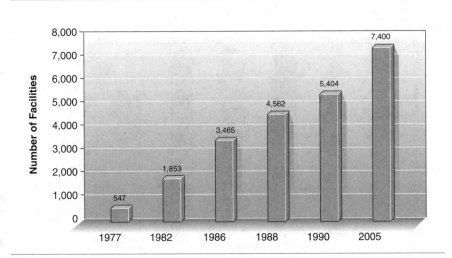

**FIGURE 15.6**
Number
of ICFMR
Facilities
(Select Years,
1977–2005)

SOURCES: Congressional Research Service 1993; CMS 2005b.

NOTE: Data intervals are irregular.

Because it provides personal care and social, therapeutic, and other services on a residential basis, the ICFMR program has higher per capita expenditures than do other Medicaid programs. In fiscal year 2001, the ICFMR per capita expenditure was $83,173 (Figure 15.7*b*), compared to the average per capita expenditure of $4,560 for all enrollees (CMS 2005a). ICFMR expenditures constitute about 4.5 percent of all Medicaid program expenditures, growing from $380 million in 1975 to $9.7 billion in 2001 (Figure 15.7*c*).

### Other Medicaid LTC Services for People with Developmental Disabilities

Medicaid has other programs that provide services to people with developmental disabilities who are not ICFMR residents. The 1981 optional HCBS waiver program was extended to people with developmental disabilities. Medicaid agencies may also fund a range of optional programs to serve people with developmental disabilities or they may pay for the care of people with developmental disabilities in nursing homes, but only if that is the most appropriate placement.

### Non-Medicaid LTC Services for People with Developmental Disabilities

Although Medicaid is the primary payer for services provided in ICFMRs, other funds support services to people with developmental disabilities. States provide separate, non-Medicaid funds to care for people with developmental

**FIGURE 15.7**

Medicaid
ICFMR
Enrollees and
Payments,
Select Years

(*a*) Number of
Medicaid
enrollees in
ICFMRs
(select years,
1975–2001).
(*b*) Medicaid
payment per
person served in
ICFMRs
(select years,
1975–2001).
(*c*) Total
Medicaid
payments for
ICFMR services
(select years,
1975–2001).

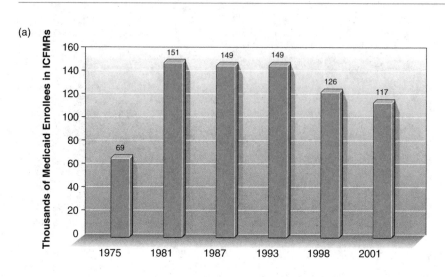

(a)

(b)

*(continued)*

disabilities, many of whom reside in small facilities that are not ICFMR-certified. States also contribute to special education funds for this population, and the federal government contributes $3.4 billion in income maintenance as well.

## LTC Services That Focus on the Elderly

In addition to the formal and informal LTC providers and the LTC programs described in the previous sections, some additional LTC demonstration programs are available specifically for elderly people in the geographic areas in which these demonstrations are located. Two of them are the Program of All-Inclusive Care for the Elderly (PACE) and social health maintenance organizations (SHMOs).

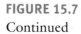

**FIGURE 15.7**
Continued

(c)

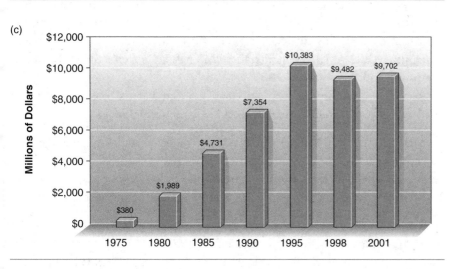

SOURCES: USDHHS 2000, 2005b.

NOTE: Data intervals are irregular.

The PACE program, modeled on San Francisco's On Lok program in Chinatown, relies on adult day care to monitor the health of frail, elderly people at risk of nursing home care and to ensure that clients obtain needed services. PACE clients are generally low-income people who are dually eligible for Medicare and Medicaid. In addition to services covered by Medicare and Medicaid, PACE clients receive vision, hearing, and dental services; meals; transportation; and nonprescription drugs (Barton, Glazner, and Poole 1995). These programs provide patients who have nursing home levels of disabilities with the support and assistive services they need in their senior residences or a community setting, thus averting the need for institutionalization.

The PACE program was first offered on a demonstration basis at 25 sites. Providers were paid a capitation rate for each enrollee, regardless of the level of frailty or type of services needed. Enrollees paid no deductibles or copayments. The 1997 Balanced Budget Act provided for limited growth in the number of PACE programs and also permitted state Medicaid programs to provide medical assistance to PACE enrollees as an optional Medicaid service. The PACE program permits most clients to continue living at home rather than be institutionalized. Medicare and Medicaid finance a comprehensive delivery system. PACE providers assume full financial risk for participants' care without limits on amount, duration, or scope of services (CMS 2005c).

**Program of All-Inclusive Care for the Elderly (PACE)**

**Social Health
Maintenance
Organizations
(SHMOs)**

To determine whether an integrated program of social and health services can maintain frail, elderly people in their homes or communities and thus avoid the need for institutionalization, and to determine the feasibility of increasing Medicare LTC benefits, the CMS has supported a SHMO demonstration in four sites since 1980.

SHMOs are financed on a prepaid, capitated at-risk basis, using three funding sources (Greenberg, Leutz, and Greenlick 1988):

1. Medicare pays 100 percent of its costs, using the adjusted average per capita cost (AAPCC) (see Chapter 7);
2. the beneficiary pays a monthly premium; and
3. Medicaid funds are a part of financing for the dually eligible Medicare and Medicaid enrollees who participate.

In addition to the acute care benefits that Medicare Parts A and B cover, which do not require copayments or deductibles for this population, SHMOs cover the following services:

- dentures;
- prescription drugs;
- optometry;
- audiometry;
- eyeglasses;
- hearing aids;
- preventive care visits;
- unlimited hospital days; and
- extended "Medicare-type" skilled nursing facilities benefits.

The chronic care benefits covered include:

- case management;
- home nursing;
- personal care;
- homemaker services;
- adult day care;
- medical transportation;
- hospice care;
- respite care; and
- chronic care in a nursing facility without a prior hospitalization.

Other services included or arranged for are home-delivered meals, electronic response systems, and chore services. The demonstration sites limit in various ways the extent of LTC services they will provide to an annual dollar amount per person, a limit on the number of nursing home days, or another limit (Barton, Glazner, and Poole 1995).

Early SHMO demonstration sites were able to reduce hospitalization rates compared with those of the non-SHMO Medicare population and to control the costs of expanded benefits (Greenberg, Leutz, and Greenlick 1988). When total costs were considered, however, all sites experienced substantial losses during the first three years of operation. By the fifth year, two projects either broke even or had net gains on a current basis and the other two had losses (Kane, Harrington, and Newcomer 1991).

The 1997 Balanced Budget Act extended the SHMO demonstration and evaluation authority until 2001 and required the secretary of the U.S. Department of Health and Human Services to submit to Congress by January 1, 1999, a plan to integrate SHMO plans as an option under the new Medicare+Choice program. Given the difficulties encountered in maintaining the viability of Medicare+Choice plans that offer only medical services, this proposed legislation has not yet occurred.

## Utilization of LTC Services

Not all people who need services from the formal LTC system are able to obtain them, as was noted in previous sections. This section reviews the utilization of formal LTC services by those who have been able to access them, beginning with home health care and then turning to home- and community-based services (HCBS) and nursing home services.

### Home Health Care
Home health care is provided to people of all ages who have insurance coverage or other resources to pay for these services, but the majority of home health care clients are Medicare beneficiaries. Utilization of home health care services focuses on the Medicare population; comparable data for other populations are limited or unavailable.

Figure 15.8 shows the percentage of Medicare home health care patients who received various levels of care or therapies in 2001: 49.7 percent received nursing care and 25.2 percent received assistance from a home health aide.

Figure 15.9*a* shows the number of Medicare beneficiaries, by age group, who received home health care services in 2001. Those in the age group 75–84 had the greatest number of beneficiaries who receive home health care. Medicare beneficiaries younger than age 65 who are Medicare-eligible because of a disability had the smallest number of home health care visits; this population comprises about 10 percent of all Medicare beneficiaries.

Figure 15.9*b* provides the demographics of Medicare beneficiaries who receive home health care by three major categorizations: gender, eligibility group (aged or disabled), and race (white or other). Because more women than men survive into older age categories and the white

**FIGURE 15.8**

Distribution of Types of Medicare Home Health Care Visits (2001)

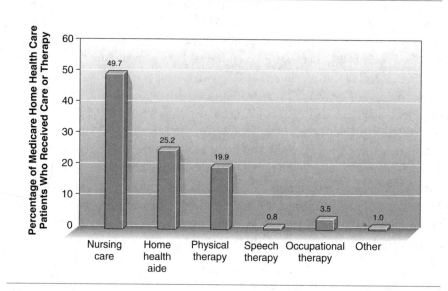

SOURCE: USDHHS 2005b.

**FIGURE 15.9**

Medicare Beneficiaries Receiving Home Health Care (2001)

(a) By age group.
(b) By gender, eligibility group, and race.

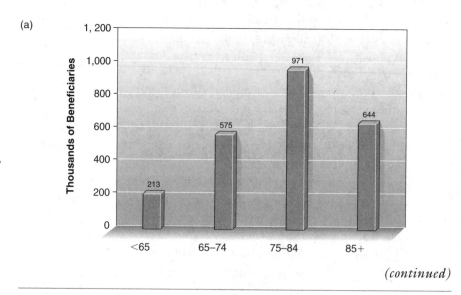

*(continued)*

population is greater than other racial and ethnic groups, it is not surprising that more females than males, more aged than disabled people, and more whites than people of other racial or ethnic groups receive home health care.

Figure 15.10, which shows the number of people served per one thousand beneficiaries, the number of visits per person served, and the

**FIGURE 15.9**
Continued

(b)

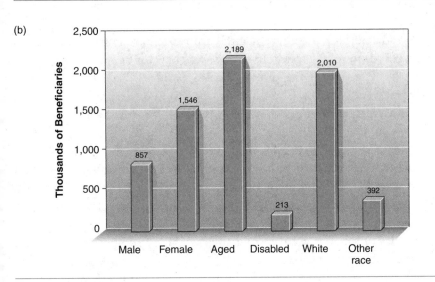

SOURCE: USDHHS 2005b.

**FIGURE 15.10**
Medicare
Home
Health Care
(Select Years,
1974–2001)

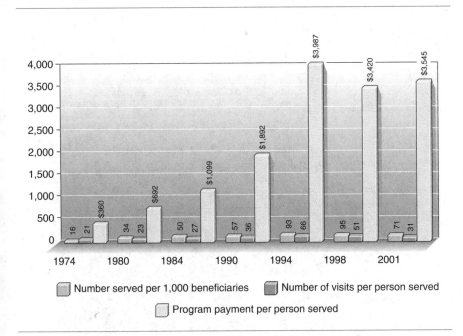

SOURCE: USDHHS 2005b.

NOTE: Data intervals are irregular.

program payment per person served, provides additional perspective on
the proportion of all Medicare beneficiaries who use home health care
services. The number of visits per person served has more than tripled in
the 27-year period covered in Figure 15.10; however, it is important to

note that the number of visits per person has dropped from the high of 66 in 1994.

Medicaid pays for home health care for children, adults, and aged and disabled people. Figure 15.11 shows the number of children and adults who received Medicaid home health care between 1975 and 2001. Figure 15.11 also shows the number of aged and disabled people who received Medicaid-reimbursed home health care for this same period.

### Home- and Community-Based Services (HCBS)

National-level information on the utilization of HCBS is difficult to obtain because state Medicaid programs, which vary widely in the services for which they reimburse, operate the HCBS waivers. Although most states have at least one HCBS waiver program that may serve all age groups, each differs in the types of services it covers and the maximum number of enrollees it can serve under each waiver.

### Nursing Home Services

Figure 15.12*a* shows the number of nursing homes available for use between 1971 and 2003. The number of nursing homes reached a high of 33,000 in 1990 and dropped to just over half that number by 2003. Mergers and consolidations account for the reduction in the number of homes. Figure 15.12*b* shows that the number of beds increased to 1.9 million in 1991,

**FIGURE 15.11**

Number of
Medicaid
Enrollees,
by Category,
Served
by Home
Health Care
(Select Years,
1975–2001)

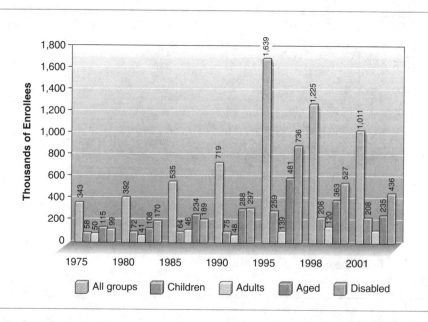

SOURCE: USDHHS 2005b.

NOTE: Data intervals are irregular.

**FIGURE 15.12**
U.S. Nursing
Home and
Related Care
Facilities
(Select Years,
1971–2003)
(*a*) Number
of U.S. nursing
home and
related care
facilities.
(*b*) Number
of beds and
residents in
nursing home
and related care
facilities.

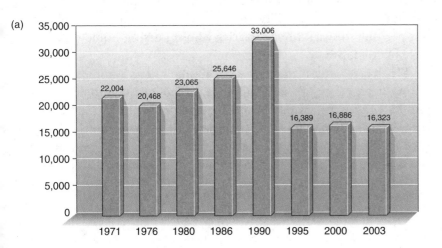

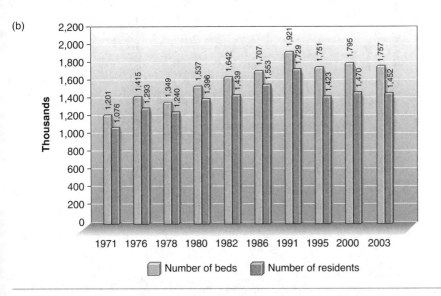

SOURCES: (*a*) USDHHS 1996, 2005a. (*b*) USDHHS 2005b.

NOTES: Facilities of 3+ beds; included skilled nursing facilities, excluded board and care homes for the developmentally disabled. Data intervals are irregular.

dropping to 1.76 million in 2003. The occupancy rate (the percentage of beds occupied) has ranged between 82 and 85 percent for the period 1995 to 2003 (USDHHS 2005a).

Data on demographic characteristics of nursing home users are incomplete. Although 41 percent of nursing home residents are never enrolled in Medicaid, the demographic information on this population is limited. Medicare is a small player in nursing home care, paying for only about

14 percent of nursing home expenditures in 2004. Figure 15.13 shows the age, gender, race, and eligibility group of the number of Medicare beneficiaries per one thousand beneficiaries whose nursing home care is paid entirely by Medicare.

Medicaid is the major payer for public nursing home care, compensating for the care of nearly 60 percent of all nursing home residents. Figure 15.14 shows the number of aged and disabled Medicaid enrollees served by nursing homes for select years between 1975 and 2001. Medicaid-eligible children and adults may also reside in nursing homes, but their numbers range from fewer than one thousand to no more than nine thou-

**FIGURE 15.13**

Demographics of Medicare Beneficiaries in Skilled Nursing Facilities, Admissions per One Thousand Beneficiaries (2001)

(*a*) By age.
(*b*) By gender, race/ethnicity, and eligibility group.

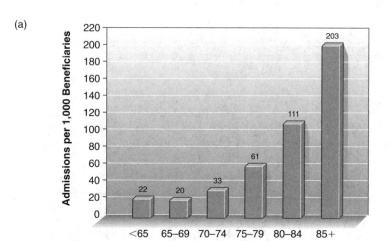

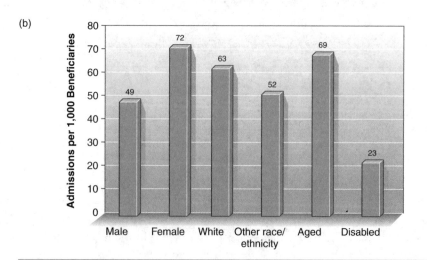

SOURCE: USDHHS 2005b.

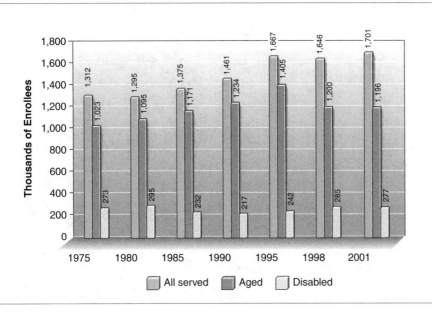

**FIGURE 15.14**
Number of
Medicaid
Enrollees, by
Category,
Served by
Nursing
Facilities
(Select Years,
1975–2001)

SOURCE: USDHHS 2005b.

NOTE: Data intervals are irregular.

sand for these years. As would be expected, aged people constitute the majority of Medicaid enrollees cared for in nursing homes.

Figure 15.15 shows the level of dependence or independence of nursing home patients, by particular ADL (mobility dependence, incontinence, and eating dependence) and by age group, for 1999. A higher proportion of nursing home residents in all age groups can feed themselves and have some mobility than are able to dress themselves.

As the population ages and demands for LTC are expected to increase, will adequate services and resources be available to meet these needs? Many clients prefer HCBS services; however, at some point, the more continuous level of care provided in a nursing home may be required by some proportion of the population.

**The Role of Nursing Home Use in Later Life**

Murtaugh, Kemper, and Spillman (1990) used 1982 to 1984 National Long-Term Care Survey data to assess the risk of nursing home use in later life. They concluded that 43 percent of individuals turning age 65 in the early 1990s have a risk of nursing home use at some point in their lives. Thirty-seven percent of those who died between 1982 and 1984 had used a nursing home. Fifty-five percent of those projected to use a nursing home will have one or more stays totaling at least one year, while 21 percent will have stays totaling five years (National Health Policy Forum

FIGURE 15.15

Nursing Home Residents Age 65+, by Functional Status (1999)

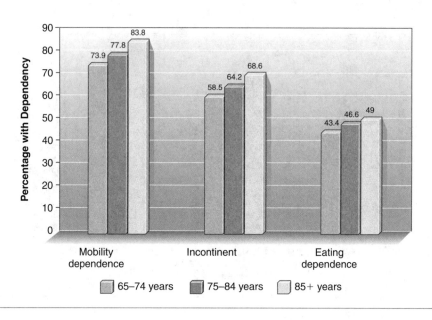

SOURCE: USDHHS 2002.

1996). This increased risk is due to the longer life expectancy of people now turning 65.

Assuming that past utilization patterns continue, more than 50 percent of the females and about 33 percent of the males who turned 65 in 1990 can expect to use a nursing home before they die. The cohort turning 65 in the year 2020 can be expected to have twice as many members who use a nursing home before they die as did the cohort who died between 1982 and 1984 (Murtaugh, Kemper, and Spillman 1990).

Given changes in the cohort sizes of the aged and disabled and in longevity, Spillman and Lubitz (2002) estimate that by the year 2010, of all estimated 2.6 million nursing home users, 44 percent will have some use, 45 percent will use the nursing home three months or longer, 24 percent will use it one year or longer, and 9 percent will use it five years or longer. By 2020, the projections for any use are 46 percent; for three months or longer, 34 percent; for one year or longer, 25 percent; and for five years or longer, 9 percent.

Research by Lakdawalla et al. (2003) on forecasting the nursing home population suggests that the several recent decades of decline in disability and institutionalization will be reversed for today's young cohorts. Lakdawalla and colleagues estimate that the future nursing home population is likely to be 10 to 25 percent higher than would be suggested by a simple extrapolation of past declines in disability. The researchers attribute some of this reversal to recent increases in obesity and asthma among young to middle-aged cohorts.

# LTC Financing

Public payers finance much of the formal LTC provided in the U.S. health services system. Table 15.4 shows major federal programs that support LTC services for the elderly and disabled, and Figure 15.16 shows the distribution of payers for nursing home and home health care. Medicare pays for only 14 percent of all nursing home care, whereas Medicaid pays for nearly half.

Medicaid, in fact, pays for the nursing home care for nearly 60 percent of all nursing home residents and for 25 percent of the home health care for all age groups, and supports other LTC services through HCBS waivers and other Medicaid services and programs. More than 33 percent of Medicaid's total expenditures are for LTC; more than 40 percent of this amount, however, is expended on the population of people younger than age 65 who have disabilities (National Health Policy Forum 1996).

Medicaid's financing of nursing home care for the aged and disabled deserves additional attention because of its volume and because of special provisions surrounding this financing. Nearly 43 percent of older people are Medicaid-eligible at the time of their admission to a nursing home. Of those persons who enter the nursing home as private-pay patients, an estimated 10 to 16 percent deplete their financial resources during their stay, and, because of their limited income and assets, become Medicaid-eligible (National Health Policy Forum 1996; Barton, Glazner, and Poole 1995). This process is called "spend-down." Medicaid has instituted some protections against spousal impoverishment, should there be a spouse physically able to remain in the couple's home; thus, the illness of one partner no longer guarantees the impoverishment of both.

Monthly charges for nursing homes in 2002 averaged $3,900 or higher (USDHHS 2002). Charges may differ by type of payer, as shown in Figure 15.17. The monthly charge for Medicare is considerably higher than the others because Medicare pays for only skilled nursing care, a much more resource-intensive level of care. Studies have shown that Medicaid patients whose payment rate may be lower than that of other clients may in some instances receive a lower quality of care (Cohen and Spector 1996).

Long-term care insurance (reviewed in Chapter 6) currently holds little promise as a major financial mechanism for LTC. In 2004, private insurance paid about 9 percent of the costs of LTC, including nursing home costs (CMS 2005a). A typical LTC policy will pay a fixed amount—between $50 and $300 per day for nursing home care and about half that for home health care (Health Insurance Association of America 2002). An inflation clause for policies purchased in advance of their anticipated use is a crucial purchase consideration. Although estimates of the proportion of those in the United States who could afford LTC insurance range from 6 to

**TABLE 15.4**

Major Federal Programs Supporting Long-Term Care Services for the Elderly and Disabled

| Program | Objectives | Fiscal Year 1993 Federal Spending: Total and LTC Only (Millions of Dollars)* | Administration | LTC Services |
|---|---|---|---|---|
| Medicare/Title XVIII of the Social Security Act | To pay for acute medical care for the aged and selected disabled | Total: $138,810 LTC: $15,800 (estimated) | *Federal:* HCFA/HHS *State:* None | Home health visits, limited skilled nursing facility services |
| Medicaid/Title XIX of the Social Security Act | To pay for medical assistance for certain low-income persons | Total: $77,367 LTC: $24,700 (estimated) | *Federal:* HCFA/HHS *State:* State Medicaid agency | Nursing home care, home- and community-based health and social services, facilities for persons with developmental disabilities, chronic care hospitals |
| Social Services Block Grant/Title XX of the Social Security Act | To assist families and individuals in maintaining self-sufficiency and independence | Total: $2,805 LTC: (not available) | *Federal:* Office of Human Development Services/HHS *State:* State social services or human resources agency; other state agencies may administer part of Title XX funds for certain groups—for example, state agency on aging | Services provided at the state's discretion, may include LTC |
| Rehabilitation Act | To promote and support vocational rehabilitation and independent living for the disabled | Total: $2,186 LTC: $54 | *Federal:* Office of Special Education and Rehabilitative Services/Department of Education *State:* State vocational rehabilitation agencies | Rehabilitation services, attendant and personal care, centers for independent living |
| Older Americans Act | To foster the development of a comprehensive and coordinated service system to serve the elderly | Total: $1,377 LTC: $765 | *Federal:* Administration on Aging/Office of Human Development/HHS *State:* State Agency on Aging | Nutrition services, home and community-based social services, protective services, and LTC ombudsman |

*Data represent total fiscal year 1993 obligations as reported in the *Budget of the United States Government, Appendix, Fiscal Year 1995,* except for estimates of Medicare and Medicaid long-term care spending. These figures are estimates for 1993 from the assistant secretary for planning and evaluation, HHS. Under the Medicaid program, states contribute an estimated $19.0 billion in support of long-term care in addition to the federal share of $24.7 billion.

NOTES: HCFA = Health Care Financing Administration; HHS = Department of Health and Human Services; LTC = long-term care.

(a)

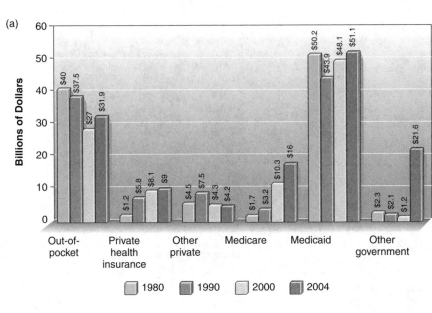

FIGURE 15.16

Financing of Long-Term Care Services, Select Years

(a) Financing of nursing home care payer (1980, 1990, 2000, 2004).
(b) Financing of home health care payer (1995, 2000, and 2004).

(b)

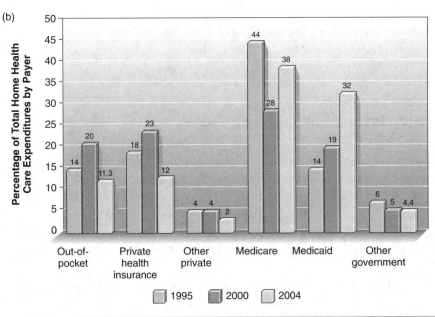

SOURCE: CMS 2005c.

**FIGURE 15.17**
Average
Monthly
Payment for
Nursing Home
Care, by Payer
(1999)

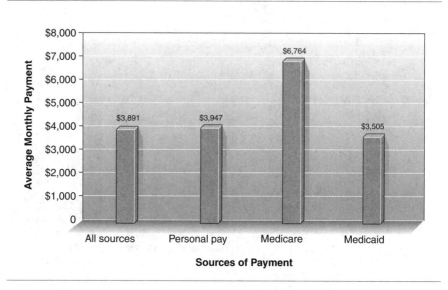

**FIGURE 15.17**
Average
Monthly
Payment for
Nursing Home
Care, by Payer
(1999)

SOURCE: USDHHS 2002.

40 percent (Harrington et al. 1991), barriers to LTC insurance remain
(Cohen and Kumar 1997).

## Policy Issues Surrounding LTC

More than 12 million Americans are estimated to need LTC services, but
not all of them receive services because of barriers—particularly financial—
to access. Coupled with this unmet need is the projected increased demand
for LTC services as life expectancy grows for people with chronic conditions, the population ages and acquires more chronic conditions, and medical technologies increase and their application broadens to save the lives of
more people.

The unmet and growing need for LTC gives rise to several policy
issues. First, what part of the health services system is, or should be, responsible for providing LTC? Second, how should LTC be financed? Third, what
organizational and other issues are linked to LTC access and utilization?

### Responsibility for LTC and LTC Financing

The questions of responsibility for providing LTC and LTC financing are difficult to disentangle. Many mistakenly believe that Medicare, because it pays
for inpatient hospital care, some physician services, and some ambulatory care
of aged and disabled people, has primary responsibility for the provision of
LTC. Although Medicare's role in providing home health care has grown dra-

matically in recent years, it pays for no other home- or community-based services, and pays for only 14 percent of all nursing home care. Although pressures to expand the Medicare role emanate from a number of sources, congressional efforts are currently focused on the implementation of the outpatient Medicare prescription drug coverage that became effective January 2006.

Medicaid is a major LTC provider through its HCBS waiver programs, payment for home health care, and its role as the primary payer for nursing home care. Established to pay for health services for low-income children, their adult caregivers, and low-income aged and disabled people, Medicaid pays for nursing home and other LTC to these populations and to people from higher-income strata who have become impoverished as a result of spending-down their resources to obtain medical care.

Few group private health insurance policies cover comprehensive LTC services. Although individual policies are available for purchase, few people buy this type of coverage because it is relatively expensive, because coverage may not include an inflation clause to deal with the likely higher costs of future care, and because of other uncertainties surrounding LTC insurance.

Providing LTC is costly because of the range of medical, nursing, assistive, social, therapeutic, residential and other services a dependent person with disabilities may need. LTC services provided in a home or community setting are likely to be less costly per person than LTC services provided in an institutional setting. The availability of services outside the institutional setting, however, swells the demand for them; dependent people who have managed with the help of family, neighbors, or friends are often eager to receive regular, formal LTC services.

## LTC Utilization Issues

The LTC infrastructure is weak at best. States individually regulate the number of nursing home beds they license. Moratoria on the construction of nursing home beds by various states as a cost-containment effort and an increase in the population of elderly resulted in a reduction in the supply of nursing home beds per one thousand elderly people between 1977 and 1985 (Murtaugh, Kemper, and Spillman 1990). Population projections indicate that an increasing proportion of the population will be at risk for nursing home use in the next several decades, suggesting that capacity-building should be occurring.

People living in rural areas may have greater difficulty accessing LTC services, particularly home- and community-based services, simply because providers may be unavailable, or because providing services to a sparse and widely scattered population may be economically infeasible. One solution to the problem of limited availability of nursing home beds in rural areas was CMS authorization, in the early 1980s, of hospital swing beds. Smaller rural hospitals in areas with few or no nursing homes may use a designated number of available beds either for acute care or LTC, depending on patient needs.

## LTC Reform

Individuals and organizations have long recognized the need for LTC reform. The U.S. Bipartisan Commission on Comprehensive Health Care reported in 1990 on its comprehensive review of the status of LTC. The commission adopted as its goal a commitment to develop recommendations "for public policies that will assure all Americans access to affordable health care coverage that allows them to obtain necessary care and assures them adequate financial protection; that will promote quality care and address problems of health care costs; and that will provide the financing required to assure access." The commission went on to make detailed recommendations on how to build universal coverage and an LTC system.

Several proposals have been fielded to prepare for the increasing need for LTC services. The Medicare Catastrophic Care Act of 1988 would have addressed a number of LTC needs, but major parts were repealed the following year because Medicare beneficiaries believed it created inequities among them. The Health Security Act of 1993 proposed to expand home- and community-based services, improve Medicaid coverage for institutional care, develop standards to improve the quality and reliability of private LTC insurance, create tax incentives to encourage people to buy LTC insurance or to help individuals with disabilities to work, and produce a demonstration study intended to pave the way toward greater integration of acute care and LTC. Congress, however, did not enact the Health Security Act.

The Physicians for a National Health Program proposed a federally mandated and funded LTC program, to be locally administered to provide all needed medical and social services to the at-risk population. They estimated additional annual expenditures of $18 to $24 billion to provide these services in 1991 (Harrington et al. 1991); more recent estimates indicate that the costs to provide LTC to all who need it could require $80 billion annually in new spending (Moon 1996). Kane (1995) recommends expanding the home care concept, expanding the use of personal care attendants (PCAs), and blurring the categorical boundaries that currently create distinct home health care, institutional care, and other LTC services.

In the absence of concerted national policy, state Medicaid programs are taking action to protect against being unduly saddled with an even larger share of providing LTC. Many governors and state legislatures, concerned about a slowing economy and other recession portents, are concertedly working to once again rein in Medicaid expenditures.

Change, even incremental change at the level of state government, is almost certain for LTC services in the short term, with the likely need for national-level action in the long term.

## Summary

Twelve million persons, nearly evenly distributed between those younger and older than age 65, need some level of LTC services. USGAO studies (2002a, 2002b) report that spending for LTC—an estimated $134 billion in 1999—could quadruple by 2050 when the baby boom population is fully vested in Medicare. Unless the preceding policy issues are addressed and resolved, this increased demand will place enormous pressure on needy individuals and their families, on public payers, and on U.S. society in general.

## Note

1. This figure is based on the charge to private-pay patients. Medicare and Medicaid each pay less than this charge for care provided to their respective beneficiaries and enrollees.

## Key Words

| | |
|---|---|
| activities of daily living (ADL) | Medicare |
| adjusted average per capita cost (AAPCC) | Medicare+Choice plans |
| adult day care | Medicare/Medicaid facility certification |
| Centers for Medicare and Medicaid Services (CMS) | omnibus budget reconciliation act (OBRA) |
| entitlement programs | personal care attendants (PCAs) |
| formal caregivers | preadmission screening |
| frail elderly | Program of All-Inclusive Care of the Elderly (PACE) |
| home- and community-based services (HCBS) | respite care |
| home health care | "sandwich generation" |
| informal caregivers | skilled nursing facility (SNF) |
| instrumental activities of daily living (IADL) | social health maintenance organization (SHMO) |
| intermediate care facilities for the mentally retarded (ICFMR) | spend-down |
| long-term care (LTC) | spousal impoverishment |
| long-term care (LTC) insurance | swing beds |
| Medicaid | U.S. Bipartisan Commission on Comprehensive Health Care |
| Medicaid waiver program | "woodwork" effect |

# References

Barton P. L., J. Glazner, and C. Poole. 1995. *Final Report: Colorado Medicaid Reform Study, Phase II, Long-Term Care*. Denver, CO: University of Colorado Health Sciences Center.

Centers for Disease Control and Prevention. 2002. "The National Nursing Home Survey: 1999 Summary." *Vital Health Statistics* 13 (152): 1–116.

Centers for Medicare and Medicaid Services. 2005a. "Highlights, National Health Expenditures, 2004." [Online information; retrieved 1/12/1006.] http://cms.hhs.gov/statistics/ nhe/historical/highlights.asp.

———. 2005b. "Intermediate Care Facilities for the Mentally Retarded (ICFMR)." [Online information; retrieved 1/17/2006.] http://new/cms/hhs.gov/CertificationandComplican/09_ICFRMs.asp.

———. 2005c. "Program of All-Inclusive Care for the Elderly (PACE)." [Online information; retrieved 1/9/2006.] www.cms.hhs.gov/PACE/.

Cohen, J. W., and W. D. Spector. 1996. "The Effect of Medicaid Reimbursement on Quality of Care in Nursing Homes." *Journal of Health Economics* 15 (1): 23–48.

Cohen, M. A., and A. K. Nanda Kumar. 1997. "The Changing Face of LTC Insurance in 1994: Profiles and Innovations in a Dynamic Market." *Inquiry* 34 (1): 50–61.

Congressional Research Service. 1993. *Medicaid Source Book: Background and Data Analysis* (a 1993 update). Washington, DC: U.S. Government Printing Office.

Coughlin, T., J. Holahan, and L. Ku. 1994. *Medicaid Since 1980*. Washington, DC: The Urban Press.

Feder, J., H. L. Komisar, and M. Niefeld. 2000. "Long-Term Care in the United States: An Overview." *Health Affairs* 19 (3): 40–56.

Friedlob, A. 1993. "The Use of Physical Restraints in Nursing Homes and the Allocation of Nursing Home Resources." Ph.D. diss., University of Minnesota, Minneapolis.

Fries, B. E. 1992. *Update RUG-III Briefing Document*. Ann Arbor, MI: University of Michigan.

Greenberg, J., W. Leutz, and M. Greenlick. 1988. "The Social Health Maintenance Organization Demonstration: Early Experience." *Health Affairs* 7 (3): 66–79.

Harrington C., C. Cassel, C. L. Estes, S. Woolhandler, and D. U. Himmelstein. 1991. "A National LTC Program for the U.S." *Journal of the American Medical Association* 266 (21): 3023–29.

Harrington C., S. Preston, L. Grant, and A. H. Swan. 1992. "Revised Trends in States' Nursing Home Capacity." *Health Affairs* 11 (2): 170–80.

Health Care Financing Administration. 2000. *Medicare and Medicaid Statistical Supplement*. Washington, DC: HCFA.

Health Insurance Association of America. 2002. *Source Book of Health Insurance Data 2002*. Washington, DC: HIAA.

Hurley, A. C., and L. Voliar. 2002. "Alzheimer's Disease: 'It's OK, Mama, If You Want to Go, It's OK.'" *Journal of the American Medical Association* 288 (18): 2324–31.

Kane, R. A. 1995. "Expanding the Home Care Concept: Blurring the Distinctions among Home Care, Institutional Care, and Other Long-Term Care Services." *The Milbank Quarterly* (73) 2: 161–86.

Kane, R. L., C. Harrington, and R. Newcomer. 1991. "Social Health Maintenance Organizations' Services, Use, and Costs, 1985–89." *Health Care Financing Review* 12 (3): 37–52.

Lakdawalla, D., D. P. Goldman, J. Bhattacharya, M. D. Hurd, G. F. Joyce, and C. W. A. Panis. 2003. "Forecasting the Nursing Home Population." *Medical Care* 41 (1): 8–20.

Manton, K. G., L. S. Corder, and E. Stallard. 1993. "Estimates of Change in Chronic Disability and Institutional Incidence and Prevalence Rates in the U.S. Elderly Population from the 1982, 1984, and 1989 National Long-Term Care Survey." *Journal of Gerontology* 48 (4): S153–S166.

Moon, M. 1996. *Long-Term Care in the U.S.* New York: The Commonwealth Fund.

Murtaugh, C. M., P. Kemper, and B. C. Spillman. 1990. "The Risk of Nursing Home Use in Later Life." *Medical Care* 28 (10): 952–62.

National Health Policy Forum. 1996. *Eligibility for Medicaid in Nursing Homes: Coverage for Indigent or Well-off Older Americans?* Washington, DC: The George Washington University.

Spillman, B. C. 2004. "Changes in Elderly Disability Rates and the Implications for Health Care Utilization and Cost." *The Milbank Quarterly* 82 (1): 157–94.

Spillman, B. C., and J. Lubitz. 2002. "New Estimates of Lifetime Nursing Home Use: Have Patterns of Use Changed?" *Medical Care* 40 (10): 965–75.

U.S. Bipartisan Commission on Comprehensive Health Care. 1990. *A Call for Action: The Pepper Commission Final Report.* Washington, DC: U.S. Government Printing Office.

U.S. Department of Commerce. 2001. *Statistical Abstract of the United States, 2001.* Washington, DC: U.S. Government Printing Office.

———. 1995. *Statistical Abstract of the United States, 1995.* Washington, DC: U.S. Government Printing Office.

U.S. Department of Health and Human Services. 2005a. *Health, United States, 2005.* Pub. No. (PHS) 05-1232. Hyattsville, MD: USDHHS.

———. 2005b. *Medicare and Medicaid Statistical Supplement 2003.* Pub. No. (PHS) 03460. Baltimore, MD: USDHHS.

———. 2002. *Health, United States, 2002.* Pub. No. (PHS) 02-1232. Hyattsville, MD: USDHHS.

———. 2000. *Medicare and Medicaid Statistical Supplement, 2000.* Pub. No. (PHS) 03386. Baltimore, MD: USDHHS.

———. 1996. *Medicare and Medicaid Statistical Supplement.* Baltimore, MD: USDHHS.

U.S. Government Accountability Office (formerly the U.S. General Accounting Office). 2003. *Long-Term Care: Federal Oversight of Growing Medicaid*

*Home- and Community-Based Waivers Should Be Strengthened.* GAO-03-576. September. Washington, DC: USGAO.

———. 2002a. *Long-Term Care: Availability of Medicaid and Home- and Community-Based Services for Elderly Individuals Varies Considerably.* GAO-02-1121. Washington, DC: USGAO.

———. 2002b. *Long-Term Care: Baby Boom Generation Increases Challenge of Financing Needed Services.* GAO-01-563T. Washington, DC: USGAO.

———. 1996. *VA Health Care: Better Data Needed to Effectively Use Limited Nursing Home Resources.* GAO/HEHS-97-27. Washington, DC: USGAO.

———. 1995. *LTC: Current Issues and Future Directions.* GAO/HEHS-95-109. Washington, DC: USGAO.

Weissert, W. G., C. M. Cready, and J. E. Pawalek. 1988. "The Past and Future of Community-Based Long-Term Care." *The Milbank Quarterly* 66 (2): 309–88.

Wolf, D. A., K. Hunt, and J. Knickman. 2005. "Perspectives on the Recent Decline in Disability in Older Ages." *The Milbank Quarterly* 83 (3): 365–95.

# TERTIARY CARE

## Introduction

Tertiary care is highly specialized and complex, and an often-costly form of care offered in inpatient settings such as children's, psychiatric, and rehabilitation hospitals, and academic health centers (AHCs). AHCs are composed of an allopathic or osteopathic school of medicine, one or more schools or programs to train allied health professionals, and a university or other teaching hospital (Shortell 1997).

The focus of this chapter is on AHCs as examples of tertiary care facilities. The chapter begins with a definition of tertiary and other forms of specialty care, outlines the range of facilities providing this level of care, and concludes with a discussion of the many policy issues facing AHCs as major tertiary care providers.

## Defining Specialty Medical Care

The definition of tertiary care is broad and centers around highly specialized, procedurally intensive inpatient care that may require a prolonged length of stay and, because of its duration and intensity, is almost certain to be costly. Examples of tertiary care include surgical procedures, such as coronary artery bypass grafts (CABGs), and also specialized diagnostic devices, such as magnetic resonance imaging (MRI) and positron emissions tomography (PET) (Blumenthal, Campbell, and Weissman 1997).

Until very recently, the term *tertiary care* described the highest and most technologic level of care available. The many advances in high-level care, however, have given rise to the term *quaternary care,* which describes high levels of care that are provided predominantly in AHCs because of the highly specialized providers required and because these services may be unprofitable for community and other hospitals to offer. Examples of quaternary care include burn units, regional trauma centers, transplant services, inpatient AIDS centers, neonatal intensive care units, and radiation therapy centers (Blumenthal, Campbell, and Weissman 1997).

## Specialty Care Providers

As knowledge of illness and disease etiology has expanded, so has the ability to specialize the care of certain conditions or disorders. Certain conditions of the complex human organism require the focus and expertise of a specialist whose experience with patients with similar conditions may contribute to improved patient outcomes. Studies by Luft (1980) and others have shown the importance of volume in maintaining provider proficiency and in achieving optimal outcomes in treating special conditions, which then suggests the centralization or regionalization of tertiary and higher levels of care.

## The AHC as a Provider of Tertiary Care

Many large community hospitals provide tertiary care and may offer as much as 90 percent of the care that an AHC can provide (Biles and Simon 1996; Mechanic and Dobson 1996). However, this section focuses on the tertiary and quaternary care provided in AHCs because several distinguishing characteristics make AHCs more than just another provider of high-level health services.

The first distinguishing characteristic of AHCs is that many of them are noted for the high levels of care they provide to indigent and uninsured patients who could not otherwise afford this level of care. AHCs provide as much as 44 percent of uncompensated inpatient care (Iglehart 1995).

AHCs are major providers of uncompensated care for several reasons. First, as major training sites of physicians and other health services providers, AHCs require an ample patient population for teaching purposes. Indigent patients with complex and multiple conditions benefit from the most advanced care and at the same time help to educate the physician and other health services provider trainees about their conditions and health status. Second, some AHCs and their teaching hospitals are public facilities, at least in part directly supported by appropriations from their sponsoring governmental entities. In return for the use of public dollars, such facilities are expected to provide a certain amount of uncompensated care. Third, because AHCs admit and care for an unusually high number of indigent patients, whose inability to pay for their care creates fiscal hardships for the facility, AHCs may be eligible for disproportionate share hospital (DSH) payments (i.e., supplemental payments) from public payers such as Medicare and Medicaid to offset some costs of caring for indigent patients.

A second characteristic that distinguishes AHCs from other specialty care providers is their educational mission. All undergraduate medical education is provided in the more than 115 AHCs or in the 13 private, freestanding medical schools that are not currently part of an AHC (Culbertson, Goode, and Dickler 1996; Bulger 1993). Nearly 60 percent of all graduate medical education is provided in AHCs (Blumenthal, Campbell, and Weissman 1997). The training of many allied health professionals, including advanced practice nurses and other levels of nurses, physician assistants, pharmacists, dentists, public health workers, and others, is centered in AHCs. AHCs are the most important trainers of the health services workforce in the United States.

A third characteristic that distinguishes AHCs from other specialty care providers is the extent and variety of research they conduct. Most clinical research and a significant proportion of basic science and biomedical research have traditionally been conducted in AHCs.

These three distinguishing characteristics of AHCs—sometimes referred to as the AHC tripartite mission of patient care and service, education, and research (what some term the "triple threat")—result in the production of both public and private goods. Public goods include the care of indigents and uninsured, health professional training, and clinical and basic science research. Private goods include clinical care, teaching, and biomedical research (Blumenthal and Meyer 1996).

AHCs produce this unique combination of goods and services through a complex, often-implicit maze of cross-subsidies. Given their reputation for providing cutting-edge care, AHCs have typically been able to charge between 15 and 35 percent more for care than other providers to support their higher costs (Blumenthal and Meyer 1996; Biles and Simon 1996). These costs include some inevitable inefficiencies resulting from AHCs' comprehensive education and training programs.

Physician education, for example, even in public AHCs, is not supported solely by state government appropriations and student tuition. Rather, the income that teaching faculty derive from the care of patients in AHC hospitals and clinics supports the costs of undergraduate medical education. This clinical income, usually channeled through one or more faculty practice plans, supports an increasing proportion of medical education, up from 7 percent in 1971 (Iglehart 1994) to 50 percent in 1994 (Biles and Simon 1996; Gallin and Smits 1997). Some clinical research also may be cross-subsidized with clinical income from faculty practice plans.

## Policy Issues Facing AHCs

A number of factors have called into question the long-term viability of AHCs. The managed care environment often challenges AHCs' ability to offer competitive pricing. In addition, while AHCs may have the latest technology and highly skilled providers, other tertiary-level facilities can legitimately make similar claims. Finally, the absence of federal or state regulation on hospital growth and development has eliminated the protective factor that may have once insulated AHCs. And AHCs are not immune from the increasing costs of doing business, particularly those related to professional education, malpractice insurance, and maintaining an up-to-date and equipped physical plant.

## AHC Costs Higher Than Other Providers

Until the evolution of an increasingly competitive health services marketplace in the 1990s, AHCs were able to maintain their comprehensive levels of care and charge payers a higher price that reflected the volume and intensity of services, and a margin to cross-subsidize the production of other public goods.

Employers and other payers, however, are increasingly scrutinizing the high costs of providing medical care and are aggressively bargaining with providers. They are much less willing to support the medical costs of groups that are not their direct beneficiaries, employees, or enrollees. Led by Medicare, they are curtailing providers' abilities to charge paying patients more to cross-subsidize the care of other groups or the production costs of other public goods.

Specialty care providers who do not produce public goods can operate more efficiently and offer lower prices to payers, thus becoming more competitive in securing patient populations than AHCs. Even populations such as Medicaid enrollees that once were considered the exclusive domain of AHCs and other public providers were in the mid- to late-1990s aggressively pursued by commercial insurers and other nonpublic providers, a 180-degree turnaround from prior years. AHCs' reputation as centers of excellence for tertiary and other specialty care results in no more than a 10 percent premium differential from other specialty care providers (Mechanic and Dobson 1996).

## Effect of Increasingly Competitive Markets on AHCs

The increasingly competitive marketplace may affect the long-term viability of AHCs. A primary focus of many AHCs, especially those in markets that are becoming increasingly consolidated or integrated and are moving toward managed competition, is to maintain an adequate patient base to support their patient care functions and to ensure an appropriate population for teaching purposes. Pursuing this priority may, at least in the short term, erode focus and resources away from AHCs' educational and research functions. One study that examined the strategies that seven major AHCs employed to maintain their competitiveness found that emphasis on education and research declined as the AHCs focused on maintaining or expanding market share (Blumenthal and Meyer 1996).

## Can AHCs Compete Effectively?

Will AHCs remain the dominant tertiary and other specialty care providers, or will growing competition in the health services market bring about substantial changes in AHCs and their tripartite mission? At the heart of this question is a larger, unresolved dilemma: Who should pay for the production of public goods?

Private markets have typically been unwilling to support the production of certain goods and services, making them by default the responsibility of the public domain. The public sector already bears some costs of medical and other health professional education. The nation's inability or unwillingness to establish a universal system of health services has placed the responsibility for health services to certain populations in the public domain. Failure to treat basic health services as a public good has left the United States in crisis (Bulger 1993).

Hill and Madara (2005) point out that AHCs' abilities to perform multiple missions—education, research, and caring for the most vulnerable populations—may be threatened by the stagnating National Institutes of Health (NIH) support for research, declining insurance reimbursements, explosive malpractice insurance costs, a crisis in government health care programs, and the growing proportion of the population that is uninsured. Cohen and Siegel (2005, 1367) add that AHCs are facing more daunting challenges than ever before in their research role, including:

> . . . high expectations by the public for a steady stream of lifesaving discoveries, news about financial conflicts of interest and scientific misconduct by researchers that threaten to erode public trust in academic institutions, tensions between the cultural norms of academe and industry that cloud their growing partnerships, obstacles to recruiting and retaining physician-scientists, constrained funding sources and increasing costs of research, and the need to transform the academic reward structure and culture to encourage collaboration and adapt to new "team science."

Moses, Their, and Matheson (2005) explored with a sample of AHC leaders their thoughts about their roles and AHC survival. AHC leaders expressed concerns regarding reimbursement uncertainties, ineffective clinical decision making, and clinical quality (mentioned in three-quarters of the interviews). They noted that their priorities included securing sufficient investment capital, revising undergraduate and graduate curricula, strengthening ties to physicians and community hospitals, attracting faculty, and meeting regulatory requirements.

A Task Force on Academic Health Centers sponsored by The Commonwealth Fund examined the future of AHCs at length. The 2003 report includes a number of suggestions for research, education, clinical care, and vulnerable populations, as well as the following recommendations regarding infrastructure and organizational responsiveness:

- AHCs should strive to be leaders in the application of information technology to improve health care.
- AHCs should develop organizational structures that are more responsive to the needs of the communities they serve.
- AHCs should dramatically improve their internal accounting capabilities and their abilities to manage the flow of funds supporting routine activities and mission-related work.
- AHCs should develop capabilities for performance measurement and improvement, and should train and lead personnel at all levels to value openness, learning, teamwork, accountability, and patient-centeredness.
- AHCs should develop mechanisms to learn about the work of other AHCs, nonacademic health care organizations, and non-health care institutions to identify best practices that may be usefully incorporated into their own activities.
- AHCs should develop mechanisms to assess continually the health care needs of their own communities and of the U.S. population more generally, and should ensure that resulting data are incorporated into strategic planning and management decisions.

The report concludes that it is difficult to envision a U.S. system without AHCs, but emphasizes the need for AHC redirection.

## Summary

Tertiary and other specialty care is currently offered in large community hospitals, in AHCs, and in specialty hospitals, such as children's, rehabilitation, and psychiatric hospitals. Highly specialized care has long been a hallmark of the U.S. health services system, and the composition of the physician workforce, where specialists outnumber generalists two to one, reflects this emphasis. The growing market influence of managed care, however, is a major force in shifting the focus of the delivery system from specialty care to primary care. This shift is creating substantial upheaval in the system, which is reflected in the major changes that AHCs, as principal tertiary and other specialty care providers, are or may soon be facing. Battling to survive in an increasingly competitive health services marketplace, many AHCs are securing their patient populations as a first line of defense. How AHCs will modify their education and research missions is not yet clear.

## Key Words

| | |
|---|---|
| academic health centers (AHCs) | faculty practice plan |
| AHC tripartite mission | magnetic resonance imaging (MRI) |
| basic science research | managed competition |
| biomedical research | Medicare |
| center of excellence | quaternary care |
| clinical research | teaching hospital |
| competition | tertiary care |
| cross-subsidies | "triple threat" |
| disproportionate share hospital | uncompensated care |
| (DSH) payments | |

## References

Biles, B., and L. Simon. 1996. "Academic Health Centers in an Era of Managed Care." *Bulletin of the New York Academy of Medicine* 73: 484–89.

Blumenthal, D., E. G. Campbell, and J. S. Weissman. 1997. *Understanding the Social Missions of AHCs.* New York: The Commonwealth Fund.

Blumenthal, D., and G. S. Meyer. 1996. "Academic Health Centers in a Changing Environment." *Health Affairs* 15 (2): 200–15.

———. 1993. "Using Academic Health Centers to Help Avoid Health Care's Next Crisis." *Journal of the American Medical Association* 269 (19): 2548–49.

Cohen, J. J., and E. K. Siegel. 2005. "Academic Medical Centers and Medical Research." *Journal of the American Medical Association* 294 (11): 1367–72.

Commonwealth Fund, The. 2003. *Envisioning the Future of Academic Health Centers.* Pub. No. 600. New York: The Commonwealth Fund.

Culbertson, R. A., L. D. Goode, and R. M. Dickler. 1996. *Organizational Models: Medical School Relationships to the Clinical Enterprise.* Washington, DC: Association of American Medical Colleges.

Gallin, J. I., and H. L. Smits. 1997. "Managing the Interface Between Medical Schools, Hospitals, and Clinical Research." *Journal of the American Medical Association* 277 (8): 651–54.

Hill, L. D., and J. I. Madara. 2005. "Role of the Urban Academic Medical Center in U.S. Health Care." *Journal of the American Medical Association* 294 (17): 2219–20.

Iglehart, J. 1995. "Rapid Changes for AMCs. Part 2." *New England Journal of Medicine* 332 (6): 407–11.

———. 1994. "Rapid Changes for AMCs. Part 1." *New England Journal of Medicine* 331 (20): 1392–95.

Luft, H. S. 1980. "The Relation between Surgical Volume and Mortality: An Exploration of Causal Factors and Alternative Models." *Medical Care* 18 (9): 940–59.

Mechanic, R. E., and A. Dobson. 1996. "The Impact of Managed Care on Clinical Research: A Preliminary Investigation." *Health Affairs* 15 (3): 72–89.

Moses, H., S. O. Their, D. H. M. Matheson. 2005. "Why Have Academic Medical Centers Survived?" *Journal of the American Medical Association* 293 (12): 1495–1500.

Shortell, S. M. 1997. "Restructuring AHCs: Values, Leadership, and Strategies." Presentation to the Association of Academic Health Centers, Washington, DC. Unpublished.

# 17

# PALLIATIVE CARE

## Introduction

Palliative care is care offered during a person's terminal illness, when no other therapeutic interventions hold promise for improvement. Palliative care may be provided by informal caregivers, such as family members in a home setting, or by formal caregivers in the patient's home or in a hospice. Hospices may be freestanding, or they may be affiliated with an inpatient hospital or a long-term care facility. This chapter focuses on formal palliative care provided in a hospice setting. The chapter begins with a definition of hospice care, identifies hospice care providers, and reviews hospice utilization. It concludes with a discussion of policy issues surrounding palliative care.

## Defining Hospice Care

Hospice care is provided to ease the pain and stress of a terminal condition when no other medical or surgical interventions are available to ameliorate the condition. Hospice care may include physicians' services; pain management and prescription drugs; nursing care; psychological counseling; short-term hospitalization; homemaker and home health aide services; physical, occupational, and speech therapy; and social services to ease the last days or weeks of life. Access to hospice care generally requires certification by a physician that the patient has a terminal condition with a life expectancy of fewer than six months.

## Hospice Care Providers

Hospice care may be provided in a patient's home, in a designated unit of a hospital or a long-term care facility, or in a freestanding hospice facility. Formal hospice care generally originates with a physician's order, which is often necessary to secure reimbursement from the payer. The physician maintains oversight of the patient, dealing with pain management, issues of nutritional intake, and physical complications that may be related to the admission diagnosis.

Day-to-day hospice care is generally provided by specially trained nurses, social workers, and therapists, who work closely with patients and their families to ensure that patients' final days of life are as comfortable as possible. In 2003, nearly 3,200 hospices were in operation in the United States, including the District of Columbia, Puerto Rico, and Guam (Matherlee 2002). The distribution of hospices varies, with the largest share (45 percent) in the South and the fewest (10.7 percent) in the Northeast. States may have as few as one hospice (South Dakota) or as many as 102 (Michigan) and 107 (North Carolina). The size of each hospice varies as well: some may have only a few beds, while others may have many (American Hospital Association [AHA] 2006).

Figure 17.1 shows the ownership status of the 3,200 hospices in the United States. Figure 17.2 shows the organizational status—whether free-standing or affiliated with another organization—of the hospices.

**FIGURE 17.1**

U.S. Hospice Ownership (2001)

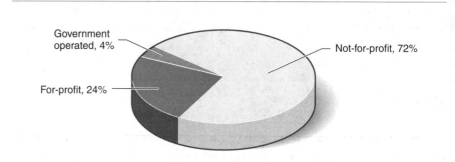

SOURCES: Matherlee 2002; National Hospice and Palliative Care Organization 2003.

NOTE: The number of hospices = 3,200.

**FIGURE 17.2**

Hospice Organizational Status (2001)

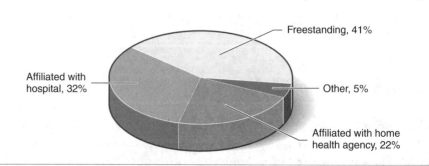

SOURCE: Matherlee 2002; National Hospice and Palliative Care Organization 2003.

NOTE: The number of hospices = 3,200.

## Utilization of Hospice Care

As is true of other health services, utilization of formal hospice care may depend on a person's health insurance coverage or other financial means. Medicare began providing hospice coverage in 1983 and pays for the majority (at least 80 percent) of formal hospice care (Christakis and Escarce 1996; Matherlee 2002). Medicaid programs have had the option since the 1985 Consolidated Omnibus Budget Reconciliation Act (COBRA) to provide hospice care to their enrollees; as of 1991, 33 state Medicaid programs provided hospice coverage, using eligibility criteria similar to those used by Medicare (Congressional Research Service 1993). Both the Medicare and Medicaid programs require their beneficiaries and enrollees who seek hospice care to waive their rights to certain other kinds of therapeutic care. Community fundraising and donations may pay for some patients' hospice care.

Figure 17.3 shows the sources of payment for hospice care in 2000. The principal admission diagnosis among patients who obtain hospice care is malignant neoplasms; 52 percent of all hospice admissions are for this condition (U.S. Department of Health and Human Services [USDHHS] 2005). Of the malignant neoplasm admissions, 12.3 percent involve the trachea, bronchus, and lung; 4.8 percent, the breast; 4.9 percent, the large intestine and rectum; and 7.7 percent, the prostate. Figure 17.4 shows that other major admission diagnoses include 6.5 percent for diseases of the respiratory system and 12.8 percent for heart disease.

Medicare is the largest payer for hospice services. Table 17.1 shows, by U.S. geographic region, the number of hospices that receive Medicare reimbursement, the average number of per-person days covered, and the Medicare payment per person in 2002. Medicare beneficiaries in hospices received an average of 52 days of care at an average per-person Medicare expenditure of $6,697.

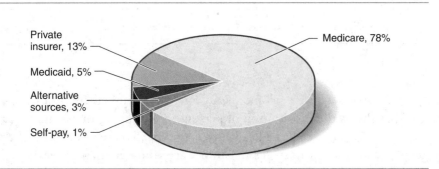

Private insurer, 13%

Medicaid, 5%

Alternative sources, 3%

Self-pay, 1%

Medicare, 78%

**FIGURE 17.3**

Sources of Payment for Hospice Care (2000)

SOURCE: Matherlee 2002.

FIGURE 17.4
U.S. Hospice
Patients,
by Primary
Admission
Diagnosis
(2000)

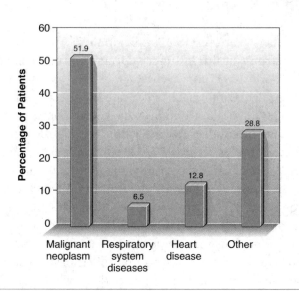

SOURCE: USDHHS 2002.

TABLE 17.1
Number
of Hospices,
Covered Days
of Care per
Person Served,
and Program
Payment per
Person Served
for Hospice
Services Used
by Medicare
Beneficiaries,
by Region
of Residence,
2002

| Geographic Region | Number of Hospices | Covered Days of Care per Person Served | Program Payment per Person Served |
|---|---|---|---|
| Northeast | 322 | 45 | $6,235 |
| Midwest | 667 | 50 | 6,150 |
| South | 858 | 63 | 7,569 |
| West | 443 | 51 | 6,833 |
| Total | 2,290 | 209 | |

SOURCE: Centers for Medicare and Medicaid Services (CMS) 2006.

Hospices care for people of any age with terminal conditions. Figure 17.5 shows the distribution of persons in four age groups—under age 65, ages 65–74, ages 75–84, and over age 85. Nineteen percent of the people who were in hospices in 2000 were younger than 65 years. The 75- to 84-year-old age group had more than double the proportion of hospice patients as did the 65- to 74-year-old age group, and the oldest

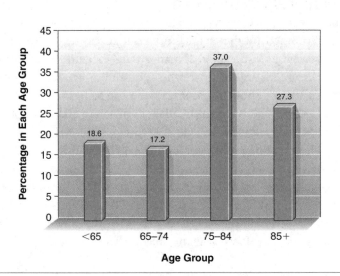

**FIGURE 17.5**
U.S. Hospice
Patients, by
Age Group
(2000)

SOURCE: USDHHS 2002.

age group (85 and older) represented more than 27 percent of hospice patients.

For Medicare beneficiaries and most Medicaid enrollees, life expectancy of six or fewer months is a criterion of hospice admission. Christakis and Escarce (1996) report that a study of Medicare hospice claims for 1990 shows that the median survival time after enrollment is only 36 days, and nearly 16 percent of the patients die within 7 days. Survival time was related to diagnosis, with the unadjusted survival after enrollment shortest for those with leukemia, lymphoma, or biliary or liver cancer, and longest for those with chronic lung disease, dementia, or breast cancer.

## Policy Issues Surrounding Palliative Care

Several policy issues surround the use of palliative care in the United States. First, do all those who need formal palliative care receive it? Second, for those who do receive formal hospice care, do they begin to receive it early enough in the course of their illness, given that the median survival rate after Medicare hospice enrollment is only 36 days? Third, how may the current interests in such issues as providing access to physician-assisted suicide affect the availability of palliative care? Each issue is briefly considered in the sections that follow.

### Access to Formal Palliative Care

Determining whether access to palliative care such as hospice services is adequate is confounded by the lack of universal access to health services and the limitations of existing data. Existing data focus on those who utilize services but are silent about those who require but cannot obtain services. Thus, little is known about the unmet need for palliative care.

What *can* be said is that as medical knowledge and technologies have helped to reduce or eradicate the causes of many diseases, particularly some communicable and contagious diseases, life expectancies have increased. With increased life expectancies comes the greater likelihood of developing one or more chronic diseases, with their varying rates of life termination. Despite many advances in health services, the human organism is mortal and does die. When the individual, the health services provider, and society can accept this fact, palliative care may, for many, become more humane and less costly.

### Is Hospice Care Initiated at the Appropriate Point in a Terminal Illness?

In their review of Medicare claims for hospice care in 1990, Christakis and Escarce (1996) found that the median survival time after admission to a hospice was 36 days, with equivalent proportions of the population under the two tails of the distribution curve: 15 percent died within 7 days, and 15 percent lived longer than 6 months. Their findings raise the question of whether admission might be occurring too late in the course of a terminal illness. Christakis and Escarce looked at hospital admissions in the 270 days prior to hospice admission and found that, although 25 percent of the patients had no hospital admission, the remaining patients averaged 1.6 hospital admissions in this period.

Termination of life differs with individuals and their many circumstances; accurately predicting the point of death is an inexact science, at best. Given the Christakis/Escarce study, however, hospice admission may occur sooner in the course of a final illness, and patients and their families may experience increased satisfaction with the care. Worthy of study is the issue of whether earlier hospice admission might also reduce expenditures for care; even though terminal patients may incur more days of hospice care, they may be able to avert one or more costly hospitalizations.

### Other Issues Regarding Palliative Care

At least two other complex and controversial policy issues relate to palliative care. The first is the matter of potentially ineffective care, and the second is the increasing discussion regarding physician-assisted suicide.

Technologic advances in the U.S. health services system have had, in recent years, a tendency to outstrip policies on how and under what circumstances such advances should be applied. The increasing ability to prolong life is not synonymous with an obligation to do so under every circumstance. Determining when extreme measures should be applied, and to whom, defies simple resolution.

**Potentially Ineffective Care**

Two fears arise from the lack of resolution about the application of advanced technologies. The first, and perhaps predominant, fear is that one will not have access to life-prolonging technologies due to a lack of health insurance coverage or personal resources to cover costs. This creates the concern that those with ample resources can be assured of every intervention, whereas those with limited or no resources may experience a reduced life expectancy.

At the other end of the spectrum, the second fear is that technologic advances may be misapplied in circumstances where there is little or no hope of the patient's recovery and return to an acceptable quality of life. Some refer to this misapplication as futile care, and a body of literature is beginning to develop around this topic. Such misapplications may further inflate health services expenditures and preclude the application of advanced technologies in circumstances where the outcome is less questionable. Society has not yet determined how to address this issue, and concern persists that it will be resolved primarily on an economic basis.

The second policy issue that may be linked to end-of-life care is that of physician-assisted suicide. The movement for physician-assisted suicide differs from right-to-die provisions, which enable a competent patient to refuse nutrition, further use of a ventilator, or other interventions that are prolonging a terminal condition. A physician-assisted suicide policy would allow individuals with a terminal condition to seek the right to suspend life-prolonging care and/or to request the assistance of a physician to terminate life when the pain and dependence created by the terminal condition become intolerable.

**Physician-Assisted Suicide**

Although the U.S. Supreme Court ruled in June 1997 that individuals do not have the right to physician-assisted suicide, most believe that this ruling does not close the debate. A Harris poll released in August 1997 found that adult Americans disagree by a two-to-one majority with the Supreme Court ruling, and more than 66 percent of those polled believe that physicians should be permitted to perform euthanasia for terminally ill patients "in severe distress" who seek help in ending their lives (Merritt 1997). The matter was once again on the docket of the U.S. Supreme Court in Fall 2005. In a January 2006 ruling, the Court upheld Oregon's right to allow physician-assisted suicide.

Oregon has had an initiative-generated physician-assisted suicide statute—the Oregon Death with Dignity Act—on its books since 1994. Between 1998 and 2004, Oregon physicians wrote 326 prescriptions for drugs to be used in assisted suicide, and 208 persons terminated their lives using these prescriptions. The Oregon Department of Human Services reports that in 2004, physician-assisted suicide was the cause of 37 deaths, about one-eighth of 1 percent of all deaths in the state (Okie 2005).

## Summary

Palliative care combines a range of medicine, nursing, and social services to assist the patient who has a terminal illness or injury. Although private health insurance may provide some coverage for palliative care—particularly hospice care—Medicare currently pays for about 80 percent of all hospice care. As the proportion of the aged population increases, along with the life expectancy of seniors, the demand for palliative care is likely to grow as well.

Several other end-of-life issues arise in discussions of palliative care, including the use of potentially ineffective care (care that cannot change the outcome and thus is a futile application) and societal interest in physician-assisted suicide to end life when the pain of a terminal illness or injury becomes intolerable. More debate is needed to help society make responsible decisions on these issues.

### Key Words

| | |
|---|---|
| Consolidated Omnibus Budget Reconciliation Act (COBRA) | physician-assisted suicide |
| | potentially ineffective care |
| hospice | right to die |
| Oregon Death with Dignity Act of 1994 | |

## References

American Hospital Association. 2006. *2006 AHA Guide to the Health Care Field.* Chicago: AHA.

Centers for Medicare and Medicaid Services (CMS) 2006. *Medicare and Medicaid Statistical Supplement, 2004.* Baltimore, MD: CMS.

Christakis, N. A., and J. J. Escarce. 1996. "Survival of Medicare Patients after Enrollment in Hospice Programs." *New England Journal of Medicine* 335 (3): 172–78.

Congressional Research Service. 1993. *Medicaid Source Book: Background and Data Analysis (1993 Update)*. Washington, DC: U.S. Government Printing Office.

Matherlee, K. 2002. "Managing Advanced Illness: A Quality and Cost Challenge to Medicare, Medicaid, and Private Insurers." National Health Policy Forum Issue Brief No. 779. Washington, DC: George Washington University.

Merritt, D. (ed.). 1997. "State Notes Update: Assisted Suicide." *State Health Notes* 18 (259): 3.

National Hospice and Palliative Care Organization. 2003. "NHPCO Facts and Figures." [Online information; retrieved 5/7/03.] www.nhpco.org/public/articles/index.cfm?cat=11.

Okie, S. 2005. "Physician-Assisted Suicide—Oregon and Beyond." *New England Journal of Medicine* 352 (16): 1627–30.

U.S. Department of Health and Human Services. 2005. *Medicare and Medicaid Statistical Supplement 2003*. Baltimore, MD: USDHHS.

———. 2002. *Health, United States, 2002*. Pub. No. (PHS) 02-1232. Hyattsville, MD: USDHHS.

# 18

# THE CARE OF SPECIAL POPULATIONS AND SPECIAL DISORDERS

## Introduction

Even in universal, comprehensive, health services delivery systems, special populations or particular physical or mental disorders may be cared for outside the unified delivery system, sometimes in a parallel system. In the United States, with its unique blend of public and private sectors, several parallel systems exist that, combined, provide health services to such special populations as the military, veterans of military service, indigenous peoples, and prisoners in correctional facilities.

The U.S. delivery system also separates the care of people with chronic mental illness from the care and treatment of people with physical ailments, despite the fact that many mental illnesses are organic in origin. This chapter examines the care of people with mental illness to illustrate the care of special disorders in the U.S. delivery system.

The chapter opens with definitions to distinguish between acute and chronic mental illness and to acknowledge the role of substance abuse and its treatment in the realm of mental illness. Mental illness care providers are then described. Utilization of treatment services, including issues of unmet need, is then addressed. Expenditures for mental health services and the principal payers for services are identified. The chapter closes with a review of policy issues surrounding the care and treatment of people with mental illness.

## Defining Mental Illness

Mental illness is not a single disorder whose symptoms range from mild to severe. It is a heterogeneous collection of unrelated disorders that affect a sizable proportion of any population (Mechanic 1987). About 15 percent of the U.S. population meets the diagnostic criteria for one or more mental disorders; such disorders vary in their effects on an individual's ability to function in society. Approximately 1 percent of the U.S population is grossly impaired by chronic mental illness, rendering them incompetent to care for themselves independently. Approximately 66 percent of those with chronic mental illness maintain a state of moderate to severe disability for at least one year (Blocke and Cournos 1990). The diagnoses most commonly linked to chronic mental illness include schizophrenia, schizoaffective disorder, and bipolar disorder. Acute mental illness differs from chronic mental illness in that it is characterized by a single episode of fairly short duration from which patients return to their optimal level of functioning.

In 2002, about 2.8 million people received hospital and residential treatment for some period of time for mental illness (U.S. Department of Health and Human Services [USDHHS] 2005). Many more people with chronic mental illness live in community settings, with family members, in group homes, in single-room-only (SRO) hotels, or on the street. Prison populations also include people with mental disorders.

Figure 18.1 depicts another perspective on persons with mental illness—those who exhibited serious psychological distress in 2002 and 2003. Persons in the 45–54 age group have the highest proportion (4.2 percent) of serious psychological distress, and the American Indian/Alaska Native has the highest rate (7.1 percent) among racial and ethnic groups. More poor persons (8.7 percent) than persons in other income categories and more women than men experience serious psychological distress.

People with developmental disabilities are not included in these estimates. Chapter 15, which reviews long-term care, contains an overview of the population with developmental disabilities, whose care is provided in

**FIGURE 18.1**
Serious Psychological Distress among Persons Ages 18 and Over (2002–03)
*(a)* By age group and gender. *(b)* By race/ethnicity. *(c)* By poverty status.

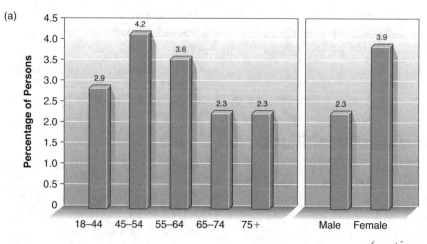

*(continued)*

FIGURE 18.1
Continued

(b)

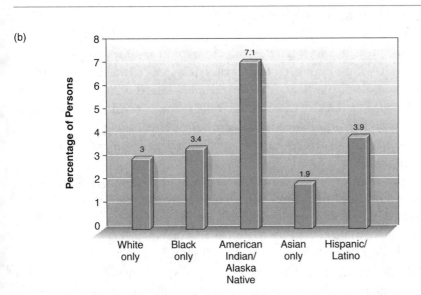

(c)

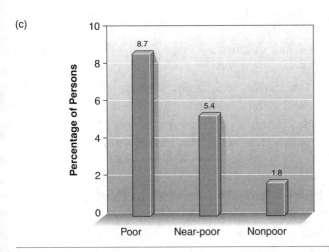

SOURCE: USDHHS 2005.

residential long-term care facilities. People with diagnoses of substance abuse, included in mental illness diagnoses, are also not included in the preceding numbers. Mental health professionals recognize the need for better data on the population with substance abuse problems. Substance abuse problems are less likely to be treated than other forms of serious mental illness, but the extent of inappropriate treatment, particularly excessive hospitalizations, appears to be substantially greater (Mechanic, Schlesinger, and McAlpine 1995).

## Mental Illness Care Providers

A range of providers, including psychiatrists who are physician specialists, psychologists, other counselors and therapists, social workers, advanced practice nurses, and others, care for the population with mental illness. The adequacy of the size of the workforce is in question (Hollingsworth 1992), given the unmet needs discussed in the sections that follow and the propensity for provider burnout in caring for this vulnerable, intensely needy population.

Several types of health services facilities provide care and treatment for mental illness. Most states still own and operate state mental institutions. General hospitals provide a significant share of inpatient care for people with mental illness. The Department of Veterans Affairs (VA) provides special psychiatric facilities for veterans of military service.

Private psychiatric institutions, many of which are members of health services systems, became increasingly visible beginning in the late 1970s and may provide both inpatient and outpatient services. The size and capacity of these facilities vary considerably.

Table 18.1 provides data for 2002 on the types and numbers of mental health treatment facilities, the number of mental health beds, and the number of beds per 100,000 civilian population. Of the specific facility types listed in the table, nonfederal general hospitals that provide psychiatric services constitute the greatest proportion (30 percent) of mental health organizations that provide inpatient treatment. The greatest proportion of beds (27 percent) is found in state and county mental hospitals.

### The Governmental Role in Providing Services to People with Chronic Mental Illness

Chronic mental illness is a psychiatric disorder that is manifest in the individual for a sustained period. People with chronic mental illness, if appropriately treated, may become or remain functioning members of a community. Serious mental illness may often be organic in nature, and its consequences are persistent and seriously disabling. The treatment and recovery options may be more limited for people with serious mental illness than for people with chronic mental illness.

Care of people with serious mental illness has long been a governmental responsibility; government often fulfilled this responsibility by institutionalizing the individual. Today, additional treatment options may permit people with serious mental illness to be cared for without institutionalization.

A significant proportion of care for people with chronic mental illness occurs in the public sector, and the origins of this locus of responsibility may help to explain why the care of mental illness has been disaggregated from the

| | Number of Mental Health Treatment Facilities | Number of Mental Health Beds | Beds per 100,000 Civilian Population |
|---|---|---|---|
| All organizations | 4,301 | 211,199 | 73.2 |
| State and county mental health hospitals | 222 | 57,263 | 19.9 |
| Private psychiatric hospitals | 253 | 25,095 | 8.7 |
| Nonfederal general hospital psychiatric services | 1,285 | 40,202 | 13.9 |
| Department of Veterans Affairs medical centers | 140 | 9,672 | 3.4 |
| Children's residential treatment | 508 | 39,049 | 13.5 |
| All other | 1,893 | 39,918 | 13.8 |

SOURCE: USDHHS 2005.

**TABLE 18.1**
Number of Mental Health Treatment Facilities and Beds for 24-Hour Residence and Treatment (2002)

care of other physical illnesses in the United States. Mental health care, unresponsive to financial incentives, has generally operated in a segmented policy world, cut off from the main dynamics of primary care (which is currently highly privatized), rather than operating as part of a public care system. Care for the seriously mentally ill is not seen as a part of the continuum of care for illness, but rather as a special, delimited problem (Hollingsworth 1992).

The care of people with mental illness was defined as a state and local governmental responsibility long before anything but the most rudimentary of personal health services was available. Initially, state and local governments shared these responsibilities, but beginning in the mid-nineteenth century, competition and rivalries between governmental units led states to assume the majority of the responsibility. Detecting a financial advantage, local governments began to redefine senility and to transfer aged people from local almshouses to state mental hospitals (Grob 1992). Thus, the public sector assumed early responsibility for serious or chronic mental illness, which was more easily recognized than other, later-defined diagnoses.

By 1930, about 80 percent of the residents of state mental hospitals were patients with chronic mental illness (Grob 1992). For many of these patients, no effective treatments were known at the time. Unable to provide effective treatment, state mental institutions often became repositories for the most seriously mentally ill. The population of residents in state mental institutions peaked at 560,000 in 1955 and then began a gradual decline as patients were transferred to other care settings.

### The Movement Toward Community Care

Deinstitutionalization—the movement of patients with chronic mental illness from state mental institutions to other care settings—did not occur overnight, and it was not the result of a single stimulus. Grob (1992), who prepared a history of mental health care in the United States, points out a number of factors that influenced deinstitutionalization.

One of the earliest factors was the distancing of psychiatrists from state mental institutions through their redefinition of concepts of mental disorders and appropriate interventions. By 1955, 80 percent of psychiatrists were employed outside of state mental hospitals. As psychiatrists left the state facilities, they were often replaced by foreign medical graduates (now called international medical graduates), who may have faced both language and cultural challenges in providing care to a dependent population.

Another factor that contributed to a shift away from state institutions to local care included a transition to psychodynamic and psychoanalytic models of therapy, a belief—based on little evidence—that community therapy was more efficacious and that early community intervention could provide a preventive function. The introduction of psychological and somatic therapies and an enhanced federal social welfare role that provided income and other assistance to people with physical and mental disabilities were other factors that contributed to deinstitutionalization.

The gradual exodus of people with chronic mental illness from state mental institutions had several consequences. First, it allowed state institutions to focus on their now much smaller patient populations and to begin to function as treatment units rather than as repositories. Second, the transition assumed that community resources would be provided to replace the services of the state institutions. The National Mental Health Act of 1946 and the Community Mental Health Center Act of 1963 were intended to strengthen community resources, but the needs were often greater than these programs could meet. Not only were the patients who had been discharged from state facilities in need of care, but the presence of community facilities introduced the availability of mental health care to a new population of users who did not have severe mental illness but who needed mental health services.

Ensuring that those with chronic mental illness had first call on community services was not part of the planning when state institutions discharged patients. In fact, the autonomous governing boards that oversaw the operation of community mental health centers often tended to overlook the needs of those with the most serious mental illness (Blocke and Cournos 1990), and established the community mental health centers to serve people with moderate mental illness who were residing and functioning in the community. Because state institutions still had fixed and operational costs, few funds could be reallocated from them to support community services. Instead, community services had to compete with state mental institutions and other entities seeking governmental support for their funding.

### Deinstitutionalization and Transinstitutionalization

Although a general public perception has been that the movement of individuals with chronic mental illness from state institutions to the community is directly responsible for the increase in the homeless population, the relationship is more complex than that. Although 33 to 40 percent of the homeless are estimated to have chronic mental illness (Hollingsworth 1992), the discharge of people with chronic mental illness from state facilities did not result in an influx of homeless people. What happened in a number of instances was not so much deinstitutionalization as transinstitutionalization (Blocke and Cournos 1990).

Many of the residents of state facilities were elderly patients with dementia, and the availability of nursing home care, supported by newly established state Medicaid programs, provided a better care alternative. Further, the Medicaid program allowed states to shift a significant share of their costs for custodial care to the federal government because federal dollars support at least 50 percent of Medicaid program expenditures.

Two additional federal welfare programs boosted the new emphasis on community mental health programs: Social Security Disability Insurance (SSDI) and Supplemental Security Income (SSI) provided income assistance to people with physical and mental disabilities. Table 18.2 compares these two programs. Because Medicaid eligibility—until the Personal Responsibility and Work Opportunity Act of 1996—was linked to such welfare programs as SSI, Medicaid soon became a primary payer for the care and treatment of people with serious mental illness, people with developmental disabilities, and qualifying people seeking general mental health services.

## Utilization of Treatment Services

When state mental hospitals were the primary treatment site for individuals with mental illness, utilization of services was framed in terms of hospital census, with the institutionalized population peaking at more than 500,000 in the mid-1950s.

The census in facilities that specialize in inpatient treatment of people with chronic mental illness averages about 150,000. A larger population of people with chronic mental illness are cared for in nursing homes. Others with chronic, serious, and more mild and moderate forms of mental illness receive care and treatment in a range of settings, including residential

**TABLE 18.2**
Comparison
of Disability
Programs
Funded by
the Social
Security
Act (SSA)

| | Social Security Disability Insurance (SSDI) | Supplemental Security Income (SSI) |
|---|---|---|
| Eligibility | Must meet SSA definition of disability; must contribute to Social Security system | Must meet SSA definition of disability; means test of income |
| Number of Persons Served | 3.6 million (1992) | ~4.5 million (1992) |
| Proportion of Expenditures | 14.4% of Medicare expenditures go to SSDI population | ~73% of Medicaid expenditures go to SSI population |
| Benefits | Cash assistance; eligibility for Medicare Part A benefits, no coverage of nonmedical services | Cash assistance, eligibility for Medicaid benefits, varied coverage for nonmedical services |
| Cost-Sharing Requirements | Medicare premium, deductible, copay | Usually limited or none |
| Program Flexibility | | Medicaid-covered services are unusually responsive to functional impairment |
| Percentage of People with Mental Impairment | 24% | 27.1% under age 65 have mental retardation, and 22.6% have mental illness |
| Duration of Participation | At least 24 months in order to become Medicare-eligible | Once eligible are unlikely to disenroll |

SOURCES: Hirsch 1994; Oberg and Polich 1988; Okpaku, Silbukin, and Schenzler 1994; and Adams, Meiners, and Burwell 1993.

NOTE: This table is taken from Barton, Glazner, and Poole 1995.

facilities, freestanding psychiatric outpatient facilities, and psychiatric units in governmental and other facilities.

Figure 18.2 provides information on the population that sought care in mental health facilities in 2002. The term *additions* indicates the new admissions, readmissions, transfers, and returns from leaves of absence to a facility. The numbers may not, therefore, represent unduplicated counts of individuals.

Utilization data do not provide a complete picture of the population with mental illness. A sizable population may not have access to diagnosis

FIGURE 18.2
Additions to
Mental Health
Facilities
(2002)

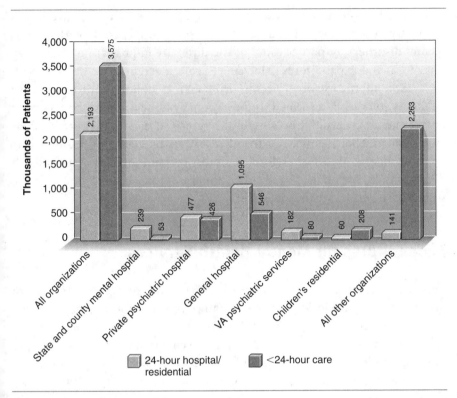

SOURCE: USDHHS 2005.

NOTE: VA = Department of Veterans Affairs.

and treatment services for mental illness. At least 15 percent of the U.S. population has no health insurance coverage, public or private, for any health services. Even though Medicaid is a major payer for services for those with mental illness, it cannot structurally fill all the gaps in the mental health care system because Medicaid access is still governed by eligibility criteria that may rule out certain at-risk populations. A sizable population has no direct access to services and, more importantly, may be too incapacitated to seek the available services.

Mechanic (1987) and other experts in mental health policy describe an "enormous, unmet need" for services, pointing out that people diagnosed with even the most evident mental illness were found to have received no mental health care of any kind in the six months prior to their diagnosis. A substantial fraction of those with mental illness are not in the system of care (Hollingsworth 1992).

Even for the population that has insured access to services for mental illness, several factors may influence the likelihood of their utilization. First, many health insurance benefit packages provide a limited number of services for acute mental health problems, but few provide comprehensive services for chronic mental illness. This limitation may be exacerbated by the movement toward managed care, in which prepaid health services providers may discourage the enrollment of people with serious mental disorders, in part because of the difficulty in projecting their likely utilization and expenditures (Mechanic, Schlesinger, and McAlpine 1995).

Second, the use of services to maintain mental health or to treat mental illness still carries a societal stigma. People who feel a need for assistance or treatment may avoid it because of the perceived risks to their status, their employment, their families, or to other aspects of their lives. Undertreatment of mental illness, therefore, is almost certain, given the difficulty in diagnosing it, the financial and other limitations in accessing care, and the stigma attached to seeking these services.

## Expenditures for Mental Health Services

Funding for mental health is more likely to come from public than from private sources. Table 18.3 shows the amount spent for care in each type of mental health facility for 2002. For specific types of facilities, the greatest amount was spent in state and county psychiatric hospitals. The low per capita expenditures for mental health services ($119 in 2002) compared to overall per capita expenditures for total health care ($4,576 in 2002) punctuates the contrast between expenditures for somatic versus mental health.

**TABLE 18.3**
Mental Health Expenditures, Percentage Distribution, and per Capita Expenditures by Type of Mental Health Organization (2002)

| | Expenditures (in Millions of Dollars) | Percentage Distribution | Amount per Capita* |
|---|---|---|---|
| All organizations | $34,302 | 100.0 | $119 |
| State and county psychiatric hospitals | 7,616 | 22.2 | 26 |
| Private psychiatric hospitals | 3,929 | 11.5 | 14 |
| Nonfederal general hospital psychiatric service | 5,179 | 15.1 | 18 |
| Department of Veterans Affairs medical centers | 1,018 | 3.0 | 4 |
| Children's residential treatment | 4,496 | 13.1 | 16 |
| All others | 12,063 | 35.2 | 42 |

SOURCE: USDHHS 2005.

*Based on the decennial census sample civilian population.

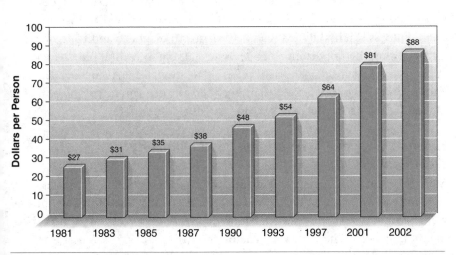

**FIGURE 18.3**

State Mental Health Agency per Capita Expenditures for Mental Health Services (Select Years, 1981–2002)

SOURCE: USDHHS 2005.

NOTE: Data intervals are irregular.

This point is further illustrated by Figure 18.3, which shows the per capita expenditures for mental health services expended by the largest provider (in terms of number of beds) of mental health services—state mental health agencies. For 2002, the per capita expenditure was $88.

## Policy Issues Related to the Care of People with Mental Illness

The care available to people with mental illness prompts the consideration of several types of policy issues, including the challenges inherent in segregating physical from mental health care, the tensions between institution-based and community treatment programs, unmet needs for treatment, the continuing stigma attached to mental illness, and the advent of managed mental health care.

### Segregation of Physical Health from Mental Health

The care of a person's physical health is seen as a continuum—from health promotion and disease prevention behaviors to therapeutic and rehabilitative functions and ultimately to palliative care. The care of a person's mental health does not follow the same model; rather, mental illness is seen as a special, delimited, and even episodic problem to be dealt with as it presents. Disease, however, does not necessarily manifest itself in this segregated fashion, and nonspecific symptomology may suggest either a physical or a mental illness.

The patient with an illness may first see a primary care provider and be treated in a general hospital, even though the ultimate diagnosis may be mental illness. Mental illness may be difficult to diagnose and to treat, thus underscoring the importance of adequate training in mental illness for generalist providers and appropriate referrals to specialists. As more is learned about disease etiology, the chasm between the treatment of physical and mental health problems may narrow.

### Tensions Between Institutional and Community Treatment Programs

Mental hospitals and mental institutions were the initial focus for the care of mental illness, although the level of care available when these institutions were being established in the mid-nineteenth century was sparse and experimental, at best. The shift of locus of care from large, often state-owned facilities to community programs in the mid-1960s was prompted by an increased awareness of civil rights, an interest in providing more humane treatment, and a perception, rather than clear evidence, that community care was more effective. Instead of replacing state-supported care, however, community care ultimately competed with state facilities for limited resources.

The shift of locus of care from mental institutions to the community is also attributed in part to the advent of neuroleptic drugs introduced in the 1950s and psychotropic drugs introduced in subsequent years. Mechanic (1987) points out that in large institutions, drugs gave treatment personnel hope and a greater sense of efficacy, which helped to facilitate this administrative change. Some drugs could blunt the most disturbing psychotic symptoms, giving families increased confidence that patient care could be managed in a community setting.

Many experts agree that both institutional and community care are important in the treatment of mental illness. For some individuals with mental illness, the protective environment of the institution remains the appropriate placement (Mechanic 1987); for others, progress is better stimulated in a smaller community program. Striking the right balance between these treatment modalities and securing adequate resources to support each are both necessary.

### Unmet Needs for the Treatment of Mental Illness

The unmet need for services for people with mental illness is significant. In addition to the unmet needs described in the preceding sections, several populations present particular concerns.

One population is the substance abusers, who often also have another mental disorder. The number of treatment facilities for substance abusers is inadequate, and the demand for such care far outpaces the resources currently committed to provide it. A second population of concern is the young schizophrenics and other seriously disturbed youth, whose conditions may be complicated by drug and alcohol use (Mechanic 1987). Access to care for any of these populations of concern is inhibited by lack of private or public insurance coverage for needed services.

## Continuing Stigma of Seeking Care for Mental Illness

Although individuals with mental illness are no longer placed in manacles and locked away from society, some would argue that attitudes have not progressed much beyond that stage. Mental illness still carries a stigma.

Treatment programs for people with mental illness may also carry a stigma. Few neighborhoods welcome group homes or other treatment facilities to the community, espousing instead the "not-in-my-backyard" (commonly referred to by its acronym, NIMBY) position. The number of effective care and treatment programs will continue to be inadequate until the stigma of mental illness can be reduced and, ideally, eradicated.

## Advent of Managed Mental Health Care

Managed care is not only a phenomenon of physical health care systems; it is making inroads into mental health care as well. Managed care has the potential to increase the availability of treatment, contain costs, and improve quality of care, but it could also result in denial of needed treatment, a decline in the quality of services provided, and cost-shifting to patients, their families, health services providers, and the community. The care of mental illness is difficult to manage because mental illness, including substance abuse, more than most other illnesses entails broad social costs that families, communities, and the legal system must bear. Chronic mental illness results in extended expenditures and costs, and the illness carries a stigma.

Despite these limitations, most mental health services are provided under some type of managed care program. At least 50 percent of state Medicaid agencies use some type of managed care—either prepaid health plans, utilization management, and/or high-cost case management—for the mental health and mental illness care services they support (Mechanic, Schlesinger, and McAlpine 1995).

The continued challenge for managed care in mental health and in other health services is to continue to provide all needed services while eliminating unneeded services. That challenge is particularly acute for mental health services, where diagnosis may be difficult, the effects of interventions are not well understood, and the populations at risk are often unable to effectively look out for their own interests.

## Summary

This chapter examines the care of people with mental illness to illustrate how the U.S. health services system deals with special disorders and special populations. People who are seriously or chronically mentally ill constitute a very diverse population. Planning services for this population is complicated by the difficulty in projecting their prognoses. The problems of mental illness are often compounded by the disadvantages of poverty and racism. Organizational barriers to effective care of people with mental illness also exist, including the absence of a clear focus of responsibility and authority for providing care, the frequent lack of effective advocacy, and discriminatory treatment of this condition in both public and private health insurance (Mechanic 1987).

### Key Words

| | |
|---|---|
| acute mental illness | Medicaid |
| additions to mental health facilities | National Mental Health Act |
| almshouses | "not-in-my-back yard" (NIMBY) |
| chronic mental illness | position |
| Community Mental Health Center Act | Social Security Disability Insurance |
| deinstitutionalization | (SSDI) |
| Department of Veterans Affairs | Supplemental Security Income |
| developmental disabilities | (SSI) |
| managed mental health services | transinstitutionalization |

## References

Adams, E. K., M. Meiners, and B. Burwell. 1993. "Asset Spend-Down in Nursing Homes." *Medical Care* 31 (1): 1–23.

Barton, P. L., J. Glazner, and C. Poole. 1995. *Final Report: Colorado Medicaid Reform Study, Phase II, Long-Term Care.* Denver, CO: University of Colorado Health Sciences Center.

Blocke, M. G., and F. Cournos. 1990. "Mental Health Policy for the 1990s: Tinkering in the Interstices." *Journal of Health Politics, Policy and Law* 15 (2): 387–411.

Grob, G. N. 1992. "Mental Health Policy in America: Myths and Realities." *Health Affairs* 11 (3): 7–22.

Hirsch, M. 1994. "Health Care of Vulnerable Populations Covered by Medicare and Medicaid." *Health Care Financing Review* 15 (4): 1–5.

Hollingsworth, E. J. 1992. "Falling Through the Cracks: Care of the Chronically Mentally Ill in the U.S., Germany, and the United Kingdom." *Journal of Health Politics, Policy and Law* 17 (4): 899–928.

Mechanic, D. 1987. "Correcting Misconceptions in Mental Health Policy: Strategies for Improved Care of the Seriously Mentally Ill." *Milbank Quarterly* 65 (2): 203–30.

Mechanic, D., M. Schlesinger, and D. D. McAlpine. 1995. "Management of Mental Health and Substance Abuse Services: State of the Art and Early Results." *Milbank Quarterly* 73 (1): 19–55.

Oberg, C., and C. Polich. 1988. "Medicaid: Entering the Third Decade." *Health Affairs* 7 (4): 83–96.

Okpaku, S., A. Silbukin, and C. Schenzler. 1994. "Disability Determinations for Adults with Mental Disorders: Social Security Administration vs. Independent Judgments." *American Journal of Public Health* 84 (11): 1791–95.

U.S. Department of Health and Human Services. 2005. *Health, United States, 2005.* Washington, DC: USDHHS.

# 19

# THE HEALTH SERVICES DELIVERY SYSTEM: MANAGED CARE

## Introduction

The preceding chapters in Part VI focus on the continuum of care—from health promotion and disease prevention to palliative care at the end of life. This chapter examines characteristics of the health services delivery system, linking earlier discussions of health system organization and financing, resource production, and economic support. The recent and ongoing shift from a fee-for-service system reimbursed through indemnity insurance to a system of managed care, in which the financing and delivery of services are integrated, is the central theme of this chapter. The backlash against managed care, a focus of recent analyses, is also addressed.

The chapter opens with a review of the many definitions for the term *managed care* and then explores the reasons for the shift in the focus of the delivery system and the expectations of many for managed care. Discussions on models of managed care, the strengths and weaknesses of managed care, and the market for managed care follow. The chapter concludes with an overview of the policy issues related to this shift from fee-for-service to managed care and the ongoing modifications in the managed care system.

## Definitions of Managed Care

David Mechanic (1994) captured a general frustration with the term *managed care* when he commented, "Managed care is used so promiscuously as to have no meaning at all." It can also be said that the term has as many referents as it has users, each holding a somewhat different notion of what the term means. *Managed care* as a term suffers from some of the same amorphousness as does the term *quality of care,* which is discussed in Chapter 20. Most would agree that at least one concept is central to the meaning of managed care: it is an integration, at some level, of the financing and delivery of health services.

In managed care, both patient utilization and provider practices are managed by an entity that has a fiduciary interest in the interactions between them. Thus, the term *managed care* serves as an umbrella for a range of organizational and reimbursement mechanisms in the U.S. delivery system.

Entities that provide managed care are sometimes referred to as managed care organizations (MCOs). Change is occurring so rapidly, with new organizational forms emerging and mutating, that defining this moving target more precisely may contribute only to the lexicon of obsolete definitions.

## The Shift from Fee-for-Service to Managed Care in the U.S. Delivery System

As does any dynamic organism, the U.S. health services delivery system has grown rapidly and incurred changes, particularly since the mid-1960s, when access to care increased for some populations and technologic advances expanded the capacity to save lives and extend life spans. Despite the growth and changes, the delivery system through the 1980s could generally be described as a public-private system in which people with social or private health insurance could autonomously seek care from the provider(s) of their choice. Providers were reimbursed for their care of individual patients on a fee-for-service basis. Other systems of care, such as prepaid care provided through certain types of health maintenance organizations (HMOs), were labeled "alternative delivery systems," part of the overall diversity of the U.S. system but relegated to the role of a minor player.

In the last 25 years, the U.S. health services delivery system has morphed from a fee-for-service system to a relatively restrictive and regulated managed care system to one in which hybridization of delivery models and the continuous introduction of new insurance products presents a definitional challenge.

### The Nature of the Delivery System Shift

To oversimplify the nature of the shift in the delivery system is tempting; oversimplification tends to classify the systems according to extremes, such as:

- Fee-for-service care focuses on individual patients, whereas managed care focuses on the health of a population.
- Fee-for-service care centers around acute care, whereas managed care emphasizes disease prevention and health maintenance.
- Fee-for-service care provides incentives for overservice, whereas managed care provides incentives for underservice.
- Fee-for-service care is largely patient-initiated, with few access barriers other than financial ones, whereas managed care controls and restricts patient access to providers.

Although these extremes harbor elements of truth, they are too polarized to serve as effective distinctions.

A better description of the essence of the initial shift may be that the focus of the delivery system is moving from the level of interactions between an individual patient and an individual provider to a focus on the comprehensive needs and care of individual patients and of a population of patients who obtain their care from the same providers. The focus thus shifts from episodic care of the individual patient, in which each episode is separately reimbursed, to holistic care of individuals and groups of individuals. Reimbursement in the latter instance may be based on episodes of care; on a fixed fee for all covered care, regardless of how much is utilized; or on another basis.

By the late 1990s, a backlash against managed care set in motion another shift. Traditional models of managed care, shown in Table 19.1 later in the chapter, began to hybridize as both providers and consumers rebelled against the restrictiveness of some aspects of managed care. The push for more choice on the parts of both parties continues to influence the ways in which services are delivered. This push also has consequences on the ability to control costs and expenditures.

## Reasons for the Shift in the Delivery System

The U.S. health services delivery system is reputed to be one of the most advanced in the world, but it is an imperfect system. Its imperfections include its lack of universal coverage, its cost and expenditure upward spirals, the increasing amount of the gross domestic product (GDP) it absorbs, and its potential for becoming the black hole of U.S. domestic economy and policy. National-level initiatives to reform the system, the most recent of which was the 1993 Health Security Act, failed in part because the price tag appeared too formidable to a partisan Congress wrestling with budget and trade deficits (Ellwood and Lundberg 1996).

Despite the failure of national-level health system reform, system changes, driven by a range of market forces, are occurring at a pace and to an extent that few prognosticators would have dared predict even 20 short years ago. What could not be accomplished using regulations over several decades, such as a reduction in excess capacity in the system, is rapidly occurring through facility mergers, acquisitions, and closures as providers, payers, and others joust for market share and survival. Books will continue to be written about the forces prompting this shift; this chapter is limited to listing some of the forces that are stimulating change and to pointing out that future change is likely, even in areas where it is not currently anticipated.

A number of forces are influencing changes in the U.S. health services delivery system. Among those discussed in the sections that follow are:

- employers' and payers' raised level of consciousness regarding the costs of providing employee health insurance;
- the perverse incentives that fee-for-service care establishes;

- the effects on utilization of self-referral, "doctor-shopping," and open access to specialists;
- the need of both private and public payers to better predict total health expenditures;
- the need for accountability of health expenditures within a society;
- the belief that optimal rather than maximal use of limited resources is more appropriate; and
- the need to increase efficiency in the system, including the appropriate use of inpatient and outpatient services and the reduction of overcapacity.

All of these forces were instrumental in shifting the focus of the delivery system to one of more rigid controls on the provision and utilization of health services, greater efforts to manage and account for costs and expenditures, and a broad-based determination to manage the interactions of providers, payers, and patients.

By 1998, however, Blendon and colleagues were reporting on the backlash against some restrictive facets of managed care. Providers felt constrained by the limited time available per patient, the inability to freely order whatever tests or procedures they deemed to be in their patients' best interests, and the controls on income dictated by certain payment arrangements. Patients rebelled at the limitations on their choices of providers, difficulties encountered in obtaining services they believed were appropriate, and the regimentation of other aspects of managed care.

**Increased Cost of Providing Employee Health Benefits**

The costs of providing employee health benefits have risen sharply in recent years, as evidenced by substantial annual premium increases through 2005 and the growing proportion of employer expenditures for health services as a share of total business revenues (see Chapter 7). Health insurance premiums experienced double-digit increases through 2005, and HMO rates rose in a commensurate fashion. Additionally, employers pay an increasing share of the total health bill: 30 percent in 2004—almost double the 16 percent total in 1965.

As employers recognized the financial consequences of the types of employee health benefits they were providing, they began to:

- organize business coalitions to increase their bargaining power with insurers;
- become self-insured rather than negotiate contracts with insurers;
- negotiate discounts with providers;
- negotiate the provision of services directly with providers, eliminating the insurance function altogether; and
- adopt a range of other cost-reducing strategies.

Moving from a passive to an aggressively active role, employers are now exerting a noticeable influence on how health services are delivered in the United States.

The fee-for-service reimbursement system, which pays separately for each care event (i.e., each physician visit, laboratory service, prescription drug, hospitalization, or other service), creates a perverse incentive to regularly provide a wide range of services, not all of which may be appropriate or needed. Ordering duplicative sets of tests, for example, each of which would be reimbursed under a fee-for-service system, may have increased each provider's flexibility but underscores the inefficiency and misuse of resources in the system. Assuming the patient is insured, the provider stands at little or no financial risk for this practice and may stand to gain financially. Some types of managed care reduce the potential for unneeded or duplicative services and thus reduce the expenditures for health services.

**Fee-for-Service Incentives**

Prior to the recent changes in the delivery system, an insured person or one who had other resources had relatively open access to health services, depending on the availability of providers. As one analyst described the previous system, health insurance provided individuals with a "hunting license" to hunt for the care they needed or desired (Feldman, Kralewski, and Dowd 1989). The insured individual thus initiated care in many instances, could directly seek care from a specialist rather than await a referral from a primary care provider (i.e., self-referral), and could "doctor-shop," switching providers to the extent that providers were available and willing to see additional patients.

**Effects on Utilization of Unconstrained Access to Care**

Consumer choice, one of the hallmarks of the U.S. system, remains a strong consumer preference, but it can also create misuse or overuse of health services. As utilization of services increases, the costs of and expenditures for services also increase, contributing to the upward spiral of health services expenditures.

The open-ended nature of health services benefits under the fee-for-service delivery system, especially evident in entitlement programs such as Medicare and Medicaid, permitted individuals to seek—and providers to provide—essentially unlimited health services, resulting in the potential for unlimited expenditures.

**The Need for Predictability and Accountability of Expenditures**

Although various cost-containment efforts were attempted, their success in curbing expenditures varied. Some efforts that did curb expenditures, such as patient cost sharing, also had adverse effects on patients' health (see Chapter 6). Open-ended systems may also compromise the ability to adequately account for utilization and expenditures in a system. Employers and public payers are among those who are seeking ways to eliminate open-ended systems and thereby increase the predictability and the accountability of their health services expenditures.

**Optimal versus Maximal Use of Resources**

In a technologically advanced health services system where providers are trained to use every intervention to save and prolong lives, there may be maximal versus optimal use of resources. Society has a difficult time acknowledging that some resources may be limited and addressing the explicit rationing of these resources. Whether or not it is acknowledged as such, medical care is already rationed by the availability and scope of health insurance and by marketplace mechanisms (Mechanic 1994). Resource use at either end of the utilization spectrum continues to be a debated issue as the delivery system undergoes transition.

**Need for Increased Efficiency in the Delivery System**

The open-ended, fee-for-service system that was a U.S. standard for decades incorporates many inefficiencies that have not resolved the problem of those without access to care and have contributed to rapidly increasing expenditures for care to those who have financial access. Among the most apparent inefficiencies are system overcapacity (including excess hospital beds), a disproportionate number of physician specialists, and duplicative and underutilized technologies.

Until recently, the laws of supply and demand that govern many other markets appeared to have little effect in achieving a balance in capacity: Hospital overcapacity led only to higher hospital charges (Drake 1997), and a disproportionate supply of physician specialists did not suppress physician incomes. Attempts to regulate capacity through initiatives such as the certificate of need (CON) program had a limited and generally short-term effect on capacity.

After years of convincing evidence that market principles did not effectively apply to much of the health services system, the market is now aggressively dealing with overcapacity in the system. Among the possible explanations of what effected this change is that care providers, anticipating an adverse regulatory environment in various system reform proposals, determined to control the system by merging and consolidating resources to reduce overcapacity. Led by Medicare, payers weighed in by constraining the ability of providers, particularly of hospitals, to cross-subsidize or cost-shift the care of unprofitable clients by charging higher prices to paying patients. The supply of physicians, fueled by generous policies on the training of international medical graduates (IMGs), became large enough that payers could divide and conquer, negotiating prices and working conditions in a previously unheard-of manner. By contrast, the current shortage in the supply of nurses is affecting capacity and patient care in an entirely different direction. The growing influence of proprietary providers at both the hospital and HMO levels is also affecting the shape of the delivery system.

## A Range of Expectations for Change in the Delivery System

The imperfections in the U.S. delivery system identified in the preceding sections generate a wide range of possible solutions, as well as expectations of patients, payers, providers, and others about these solutions. Many of the solutions have been identified as *managed care solutions*, and the term has been vested with more promise than it is likely to deliver. Among the range of expectations of managed care are that it will:

- rationalize the use of resources, avoiding overuse or underuse;
- provide greater accountability at all levels;
- enable a more accurate prediction of health expenditures;
- contain and/or reduce health expenditures;
- shift the focus of the delivery system from acute care and crisis intervention to disease prevention and health maintenance;
- reduce physician practice variations; and
- ensure better outcomes of care.

Several models of managed care and their likelihood in meeting some of the preceding expectations are examined in the sections that follow.

# Models of Managed Care

Many kinds of organizations fit under the umbrella of managed care. This section describes some better-known models and introduces some of the more recent developments. New models or variations of models are emerging; some will flourish, and others will adapt to changing circumstances, while still others will not survive. The appearance of models of managed care seems much like using a kaleidoscope: the elements, or participants, remain constant, but a slight turn of the glass introduces a new pattern or model.

Table 19.1 provides a summary of some of the early, traditional managed care models, including information on provider payment mechanisms, provider incentives, enrollee incentives, cost-saving mechanisms, and risk assumption. Enough hybridization and alteration has occurred among these models that Table 19.1 now serves principally as a snapshot of the origins of models of managed care.

## Prepaid Group Practice (PGP)

The prepaid group practice (PGP) was recommended as the most effective care delivery system as early as 1932 in the report of the Committee on the Costs of Medical Care (CCMC), a self-formed committee to study the economics of medical care. The PGP is an early model of managed care. Insurers, employers, or other parties contract with either a single specialty physician group or, more usually, a multispecialty physician group to

**TABLE 19.1** Managed Care Models

| Model | Description | Provider Payment Mechanisms | Provider Incentives | Enrollee Incentives | Cost-Saving Mechanisms | Risk Assumptions | Comments |
|---|---|---|---|---|---|---|---|
| HMO (staff model) | Medical care delivery through salaried employee physicians who provide a specific set of services to a defined population | Salary; physicians are employees of the HMO | • Defined patient population<br>• No claims processing<br>• Low/no start-up costs for new physicians | • Comprehensive range of services for a fixed price<br>• Coverage of primary care and preventive services<br>• Community rate-based premiums | • Utilization review<br>• Provider bonuses based on productivity and meeting utilization targets<br>• Education of providers and patients<br>• Gatekeeping | HMO | Concerns voiced about incentives to underutilize in a capitated system |
| HMO (group model) | Medical care delivery through a medical group practice contracted to provide a specific set of services to a defined population | Capitation for group; salary or FFS reimbursement for participating physicians | • Defined patient population<br>• No/few claims processing<br>• Low/no start-up costs for new physicians | • Comprehensive range of services for a fixed price<br>• Coverage of primary care and preventive services<br>• Community rate-based premiums | • Utilization review<br>• Provider bonuses<br>• Prior approval<br>• Financial incentives through withholding accounts<br>• Education<br>• Gatekeeping | HMO and group | Concerns voiced about incentives to underutilize in a capitated system |

| | Definition | Reimbursement | Advantages to providers | Benefits to enrollees | Cost control mechanisms | Who bears risk | Comments |
|---|---|---|---|---|---|---|---|
| HMO (IPA/network model) | Medical care delivery through a panel of contracted providers for the provision of a specific set of services to a defined population | FFS reimbursement capitation | • Can accept patients from multiple plans and/or retain indemnity patients<br>• Rapid claims turnaround<br>• Increased pool of patients<br>• Some flexibility in referral | • Comprehensive range of services for a fixed price<br>• Coverage of primary care and preventive services<br>• Community rate-based premiums<br>• Greater likelihood of maintaining patient-provider relationship | • Utilization review<br>• Prior approval<br>• Financial incentives through withholding accounts<br>• Gatekeeping | Purchasers | • Until the advent of POS options, IPAs were the fastest-growing HMO model.<br>• The generalist-to-specialist ratio can affect cost savings (i.e., greater ratio of specialists reduces cost savings).<br>• Capitated forms are more effective in reducing costs. |
| PPO | Contractual arrangement between a panel of providers and purchasers of health services for the provision of a specific set of services to enrollees | Discounted FFS reimbursement | • Patients form multiple plans<br>• Increased patient pool<br>• Rapid claims turnaround<br>• Low financial investment | • Reduced cost sharing for within-plan use<br>• Expanded benefits<br>• Partial coverage for out-of-plan use<br>• Reduced premiums | • Utilization review<br>• Prior approval<br>• Selective contracting of cost-efficient providers<br>• Discounted reimbursements<br>• Movement toward gatekeeping | Purchasers | Potential for monopoly if purchaser becomes very large |
| EPO | Contractual arrangement between a panel of providers and purchasers of health services for the provision of a specific set of services to enrollees | Discounted FFS | • Increased pool of patients<br>• Rapid claims turnaround<br>• Low financial investment | • Low/no cost/sharing<br>• Expanded benefits<br>• Reduced premiums | • No out-of-plan reimbursements<br>• Utilization review<br>• Prior approval<br>• Selective contracting of cost-efficient providers<br>• Discounted reimbursements | Purchasers | Most states' insurance regulations prohibit restrictions on access to providers as it constitutes "restraint of trade" |

(continued)

**TABLE 19.1** Managed Care Models Continued

| Model | Description | Provider Payment Mechanisms | Provider Incentives | Enrollee Incentives | Cost-Saving Mechanisms | Risk Assumptions | Comments |
|---|---|---|---|---|---|---|---|
| POS model | Subscriber chooses provider at the point of service rather than upon enrollment into the plan | Varied | Potential to attract a broader range of subscribers | Flexibility to choose provider | | | |
| PSO | Joint ventures between physicians, hospitals, and other providers | Capitation | Guaranteed panel of patients | | May reduce or eliminate insurance or other costs | Provider | |
| SHMO | Medicare demonstration combines social and health services for frail elderly | Capitation | Ability to provide more comprehensive and continuous services, both social and health | • Availability of additional services • Potential avoidance of institutionalization | • Deferred institutionalization • Reduced rates of hospitalization | Provider | |
| Integrated Delivery System/ Network | Network of services to a defined population | Varied | Maintain panel of patients | Broader choice of provider | | Provider | |

SOURCE: Barton, Bondy, and Glazner 1993.

NOTES: EPO = exclusive provider organization; FFS = fee for service; HMO = health maintenance organization; IPA = independent practice association; POS = point-of-service plan; PSO = provider-sponsored organization; SHMO = social health maintenance organization.

provide a predetermined range of benefits or services to a specific population for a fixed price. Early PGPs include Ross-Loos, established in Los Angeles in the 1920s, and Kaiser Permanente, established on the West Coast in the 1930s. Providers may have been at risk for providing care (i.e., the full extent of covered benefits had to be provided), regardless of whether the cost of those benefits to the provider exceeded the preestablished payment rate.

## Health Maintenance Organizations (HMOs)

PGPs were the precursors for the health maintenance organizations (HMOs) that began to appear in the early 1970s. The HMO was an outgrowth of congressional frustration with the uncontrolled utilization and expenditures for the Medicare program (Ellwood and Lundberg 1996), and was proposed to officials in the Nixon administration as a way to address both issues. The result was the 1973 Health Maintenance Organization Act, which established federal standards for HMOs and required employers of a certain size that offered health insurance to their employees to offer at least one HMO. Large corporations that purchased employee health services from HMOs were a major influence in shaping the present marketplace (Ellwood and Lundberg 1996). HMO plans constituted 23 percent of the health plan market in 2003 (U.S. Department of Health and Human Services [USDHHS] 2005).

Several different initial HMO models include the group model, the staff model, the independent (sometimes referred to as individual) practice association, and the network model. All are distinguished by the following characteristics:

- To varying degrees, each model combines the delivery of care with its financing.
- An HMO assumes a contractual responsibility to provide or assure the delivery of a stated range of health services, including at least ambulatory and inpatient care.
- An HMO serves a population defined by enrollment in a plan.
- Subscriber enrollment is generally voluntary but may be mandated by the payer.
- The subscriber and/or the payer pays a fixed monthly or annual premium that is independent of the utilization of services.
- The HMO assumes at least part of the financial risk in the provision of covered services.

The following characteristics of each model may help to distinguish them. What is important to remember, however, is that a process of hybridization is occurring among these and other models of managed care that blurs their once-sharp distinctions.

**Group Model HMO**   In a group model HMO, a single, large, multispeciality group practice is either the sole or a major source of care for the HMO enrollees. The group may have existed before the corporately distinct HMO entity formed, but it has an exclusive contract only with the one HMO. Some groups also see fee-for-service or preferred provider organization (PPO) patients; others are not permitted to do so. Because of the similarity with the staff model HMO, the term *staff/group model HMO* is often used to denote these large HMOs (Weiner and de Lissovoy 1993).

**Staff Model HMO**   In a staff model HMO, the majority of enrollees are cared for by physicians who are on the HMO staff. Although these physicians may be involved in risk-sharing arrangements, a majority of their income usually is derived from a fixed salary. The group-cooperative, consumer-controlled HMOs are usually staff model plans. Because the physicians in this type of HMO are also organized into groups, the term *group/staff model* is used to encompass both this and the group model HMO (Weiner and de Lissovoy 1993).

**Independent Practice Association (IPA)**   The independent practice association (IPA), sometimes referred to as the individual practice association, is an open-panel type of HMO in which individual physicians or small group practices contract to provide care to enrolled members. The primary care physicians may be paid by capitation or fee-for-service with a "withhold" risk-sharing arrangement. The withhold mechanism establishes a reserve fund that can be used to cover unanticipated costs of care; unused funds are then redistributed to providers at the close of the contract period. In the event of a shortfall, providers are expected to make up the differences from their allocations.

An IPA entity may be legally distinct from the HMO entity with which the member enrolls. Physicians participating in IPAs retain their right to treat non-HMO patients on a fee-for-service basis (Weiner and de Lissovoy 1993).

**Network Model HMO**   In a network model HMO, a network of two or more existing group practices contracts to care for the majority of patients enrolled in an HMO plan. A network model HMO may also contract with individual providers in a fashion similar to an IPA. Providers contracting with a network model HMO are usually free to serve fee-for-service patients as well as those enrolled in other HMOs and PPOs (Weiner and de Lissovoy 1993).

### The Social Health Maintenance Organization (SHMO)

The social health maintenance organization (SHMO) is a Medicare demonstration project to determine the feasibility of combining social, health, and medical services under one capitation payment. See Chapter 15 for a more thorough examination of the SHMO.

## *Preferred Provider Organization (PPO) and Exclusive Provider Organization (EPO)*

Until the early 1980s, the models described in the preceding sections constituted the realm of managed care. Discontent with the imperfections of the delivery system led to the introduction of another model, the preferred provider organization (PPO), and to a variant, the exclusive provider organization (EPO).

The PPO is a type of integrated delivery system in which the PPO entity acts as a broker between the purchaser of care and the provider. In a PPO, consumers have the option to either use or not use the preferred providers available within the plan. Consumers are channeled toward in-plan providers through the use of lower cost sharing and greater benefit coverage. In return for patient referrals, providers agree that their care will be managed. Providers are usually paid a discounted fee-for-service payment, and they do not participate in financial risk sharing. In 2001, PPO plans constituted 48 percent of the health plan market (Health Insurance Association of America [HIAA] 2002).

EPOs are a type of PPO in which patients must exclusively use the providers within the PPO, although they may pay out-of-pocket to see out-of-plan providers (Weiner and de Lissovoy 1993).

Although a PPO gives consumers greater choice than the staff model HMO, for example, its ability to control expenditures is limited by the level of discount that can be negotiated with providers. This limitation helped to give rise to another variant—the point-of-service (POS) model, discussed in the next section.

Hurley, Strunk, and White (2004) discuss "the puzzling popularity of the PPO," noting that more than 100 million people (over half of the people in the United States with private health care benefits) receive their care through a PPO. They note that the many forms that a PPO can take contribute to the confusion about this model of managed care and add that the embracing of PPOs was more a flight from the restrictions feared to be inherent in HMOs than an appeal of PPO features.

## *Point-of-Service Model*

The point-of-service (POS) model is a hybridized managed care plan that offers consumers a choice of options at the time they seek services, rather than at the time they choose to enroll in a health plan (Weiner and de Lissovoy 1993). The POS model was a fast-growing model of managed care through the 1990s (Drake 1997), principally because it offers the subscriber flexibility in choice of providers. Choice is considered a key to promoting quality (Stauffer 1997). Consumers who choose POS plans are likely to have higher cost sharing in the form of deductibles, co-insurance, and copayments but may elect this coverage because it ensures freedom of choice of provider.

Although HMOs introduced the POS model as a way to maintain their competitiveness, the POS is not the ultimate organism in this evolutionary process. Recent innovations include integrated delivery networks and provider-sponsored organizations.

### Integrated Delivery Networks

Integrated delivery networks, sometimes called organized delivery systems, integrate a variety of health services organizations to deliver a broad array of health services across the continuum of care in a cost-effective manner. Shortell et al. (1993) define an organized delivery system as "a network of organizations that provides or arranges to provide a coordinated continuum of services to a defined population and is willing to be held clinically and fiscally accountable for the outcomes and the health status of the population served."

The integration of health organizations may be vertical or virtual (Robinson and Casalino 1996). Vertical integration gathers hospitals, medical groups, and other delivery system elements under one umbrella with a unity of purpose and control. It also creates substantial pressure for capital funds for acquisition purposes. Two weaknesses are inherent in the vertical integration approach to developing organized delivery systems: the incentive system becomes lessened or weakened by the organizational hierarchy that is established, and influence costs, which are the effects of internal struggles over the control of resources, increase greatly.

Virtual integration achieves coordination on a contractual basis. This type of organized delivery system has more autonomy to adapt to changing environmental circumstances because it is unencumbered by a large-salaried workforce and the need to maintain hierarchies or the bureaucratic structures that seem inevitable in a vertically integrated organization.

### Provider-Sponsored Organizations (PSOs)

Provider-sponsored organizations (PSOs) are variants of integrated networks. The PSO label appears to be eclipsing that of the integrated network; the concepts are so similar that differentiating between them is difficult.

PSOs, sometimes called provider-sponsored networks (PSNs), are provider affiliations organized to offer both health insurance and health services to local or regional populations to counterbalance the growing market power of national and regional health plans and insurers (National Health Policy Forum [NHPF] 1996).

Organizationally, PSOs may range from loose affiliations of physicians to highly integrated networks of physicians and hospitals. They sell services to a variety of purchasers, including individuals, other PSOs, HMOs, traditional insurance companies, employer health plans, and governmental agencies, and accept a range of payment mechanisms, from fee-for-service to full capitation (NHPF 1997).

Depending on how they are structured, PSOs bear some financial risk for the services they contractually provide. Although PSOs may contract with health plans and insurers, they are seen by many as end runs around the traditional delivery and financing arrangements, bypassing plans and insurers to contract directly with private and public health services purchasers for the care of specific populations (NHPF 1996).

A type of PSO organized to provide care to Medicare beneficiaries (except those with end-stage renal disease), is described in the 1997 Balanced Budget Act (PL 105-33) as a public or private entity that:

- is established or organized and operated by a health services provider or group of affiliated health services providers;
- provides a substantial proportion of contractually specified health services items and services directly through the provider or affiliated providers; and
- with respect to the affiliated partners, shares directly or indirectly in substantial financial risk in the provision of such items and services and has at least a majority financial interest in the entity.

The Balanced Budget Act envisioned the PSO as a primary mechanism for hospitals and physicians to offer health insurance or health benefits coverage to Medicare beneficiaries as a Medicare+Choice health plan. Under this act's provisions, PSOs would be licensed by states and certified by the Centers for Medicare and Medicaid Services (CMS) as eligible to provide care to Medicare beneficiaries as an alternative to fee-for-service care.

Another type of PSO—the physician-hospital organization (PHO)—was in the policy spotlight in the early 1990s. PHOs are joint ventures between a hospital(s) and its medical staff to contract with HMOs or self-insuring employers to provide services to an enrolled population. PHOs typically assume risks for services they provide under a capitation arrangement. In the mid-1990s, many large hospitals created or planned to create such entities, but interest in this type of organization appears to have waned (see Chapter 9).

### Other Models of Managed Care

Other models of managed care, including tiered benefit packages and consumer-directed health plans, are addressed in Chapter 6.

## Strengths and Weaknesses of Managed Care

Managed care offers both strengths and weaknesses as the mainstream system of health services delivery in the United States. Strengths or accomplishments attributed to managed care include:

- slowing of health services expenditures in the early 1990s (Ginzberg and Ostow 1997);
- lower hospital admission rates, shorter hospital lengths of stay (LOS), less use of expensive procedures and tests, mixed results on outcomes, somewhat lower consumer satisfaction with services but higher satisfaction with costs (Miller and Luft 1994);
- creation of new organizations to allocate money and talent in a rational way (Ellwood and Lundberg 1996);
- development of reliable and pervasive tools for measuring some health outcomes (Ellwood and Lundberg 1996);
- growing consensus on the importance of preventive services (Ellwood and Lundberg 1996);
- incorporation of the best clinical practices into guidelines (Ellwood and Lundberg 1996);
- initial public reporting mechanisms regarding quality of care (Ellwood and Lundberg 1996);
- information systems that support, monitor, and provide feedback on the effects of health services (Ellwood and Lundberg 1996);
- potential, if responsible, administrative safeguards that are applied to function as a more reasonable way of determining appropriate treatment than market mechanisms (Mechanic 1994);
- efforts to eliminate waste and redundancy in the system (Kassirer 1997); and
- greater attention to management of chronic diseases (Kassirer 1997).

Weaknesses or failures of managed care that analysts have noted include:

- reduced power resulting in physicians and hospitals protecting their professional and economic interests and acting independently in the interests of their patients (Ginzberg and Ostow 1997);
- lack of principles of accountability to the public for health quality (Ellwood and Lundberg 1996);
- inability to reduce national health expenditures despite some ability to reduce costs and offer value for money (Enthoven 1993b);
- unevenness of utilization review performed by review firms as a carve-out function; such firms may not review practices that could improve agency accountability, may underutilize methods to educate providers, and may not effectively use appeals mechanisms (Schlesinger, Gray, and Perreira 1997);
- forced choices physicians must make between the best interests of their patients and their own economic survival (Kassirer 1997);

- lag of regulations to protect the delivery of care, leaving the "amoral and impersonal mechanisms of the market" to determine how care is delivered (Kassirer 1997);
- potential for underservice exemplified by such practices as "drive-through deliveries," short inpatient hospital stays for childbirth mandated by some managed care organizations (Drake 1997; Ginzberg and Ostow 1997) (these short stays have since been precluded by overriding national regulations);
- lack of information systems, which makes evaluating the contents of care difficult (Ellwood and Lundberg 1996); and
- employers being placed in a decision-making position in health services when their preference is to offer information, options, and partial support for health benefits. It has altered the core functions of insurers from predicting cost trends and establishing premiums accordingly to accepting the prices offered by purchasers and seeking to hold expenditures beneath these limits. Physicians and hospitals no longer wish to fulfill the dual roles as agents for society and for the individual patient of managing costs as well as quality (Robinson 2001).

Each list will lengthen as experience with managed care continues. Several important caveats about the previous lists must be noted:

- What some see as strengths, others see as weaknesses (e.g., the status of information systems).
- Many of these same statements could be applied to a fee-for-service delivery system; the observation may reference some but not all forms of managed care, given the considerable variation in models of managed care discussed earlier.
- Much of the research on managed care focuses on the staff model HMO with salaried physicians, most of which are organized as not-for-profit organizations (Woolhandler and Himmelstein 1995; Mechanic 1994). Such research findings may be applied, in error, to other forms of managed care.

Regardless of the various models' strengths and weaknesses, what is clear is that managed care in all its various forms has displaced fee-for-service as the mainstream reimbursement system. The pendulum appears now to be swinging away from the most restrictive managed care models to those that permit the subscriber greater choice and flexibility. In a tight economy, however, employers who provide health insurance still have the advantage of choosing more rather than less restrictive plans because more restrictive plans are often less expensive.

## Managed Competition

Managed care is still a "work in progress," according to many (Ellwood and Lundberg 1996). Managed competition, a refinement of the managed care concept, was proposed in the late 1980s by the Jackson Hole Group, analysts and policy leaders including, among others, economist Alain Enthoven and Paul Ellwood (a pioneer in the HMO concept). Managed competition is a purchasing strategy to obtain maximum value for both consumers and employers. Central to the managed competition concept is the role of the sponsor, a health insurance purchasing cooperative (HIPC), which purchases health services coverage for a large group of subscribers, and in so doing, structures and adjusts the market to overcome attempts by insurers to avoid price competition (Enthoven 1993a). Thus, managed competition incorporates elements of price competition and market regulation.

Competition occurs among large health plans. Regulation is instituted to prevent efforts to avoid price competition. The 1993 Health Security Act relied heavily on the concepts of managed competition. Despite Congress's failure to pass this act, principles and adaptations of the managed competition concept are evident in many health services markets today (Schlesinger 1997; Luft 1996; Zwanziger and Melnick 1996).

## Managed Care Market Share

Managed care has become the mainstream delivery system in the United States. By 2000, 92 percent of the population with employer-sponsored health insurance was enrolled in some form of managed care, including POS plans. Nearly 60 percent of Medicaid enrollees were enrolled in managed care plans, including Medicaid's Primary Care Case Management (PCCM) plans operated by state Medicaid agencies (Gauthier and Rogal 2001). Seventeen percent of Medicare beneficiaries were enrolled in Medicare+Choice plans, Medicare's managed care option (CMS 2002), now known as Medicare Advantage plans.

Most states are aggressively seeking to enroll a larger proportion of their Medicaid populations into a form of managed care. All but two states, Alaska and Wyoming, have some type of managed care for enrollees (CMS 2002). A number of Medicare+Choice plans began withdrawing from the program as early as 1999 (NHPF 2001), contending that provider payment was inadequate to support the services provided. In 2002, 58 Medicare+Choice contracts indicated plans to either withdraw from the program (22 plans) or to reduce their services (36 plans). This left the total of Medicare beneficiaries affected by plan withdrawal over a four-year period at 2.2 million persons (NHPF 2001). The 2002 Medicare Prescription Drug

Improvement and Modernization Act created a new Part C, replacing Medicare+Choice plans with Medicare Advantage plans.

The growth of managed care is not yet evenly distributed but rather is concentrated in certain areas. The Minneapolis–St. Paul area and the entire state of Minnesota have a high concentration of managed care organizations and broad coverage of Minnesota's population. In California, managed care clearly dominates the delivery system: half of those with private health insurance are in HMOs, and the other half are in PPOs; about one-third of Medicare beneficiaries are in HMOs; and more than half of the Medicaid enrollees are in HMOs (Robinson and Casalino 1996). Other high concentrations occur where sufficient populations of consumers or subscribers and an adequate to excessive supply of health services providers and facilities exist.

The growth of managed care is not evenly distributed across all models. Enrollment in staff and group model HMOs has slowed, influenced in part by the domination of self-insured organizations, which account for 45 percent of the coverage to employees with health insurance (Cunningham 1997). The growth rate for IPAs—until recent years the fastest growing among the various models of managed care (Kane, Turnbull, and Schoen 1996)—was eclipsed by that of POS models by 2001 (HIAA 2002). The backlash against managed care has resulted in movement away from restrictions on both providers and consumers and toward more choice and individual decision making for both parties. The consumer-directed health plans that began emerging in the early 2000s are an indicator of yet another transition in the delivery system.

Some types of managed care appeal to subscribers because of a greater range of provider choices. Figure 19.1 shows the growth rate of enrollees in various managed care models of employer-sponsored health insurance plans for 1996 and 2001. Figure 19.2 shows the growth rates for Medicaid enrollees in managed care between 1991 and 2003.

The number of HMO plans was 652 in 1997 but declined to 412 by 2004 (USDHHS 2005). The same phenomenon occurring in the hospital industry is apparent among HMOs: acquisitions, mergers, and consolidations are reducing the number of players, resulting in fewer but larger and more powerful organizations. Many of these organizations are regional or national in scope. The large size of these organizations raises concerns among some, who fear that "merger mania" may create organizations that are too big to fail—that is, organizations that enroll such a significant part of the population that, should they get overextended, governments might have to bail them out to protect the health and welfare of the population (Fuchs 1997).[1]

The growth of managed care organizations and the market share they represent also are not evenly distributed between proprietary and not-for-profit organizations. Although many of the first-established HMOs were created as not-for-profit organizations, the growth has been among proprietary HMOs. Whether this growth in the proprietary sector serves the delivery

**FIGURE 19.1**

Enrollment in Employer-Sponsored Health Plans (1996 and 2001)

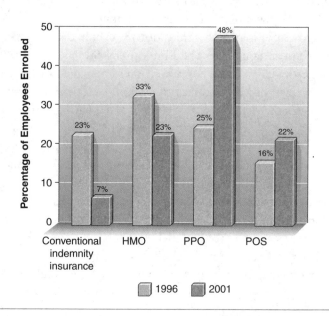

SOURCE: Health Insurance Association of America 2002. Used with permission from America's Health Insurance Plans (formerly the Health Insurance Association of America).

**FIGURE 19.2**

Number and Percentage of Medicaid Beneficiaries Enrolled in Managed Care (1991–2003)

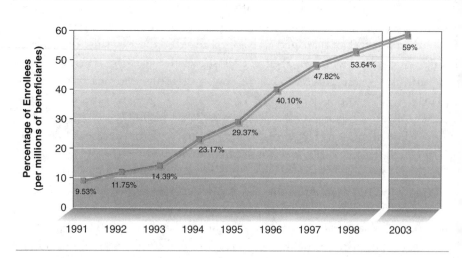

SOURCES: CMS 2000; U.S. Government Accountability Office (USGAO) 2005.

NOTE: June 30th reporting date for each year. Prior to 1996, state-reported managed care data may include duplicated enrollment.

system well is still being debated. Concerns have been raised about the willingness of proprietary organizations to support the production of such public goods as health professional education, research, and care of indigent populations (Lawrence, Mattingly, and Ludden 1997; Ginzberg and Ostow 1997).

## Medicare and Medicaid Managed Care

Medicare and Medicaid managed care constitutes a special part of the managed care market and generates issues specific to the care of vulnerable populations. The Medicare program has permitted managed care options from the outset and introduced a risk-sharing contract option in 1972.[2] Managed care plans that participate in the CMS risk contract program receive a capitation payment equivalent to 95 percent of the adjusted average per capita cost (AAPCC). The 1997 Balanced Budget Act provided for the establishment of a range of managed care plans under the Medicare+Choice program. The Medicare Advantage program that replaced Medicare+Choice is revising the types of plans available to beneficiaries. As of August 2004, 12 percent of Medicare beneficiaries (4.6 million persons) were enrolled in managed care plans (USGAO 2005).

Enrollment in Medicaid managed care programs has traditionally occurred primarily through Medicaid 1915 and 1115 waivers that permit managed care. The 1981 Omnibus Budget Reconciliation Act (OBRA) authorized the option for Primary Care Case Management (PCCM) programs to be established by state Medicaid programs. The PCCM program initially paid providers a $3 per member per month administrative fee to enroll Medicaid eligibles and ensure that they received the care they needed, including referrals to specialists. Medical services provided were usually paid on a fee-for-service basis. Twenty-nine state Medicaid programs had PCCM options in 2001 (Sprague 2001). Some states have augmented the monthly administration fee; others have expanded the PCCM model to include the management of specific diseases, such as diabetes.

The 1997 Balanced Budget Act, however, gives states more flexibility in developing managed care programs. Mandatory managed care may be implemented by amending the state's Medicaid State Plan, which generally requires action by a state's legislature, rather than by seeking a waiver, which requires CMS approval and must be periodically renewed. This act also authorized a PCCM-like demonstration program to be offered to Medicare beneficiaries in select regions of the country. The CMS selected and funded 15 such sites in early 2001, but the program has not yet been evaluated.

By 2000, all states but Alaska and Wyoming had implemented some kind of Medicaid managed care. By 2003, 59 percent of all Medicaid enrollees received their health services through some type of managed care, compared with less than 10 percent in 1991 (USGAO 2005). Future enrollment growth will depend on Medicaid's ability to identify managed care programs that can appropriately care for vulnerable populations with significant physical and mental disabilities.

## Policy Issues Surrounding Managed Care

Because managed care is a work in progress, the list of policy issues surrounding it is also dynamic. This chapter cannot begin to do justice to the universe of issues regarding managed care but briefly discusses those related to physician practice, enrolled populations, quality of care, regulation, and cost containment.

### Physician Practice

The pervasiveness of managed care suggests that few physicians have the luxury of avoiding participation. In fact, the majority of physicians have entered into at least one contractual agreement with managed care entities. In 2001, more than 90 percent of physicians worked with at least one managed care contract (Strunk and Reschovsky 2002).

**Gag Rules**  Managed care requires a practice style and orientation that is different from what physicians trained prior to the 1990s are accustomed to. Physicians have traditionally been trained to function as the patient's advocate, helping the patient to navigate the complex delivery system to obtain appropriate care. Most believe that maintaining the advocacy role is essential (Mechanic 1994; Ginzberg and Ostow 1997), but physicians' advocacy for a patient may put them on a collision course with a managed care organization's practice guidelines. As a result, some managed care organizations have issued—either as a part of their contract with a physician or as a separate policy statement—what have come to be referred to as gag rules. A gag rule is defined as:

- a contractual provision between a plan and providers that limits information, advice, and counsel that a provider may give a patient;
- an anticriticism provision that prohibits a provider from making any communication that may adversely affect confidence in the health plan; and
- any health plan practice that inhibits open communication between a physician and a patient (Etheredge and Jones 1997).

Congress came close to passing a prohibition against gag rules in 1996, and several states have passed or are considering passing such laws.

**Physician Autonomy**  The type of managed care system in which they practice may affect physicians' autonomy of practice in the use of specialty services, physician referrals, drugs and devices, and other technologies. To contain expenditures, physicians have to control utilization of services. What constitutes appropriate utilization is still being widely debated.

While a delivery system based on fee-for-service reimbursement is conducive to the overutilization of services, the specter that haunts many who are apprehensive of managed care is the potential for underutilization of needed services as a way to contain expenditures. Physicians fear being "squeezed between their patients and their employers" regarding a patient's needs and the managed care plan's guidelines on utilization (Kassirer 1997).

### Enrolled Populations

Managed care changes the ways in which patients seek and obtain care. Among these changes are the narrowing of consumer choice of provider; the predisposition of consumers to select plans that best match their self-assessed health status (selection bias); the often involuntary turnover in plans, which affects continuity of care; and the satisfaction levels that consumers express about managed care. Managed care has also changed the ways in which services are delivered and has prompted the conceptualization of new delivery forms. One such conceptualization is the development of HMOs that specialize in the care of particular populations, such as persons with disabilities.

**Consumer Choice**

Managed care organizations, particularly those that developed from the prepaid group practice (PGP) model, have made some consumers wary because their choice of provider is limited to those on the managed care organization's provider panel. Aged people or people with chronic conditions or severe physical or mental disabilities may avoid managed care enrollment if their preferred caregivers are not empanelled (Hellinger 1995). The demand for choice, a central tenet of U.S. society, led first to the development of PPOs and POS plans to address this demand, and more recently, to the emergence of consumer-directed health plans.

**Selection Bias**

Adverse selection occurs when people with the greatest anticipated health services needs flock to the managed care organization that offers the richest benefit package, thus ensuring higher service utilization and expenditures for this plan. Robinson and Gardner (1995) studied adverse selection among multiple competing HMOs and found that utilization was based not solely on epidemiologic factors but also on certain organizational and economic factors in particular health plans. Their findings contradict the popular belief that HMOs attract only the younger, healthier enrollees.

Hellinger (1995), who looked at selection bias in HMOs and PPOs, found that all plans that restrict the enrollee's choice of provider (i.e., group practice HMO, staff HMO, IPA HMO, and EPO) enjoy favorable selection among the nonelderly and the elderly, in part because individuals who want to retain provider choice do not enroll in these plans. The increasing focus on more consumer choice and greater flexibility is likely to affect the issue of selection bias, particularly if consumers choose less restrictive options.

One way to reduce selection bias would be to consider the development of specialized HMOs for people with disabilities; such HMOs would be staffed appropriate to enrollees' needs and include a payment rate reflecting an enriched benefit package (Mechanic 1994). These HMOs might be the only way to secure additional Medicaid enrollment because a majority of the healthiest enrollees are already in a managed care system. Creating a reimbursement system that can attract providers to this kind of a delivery system remains a challenge.

**Turnover**    Subscriber turnover in managed care plans is a significant issue, affecting the continuity of care provided and received, and potentially influencing the organization's incentives to maintain a long-term perspective on individual and population health status. According to a mid-1990s study of managed care (The Commonwealth Fund 1995), working Americans change health plans frequently, and most of this change is involuntary because the employer drops one or more plans, replacing them with new plans that offer the employer a better deal. It is not yet clear where the consumer-directed health plan movement will lead. Employers may be looking at this option as a vehicle for shifting more costs to employees. The vitality of the labor market can also influence the nature and range of health benefit plans offered to employees.

**Customer Satisfaction**    Although the proportion of the population receiving health services from a managed care system is growing, patient satisfaction with managed care varies.

One study of the patient's perspective on managed care compared satisfaction between managed care enrollees and those who received care in a fee-for-service system (The Commonwealth Fund 1995). Managed care enrollees reported lower satisfaction levels than their fee-for-service counterparts along the following dimensions: plan attributes, overall plan, quality of services, ease of changing physicians, choice of physicians, access to specialty and emergency care, and waiting time for appointments.

Those enrolled in managed care plans who were not afforded a choice of health plan had higher dissatisfaction levels than people enrolled in managed care who had been able to choose among health plans. The type of managed care plan in which respondents were enrolled also affected their satisfaction level.

In the sample population surveyed, enrollees rated group and staff HMOs similarly overall to ratings by enrollees in fee-for-service plans. Independent practice associations (IPAs) were associated with slightly higher dissatisfaction levels; network/mixed-model HMOs and PPO plans received the highest dissatisfaction ratings. Ratings for overall quality of service varied widely across the models of managed care as well. In at least one area—out-of-pocket costs—consumers indicated higher satisfaction with managed care plans as a group than did people in fee-for-service care (Davis, Schoen, and Sandman 1996).

Miller and Luft (1994, 1997, and 2002) have tracked HMO plan performance, including patient satisfaction, since research reports began appearing in the literature in 1980. They have noted changes in patient satisfaction over time. In their earlier studies, greater satisfaction with financial aspects of HMO plans, compared to fee-for-service plans, was seen as a trade-off for less satisfaction with nonfinancial aspects. This trade-off could not be clearly seen in their 2002 study.

Some of the "backlash" against managed care described by Blendon et al. (1998) involves consumers' frustration with what they perceive as restrictions that inhibit their access to care and some diminution of quality. The Center for Studying Health System Change studied consumer attitudes toward the health services system  and found a slight increase in consumer confidence in the system and trust in physicians between 1997 and 2002 but noted strong evidence of continued public concern about the influence of health plans on medical decision making (Reed and Trude 2002). The development of new types of plans and insurance products, which offer an opportunity to migrate away from more restrictive options, suggests that consumers are still experiencing unrest and dissatisfaction.

## Quality of Care

Does the quality of care under managed care differ from that under fee-for-service care? Fearful of managed care's incentives for underservice, critics have proffered dire predictions about the inferiority of care under managed care systems. Lumping together many different kinds of organizations and the care they provide under the umbrella of managed care is clearly inappropriate with regard to quality of care. As noted, many of the findings about quality of care in managed care systems pertain to long-established prepaid group practice (PPG) organizations; some of the more recent managed care models have not been around long enough for definitive conclusions about quality to be drawn.

Fuchs (1997) notes that the pursuit of quality has had little role in the spread of managed care. Many analysts are maintaining a watchful wait, conceding that there is as yet little or no evidence to suggest that the quality of managed care is inferior to that of fee-for-service care (Ellwood and Lundberg 1996; Kassirer 1995) and emphasizing that monitoring health outcome performance must be a crucial element of any health services delivery system (Miller and Luft 1994).

Miller and Luft examined the differences between models of managed care—typically HMOs—and fee-for-service care in three iterative studies (1994, 1997, 2002). Their 1994 study showed that quality of care in HMOs was not substandard when compared to fee-for-service care. They found the quality distinctions between the two more difficult to interpret in their 1997 study but concluded that the evidence did not support fears that HMOs uniformly led to worse quality of care than that provided in fee-for-service settings. They added, however, that their data on quality were collected before the 1992 round of cost cutting began. Miller and Luft's 2002 study concluded that both types of plans (HMO and fee-for-service) provide roughly comparable quality of care and that HMOs somewhat lower the use of hospital and other expensive resources.

Concerns about quality appear to be on the increase. The Institute of Medicine's (IOM) seminal studies on quality, the advent of the Leapfrog Group and its interest in quality, the quality measures developed and implemented for the Health Plan Employer Data and Information Set (HEDIS®), and the use of the Consumer Assessment of Healthcare Providers and Systems (CAHPS®) hospital survey are indicators of this renewed emphasis (see Chapter 20).

### Regulation

Although the market influence on the delivery of health services has clearly grown in recent years, is the delivery of health services to be controlled entirely by market forces as is any other commodity? Views on this issue vary, but many long-established health services researchers and analysts believe that some regulation of the delivery system is necessary. Even the managed competition concept, which emphasizes price competition, also incorporates regulatory mechanisms to control entities that would attempt to avoid price competition.

Kassirer (1995) suggests that the fundamental question of managed care is whether health services should be subjected to the values of the marketplace. Fuchs (1997) points out that social control of medicine requires professional norms, market competition, and governmental regulation. Mechanic (1994) calls for both state and federal regulation of managed care. Ginzberg and Ostow (1997) call for regulatory control in managed care to protect patients. Zwanziger and Melnick (1996) cite the need for a governmental role to protect competition in health services markets and also to ensure that access to and quality of care are not adversely affected in managed care plans.

In a retrospective of Paul Starr's *The Social Transformation of American Medicine* more than two decades ago, in which Starr forecasts the corporatization of the delivery system, Havighurst (2004) notes that Starr's book came "at the turning point in the history of American health policy when government was beginning to shut down the regulatory experiments of the 1970s and to set off in pursuit of other, especially private, solutions to the chronic problem of rising costs." Such solutions are still being conceptualized and implemented; not enough time or experience has occurred to afford meaningful evaluation.

## Cost Containment under Managed Care

A primary motivation in the development of managed care was to contain costs of and expenditures for health services. What does the evidence show? The following list summarizes the findings, but many of the findings are specific to a particular type of managed care organization—principally, the prepaid group practice (PGP).

- In a study of managed care in California, Robinson (1996) found that hospital expenditures grew 44 percent less rapidly in markets with high HMO penetration between 1983 and 1993.
- During the period 1985 to 1993, hospitals in areas with high rates of HMO penetration and growth had a slower rate of growth in expenses than hospitals in low-penetration areas (Gaskin and Hadley 1997).
- Zwanziger and Melnick's (1996) study of managed care in California and Minnesota concluded that managed care appeared to have controlled costs.
- Managed care has reduced spending by reducing services to patients, providing services more efficiently, and squeezing incomes of physicians and other health services providers (Fuchs 1997).
- HMOs in areas with more competitors have lower premiums than HMOs established in less competitive areas (Feldman, Wholey, and Christianson 1996).
- Managed care growth in the 1980s led to a slowing of expenditures in the early 1990s, but whether this slowing is a one-time event or the beginning of a trend is not clear (Ginzberg and Ostow 1997).
- Selective contracting with providers (i.e., permitting only those who meet certain standards to provide care to defined populations) is an effective cost-containing strategy (Drake 1997).
- A study of managed care plan performance found that, compared with indemnity plans, HMOs had somewhat lower hospital admission rates, shorter lengths of stay, and less use of expensive procedures and tests (Miller and Luft 1994).

The effects of managed care on health services costs and expenditures will continue to be one of the most significant questions about the U.S. health services delivery system.

## Summary

The shift from a fee-for-service to a managed care delivery system continues to substantially affect all participants. Physicians and other providers are required to practice in new ways, and some experience declining incomes; their satisfaction levels with these changes remain mixed. Hospitals and other facilities experienced changes as downsizing and other reductions in capacity occurred in the late 1990s, but capacity development again appears to be on the rise. Payers for health services are exerting greater influence on how the delivery system is shaped. Consumers are also accommodating to changes in the traditional ways in which they have sought and obtained care. The extent of change indicates that the system has not yet reached equilibrium.

Nowhere are the changes in the U.S. health services system more evident—and more constant—than in the area of managed care. The various experiments to integrate the financing and delivery of health services have provided a laboratory for study of the alternating emphases on access to, costs and expenditures for, and quality of health services. The movement toward managed care was principally motivated by the need to reduce costs for care, and was embraced by various payers as the solution to the unchecked rise in health services expenditures. Managed care was also seen, at least in the case of Medicaid's Primary Care Case Management (PCCM) program, as a way to systematically increase access to care for Medicaid enrollees.

What seemed an inexorable movement of the entire delivery system toward managed care in the mid-1990s has now become a stepping back and reexamination of this initiative. The "managed care backlash" discussed by Blendon and associates in 1998 indicated that consumers were frustrated with difficulties in accessing providers, concerned about the quality of care they were receiving, and dissatisfied that their costs were not being reduced or contained. Providers were frustrated about the constraints placed on them in the provision of care they deemed best, limited time with patients, potential financial penalties if they referred patients to specialty care, and the need for payer authorization before certain procedures or services could be provided. Additionally, providers also faced changes in their incomes as their risk for providing services increased with each new contract. Payers for care, seeking ways to reduce their expenditures, had to contend with shifting alliances among providers, hybridization of service plans and models of care, and subscribers or employees (in the case of self-funded companies) who expressed their dissatisfaction with their health services plans. A strong economy and a tight labor market in the late 1990s and into the year 2000 required employers, in particular, to reconsider the entire issue of employee health benefits.

The obituary for managed care as a political, if not a financial, failure has already been written (Robinson 2001). Robinson concludes that "after a turbulent decade of trial and error, [the managed care] experiment can be characterized as a partial economic success and a total political failure." He then examines which entity—the physician, the insurer, the employer, the government, or the consumer—is best suited to balance resources and expectations "in the brave new world after managed care." His prediction seems to be realized, at least as evidenced by the consumer-directed health plan movement.

It can be argued that the announcement of managed care's demise is premature. At this stage in an ever-changing environment, however, it can at least be concluded that what was once perceived as a wholesale movement toward rationalizing access to services (and what some would describe as rationing services) and thereby containing costs has not provided the hoped-for panacea. Rather, concerns about quality, as well as access and costs, have engendered a push of the pendulum away from proscription and toward moderation. A constant, and constantly changing, factor that influences the delivery system is the strength of the economy. When jobs are at stake in a weak economy, employees have less room to demand increased flexibility in health plans, particularly when such increases generally translate to increased costs to both the employer and the employee. Few would argue that a full-scale return to the fee-for-service reimbursement system is likely, but most would agree that changes in how health services are organized, financed, and delivered in the United States will continue.

## Notes

1. The concern about organizations too big to fail is not without foundation. In the early 1970s in California, a number of managed care organizations were created—at least on paper—to serve the MediCal (California's Medicaid) population. When these organizations were unable to meet their service commitments, state government had to step in to ensure care for this population. This debate stimulated federal government regulations as part of the 1976 HMO amendments that prohibited any federally qualified HMO's enrollment of Medicaid enrollees or Medicare beneficiaries to exceed 50 percent of total enrollment. This proportion was revised upward to 75 percent by the provisions of the 1981 OBRA. The Medicare+Choice plans established by the 1997 Balanced Budget Act, however, are composed entirely of Medicare beneficiaries.

2. Under Medicare's initial authority for paying HMOs for care to Medicare beneficiaries, HMOs could choose a risk option, which limited their profit potential and made them fully liable for losses, or a cost-based option. The risk option had little appeal to providers, and the cost-based option lacked strong financial incentives to reduce

unnecessary care and to deliver care efficiently. Consequently, a 1982 legislative change, which established a fixed monthly payment—the adjusted average per capita cost (AAPCC) rate—made Medicare risk contracts more attractive to providers (USGAO 1997b).

## Key Words

| | |
|---|---|
| adjusted average per capita cost (AAPCC) | Kaiser Permanente |
| alternative delivery system | managed care |
| backlash against managed care | managed care organization (MCO) |
| Balanced Budget Act of 1997 | managed competition |
| capitation | Medicaid |
| carve-out function | Medicare |
| Centers for Medicare and Medicaid Services (CMS) | Medicare+Choice plans |
| certificate of need (CON) program | Medicare risk-sharing HMOs |
| Committee on the Costs of Medical Care (CCMC) | network model HMO |
| competition | not-for-profit organization |
| cost containment | omnibus budget reconciliation act (OBRA) |
| cost sharing | organized delivery system |
| discounted fee-for-service payment | patient satisfaction |
| drive-through delivery | physician-hospital organization (PHO) |
| exclusive provider organization (EPO) | point-of-service (POS) plan |
| fee-for-service delivery system | preferred provider organization (PPO) |
| gag rules | prepaid group practice (PGP) |
| gross domestic product (GDP) | prepaid health plan |
| group model HMO | provider service networks (PSN) |
| health insurance purchasing cooperative (HIPC) | provider-sponsored organization (PSO) |
| health maintenance organization (HMO) | rationing |
| Health Maintenance Organization Act | regulation |
| Health Security Act | risk |
| hybrid organization | Ross-Loos PGP |
| indemnity health insurance | selection bias |
| independent practice association (IPA) | selective contracting |
| integrated delivery network/system | self-insured business |
| international medical graduate (IMG) | self-referral |
| Jackson Hole Group | staff model HMO |
| | turnover |
| | utilization review |
| | vertical integration |
| | virtual integration |

# References

Barton, P. L., J. Bondy, and J. Glazner. 1993. *Colorado Medical Reform Study.* Denver, CO: University of Colorado Health Sciences Center.

Blendon, R. J., M. Brodie, J. M. Benson, D. E. Altman, L. Levitt, T. Hoff, and L. Huzick. 1998. "Understanding the Managed Care Backlash." *Health Affairs* 17 (4): 80–94.

Centers for Medicare and Medicaid Services. 2002. *Medicare and Medicaid Statistical Profile, 2002.* Baltimore, MD: CMS.

———. 2000. *A Profile of Medicaid, 2000 Chartbook.* [Online information; retrieved 3/28/02.] www.cms.gov.

Commonwealth Fund, The. 1995. *Managed Care: The Patient's Perspective.* New York: The Commonwealth Fund.

Cunningham, R. 1997. "Hybrids Take Center Stage as New Phase in Cost War Looms." *Medicine and Health* 51 (14): S1–S4.

Davis, K., C. Schoen, and D. R. Sandman. 1996. "The Culture of Managed Care: Implications for Patients." *Bulletin of the NY Academy of Medicine* 73 (1): 173–83.

Drake, D. F. 1997. "Managed Care: A Product of Market Dynamics." *Journal of the American Medical Association* 227 (7): 560–63.

Ellwood, P. M., and G. D. Lundberg. 1996. "Managed Care: A Work in Progress." *Journal of The American Medical Association* 276 (13): 1083–86.

Enthoven, A. C. 1993a. "The History and Principles of Managed Competition." *Health Affairs* 12 (Supplement): 4–48.

———. 1993b. "Why Managed Care Has Failed to Contain Health Costs." *Health Affairs* 12 (3): 27–43.

Etheredge, L., and S. B. Jones. 1997. "Consumers, Gag Rules, and Health Plans: Strategies for a Patient-Focused Market." Research Agenda Brief. Washington, DC: The George Washington University.

Feldman, R., J. Kralewski, and B. Dowd. 1989. "Health Maintenance Organizations: The Beginning or the End?" *Health Services Research* 24 (2): 191–211.

Feldman, R., D. Wholey, and J. Christianson. 1996. "Economic and Organizational Determinants of HMO Mergers and Failures." *Inquiry* 33 (2): 118–32.

Fuchs, V. R. 1997. "Managed Care and Merger Mania." *Journal of the American Medical Association* 277 (11): 920–21.

Gaskin, D. J., and J. Hadley. 1997. "The Impact of HMO Penetration on Hospital Cost Inflation, 1985–1993." *Inquiry* 34 (3): 205–16.

Gauthier, A. K., and D. L. Rogal. 2001. *The Challenge of Managed Care Regulation: Making Markets Work?* Washington, DC: Academy for Health Services Research and Health Policy.

Ginzberg, E., and M. Ostow. 1997. "Managed Care—A Look Back and a Look Ahead." *New England Journal of Medicine* 336 (14): 1018–20.

Havighurst, C. C. 2004. "Star on the Corporatization and Commodification of Health Care: The Sequel." *Journal of Health Politics, Policy, and Law* 29 (4, 5): 947–67.

Health Insurance Association of America. 2002. *Source Book of Health Insurance Data 2002.* Washington, DC: HIAA.

Hellinger, F. J. 1995. "Selection Bias in HMOs and PPOs: A Review of the Evidence." *Inquiry* 32 (2): 135–42.

Hurley, R. E., B. C. Strunk, and J. S. White. 2004. "The Puzzling Popularity of the PPO." *Health Affairs* 23 (2): 56–68.

Kane, N. M., N. C. Turnbull, and C. Schoen. 1996. *Markets and Plan Performance: Summary Reports on Case Studies of IPA and Network HMOs.* New York: The Commonwealth Fund.

Kassirer, J. P. 1997. "Is Managed Care Here to Stay?" *New England Journal of Medicine* 336 (14): 1013–14.

———. 1995. Managed Care and the Morality of the Marketplace. *New England Journal of Medicine* 333 (1): 50–52.

Lawrence, D. M., P. H. Mattingly, and J. M. Ludden. 1997. "Trusting in the Future: The Distinct Advantage of Nonprofit HMOs." *Milbank Quarterly* 75 (1): 5–10.

Luft, H. S. 1996. "Compensating for Biased Selection in Health Insurance." *The Milbank Quarterly* 64 (4): 566–91.

Mechanic, D. 1994. "Managed Care: Rhetoric and Realities." *Inquiry* 31 (2): 124–28.

Miller, R. H., and H. S. Luft. 2002. "HMO Plan Performance Update: An Analysis of the Literature, 1997–2001." *Health Affairs* 21 (4): 63–86.

———. 1997. "Does Managed Care Lead to a Better or Worse Quality of Care?" *Health Affairs* 16 (5): 7–25.

———. 1994. "Managed Care Plan Performance Since 1980." *Journal of the American Medical Association* 271 (19): 1512–19.

National Health Policy Forum. 2001. *Reconsidering Medicare+Choice: What Options Remain?* Washington, DC: The George Washington University.

———. 1997. *The Medicare Risk Contract Game: What Rules Should PSOs Play By?* Issue Brief No. 702. Washington, DC: The George Washington University.

———. 1996. *Trends in Health Network Development: Community and Provider Incentives in a Managed Care Environment.* Issue Brief No. 690. Washington, DC: The George Washington University.

Reed, M. C., and S. Trude. 2002. "Who Do You Trust? Americans' Perspectives on Health Care, 1997–2001." Tracking Report No. 3. Washington, DC: Center for Studying Health System Change.

Robinson, J. C. 2001. "The End of Managed Care." *Journal of the American Medical Association* 285 (20): 2622–28.

———. 1996. "Decline in Hospital Utilization and Cost Inflation under Managed Care in California." *Journal of the American Medical Association* 276 (13): 1060–64.

Robinson, J. C., and L. P. Casalino. 1996. "Vertical Integration and Organizational Networks in Health Care." *Health Affairs* 15 (1): 7–22.

Robinson, J. C., and L. B. Gardner. 1995. "Adverse Selection among Multiple Competing Health Maintenance Organizations." *Medical Care* 33 (12): 1161–75.

Schlesinger, M. 1997. "Countervailing Agency: A Strategy of Principled Regulation under Managed Competition." *The Milbank Quarterly* 75 (1): 35–87.

Schlesinger, M. J., B. H. Gray, and K. M. Perreira. 1997. "Medical Professionalism under Managed Care: The Pros and Cons of Utilization Review." *Health Affairs* 16 (1): 106–24.

Shortell, S. M., R. R. Gillies, D. A. Anderson, J. B. Mitchell, and K. L. Morgan. 1993. "Creating Organized Delivery Systems: The Barriers and the Facilitators." *Hospital and Health Services Administration* 38 (4): 447–66.

Sprague, L. 2001. "Primary Care Case Management: Lessons for Medicare?" National Health Policy Forum Issue Brief No. 768. Washington, DC: National Health Policy Forum.

Stauffer, M. 1997. *Point of Service.* Washington, DC: National Conference of State Legislatures, Policy Training Service.

Strunk, B. C., and D. J. Reschovsky. 2002. "Kinder and Gentler: Physicians and Managed Care, 1997–2001." Tracking Report, No. 5. Washington, DC: Center for Studying Health System Change.

U.S. Department of Health and Human Services. 2005. *Health, United States, 2005.* Washington, DC: USDHHS.

U.S. Government Accountability Office (formerly the U.S. General Accounting Office). 2005. *Medicaid Managed Care: Access and Quality Requirements Specific to Low-Income and Other Special Needs Enrollees.* GAO-05-44R. December 2004. Washington, DC: USGAO.

———. 1997a. *Medicaid Managed Care: Challenge of Holding Plans Accountable Requires Greater State Effort.* GAO/HEHS-97-86. Washington, DC: USGAO.

———. 1997b. *Medicare HMO Enrollment: Area Differences Affected by Other Than Payment Rates.* GAO/HEHS-97-37. Washington, DC: USGAO.

Weiner, J. P., and G. de Lissovoy. 1993. "Razing a Tower of Babel: A Taxonomy for Managed Care and Health Insurance Plans." *Journal of Health Politics, Policy and Law* 18 (1): 75–103.

Woolhandler, S., and D. U. Himmelstein. 1995. "Extreme Risk—The New Corporate Proposition for Physicians." *New England Journal of Medicine* 333 (25): 1706–08.

Zwanziger, J., and G. A. Melnick. 1996. "Can Managed Care Plans Control Health Care Costs?" *Health Affairs* 15 (2): 185–99.

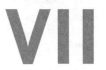
# MEASURING OUTCOMES
# OF THE DELIVERY SYSTEM

# 20

# ISSUES IN QUALITY OF CARE

## Introduction

The U.S. health services system is often discussed as having three major dimensions: access to care, costs of and expenditures for care, and quality of care. Analysts differ in their views about the extent of success in striking the appropriate balance among these dimensions in the U.S. system. The pattern, however, may be seen as a continuous shift in focus among the three dimensions. Instead of being equally balanced, each dimension has its day in the sun; action on the part of one dimension is followed by reaction from the other two.

The Great Society days of the mid-1960s, for example, focused resources on increasing access to care through a variety of governmental programs, such as Medicare and Medicaid. As access increased, so did expenditures for care, so that in the early 1970s, the focus was on ways to reduce expenditures and control costs through such programs as the Economic Stabilization Program (ESP), which froze hospital salaries and wages, and the professional standards review organizations (PSROs), which began to scrutinize and make recommendations about Medicare inpatient hospitalizations. A primary focus on costs soon generated concerns about quality of care (i.e., are the corners being cut to reduce expenditures having an adverse effect on quality of care?).

Although at least one early twentieth-century pioneer was concerned about quality-of-care issues, a focus on quality of care is relatively recent in the U.S. system, with major initiatives and research dating from the 1970s. Analyzing the quality of care is an inexact science at best, but the newness of the science and the current imprecision in many areas only underscore the need for greater—rather than diminished—focus on quality-of-care issues.

This chapter first examines working definitions of quality of care and related concepts and then reviews the development of the focus on quality of care in the U.S. system. Major quality-of-care initiatives, such as total quality management (TQM) and continuous quality improvement (CQI) in health services, are described, and various programs and instruments to measure quality of care are identified. An examination of initiatives to regulate or control the quality of health services provided in the United States follows. The chapter closes with comments on quality-of-care policy issues.

## Quality of Care: Working Definitions

One reason the study of quality of care is a new science is that operationalizing a definition of "quality" remains a challenge. The concept embodies a degree of relativity and a range of perspectives from which the concept can be assessed (e.g., the provider, the patient, the payer, and the delivery system).

### What Is Quality?

Several definitions of *quality* have been offered and implemented in recent years. Avedis Donabedian, a contemporary leader whose work helped shape the current understanding of quality, defined high quality of care as "that kind of care which is expected to maximize an inclusive measure of patient welfare, after one has taken account of the balance of expected gains and losses that attend the process of care in all its parts" (Donabedian 1980). In 1984, the American Medical Association (AMA) defined high quality of care as care "which consistently contributes to the improvement or maintenance of quality and/or duration of life" (AMA Council of Medical Service 1986). In 1990, the Institute of Medicine (IOM) declared that quality "consists of the degree to which health services for individuals and populations increase the likelihood of desired health outcomes and are consistent with current knowledge" (Lohr 1990). This chapter subscribes to the IOM definition of quality of care.

An important exclusion from this chapter's discussion of quality of care is the concept of quality of life. Quality of life is unquestionably related to quality of care but constitutes a separate study area. The works of Gill and Feinstein (1994) and others explore quality-of-life issues, instruments, and measurement.

### Quality Assessment, Quality Improvement, and Quality Assurance

The study of quality of care encompasses at least three foci: quality assessment, quality improvement, and quality assurance. The use of these terms and the understanding of their interrelationships vary; the definitions that follow indicate how the terms are used in this book.

*Quality assessment* measures the essential elements of quality of care (i.e., the technical proficiency with which care is rendered and the interpersonal interactions of the physician and the patient in the care process) and the outcomes of that care. Measurement is a key component of the assessment process. The concept of *quality improvement* has been borrowed from industry and is composed of the set of techniques for continually studying and improving the delivery of health services and products to meet the needs and expectations of the customers requiring those services and products. The term *customers* reflects the industrial origins of this concept, and the use of this term in place of the more familiar term *patients* or the slightly less inflammatory term *users* remains controversial with many in the health services system. *Quality assurance* embraces the full cycle of activities and systems for maintaining the quality of patient care.

## Development of a Quality Focus in the U.S. System

Although a systemwide focus on quality of care is a relatively recent phenomenon within the U.S. health services system, at least one turn-of-the-twentieth-century pioneer was consumed with the issue. Ernest Amory Codman, a physician born in Boston in 1869, became interested early in his medical career in what he termed the "end result idea." Codman described his end result idea as "merely the commonsense notion that every hospital should follow every patient it treats, long enough to determine whether or not the treatment has been successful, and then to inquire 'if not, why not?' with a view to preventing a similar failure in the future" (Donabedian 1989). Codman's vision included the establishment of an "efficiency" committee in every hospital to review unsatisfactory results and to recommend both educational and punitive actions in instances of failure. Although Codman preferred the term *efficiency* to the term *quality,* his end result assessment approximates current ideas about quality monitoring and assurance (Donabedian 1989).

It was not until the 1970s that a concerted focus on quality of care could be detected in the U.S. system. Early leaders in the field of quality of care include John Wennberg, Avedis Donabedian, and Robert Brook. Wennberg and his colleague Gittelsohn (1973), in a study of ten surgical procedures in 13 Vermont hospital areas, observed wide variation in practice patterns among community physicians and hospitals. They concluded that resource input, utilization of services, and expenditures varied widely among neighboring communities and that variations in utilization indicated considerable uncertainty about the effectiveness of different levels and specific kinds of aggregate health services.

In a subsequent study, Wennberg and Gittelsohn (1982) found in their analyses of surgical procedures among six states (Connecticut, Maine, Massachusetts, New Hampshire, Rhode Island, and Vermont) that the amount and the cost of hospital treatment in a community have more to do with the number of physicians there, their medical specialties, and the procedures they prefer than with the health of the residents.

Donabedian's work (1980) in defining quality of care and shaping the ways in which it is measured is seminal in the field. Donabedian first articulated the concepts of structural, process, and outcome measures of quality. Structural measures consider the characteristics of the system, such as the number, type, size, and location of hospitals; the number and qualifications of health services providers; and other system amenities.

Structural measures are the most tangible and most easily identified; they often reveal more about access to care than about the quality of care received. Process measures consider the components of the interaction between the physician or other type of health services provider and the patient, focusing on the technical quality of care and the interpersonal interactions among the participants. Outcome measures concentrate on the patient's subsequent health status following an intervention. Outcomes are the least tangible, and often most difficult, aspect of quality of care to measure.

Brook and various colleagues began work on quality of care in the early 1970s, focusing first on the issue of immunizations that were administered to Medicaid enrollees as part of New Mexico's Experimental Medical Care Review Organization (EMCRO), a predecessor to the PSRO, peer review organization (PRO), and quality improvement organization (QIO) programs (Brook and Williams 1976). They found that a small number of physicians were responsible for a sizable proportion of improperly administered injections. Through targeted physician education and sanctions in the form of physician payment denials, the inappropriate use of injections was substantially corrected. Work on the appropriateness of services and procedures under specific circumstances followed (Brook et al. 1986; Park et al. 1986; Kosecoff, Chassin, and Fink 1987; Kahn et al. 1988), as did work on practice guidelines and other aspects of quality of care (Brook 1989).

### Importance of Data in Assessing Quality of Care

Effectively evaluating quality of care is dependent to a large extent on the types of data available or collected for this purpose. The most readily available data about health services interventions are administrative or claims data, which include information about the encounter (i.e., time, place, duration); the charges for the encounter (i.e., what was billed to the payer, which may have limited relationship to the costs of the encounter); the diagnosis; the provider's name and specialty; and basic demographic data on the patient.

Not surprisingly, early quality-of-care evaluations thus focused on what could be most easily measured, including the patient's utilization and the provider's practice profile. The principal limitation of using administrative data for quality-of-care studies is that the studies provide little or no clinically meaningful data by which to evaluate the care rendered. To augment administrative data, researchers use the patient's chart (a useful but labor-intensive and expensive data source), surveys to providers and patients, audio- and videotapes of encounters, and other research methodologies.

Table 20.1 identifies data sources for obtaining quality-of-care information. Siu and his colleagues (1991) evaluated the medical record, a report from the patient, and administrative data to measure access to care, utilization, interpersonal aspects of care, technical aspects of care, outcomes of care, and other dimensions.

**TABLE 20.1** Data Sources for Obtaining Quality-of-Care Information

| Variable | Medical Record | Patient Report | Administrative Data |
|---|---|---|---|
| Access to care | Data on frequency of visits only | May be best source of information | Data on frequency of visits only |
| Use of services | Adequate, but data may need to be obtained from several types of records | Possible, but information may lack details on dates and frequency | If available, may be the best source for covered services |
| Symptoms | Limited data, generally on most important symptoms | May be best source of information | Not useful |
| Interpersonal aspects of care | Limited data | May be best source of information | Not useful |
| Technical aspects of care | Data may be available only on most important processes | Patients may be good reporters, but recall of past visits is untested | Not useful |
| Diagnostic tests | Good source, particularly for abnormal test results, but hospital records may miss data on outpatient tests | Patients recall testing in general terms but may not know details | If available, may be best source of data, although test results will not be available |
| Medications | Good source for important drugs; other drugs may not be recorded | Fair source of information on current medications | If available, may be good source for certain types of medications |
| Patient education | May not be documented | May be best source of information | Not useful |
| Outcomes of care | Useful for some outcomes, but data on many outcomes are frequently missing, and functional status is generally missing | Richest source of data on patient function | Useful for assessing mortality and other selected outcomes likely to be recorded on claims |

SOURCE: Siu et al. 1991. Copyrighted and published by Project HOPE/*Health Affairs*. The published article is archived and available online at www.healthaffairs.org.

Based in large part on available data, trends in quality assessment can be observed (Chassin 1996). The concern with quality of care in the 1960s took the form of increasing access through Medicare for specific populations, such as the elderly and disabled, and through Medicaid for low-income children and their caregivers. In the 1970s, physician peer review, mandated by the Medicare program, was in the quality spotlight. The 1980s ushered in a focus on quality assurance, whereas public report cards were one hallmark of the concern with quality of health services in the 1990s. With the turn of the twenty-first century, analysts are assessing whether health services, particularly medical technologies, are underused, misused, or overused and the quality implications for each scenario. The need for better ways to measure quality remains a challenge.

## Measuring Outcomes of Care

Much of the current emphasis on quality of care focuses on the measurement of outcomes, via the field of outcomes research, predicated on the belief that the ultimate patient outcome should receive the primary scrutiny in examining quality of care. Congress established the Agency for Healthcare Research and Quality (AHRQ), formerly the Agency for Health Care Policy and Research (AHCPR), in 1989 within the U.S. Department of Health and Human Services (HHS) to be the federal government's focal point for effectiveness and outcomes research (U.S. General Accounting Office [now known as the U.S. Government Accountability Office—USGAO] 1995). The AHRQ supports a range of outcomes research activities, including:

- a focus on evidence-based practice, with 60 evidence reports on a variety of clinical topics generated by 13 evidence-based health centers by mid-2002;
- a Center for Outcomes and Effectiveness Research, whose portfolio includes the support of patient outcome research teams (PORTs), a Pharmaceutical Outcomes Research Program, and the support of Minority Health Research Centers;
- a technology assessment function (discussed in Chapter 10);
- support of the U.S. Preventive Services Task Force; and
- support of the National Guidelines Clearinghouse.

The AHRQ's development of clinical practice guidelines was an exhaustive—and sometimes controversial—assessment of the state-of-the-art for a given procedure and the issuance of guidelines for the optimal performance of this procedure. The AHRQ first conducted an extensive critical review of the literature and then convened a panel of 15 to 20 clinicians and other experts, and at least one consumer representative, to evaluate their findings and to issue guidelines for the use of practicing physicians. Table 20.2 lists the 18 guidelines issued between 1992 and 1996. These

- Acute pain management: operative or medical procedures and trauma
- Urinary incontinence in adults: update
- Pressure ulcers in adults: prediction and prevention
- Cataracts in adults: management of functional impairment
- Depression in primary care: detection, diagnosis, and treatment
- Sickle-cell disease: screening, diagnosis, and management
- Evaluation and management of early HIV infection
- Benign prostatic hyperplasia: diagnosis and treatment
- Management of cancer pain
- Unstable angina: diagnosis and management
- Heart failure: evaluation and care of patients with left ventricular systolic dysfunction
- Otitis media with effusion in young children
- Quality determinants of mammography
- Acute low-back problems
- Treatment of pressure ulcers
- Poststroke rehabilitation
- Cardiac rehabilitation
- Smoking cessation

**TABLE 20.2**
AHRQ-
Sponsored
Clinical
Practice
Guidelines,
List of Topics

SOURCE: Agency for Healthcare Research and Quality 2001b.

guidelines are currently archived because time and new developments have outdated many of them, but they can be accessed on the AHRQ's web site (www.ahrq.gov/).

Any proscriptive process generates criticism, and the AHRQ's development of clinical practice guidelines was no exception. Among the criticisms directed at the AHRQ were the following (USGAO 1995):

- The guideline topics are too broad, increasing the difficulty in achieving specificity.
- The texts are too lengthy and require too much time to read and absorb.
- The guidelines generally do not include specific information about the cost-effectiveness of alternative approaches.

The AHRQ ceased the development and dissemination of its own guidelines in 1996 but maintains the National Guideline Clearinghouse, which can be accessed at the AHRQ's web site.

Although the AHRQ assumed the federal-level leadership in the development of clinical practice guidelines for a limited time, it was not the sole force in this endeavor. Two other federal organizations participate in the development and issuance of guidelines: the National Institutes of Health (NIH) and the Centers for Disease Control and Prevention (CDC).

In addition, an estimated 75 nongovernment organizations have issued thousands of guidelines (USGAO 1995), although many of these are institution-specific and likely to be somewhat limited in their general utility.

### Adverse Events as an Outcome Measure

The AHRQ and other organizations, including the Institute of Medicine, have become concerned about poor outcomes—adverse events—that may result in a patient's death. In 2000, the IOM issued what has become a seminal report on matters of patient safety, particularly in the inpatient hospital setting. It reported that more than one million preventable adverse events occur each year in the United States, of which 44,000 to 98,000 are fatal (Kohn, Corrigan, and Donaldson 2000). Much debate has ensued about the exact number of such events, but many would conclude that the matter is not trivial. Leape (2002) discusses voluntary and mandatory external reporting systems, identifies how such systems could be improved, and considers the potential for a national voluntary reporting system for adverse events.

### Other Quality-of-Care Activities

Efforts to advance the science of measuring quality of care have included other activities worthy of note, even if they cannot be fully explored in this chapter. Among these activities are practice profiling (Kassirer 1994), the use of criteria mapping (Greenfield et al. 1975), and achievable benchmarks (Shaneyfelt 2001).

## Major Quality-of-Care Initiatives

Although interest in quality of care has broadened in recent years from the providers and the regulators to the users of care, payers for care, and others, large-scale quality-of-care initiatives have been few.

### Total Quality Management and Continuous Quality Improvement

Within the last two decades, researchers interested in quality of care have adapted principles of industrial control—most notably those of W. Edwards Deming (1986)—to the health services field. Two related movements—total quality management (TQM) and continuous quality improvement (CQI)—illustrate the adaptation to the health services system of findings from other disciplines. TQM and CQI are discussed together (TQM/CQI) because they are interrelated and based on five principles (Shortell et al. 1995):

1. a focus on underlying organizational processes and systems as causes of failure rather than blaming individuals;
2. the use of structured problem-solving approaches based on statistical analysis;

3. the use of cross-functional employee teams;
4. employee empowerment to identify problems and opportunities for improved care and to take the necessary action; and
5. an explicit focus on both internal and external customers.

TQM/CQI differs from traditional quality assurance in a number of ways. One of the most important differences is the TQM/CQI focus on understanding and improving underlying work processes and systems, in contrast to the emphasis of traditional quality assurance on correcting after-the-fact errors of individuals (Shortell et al. 1995).

### Consumer Assessment of Healthcare Providers and Systems (CAHPS®)

In the late 1990s, the AHRQ, in collaboration with the Centers for Medicare and Medicaid Services (CMS), funded the Consumer Assessment of Health-care Providers and Systems (CAHPS®) project to help consumers identify the best health care plans and services for their needs. A CAHPS hospital survey was developed and implemented to periodically measure hospital care from the patient's perspective. Results are intended to help hospitals improve their performance in areas identified as consumer concerns.

### Leapfrog Group

The Leapfrog Group was established by a number of large employers and public purchasers in 2000 to attempt to consolidate the purchaser voice and stimulate consumers and clinicians to improve health care quality (Galvin et al. 2005). The impetus was to help hospitals make leaps in quality and safety by fostering participation in computerized physician order entry (CPOE). Diffusion of some Leapfrog initiatives has been slower than anticipated, and their effects have been difficult to measure. Nonetheless, analysts see the Leapfrog Group as a market catalyst that is shaping purchasers' awareness of value purchasing when it comes to health benefits (Galvin et al. 2005).

### Pay for Performance (P4P)

Pay for performance (P4P) is yet another initiative to stimulate improvements in quality of care. P4P is directed not only to inpatient care but also to outpatient care. Its intent is to link the reimbursement for health benefit programs to improved outcomes, based on established goals for improvement (see Chapter 7).

## Measuring Quality of Care

Quality of care is measured many ways. In a series of articles on quality of care, Brook, McGlynn, and Cleary (1996) identify five major methods of quality assessment that use either or both process and outcome data. The first three methods are implicit (i.e., no prior agreements about what constitutes good or poor quality exist), and each method centers around a key question:

1. Was the process of care adequate?
2. Could better care have improved the outcome?
3. Considering both the process and outcome of care, was the overall quality of care acceptable?

The fourth method uses explicit process criteria to evaluate the provision of care so that, for specific conditions, an expert evaluates the care that was provided against the care that should have been provided. The result is expressed as a proportion of the criteria that were met. The fifth method uses explicit a priori criteria to determine whether the observed results of care are consistent with the outcome predicted by a model that has been validated on the basis of clinical judgment and scientific evidence.

A range of instruments has been designed and validated to measure various aspects of quality of care. This overview cannot begin to do justice to the many instruments but will briefly describe patient satisfaction instruments, the Health Plan Employer Data and Information Set, and other report cards to illustrate some currently available instruments.

## Patient Satisfaction

One way to measure quality of care is to ask patients about their perceptions of the care they received. The most common way to obtain this measure is to use a patient satisfaction survey instrument, administered in person, over the phone, through the mail, or by computer. Patient satisfaction surveys can provide information on underuse, interpersonal aspects of care, and expectations and preferences (Lohr 1990). Among others, Davies and Ware (1988) have pioneered the development of valid and reliable patient-assessment instruments.

Patient satisfaction is being assessed by Medicare beneficiaries through the CAHPS project, initiated in 1995 by the AHRQ. Used by some Medicaid programs and other public and private employers as well, the CAHPS survey, administered by mail or telephone, asks plan subscribers about their views on a number of access to services and provider communication issues. The 2000 survey found that (AHRQ 2001a):

- overall, managed care enrollees rate their health care highly and report positive experiences with their care;
- Medicaid, Medicare, and commercial enrollees rate their care differently; and
- average ratings and reports by enrollees vary across managed care plans.

## Health Plan Employer Data and Information Set (HEDIS)®

As employers and other payers for care became aware of the growing costs of providing employee health benefits, they began to seek more information about the differences among health plans, particularly prepaid managed care plans such as HMOs, available to their employees.

Comparing competing plans may be difficult because of the variations in benefit coverage, cost sharing, prior authorization, and other requirements. To alleviate the comparison difficulties, the National Committee for Quality Assurance (NCQA) developed the Health Plan Employer Data and Information Set (HEDIS®), issuing the first version (version 1.0) in 1991. Special versions have been developed for Medicaid and Medicare. Some refer to HEDIS as a type of report card; other report cards are discussed in the section that follows.

HEDIS relies principally on administrative data to measure six dimensions of prepaid managed care plans: quality management, physicians' credentials, members' rights and responsibilities, preventive health services, utilization management, and medical records. HEDIS incorporates more than 60 performance indicators to assist in the measurement of quality of care, access to and satisfaction with care, use of services, plan finances, and plan management. Of the nine indicators of quality of care, one (low birth weight) focuses on an outcome, and a second (hospitalization rates for patients with asthma) focuses on a proxy for an outcome (Iglehart 1996). The remainder focus on access to preventive services. Table 20.3 summarizes the 2002 HEDIS measures and indicates whether they apply to Medicaid, commercial, or Medicare product lines.

## Other Report Cards

Borrowing from the evaluation of a student's performance in school, some health services associations, professional organizations, and citizen interest groups have begun issuing report cards that grade the performances of health facilities, health plans, and health systems. The CMS was one of the first to use the report card concept; from 1987 to 1992, the CMS issued annual reports on the observed and expected mortality rates in each hospital that performed coronary artery bypass graft (CABG) surgery (USGAO 1995). The CMS was criticized for issuing these reports because the media generally did not understand the case-mix of patients in a hospital and thus often oversimplified the data by generating a "best-to-worst" hospital list based on the reported rates alone.

In 1991, California mandated the development of report cards for all hospitals licensed in the state; Ohio and Pennsylvania have similar laws that mandate public dissemination of quality performance data on health institutions (Gudin 1997). Other states have initiated and ultimately repealed

**TABLE 20.3**
HEDIS
2002 Summary
Table of
Measures,
Product Lines,
and Changes

| HEDIS 2002 Measures | Applicable to | | |
|---|---|---|---|
| | Medicaid | Commercial | Medicare |
| Childhood immunization status | X | X | |
| Adolescent immunization status | X | X | |
| Breast cancer screening | X | X | X |
| Cervical cancer screening | X | X | |
| Chlamydia screening in women | X | X | |
| Controlling high blood pressure | X | X | X |
| Beta-blocker treatment after a heart attack | X | X | X |
| Cholesterol management after acute cardiovascular events | X | X | X |
| Comprehensive diabetes care | X | X | X |
| Use of appropriate medications for people with asthma | X | X | |
| Follow-up after hospitalization for mental illness | X | X | X |
| Antidepressant medication management | X | X | X |
| Advising smokers to quit | X | X | X |
| Flu shots for adults ages 50–64 | | X | |
| Flu shots for older adults | | | X |
| Pneumonia vaccination status for older adults | | | X |
| Medicare health outcomes survey | | | X |
| Adults' access to preventive/ ambulatory health services | X | X | X |
| Children's access to primary care practitioners | X | X | |
| Prenatal and postpartum care | X | X | |
| Annual dental visit | X | | |
| Availability of language interpretation services | X | X | X |
| HEDIS/CAHPS 2.0H adult survey | X | X | |
| HEDIS/CAHPS 2.5H child survey | X | X | X |
| Practitioner turnover | X | X | X |
| Years in business/total membership | X | X | X |
| Frequency of ongoing prenatal care | X | | |
| Well-child visits in the first 15 months of life | X | X | |
| Well-child visits in the third, fourth, fifth, and sixth years of life | X | X | |
| Adolescent well-care visit | X | X | |

(*continued*)

TABLE 20.3
Continued

| HEDIS 2002 Measures | Applicable to | | |
|---|---|---|---|
| | Medicaid | Commercial | Medicare |
| Frequency of selected procedures | X | X | X |
| Inpatient utilization—general hospital/acute care | X | X | X |
| Ambulatory care | X | X | X |
| Inpatient utilization—nonacute care | X | X | X |
| Discharge and average length of stay —maternity care | X | X | |
| Cesarean section | X | X | |
| Vaginal birth after cesarean (VBAC) rate | X | X | |
| Births and average length of stay, newborns | X | X | |
| Mental health utilization— inpatient discharges and average length of stay | X | X | X |
| Mental health utilization—percentage of members receiving services | X | X | X |
| Chemical dependency utilization— inpatient discharges and average length of stay | X | X | X |
| Chemical dependency utilization— percentage of members receiving services | X | X | X |
| Outpatient drug utilization | X | X | X |
| Management of menopause | | X | |
| Board certification/residency completion | X | X | X |
| Practitioner compensation | X | X | X |
| Arrangements with public health, educational, and social service organizations | X | X | X |
| Total enrollment by percentage | X | X | X |
| Enrollment by product line (member years/member months) | X | X | X |
| Unduplicated count of Medicaid members | X | | |
| Diversity of Medicaid membership | X | | |
| Weeks of pregnancy at time of enrollment in the MCO | X | | |

SOURCE: National Committee on Quality Assurance 2001.

NOTES: CAHPS = Consumer Assessment of Healthcare Providers and Systems; HEDIS = Health Plan Employer Data and Information Set; MCO = managed care organization.

similar initiatives; Colorado established its Health Data Commission in the early 1980s but repealed it in 1996.

Institutional report cards have had a mixed reception. What is not clear is whether the availability of this information influences individuals any more than other information sources. Hospital report cards are reported to be less influential than the advice of family members or recommendations from personal physicians. The use of hospital report cards raises concerns that hospitals may transfer high-risk patients to maintain satisfactory ratings or that providers may become increasingly wary of high-risk cases because of their implications for boosting a facility's mortality rates (Gudin 1997).

The American Public Health Association (APHA) issued its first report card on the public health of the nation in 1992. The APHA assessed public health on a state-by-state basis, measuring:

- medical care access;
- the health of the environment;
- the health of neighborhoods;
- the healthy behaviors of the state's population; and
- the extent of community health services, measured by governmental per capita spending for health, for sewage and sanitation services, and for public health workers.

The APHA's report card was issued as a benchmark for health measures and to raise consciousness about the need to refocus the U.S. system from its treatment orientation to a preventive services orientation (APHA 1992).

Infection-control report cards are one of the most recent advents in this field (Weinstein, Siegel, and Benjamin 2005). Although report cards for nosocomial infections are still in the development and testing phases, current report cards focus on three kinds of common infections associated with high morbidity and mortality that are likely to be controllable: those associated with central venous catheters, surgical-site infections, and ventilator-associated pneumonia. An initial focus is on linking process with outcome measures to gauge quality of care for these three types of infections.

## Monitoring and Regulating Quality of Care

### Monitoring Quality of Care

Quality of care can be monitored at many levels, from the individual provider to a national-level organization. Two national organizations that monitor quality of care are the Joint Commission on Accreditation of Healthcare Organizations (JCAHO) and the National Committee for Quality Assurance (NCQA).

The JCAHO was established in 1951 as an arm of the American Hospital Association (AHA), initially to set standards for the operation and accreditation of hospitals, and more recently to provide these same services to nursing homes and other health services organizations. Participation in the JCAHO is voluntary, but states may link their facility licensure requirements to JCAHO participation, or payers may link their reimbursement to facilities that have attained JCAHO accreditation.

The JCAHO has established performance standards and quality indicators that facilities must meet; regular site visits by JCAHO teams assess facility compliance with these standards.

The National Committee for Quality Assurance (NCQA) was established in 1979 by the American Managed Care and Review Association and the Group Health Association of America and became an independent entity in 1990 (Iglehart 1996). The NCQA focuses on the quality of care provided in managed care plans, particularly in prepaid health plans such as HMOs, and is the leading accreditor of managed care plans. The NCQA is concentrating on including more preferred provider organizations (PPOs) and other forms of managed care under its quality assurance umbrella. The HEDIS instrument noted earlier was developed and implemented by the NCQA.

## Regulating Quality of Care

In a free-market system, failures in the market are often dealt with through regulation. The U.S. system has an uneven, and not entirely successful, history of trying to regulate access to care, costs of and expenditures for care, and quality of care. Regulating quality of care is a relatively recent endeavor, given the newness of the focus on quality. Efforts to regulate quality may be based on concerns about growing expenditures for care. Distinguishing between concerns about costs and quality is not always the straightforward task it may appear to be; this issue is discussed further later in the chapter as a policy consideration about quality of care.

In 1972, Congress mandated one of the initial efforts to regulate quality of care through an amendment to the Medicare title of the Social Security Act that established the professional standards review organizations (PSROs). The increasing hospitalization rates of Medicare beneficiaries, the growing number of surgical procedures done on them, their longer lengths of stay, and an awareness of the variations in physician practice patterns stimulated the authorization of PSROs, which were charged with conducting peer reviews of Medicare inpatient hospitalizations. PSROs could be established for medical marketplaces; that is, they did not have to conform to state boundaries, but all areas of a state had to be covered by a PSRO.

The PSRO structure proved to be weak and unsatisfactory. PSROs could cover multiple states or parts of multiple states; therefore, they often had to accommodate to multiple state health professional and facility licensure requirements in their reviews. Decisions about the quality, necessity, and cost-effectiveness of care were based on local standards of practice, which varied widely. PSROs focused primarily on the quality of care that Medicare inpatients received, but some congressional leaders believed that PSROs needed to expand their focus to other populations and contract with private businesses for utilization review and other quality assessment functions.

With the 1982 Tax Equitability and Fiscal Responsibility Act (TEFRA), Congress replaced the PSROs with peer review organizations (PROs). PROs had to conform to state boundaries, although a PRO could include several states. Like their predecessors, PROs were charged with reviewing Medicare inpatient hospitalizations to determine their medical necessity and appropriateness, cost-effectiveness, and whether care of sufficient quality was rendered. PROs were also required to take regional and national practice norms into account in their decisions.

PROs engaged in preadmission review, review of the outlier cases of diagnosis-related groups (DRGs), retrospective review, and validation of the use of the appropriate DRGs. The review role was expanded to ambulatory surgical centers (ASCs), home health agencies, and skilled nursing facilities (SNFs). PROs also were encouraged to contract with other payers, such as Medicaid, to provide utilization review services for them.

PROs have not remained untouched by controversy. An Institute of Medicine (IOM) report in 1990 described PROs as too adversarial and punitive and recommended structural changes (Lohr 1990), which the Health Care Financing Administration (HCFA) rejected. Within two years, however, the HCFA, now known as the Centers for Medicare and Medicaid Services (CMS), began to reshape the PROs along the lines envisioned by the IOM, intending "to move from dealing with individual clinical errors to helping providers improve the maintenance of care" (Sprague 2002). The Health Care Quality Improvement Program (HCQIP) was created, and PROs eventually became known as quality improvement organizations (QIOs).

QIOs, according to their legislative authority under Title XVIII of the Social Security Act, are to:

- improve the quality of care for beneficiaries by ensuring that beneficiary care meets professionally recognized standards of health care;
- protect the integrity of the trust fund by ensuring that Medicare only pays for services and items that are reasonable and medically necessary and that are provided in the most appropriate (for example, economical) setting; and
- protect beneficiaries by expeditiously addressing individual cases, such as beneficiary complaints, provider-issued notices of noncoverage, Emergency Medical Treatment and Active Labor Act (EMTALA) violations related to patient "dumping," and other statutory responsibilities (Sprague 2002).

QIOs have concentrated their quality improvement activities in six areas: acute myocardial infarction, breast cancer, diabetes, heart failure, pneumonia, and stroke. In the 2002 funding cycle, QIOs were expected to continue to work on national and local quality improvement projects, collaborate with Medicare Advantage organizations on quality improvement projects, continue to address payment error reduction, and perform other mandatory duties. The challenge to QIOs is to balance their collaborative role—working on quality improvement programs with hospitals and other providers—with their role of being a regulatory body that enforces certain standards.

## Quality-of-Care Policy Issues

Three of the many policy issues that surround the study of quality of care are briefly discussed here:

- the carrot or the stick approach in quality assessment,
- provider attitudes toward quality assessment, and
- frequent blurring of the lines between issues of cost and quality.

### The Carrot or the Stick Approach in Quality Assessment

An ongoing debate in the assessment of quality of care is whether errors in practice are best remedied through education or through sanction. Because the practice of medicine remains as much an art as a science, standards may be imprecise or highly variable, which suggests that education is the better approach.

One reason for the recent interest in quality improvement is an effort to move the focus on quality away from blaming the individual to an understanding of the processes and systems that cause failure. Explicit and abusive practices may occur, however; in such instances, many would favor the use of sanctions to deter poor-quality practice.

### Provider Attitudes Toward Quality Assessment

Health services providers agree about the importance of providing the best quality of care possible. Less agreement exists about how high-quality care can be rendered and measured, with a fair amount of skepticism from the medical community that current emphases on quality are really directed at improving patients' health. Chassin (1996) notes several reasons for this skepticism:

- The emphasis of many quality assurance efforts seems to be more on document and credential reviews than on improved patient outcomes.
- There is a dearth of evidence that quality assurance programs actually do anything to improve patient outcomes.
- Many initiatives labeled as quality concerns are really aimed at cost containment or at marketing.

Skepticism may diminish as new tools and measures (e.g., practice guidelines, the calculation of risk-adjusted outcomes, or the ability to understand how errors creep into practice) are more widely disseminated and applied.

### Distinguishing Between Concerns about Quality and Health Services Costs

Concerns about health services costs and quality often overlap and may sometimes appear inextricably tangled. This blurring of boundaries, when cost containment initiatives are masqueraded as concerns about quality, contributes to provider cynicism. Efforts to contain or reduce health services costs frequently give rise to concerns that quality may be compromised.

Table 20.4 provides examples of concerns about quality of care that have been stimulated by measures to reduce health services expen-

**TABLE 20.4**
Concerns about Quality of Care Related to Cost-Containment Initiatives

| Cost-Containment Initiative | Quality-of-Care Concerns |
|---|---|
| Reduction of insurance coverage for patients (denial of coverage, reduction in benefits, increased cost sharing) | Coverage will be eliminated for needed services, or patients will jeopardize health by deferring care because of increased cost-sharing requirements. |
| Organization of providers into competing managed care organizations | Patients will lose access to their preferred provider; patients will lose access to needed specialty care. |
| Development of specialized forms of coverage for particular high-cost illnesses | Patients' basic insurance coverage will exclude this special care; patients in need of this care may be unable to afford the premiums or the copays. |
| Reduction in payments to providers | Providers will reduce or eliminate their provision of affected services or procedures to patients who still require them. |
| Development of provider incentives for financial risk-sharing | Providers will underserve patients in order to remain within their profit margin. |
| Increase in the authority of primary care physicians over the provision of specialty care | Primary care gatekeepers will inhibit or deny needed access to specialty care. |
| Implementation of utilization review (UR) procedures | Potential sanctions for overutilization may deter the ordering of needed services or procedures. |
| Development of provider profiles | Providers may be inhibited in ordering needed services or procedures for a patient if such is outside a prescribed norm. |

NOTE: The categories of cost containment initiatives were adapted from data published in Blumenthal 1996.

ditures. Although more quality issues appear to stem from overuse rather than underuse of services (Berwick 1996), concerns about underservice, particularly as related to managed care's more predominant role in the delivery system, where fears of underservice remain, continue to abound. These concerns underscore the challenge in balancing access to, costs of and expenditures for, and quality of care. One researcher (McNeil 2001) raises concerns about the potential for too quickly dismissing underuse as an issue. McNeil points out that all three types of use are related to uncertainty and rising health services costs. Underuse in particular stems from uncertainty as well as from financial arrangements and incentives that have been structured around utilization and are often based on old and thus inaccurate data. She recommends a series of steps to generate and disseminate more accurate and timely data to help with utilization decisions.

## Summary

Expanding access to health services and controlling expenditures have often overshadowed a focus on the quality of services provided. As abilities to better define and measure quality have increased, so has interest in knowing more about quality of care, particularly the outcomes of an intervention. An increased focus on quality ideally leads to more optimal resource allocation as less effective interventions are replaced by those of established efficacy.

## Key Words

administrative data

adverse events

Agency for Health Care Policy and
    Research (AHCPR)

Agency for Healthcare Research and
    Quality (AHRQ)

ambulatory surgical centers (ASC)

American Medical Association
    (AMA)

American Public Health Association
    (APHA)

appropriateness of care

Brook, Robert H.

case-mix

Centers for Disease Control and
    Prevention (CDC)

claims data

clinical practice guidelines

Codman, Ernest A.

computerized physician order entry
    (CPOE)

Consumer Assessment of Healthcare
    Providers and Systems (CAHPS)

continuous quality improvement
    (CQI)

criteria mapping

Deming, W. Edwards

Donabedian, Avedis

Economic Stabilization Program (ESP)

Emergency Medical Treatment and
    Active Labor Act (EMTALA)

end result idea

| | |
|---|---|
| *Experimental Medical Care Review Organization (EMCRO)* | *practice profiling* |
| | *practice variation* |
| *Health Care Financing Administration (HCFA)* | *preadmission review* |
| | *preferred provider organization (PPO)* |
| *health maintenance organization (HMO)* | *process measures* |
| | *professional standards review organization (PSRO)* |
| *Health Plan Employer Data and Information Set (HEDIS)* | *quality* |
| *home health agency* | *quality assessment* |
| *Institute of Medicine (IOM)* | *quality assurance* |
| *Joint Commission on Accreditation of Healthcare Organizations (JCAHO)* | *quality improvement* |
| | *quality improvement organization (QIO)* |
| *Medicare* | *quality of life* |
| *Medicare+Choice* | *report cards* |
| *National Committee for Quality Assurance (NCQA)* | *retrospective review* |
| | *skilled nursing facilities (SNFs)* |
| *National Institutes of Health (NIH)* | *structural measures* |
| *outcome measurement* | *Tax Equity and Fiscal Responsibility Act (TEFRA) of 1982* |
| *outcomes research* | |
| *outlier review* | *total quality management (TQM)* |
| *patient outcome research teams (PORTs)* | *U.S. Preventive Services Task Force* |
| | *utilization review* |
| *patient satisfaction* | *Wennberg, John* |
| *Peer Review Organization (PRO)* | |

## References

Agency for Healthcare Research and Quality. 2001a. *Annual Report of the National CPHPS® Benchmarking Database 2000.* Rockville, MD: AHRQ.
————. 2001b. "Centers and Topics." [Online information; retrieved 7/15/02.] www.ahrq.gov/clinic/epc/.

American Medical Association Council of Medical Service. 1986. "Quality of Care." *Journal of the American Medical Association* 256: 1032–34.

American Public Health Association. 1992. *America's Public Health Report Card.* Washington, DC: APHA.

Berwick, D. M. 1996. "Part 5: Payment by Capitation and the Quality of Care." *New England Journal of Medicine* 335 (16): 1227–31.

Blumenthal D. 1996. "The Origins of the Quality-of-Care Debate." *New England Journal of Medicine* 335 (15): 1146–49.

Brook, R. H. 1989. "Practice Guidelines and Practicing Medicine: Are They Compatible?" *Journal of the American Medical Association* 262 (21): 3027–30.

Brook, R. H., M. R. Chassin, A. Fink, D. H. Solomon, J. Kosecoff, and R. E. Park. 1986. "A Method for the Detailed Assessment of the Appropriateness of Medical Technology." *International Journal of Technology Assessment* 2 (1): 53–63.

Brook, R. H., E. A. McGlynn, and P. D. Cleary. 1996. "Part 2: Measuring Quality of Care." *New England Journal of Medicine* 335 (13): 966–70.

Brook, R. H., and K. N. Williams. 1976. "Effect of Medical Care on the Use of Injections: A Study of the New Mexico Experimental Medical Care Review Organization." *Annals of Internal Medicine* 85 (4): 509–15.

Chassin, M. R. 1996. "Part 3: Improving the Quality of Care." *New England Journal of Medicine* 335 (14): 1060–63.

Davies, A. R., and J. E. Ware. 1988. "Involving Consumers in Quality of Care Assessment." *Health Affairs* 7 (1): 33–48.

Deming, W. E. 1986. *Out of Crisis.* Cambridge, MA: Massachusetts Institute of Technology.

Donabedian, A. 1989. "The End Results of Health Care: Ernest Codman's Contribution to Quality Assessment and Beyond." *The Milbank Quarterly* 67 (2): 322–61.

———. 1980. *Explorations in Quality Assessment and Monitoring. Vol. I. The Definition of Quality and Approaches to Its Assessment.* Chicago: Health Administration Press.

Galvin, R. S., S. Delbanco, A. Milstein, and G. Belden. 2005. "Has the Leapfrog Group Had an Impact on the Health Care Market?" *Health Affairs* 24 (1): 228–33.

Gill, T. M., and A. R. Feinstein. 1994. "A Critical Appraisal of Quality-of-Life Measurements." *Journal of the American Medical Association* 272 (8): 619–26.

Greenfield, S., C. E. Lewis, S. H. Kaplan, and M. B. Davidson. 1975. "Peer Review by Criteria Mapping: Criteria for Diabetes Mellitus." *Annals of Internal Medicine* 83 (6): 761–70.

Gudin, M. 1997. "Hospital Report Cards: Pass, Fail, or Incomplete?" *State Health Notes* 18 (254): 1, 6.

Iglehart, J. K. 1996. "The National Committee for Quality Assurance." *New England Journal of Medicine* 335 (13): 995–99.

Kahn, K. L., J. Kosecoff, M. R. Chassin, M. F. Flynn, A. Fink, N. Pattaphongse, D. H. Solomon, and R. H. Brook. 1988. "Measuring the Clinical Appropriateness of the Use of a Procedure: Can We Do It?" *Medical Care* 26 (4): 415–22.

Kassirer, J. P. 1994. "The Use and Abuse of Practice Profiles." *New England Journal of Medicine* 330 (9): 634–35.

Kohn, L. T., J. M. Corrigan, and M. S. Donaldson. 2000. *To Err Is Human: Building a Safer Health System.* Washington, DC: National Academy Press.

Kosecoff, J., M. R. Chassin, and A. Fink. 1987. "Obtaining Clinical Data on the Appropriateness of Care in Community Practice." *Journal of the American Medical Association* 258 (18): 2538–42.

Leape, L. L. 2002. "Reporting of Adverse Events." *New England Journal of Medicine* 347 (20): 1633–38.

Lohr, K. N. 1990. *Medicare: A Strategy for Quality Assurance.* Washington, DC: National Academy Press.

McNeil, B. J. 2001. "Hidden Barriers to Improvement in the Quality of Care." *New England Journal of Medicine* 345 (22): 1613–20.

National Committee on Quality Assurance. 2001. "The State of Managed Care Quality." [Online information; retrieved 7/15/02.] www.ncqa.org/somc2001/.

Park, R. E., A. Fink, R. H. Brook, M. R. Chassin, K. L. Kahn, N. J. Merrick, J. Kosecoff, and D. H. Solomon. 1986. "Physician Ratings of Appropriate Indications for Six Medical and Surgical Procedures." *American Journal of Public Health* 76 (7): 766–72.

Shaneyfelt, T. M. 2001. "Building Bridges to Quality." *Journal of the American Medical Association* 286 (20): 2600–01.

Shortell, S. M., J. L. O'Brien, J. M. Carman, R. W. Foster, E. F. Hughes, H. Boerstler, and E. J. O'Connor. 1995. "Assessing the Impact of Continuous Quality Improvement/Total Quality Management: Concept vs. Implementation." *Health Services Research* 30 (2): 377–401.

Siu, A. L., E. A. McGlynn, H. Morgenstern, and R. H. Brook. 1991. "A Fair Approach to Comparing Quality of Care." *Health Affairs* 10 (2): 62–75.

Sprague, L. 2002. "Contracting for Quality: Medicare's Quality Improvement Organizations." National Health Policy Forum Issue Brief No. 774. Washington, DC: The George Washington University.

U.S. Government Accountability Office (formerly the U.S. General Accounting Office). 1995. *Health Care: Employers and Individual Consumers Want Additional Information on Quality.* GAO/HEHS-95-201. Washington, DC: USGAO.

Weinstein, R. A., J. D. Siegel, and P. J. Benjamin. 2005. "Infection-Control Report Cards—Securing Patient Safety." *New England Journal of Medicine* 353 (3): 225–27.

Wennberg, J., and A. Gittelsohn. 1982. "Variations in Medical Care among Small Areas." *Scientific American* 246 (4): 120–34.

———. 1973. "Small Area Variations in Health Care Delivery." *Science* 192 (4117): 1102–08.

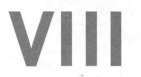
# FUTURE DIRECTIONS
# OF THE DELIVERY SYSTEM

# CONTINUING CHANGE IN THE U.S. HEALTH SERVICES DELIVERY SYSTEM

## Introduction

Despite the failure of proposed governmental reforms in the early 1990s, the health services system continues to change—often in ways and to degrees that are essentially unparalleled in its history. This chapter attempts to capture these changes and to illustrate the dynamic nature of the system and its interdependent components. Four aspects of this change are considered:

1. What is changing among the system components in access to, costs and financing of, and quality of services?
2. Why are these changes occurring?
3. What are the effects of changes on patients, providers, payers, and insurers?
4. In what parts of the system are changes likely to continue?

## What Is Changing in the U.S. Health Services Delivery System?

The extent of change occurring in the U.S. health services delivery system can readily be seen by examining changes in the major dimensions of access to, costs and financing of, and quality of services. Key changes to each are briefly reviewed in the sections that follow.

### Financing Changes

Of the five major components of the Roemer model of a health services system—management, administration, resources, economic support, and the delivery system—change is most evident in the economic support component, particularly in how services are financed. Financing changes directly affect the ways in which health services are delivered.

Public sources of health insurance such as Medicare continue their gradual climb as the dominant financing source for health services. Given the aging of the population and longer life spans, this trend is likely to continue. Beginning in 2016, the outlays (expenditures) for Medicare Part A are expected to exceed the revenues coming in to support this program. Although a strong economy through the 1990s forestalled the projected bankruptcy of the Part A trust fund until 2029 (the currently projected date), one cannot look only at the Hospital Insurance (Part A) side of Medicare (Wilensky 2001; U.S. General Accounting Office [now known as the U.S. Government Accountability Office—USGAO] 2001). Part B, Supplemental Medical Insurance, currently constitutes 40 percent of Medicare's expenditures. Only one-quarter of the financing of Part B comes from beneficiary premiums; the remaining 75 percent comes from federal general funds.

The hoped-for tourniquet to Medicare's increasing expenditures—Medicare+Choice—has increased rather than stemmed the flow because of flaws in its payment structure (as well as flaws in the Medicare fee-for-service payment structure). Whether the Medicare Advantage program, which replaced the Medicare+Choice program in 2003, will be able to contain expenditures, is not yet known. Adding a prescription drug benefit for Medicare beneficiaries, as the Medicare Prescription Drug Improvement and Modernization Act (MMA) of 2003 did, will considerably boost Medicare's expenditures. The debate is over how fast and how high these expenditures will grow.

Expenditure increases in any of the other public payment sources—including Medicaid, Veterans Affairs, TRICARE, and Indian Health Service—will likely add to the dominance of the public sector as the largest source of financing of health services.

Other changes in financing include increased out-of-pocket payments by consumers as:

- payers shift more of their costs for providing health insurance to their employees by raising deductibles and increasing copayments;
- individuals pay more for services not covered by their plans; and
- those without insurance must cover the full cost of services if they have any means to do so.

Changes in the way services are reimbursed comprise another aspect of the financing of health services. The 1990s ushered in a fast-paced movement away from fee-for-service financing and toward a range of managed care payment mechanisms, including capitation and discounted fee-for-service.

What has been increasingly referred to as the "backlash against managed care" (Blendon et al. 1998)—in which consumers, providers, employers, and others have expressed frustrations with various facets of managed care—indicates a move away from capitation as a payment mechanism for the receipt of a predetermined set of services to a specific population. The likelihood of a wholesale return to the fee-for-service payment system seems slim, at best; the cost-increasing incentives inherent in such a system argue against it.

New approaches, such as defined contribution and premium support, are under consideration. Defined contribution means that a payer would provide a standard dollar amount of health benefits to all subscribers; individuals who wanted more benefits than could be purchased with the defined contribution would be responsible for paying for them out-of-pocket. This approach could conceivably alter the taxable status of employer-sponsored benefits. Similarly, a premium support, widely discussed as an alternative by the late-1990s National Bipartisan Commission on the Future of Medicare, would provide a standard premium amount for beneficiaries with which to purchase inpatient and outpatient benefits. Beneficiaries who wanted greater benefits would be responsible for their cost. A more recent move is the consumer-directed health plan, in which consumers seek a greater role in determining what benefits are provided, what providers are included, and other matters of plan design. As consumer choice widens, however, the ability to control costs and expenditures erodes.

Benefit packages are also likely to change. The three-tiered approach to prescription drug coverage now serves as a model for other benefits. In the three-tiered approach, health plans cover a generic drug (tier one), increase the copayment or co-insurance for a brand-name drug (tier two), and refuse to pay any part of the cost of drugs not listed on their specific formulary (tier three). Benefit packages have begun to emulate this approach.

Despite the turmoil in the financing picture, one can safely conclude that:

- consumers are likely to be paying more for their care;
- reductions in covered benefits and/or increased copayments and co-insurance in benefit packages are likely;
- public and private payers will be pressing for ways to curb their increasing outlays for health benefits, whether through a defined contribution, premium support, or the development of new insurance products, such as health savings accounts (HSAs) or other approaches; and
- payment mechanisms are likely to lie between the extremes of fee-for-service and capitation.

## Delivery System Changes

The move toward integrated systems of care delivery heralded by the managed care movement throughout the 1990s has halted. Alliances and networks—in some cases, hurriedly constructed to respond to market changes—are being dismantled. The frenzy in buying up medical practices to ensure access to a patient population as well as the fervor of the medical practice management movement have abated. In some instances, the hoped-for profit in these endeavors simply could not be realized; administrative systems could not be further tightened without jeopardizing the practice's operations, which then resulted in negative changes in patient flows.

The streamlining and belt-tightening in some venues of the health services system resulted in reduced capacity in some areas. Hospitals closed beds—and even units and wings—as they merged with other hospitals or became just one of many other players in a larger system. These closures resulted in workforce reductions, and workers such as nurses sought other employment opportunities, sometimes outside the health services system. The surplus of some health professions, including physician specialists, brought about at least temporary changes in the educational system, with some medical schools altering their curricula to focus on the training of generalist physicians. Inability to effectively forecast and train appropriate numbers of all types of providers, however, often results in today's surplus becoming tomorrow's shortage.

Analysts are considering the issue of capacity and indicating that the pendulum may need to swing back to a restoration or increase of capacity in some instances. The Center for the Study of Health System Change points out the serious undercapacity of hospital emergency departments (Ginsburg 2001), where emergency transport systems may have to contact multiple hospitals before finding one that can receive emergency cases. The misuse of hospital emergency departments is certainly a contributing factor, motivating a number of hospitals to install a nurse or other health professional to rigorously screen those seeking emergency department care. Individuals with nonemergency conditions are referred to other sources of care to protect the use of increasingly limited resources.

Two other changes across parts of the delivery system merit comment. Some major managed care organizations have recently curtailed the use of prior authorizations for some services, finding that prior authorizations are not cost-effective. Others have reevaluated their gatekeeping functions and determined that they did not substantially change the use of specialty services (Ferris et al. 2001), whereas in some models of managed care, gatekeeping still serves an important purpose (Lawrence 2001). Although these changes in prior authorizations and gatekeeping may have alleviated some of the stresses that consumers and providers were experiencing with managed care, they were not, in themselves, sufficient to counterbalance the backlash against managed care.

### Changes in Access

The full effects of legislation intended to increase access—the Health Insurance Portability and Accountability Act (HIPAA) of 1996, the Mental Health Parity Act (MHPA) of 1996, and the State Children's Health Insurance Program (SCHIP) of 1997—are not yet completely known. HIPAA's provisions include ways to encourage the offering of health insurance in small businesses, but the strength of the economy as much as any factor influences small business insurance offerings. Despite the MHPA's stipulations that coverage for mental health treatment should be equivalent to that for physical health, early studies have found that parity does not yet exist (USGAO 2000). Further, this act's authorization expired September 30, 2001; reauthorization or replacement legislation has been proposed but not yet enacted. Although the SCHIP is getting closer to enrolling a higher proportion of eligible children, many states had difficulty in spending their federal matching funds in the early years of the program, and enrollment of eligible children still remains below projections in some states.

The proportion of the population without health insurance for part or all of a year has not dropped below its 15 to 20 percent average, even in the strong economy and increased prosperity for much of the population experienced in the United States through the 1990s. As the economy experiences a downturn, the proportion of the population without health insurance will almost certainly increase. A larger proportion of those who are offered employer-sponsored insurance refuse it, due to its costs to the individual or for other reasons. Nonetheless, a sizable part of the population that might wish to be insured cannot obtain insurance. Without universal access, the current patchwork of public and private health insurance will never cover many who need the kind of care available only with health insurance. Indeed, economist Uwe Reinhardt (2003) has little optimism that, barring some cataclysmic event, universal access will ever be achieved in the United States.

The declining number of hospital emergency departments and the increased stringency in screening those who seek emergency care for nonurgent conditions will continue to limit access to persons who have no other designated source of care. The current nursing shortage contributes to this limitation, and the 2003 Supreme Court ruling that limits the number of hours that medical residents may expect to be attending or on call may also have an effect on access.

One additional change in the world of managed care is that some managed care organizations (MCOs) are rethinking their use of gatekeeping. In many MCOs, primary care physicians served as gatekeepers, blocking patients from self-referral to specialists and requiring their prior review and approval of such referrals. This practice has frustrated consumer and provider alike, so much so that MCOs such as Harvard Vangard Medical Associates have reduced or eliminated this practice (Ferris et al. 2001).

## Changes in Quality

Is quality of care better today than it was just a few years ago? Increasing attention is being paid to quality, and efforts to better measure the outcomes of care have increased. The Agency for Healthcare Research and Quality (AHRQ) is supporting research in evidence-based health services, reorienting providers to reexamine their standards of care and to seek scientific evidence, where available, for their diagnosis and treatment decisions. The Centers for Medicare and Medicaid Services (CMS) has redirected its peer review organizations (PROs) from retrospective review of care and attendant sanctions to become quality improvement organizations (QIOs). QIOs work with providers to improve the quality of care, changing their focus from the cause of the problem (or the perpetrator) to ways to continuously improve performance and generate better patient outcomes.

Concerns remain about the quality of care provided. A study of inpatient quality of care by RAND researchers indicates that only about 55 percent of inpatients get the physician and nursing care that their condition requires (Asch et al. 2006). Despite agreed-to guidelines and protocols for care, adherence is not uniform. The RAND study also indicates that gender and race/ethnicity differences do not have much influence on the appropriateness of the level and type of care provided.

The Institute of Medicine (IOM) and individual researchers have identified a wide range of adverse events, particularly in inpatient settings, that indicates that many medical errors that result in disability or death could have been avoided (Kohn, Corrigan, and Donaldson 2000; Leape 2002). The absence of a patients' bill of rights, which would allow patients to bring claims of adverse actions against MCOs, frustrates those who seek to redress such grievances through the legal system. The U.S. Supreme Court, in its 2005 session, upheld the limits on the ability of individuals to bring legal action against MCOs.

For all the criticism leveled at MCOs, some researchers are concerned that the dismantling of managed care may remove an important platform from which to measure quality (Ginsburg 2001). The enrollment of specific populations into MCOs, even though turnover existed in these enrollments, permitted the study of diagnosis, treatment, and outcomes in a more concentrated and systematic way than may be possible with new delivery systems. Losing the ability to look at the health of subpopulations, which was possible by looking at MCO enrollees, may at least in the short term weaken the ability to develop, implement, and evaluate new measures of the quality of care.

## Why Are Changes Occurring in the Health Services System?

No one factor or event can account for the unrest and impending changes in the U.S. health services system. The move away from a fee-for-service system and toward managed care was about containing health expenditures as much as it was about rationalizing the use of health services. Although on several fronts some of the cost and expenditure goals were attained, these results came at the price of general frustration with managed care on the parts of most of its participants. Providers became frustrated at the controls placed on their practice styles and their loss of autonomy in determining what was best for their patients. Consumers became frustrated with their lack of choices and by new requirements that they interact with the system in very circumscribed ways. Employers who provided health insurance for their workers became frustrated that their costs for this benefit were not being contained (and have recently started to again escalate) and that their employees were unsatisfied with the coverage options provided. Although many report satisfaction with the care they receive (Miller and Luft 1994, 1997), this satisfaction becomes overshadowed by the general sense of disgruntlement that seems pervasive (Miller and Luft 2002; Robinson 2001).

Demographics—particularly, the aging of the population—and projections of increased demand for services, will continue to prompt some changes in the delivery system. New technologies, whether from stem cell research or other promising lines of inquiry, will also stimulate delivery system changes.

Given this society's historic distaste for a complete overhaul of the system and/or replacement with another form, can incremental change address the current levels of perceived frustration and disgruntlement? The status of the U.S. economy is one of the most important factors that affects change. If the economy's rebound remains slow, retrenchment of payers, in particular, may continue, and the potential for growth in coverage or services is likely to be curtailed.

## What Are Some Effects of Change on System Participants?

No one is immune to the changes occurring in the U.S. health services system, and the full extent of these changes is not yet known. This section reviews a sample of the effects that are being observed on some major participants: the patient or consumer, the provider, the payer, and the insurer.

### Consumers of Health Services

Consumers remain divided into two camps: those who have regular access to health services because they are covered by private or public health insurance and those who by choice or by circumstances do not have public or private health insurance and therefore have more limited and irregular access to comprehensive care.

Insured individuals may experience a range of effects from changes in the delivery system. They may be forced to change providers because their employer changes health plans, resulting in turnover in the panel of providers associated with the plans. They may be offered an increased benefit package as an inducement to join a particular, often more restrictive, plan. Cost sharing (i.e., higher premiums, deductibles, copayments, and co-insurance) may increase. Coverage of dependents may decrease, or the insured individual may need to pay more to maintain dependent coverage.

Consumers who have pushed for more say in the design of health benefit packages may be faced with new choices whose long-term consequences are not clear. HSAs may appeal to the healthy worker who has experienced few health expenditures and does not anticipate a change in expenditures. But wide-scale choice of any HSA option may erode the employer-sponsored health insurance system. Is that a good change—or one that is not so good? It is just too early to call this play.

The person who is without health insurance because of financial or other barriers may find accessing care to be increasingly difficult. The flexibility that individual or small group providers once had to render uncompensated care has diminished. Safety-net providers, such as public and teaching hospitals, are scrambling for their financial survival and thus are trying to retain paying patients. Their margins for providing unpaid care, never generous at best, are shrinking as the level of disproportionate share hospital (DSH) payments is subject to pressure from other demands on the federal budget.

## Providers of Health Services

The span of changes in the delivery system in recent years has affected providers in various ways. Moving the provision of major services from an inpatient to an outpatient basis influenced the need for primary care providers and midlevel practitioners. For some providers, particularly for some physicians, the move into integrated networks and more managed systems of care created a sense of frustration with controls over their time to see patients, their ability to provide or refer patients to the full range of services they believed were required, and their general loss of autonomy. The current nursing shortage has been attributed to several causes, including the aging of the workforce and the increased demands placed on nurses in inpatient settings where the caseload now consists of the most seriously ill patients. Changes in the system also spawned an entirely new type of health professional—the hospitalist, a physician whose locus of care is the hospital, where he or she provides the inpatient care for members of specific health plans. Long-established but only recently acknowledged providers of complementary and alternative medicine (CAM) are likely to continue to play a significant role in the U.S. delivery system.

Provider payment has to be recognized as a continued sore spot among many health providers. Payers, both private and public, continue to try to contain expenditures by reducing provider payments. At the high point of managed care, many providers found that they had negotiated payment rates that were well below their costs of providing care. Their options were to absorb the extra costs, get out of such contracts as soon as possible, or in some cases, to forfeit their practices because their expenses significantly exceeded their revenues. Decreases in Medicare's payment to physicians have prompted some to refuse to add more Medicare beneficiaries to their patient panels. Provider payment remains an issue in state Medicaid and in some state SCHIP programs.

## Health Services Payers

Health services payers include employers who provide health insurance coverage, payers of public insurance such as Medicare, and payers of other governmental programs, such as Medicaid. Consumers are also payers. (Some effects of system changes on consumers are noted in previous sections.)

Payers in both public and private health services delivery systems are frustrated at the increasing amount of time and money required to provide health insurance or health services coverage to the populations for which they are responsible. The strength of the economy influences the ability of providers to offer benefits. In a strong economy, private payers for health services may offer richer benefit packages, even at a loss to their bottom line, to retain a competitive workforce. In a weaker economy, the payer may call more of the shots; employees in need of job security are in a weaker bargaining position about their health benefits. Public payers may benefit from a strong economy either because the economy is swelling the trust funds used to pay for care (Medicare) or keeping people in the workforce and off of public assistance rolls (Medicaid). In this cycle of a wartime economy that is attempting to rebound, as well as increasing costs to provide care, both public and private payers are considering increased cost sharing. Interest in a defined contribution or premium support mechanism for providing health benefits also seems to be increasing. Many payers are scrutinizing new health insurance products such as HSAs as they consider what kinds of benefit packages to offer.

## Health Insurers

Health insurers, sometimes viewed as the villains in the health services melodrama, are again seeking double-digit increases in premiums to cover the costs incurred in paying for covered services. Insurers are examining the alliances and coalitions into which they have entered in recent years. They are designing new benefit packages or coverage approaches to respond to the unrest in the current insurance market.

Private insurance continues to look for ways to reduce its risk in coverage. One new option under consideration is high-deductible catastrophic coverage, which covers catastrophic events following the payment of a higher deductible than is charged under contemporary plans and which also provides an annual allowance so that the subscriber can pay for both insured and uninsured services. The unspent annual allowance may be carried forward to pay for care in future years but cannot be transferred to a future employer (Ginsburg 2001). HSAs are a variant on this type of coverage.

## Likelihood of Future Change

Change is likely to be the constant in the U.S. health services system. No viable solution has yet been offered for the problem of the uninsured.

Medicare is the most prominent of public insurers, and calls for its reform continue. Analysts who have long studied Medicare and who also have been responsible for overseeing it argued that the payment structure and other program aspects should be reformed before grafting on a prescription drug benefit (Vladeck 2001; Wilensky 2001). Those reforms did not occur, and outpatient prescription drug coverage for Medicare beneficiaries became a reality on January 1, 2006, following the passage of the Medicare Prescription Drug Improvement and Modernization Act (MMA) of 2003.

Increased cost sharing by persons with private or public health insurance is high on the list of likely changes in the U.S. delivery system. Ginsburg (2001) raises the concern about the ability of future cost sharing to address increases in expenditures that are driven by a relatively small number of people with serious chronic and other conditions (see Chapter 7).

These and other changes are stimulating a reexamination of many long-held values and long-debated issues in U.S. culture, including:

- the importance of freedom of choice,
- the emphasis on efficiency over equity,
- the debate over whether every individual should have access to at least a basic set of health benefits, and
- the extent to which a focus on controlling access and containing expenditures jeopardizes the provision of high-quality services.

## Key Words

adverse events
Agency for Healthcare Research and Quality (AHRQ)
backlash against managed care
business coalitions
capitation

Centers for Medicare and Medicaid Services (CMS)
co-insurance
copayments
cost sharing
deductible

disproportionate share hospital (DSH) payments

fee-for-service payment

gatekeeping

Health Insurance Portability and Accountability Act (HIPAA)

health savings accounts (HSAs)

Institute of Medicine (IOM)

Medicaid

Medicare

Medicare+Choice

Medicare Prescription Drug Improvement and Modernization Act of 2003

Medicare trust funds

Mental Health Parity Act

midlevel practitioners

National Bipartisan Commission on the Future of Medicare

patient satisfaction

patients' bill of rights

premium

prior authorization

quality improvement organizations (QIOs)

State Children's Health Insurance Program (SCHIP)

# References

Asch, S. M., E. A. Kerr, J. Keesey, J. L. Adams, C. M. Setodji, S. Malik, and E. A. McGlynn. 2006. "Who Is at Greatest Risk for Receiving Poor-Quality Health Care?" *New England Journal of Medicine* 354 (11): 1147–56.

Blendon, R. J., M. Brodie, J. M. Benson, D. E. Altman, L. Levitt, T. Hoff, and L. Huzick. 1998. "Understanding the Managed Care Backlash." *Health Affairs* 17 (4): 80–94.

Ferris, T. G., Y. Chang, D. Blumenthal, and S. D. Pearson. 2001. "Leaving Gatekeeping Behind—Effects of Opening Access to Specialists for Adults in a Health Maintenance Organization." *New England Journal of Medicine* 345 (18): 1312–17.

Ginsburg, P. B. 2001. *Navigating a Changing Health System*. Washington, DC: Center for Studying Health System Change.

Kohn, L. T., J. M. Corrigan, and M. S. Donaldson. 2000. *To Err Is Human: Building a Safer Health System*. Washington, DC: National Academy Press.

Lawrence, D. 2001. "Gatekeeping Reconsidered." *New England Journal of Medicine* 345 (18): 1342–43.

Leape, L. L. 2002. "Reporting of Adverse Events." *New England Journal of Medicine* 347 (20): 1633–38.

Miller, R. H., and H. S. Luft. 2002. "HMO Plan Performance Update: An Analysis of the Literature, 1997–2001." *Health Affairs* 21 (4): 63–86.

———. 1997. "Does Managed Care Lead to Better or Worse Quality of Care?" *Health Affairs* 16 (5): 7–25.

———. 1994. "Managed Care Plan Performance Since 1980: A Literature Analysis." *Journal of the American Medical Association* 271 (19): 1512–19.

Reinhardt, U. E. 2003. "Is There Hope for the Uninsured?" *Health Affairs Web Exclusive,* August 27, 2003. http://content.healthaffairs.org/cgi/reprint/hlthaff.w3.376v1.pdf

Robinson, J. 2001. "The End of Managed Care." *Journal of the American Medical Association* 285 (20): 2622–78.

U.S. Government Accountability Office (formerly the U.S. General Accounting Office). 2001. *Higher Expected Spending and Call for New Benefits Underscore Need for Meaningful Reform.* GAO-01-539T. Washington, DC: USGAO.

———. 2000. *Mental Health Parity Act: Despite New Federal Standards, Mental Health Benefits Remain Limited.* GAO/HEHS-00-95. Washington, DC: USGAO.

Vladek, B. C. 2001. "Learn Nothing, Forget Nothing—the Medicare Commission Redux." *New England Journal of Medicine* 345 (6): 456–58.

Wilensky, G. R. 2001. "Medicare Reform—Now Is the Time." *New England Journal of Medicine* 345 (6): 458–62.

# GLOSSARY OF KEY WORDS

## A

**academic health center (AHC)**—A tertiary care center that combines clinical, educational, and research activities. Many AHCs are affiliated with schools of medicine or osteopathy, as well as with schools for other health professions. Quaternary or quintenary services are most likely to be provided at AHCs.

**access to care**—The ability to overcome financial, geographic, cultural, temporal, and other barriers to obtain health services.

**accreditation**—The process by which an institution or educational program, for example, is evaluated against standard criteria to determine the extent to which it meets or exceeds these criteria. The process is intended to ensure quality of performance and outcome.

**activities of daily living (ADLs)**—A functional assessment scale of the ability of an individual to perform key activities, such as toileting, transferring from a bed to a chair, dressing, and eating.

**actuary**—An accredited insurance statistician who calculates premium rates, reserves, and dividends.

**acuity index method**—One of several measures of the severity of an illness or disease.

**acute care**—Inpatient diagnostic and short-term treatment of patients.

**acute mental illness**—Mental illness characterized by a single episode of fairly short duration from which patients return to their optimal level of functioning.

**Acute Physiology and Chronic Health Evaluation (APACHE)**—One of several instruments used to measure health status and severity of illness.

**additions to mental health facilities**—The new admissions, readmissions, transfers, and returns from leaves of absence to a mental health facility.

**adjusted average per capita cost (AAPCC)**—An estimate of the average cost incurred by Medicare per beneficiary in the fee-for-service system, adjusted by county for geographic cost differences related to age, sex, disability status, Medicaid eligibility, and institutional status.

**Administration for Children and Families (ACF)**—A major programmatic unit within the U.S. Department of Health and Human Services (the Ministry of Health equivalent for the United States) that oversees programs that address health and welfare of children and family units.

**administrative costs**—Costs for marketing, enrollment, customer service, and claims processing for health insurance.

**administrative data**—Insurance claims data that provide a basis for determining utilization of health services by gender, age, and other variables.

**administrative load**—The cost of insuring an individual or population, including risk assessment, marketing, and claims processing.

**Administrative Procedures Act (APA)**—Federal legislation that, among other topics, provides a rule-making process in which proposed federal regulations are printed in the *Federal Register* for comment and in their final form.

**administrative services only (ASO)**—A contract between an insurer (or its subsidiary) and a group employer, eligible group, trustee, or other party in which an insurer provides certain administrative services. These services may include actuarial support, benefit design, claims processing, data recovery and analysis, benefit communication, financial advice, medical care conversions, data preparation for government reports, and stop-loss coverage.

**adult day care**—A form of long-term care in which adults with impairments are cared for, often in a residential setting, during the workday and then are returned to the usual source of care (often a family member's home) at the end of the workday.

**advanced practice nurses (APNs)**—Nurses who specialize in an area of clinical practice. Nurse practitioners are types of APNs, and they specialize in pediatrics, geriatrics, family medicine, women's health, and other areas.

**adverse events**—Inferior outcomes of medical care, resulting in injury or death to the patient.

**adverse selection**—The systematic selection by high-risk consumers of insurance plans with greater degrees of coverage. Insurers who offer these plans end up with insured persons who incur greater-than-average costs.

**Agency for Healthcare Research and Quality (AHRQ)**—The federal agency that funds outcomes research. Formerly, the Agency for Health Care Policy and Research.

**AHC tripartite mission**—The three-pronged mission of academic health centers (AHCs) that includes education, clinical services, and research.

**Aid to Families with Dependent Children (AFDC)**—Cash assistance program that covered, through 1996, single-parent families and two-parent families with an unemployed principal earner. All recipients of AFDC received Medicaid automatically. Each state set its own income limits for AFDC. The 1996 Personal Welfare and Work Responsibility Act replaced the AFDC program with the Temporary Assistance to Needy Families (TANF) program.

**allied health provider**—Physical therapists, social workers, respiratory therapists, medical technologists, and other categories of health professionals who at some level provide health services to patients.

**allopathic physician**—A physician trained to make use of all measures proven to be of value in the prevention or treatment of diseases.

**almshouses**—A colonial-era facility for the poor and indigent that was supported by the alms (money or goods) given to care for the poor.

**alternative delivery system**—Until the mid-1990s, managed care in its various forms was considered the alternative delivery system, meaning it was an alternative to fee-for-service (FFS) care. Most today would conclude that the FFS system has become the alternative to managed care.

**ambulatory care**—Care for episodic and chronic conditions and for health maintenance.

**ambulatory surgical center (ASC)**—Center that provides surgical services that do not require an inpatient hospital stay. Medicare pays an institutional fee for use of an ASC for certain approved surgical procedures. Medicare will also pay for physician and anesthesia services that are provided for these procedures.

**American Red Cross**—One of a range of voluntary health agencies that has identified a niche in the multifaceted U.S. health services system. The American Red Cross has established a role in maintaining the nation's blood supply and in assisting with the health of populations during natural disasters, such as tornadoes or earthquakes.

**Americans with Disabilities Act (ADA) of 1990**—Legislation to ensure that persons with physical or mental impairments are provided reasonable access to health services.

**antitrust**—Describes laws and regulations that preclude any one provider from establishing a monopoly that interferes with open and unrestricted commerce.

**appropriateness of care**—A field of inquiry to determine whether the health services rendered to a patient are the proper services, in the correct amount and duration, for that patient's health status.

**assistive technology device**—A device such as a computer or speech board that permits individuals with a disability to communicate or enhance their functional abilities in other ways.

**association health plans (AHPs)**—Group health insurance plans created by professional associations or groups such as Chambers of Commerce that permit small businesses to obtain employee health insurance coverage for better prices than they could obtain as individual small businesses.

**average length of stay (ALOS)**—Numbers of days a patient stays in the hospital for a given condition. The ALOS varies by geographic area in the United States, due in part to variations in practice.

# B

**baby boomer**—A person born in the United States in the post–World War II population explosion between 1946 and 1964.

**backlash against managed care**—Negative reactions of consumers and providers to restrictions and reductions in choice within managed care plans.

**backward integration**—A type of vertical integration in a health services system in which the hospital or other central organization moves toward the supplier.

**bad-debt care**—Care that providers, particularly hospitals and physicians, are forced to write off as bad debt because the person incurring the care is unable or unwilling to pay for the care received. Other terms for this phenomenon include *charity care* and *uncompensated care*.

**Balanced Budget Act of 1997**—The Omnibus Budget Reconciliation Act for 1997. It introduced many changes into the U.S. health services system, including the State Child Health Insurance Plan (SHCIP) and Medicare+ Choice plans as the new Part C of Medicare. It also required prospective payment for more of Medicare's services, such as home health care and skilled nursing, and established Medicare payment changes (principally reductions) to other providers of care.

**basic science research**—Usually laboratory-based research, often at the molecular level, that provides the information necessary for the exploration of clinical research.

**behavioral health**—Types of health behaviors (or unhealthy behaviors) that directly influence health status. Substance abuse and mental health status are included in the studies of behavioral health.

**behavioral health organizations (BHOs)**—A health services delivery organization that focuses its treatment on substance abuse and mental illness diagnoses.

**"big-ticket" versus "little-ticket" technology**—Health services technology can be a driving force in the increase in costs and expenditures. The effects of "big-ticket" items—new forms of diagnostic imaging, for example—are easily discernible. Smaller-priced technologies, however, may also have an effect on costs and expenditures—in part, because they may be used much more frequently.

**biomedical research**—Basic and applied research into the cause and nature of illness and disease.

**birthing centers**—Centers that may be established outside the hospital inpatient setting as a business carve-out, intended not only as specialty centers but also marketed as more comfortable and hospitable places in which to give birth. To retain this important part of the health services market, many hospitals established their own on-premises centers.

**black lung program**—A federal program established to provide health services to coal miners, particular in the Appalachian area, who were likely to be uninsured and suffering from this occupational-related respiratory disease.

**block grants**—A form of intergovernmental assistance whereby grant-in-aid programs are grouped into funding blocks. Often, the block grant funding amount is less than the combined amount of the individual programs it groups together, and fewer "strings," or governmental requirements, may be associated with a block grant. The 1981 OBRA of the Reagan administration greatly reduced the number of individual program grants in health, blocking them into four major groups: prevention; maternal and child health; alcohol, drug abuse, and mental health; and primary care.

**Blue Cross**—An early provider of group health insurance plans, it has evolved into a national association of hospital plans (Blue Cross) and physician services (Blue Shield) plans. Those Blue Cross plans that remain not-for-profit are likely to have relief from certain provisions that state governments require of other insurers doing business in their states. In recent years, a number of Blue Cross plans have converted from not-for-profit to proprietary plans.

**Blue Shield**—A type of insurance developed in the 1930s to cover the costs of physician office visits and other kinds of outpatient care (see *Blue Cross* for the coverage of inpatient care).

**board certification**—The process by which physician specialists are examined and determined to have met the academic and clinical standards of their specialty.

**breakthrough technologies**—Technologies that significantly alter the way in which specific types of health services are provided. Successful organ transplantation may be considered one type of breakthrough technology. Breakthrough technologies are considered to be at the other end of the spectrum from halfway technologies, an example of which is kidney dialysis.

**business coalitions**—Coalitions created by employers and other business leaders who seek to more efficiently provide health insurance or services to their employees. The power of group negotiation, purchasing, and other standard setting is used to contain costs and expenditures.

## C

**capital expenditure review**—A review of a health services facility's proposed capital expenditure above a certain threshold as one way to try to contain health costs and expenditures. It was motivated by the recognition that unnecessarily duplicative capacity increased costs and expenditures, which were passed along to the payer, whether that was an employer who sponsored health insurance and/or the individual who received the services.

**capitation**—(1) A payment system used in managed care in which the provider is paid a fixed, predetermined amount on a regular basis (usually monthly) for the provision of all covered benefits to the insured individual. The provider is at risk if the beneficiary uses more than the projected level of services. A capitation rate can be adjusted for specific patient characteristics, such as age and sex. (2) The basis on which the federal government provides support for the training of health professionals (i.e., grants made to colleges and universities based on the number of students to be trained in a profession).

**capitation grants**—Federal funds provided as early as the 1940s through the early 1980s to schools of medicine, nursing, dentistry, pharmacy, and veterinary medicine to encourage their expansion and production of a greater number of graduates ready to practice in these areas. Schools received a per capita payment for each health professions student they enrolled.

**carve-out function**—A separation of a certain type of service—often, mental health services, for example—from a basic insurance benefit package. Carved-out services may then be received from only a limited and specific set of providers as one way to manage utilization and costs.

**case-mix**—An analysis of age, gender, health status, and other factors that may distinguish one group of patients, and their utilization of health services, from other groups.

**center of excellence**—A designation for a unit that provides a particular set of services—such as heart transplantation, for example—to recognize that the process and outcomes of care are superior to those of similar centers.

**Centers for Medicare and Medicaid Services (CMS)**—The federal agency within the U.S. Department of Health and Human Services responsible for Medicare, Medicaid, and the State Children's Health Insurance Program (SCHIP). Formerly, the Health Care Financing Administration.

**certificate of need (CON) program**—Established by the 1974 National Health Planning and Resources Development Act as a capital expenditure review program for hospitals, nursing homes, and other health services facilities. States that did not implement CON programs by established dates risked the loss of a range of other federal funds. This provision of federal law was repealed in 1986, although some states have elected to retain a modified form of this program, principally to govern the growth of nursing homes.

**certification**—The process by which health services facilities or health professions are deemed to have met national standards. Medicare has a certification process required of any facility that wants to be reimbursed for the care of Medicare beneficiaries. Certain health professions may require periodic certification and recertification to ensure that its practitioners remain current with the tenets of their profession.

**CHAMPUS Reform Initiative**—An effort in the early 1990s to change the military's Civilian Health and Medical Program of the Uniformed Services health services system from an indemnity to a managed care focus in an effort to reduce costs and expenditures.

**charity care**—Health services provided by an institution or a health services provider to an individual who is usually uninsured and unable to pay for these services. The 1946 Hill Burton Construction Act required recipient hospitals to provide a certain amount of charity care in order to receive federal construction funds. This type of care is also referred to as bad-debt or uncompensated care.

**cherry picking**—The act of choosing only the healthiest enrollees in an insurance plan, for example, as a way to reduce the insurer's risk and potentially increase its profits.

**chronic disease care**—Ongoing care provided to a patient of any age who suffers from one or more chronic conditions, such as diabetes, heart disease, or mental impairments. This level of care differs from acute or episodic care rendered for an event that may be infrequent but potentially catastrophic, such as a cerebral vascular event or an accidental injury.

**chronic mental illness**—A persistent and ongoing mental impairment that may be treatable, permitting the patient to live normally in a community setting.

**claims data**—Databases that include the utilization of services, charges, and other data on a group of insured persons.

**claims processing**—The processing of a request for payment for health services to an insured person by the entity providing the service.

**Clayton Act**—One of several pieces of federal legislation intended to protect against antitrust arrangements by health services facilities and providers.

**clinical practice guidelines**—Guidelines developed by provider organizations, professional societies, and others to prescribe how a particular clinical intervention should be conducted in terms of its process and outcome.

**clinical research**—Research related to the care and treatment of patients with illness or disease. Clinical research depends on basic research to provide the scientific basis for exploring illness and disease.

*Code of Federal Regulations (CFR)*—The compilation of all federally issued regulations, including those pertaining to health services.

**co-insurance**—The percentage share of medical bills that a beneficiary must pay. The portion of reimbursable hospital and medical expenses, after subtraction of any deductible, that an insurer does not cover and for which the beneficiary is responsible.

**commercial health insurance**—Insurance provided by private-sector vendors and thus differentiated from public or social insurance. The Blue Cross plans, until they began to convert to proprietary plans, were usually not considered commercial plans.

**Committee on the Costs of Medical Care (CCMC)**—A committee of providers, legislators, policy makers, and others convened in the late 1920s to consider ways to contain the costs of providing medical care. The farsighted committee recommended the use of prepaid care, a recommendation not broadly implemented until nearly 50 years after its reports were issued.

**community health center**—A federally funded organization that provides primary care health care, often on a sliding-fee scale. Community health centers are often located in urban settings. They are now combined, in terms of funding and the provision of services, with migrant health centers.

**community hospital**—A classification of hospital that indicates a facility, usually a not-for-profit hospital, that is developed in and operated by the community.

**Community Mental Health Center Act of 1964**—Legislation that provided federal funds to establish treatment centers in the community for chronic mental illnesses. It was envisioned that these centers would support the treatment of patients being released from state and other mental institutions by the wave of deinstitutionalizations that began in the early 1970s; the capacity of and funding for these community centers were insufficient to meet these needs.

**Community and Migrant Health Center Program**—Two separate programs established as part of the Great Society of the mid-1960s and later merged into one program to provide health services at low or no cost in underserved metropolitan and rural areas to qualifying individuals.

**community rating**—A method of setting insurance premiums for health services coverage. In this method, the risk is spread across all community members and each pays the same premium, unadjusted for individual health status.

**competition**—An underlying tenet of a free market system, in which economic decisions are determined to be most efficient if they are made in a competitive environment. When competition does not work in the market, decision makers often turn to regulation to correct the market.

**complementary and alternative medicine (CAM) providers**—Nontraditional providers of health services, such as chiropractors, acupuncturists, and herbalists.

**Comprehensive Health Planning (CHP) Act of 1966**—Great Society legislation intended to give states and regions within those states the responsibility for (1) assessing their needs for health services, (2) planning to obtain needed services and eliminating unnecessarily duplicative services, and (3) beginning to respond to the increase in health services costs and expenditures that was resulting from increased access to health services.

**computerized physician order entry (CPOE)**—An electronic means for physicians to input their prescriptions and other orders for patient services. The intent is to reduce errors that may result from unclear handwritten instructions and to expedite the receipt of the orders at their proper destination. Increasing patient safety is the major motivation for this approach.

**Computerized Severity Index**—One of a range of instruments to determine the severity of a patient's illness.

**concurrent review**—A process of ongoing review while the patient is undergoing treatment in the hospital to certify the length of stay that is appropriate for the approved admission.

**Consolidated Omnibus Budget Reconciliation Act (COBRA) of 1985**—That year's annual omnibus budget reconciliation act. This particular act is important for establishing a way that insured individuals and their dependents, who lost their coverage through loss of a job or because of divorce from or the death of the insured, could retain their group coverage policy for a period of time as long as they paid a premium rate established by this act.

**consumer protection**—A governmental regulatory role to protect the consumer from goods or services (such as medications and devices) that could be injurious or harmful to health.

**continuous quality improvement (CQI)—** A focus on correcting errors without an undue focus on assigning blame, with a goal of ongoing improvement in the quality of the service rendered or the product being produced.

**continuum of care—**An ideal view of systematic and continuous health services needed and rendered, beginning with healthy prenatal care and continuing to provision of the appropriate level of care until the end of a life.

**contract research organization (CRO)—** A freestanding research organization, often a proprietary organization, that contracts or subcontracts with governmental and other entities, including pharmaceutical manufacturers, to conduct research such as clinical trials for a new drug or other biomedical development.

**copayments—**Flat fees that insured persons must pay for a particular unit of service, such as an office visit, emergency room visit, or the filling of a prescription.

**cost—**The amount spent to produce a good or service.

**cost containment—**A range of initiatives aimed at providers of services, payers for services, and users of services to help reduce the costs of care and ultimately the overall expenditures for health services. See Table 7.6.

**cost of/expenditures for care—**Terms that are often used interchangeably to refer to the amounts spent to produce a good or a service (cost of care) and the amounts spent for goods and services (expenditures for care).

**cost-saving technologies—**The introduction of technologic approaches that provide services in more cost-effective ways.

**cost sharing—**The generic term that includes copayments, co-insurance, and deductibles; also, out-of-pocket payments.

**cost shifting—**An action by the provider of health services to shift the costs of care from a low-paying or nonpaying source to a payer with deeper pockets in order to cover the costs of providing services. The costs of providing health services to uninsured persons, for example, were covered in part by charging a higher rate to insured persons.

**Council for Education in Public Health (CEPH)—**The national body that accredits all schools of public health and programs in public health that are based in other academic settings, such as schools of medicine.

**Council on Graduate Medical Education (COGME)—**Authorized by Congress in 1986 to provide an ongoing assessment of physician workforce trends, training issues, and financing policies, and to recommend appropriate federal and private-sector efforts to address identified needs.

**cream skimming—**See *cherry picking*.

**criteria mapping—**A method developed by Sheldon Greenfield and others to assess quality of care.

**critical access hospital (CAH)—**A Medicare payment category for smaller, often rural, hospitals. The designation is intended to acknowledge the differences in patient volume and service delivery that often occur in such hospitals and to avoid penalizing them financially when they do not and cannot provide services in the same way as do larger hospitals.

**crossover population—**As used in the field of health services, generally refers to Medicare beneficiaries who, by virtue of their low incomes, are also eligible for certain Medicaid services. About 16 percent of Medicare beneficiaries are considered the crossover population; they are sometimes referred to as *dually eligible*.

**cross-subsidization—**Establishing charges for health services in such a way that higher charges can be set for some services in order to cover the costs of a less-profitable service, or higher charges may be set for some services to cover the costs of services for which little or no payment is made. Facilities may use revenues from a higher profit center to cover the costs of a service or center that is not recouping its costs.

## D

**debt financing**—Borrowing funds, to be paid back with interest, as a way to finance an endeavor.

**deductible**—A specified amount of spending for health services for which an individual or a family is responsible before their health insurance coverage becomes effective.

**defensive medicine**—The provision of medical services and treatments that may not necessarily be clinically justified but that are provided as evidence that every possible treatment was offered in order to avoid malpractice actions.

**defined benefit**—An approach to providing health insurance based on an established and specific set of services, and only those services, that are covered by a particular insurance plan.

**defined contribution**—As one way to give employees greater responsibility for health services decisions, employers may provide a fixed allowance per employee for that employee's purchase of health insurance, rather than providing specific health insurance policies from which the employee chooses.

**deinstitutionalization**—A movement in the early 1970s to remove persons with chronic mental illnesses from state and other long-term institutions and place them in the community. It was assumed, wrongly in some cases, that community mental health centers would be available to provide the care these individuals needed, but the transition in many instances was not carefully managed, and anticipated resources were not always available.

**Dependents Medical Care Program**—One of several predecessor programs to CHAMPUS that provided health services to the dependents of active-duty military personnel.

**deregulation**—The move in certain sectors, including parts of the health services sector, to allow the principles of the free market to govern the provision of goods and services and to remove governmental regulations that

had been placed to control some part of the provision of goods and services.

**determinants of health**—The model used by Milton Roemer and others to demonstrate that health status is not entirely determined by available health services. Genetics, education, income, geographic location, race and ethnicity, and many other factors influence health status.

**developmental disabilities**—Physical or mental conditions that may impair an individual's ability to function fully and independently in society.

**diagnosis-related groups (DRGs)**—A classification system that categorizes patients into groups that are clinically coherent and homogeneous with respect to inpatient short-stay hospital resource use.

**direct graduate medical education (DGME) payments**—A part of Medicare's payment to hospitals and managed care organizations that participate in the specialty training of physicians.

**disability-adjusted life years (DALYs)**—A measure of health status that incorporates aspects of both morbidity and mortality.

**disability days**—A measure of functional status in which the number of days that one is able to perform work, go to school, or engage in other usual functions is compromised by some physical or mental disability.

**disability insurance**—Short- or long-term insurance an individual may purchase to protect against loss of income related to a disabling injury or illness.

**discounted fee-for-service payment**—A payment mechanism that pays the provider less than the established fee-for-service payment as one way to reduce costs and expenditures. Providers who accept such payment may be basing their acceptance of reduced payment on the potential for increasing the volume of services provided.

**discretionary funds**—Funds that have not been committed to an entitlement program and may be used at the agency's discretion to address new needs and problems. Entitlement programs such as Medicare and Medicaid have reduced the availability of discretionary funding for other kinds of health programs at the federal and state levels.

**disease**—The presence of pathology that compromises the health of an individual.

**disease prevention**—Averting the onset of disease through such preventive measures as health screenings and maintaining good health practices in physical activity and nutrition.

**disease staging**—Assessing the progression of a disease by comparing its manifestation in a patient with known stages. Cancer is one disease for which stages have been defined.

**disproportionate share hospital (DSH) payments**—Payments provided principally by Medicare and Medicaid to hospitals and some other providers that serve a relatively large volume—a disproportionate share—of low-income persons. Examples are public hospitals, inner-city hospitals, and some academic health centers.

**downsizing**—The act of reducing capacity as one way to reduce the costs of providing services.

**"dread disease" insurance policies**—Disease-specific insurance policies that cover the insured for one specific disease, such as cancer.

**drive-through delivery**—The label given the 1990s movement to reduce the amount of inpatient hospitalization for childbirth. Federal laws have been established to protect mothers and infants from discharge before it is medically advisable to do so.

**Drug Enforcement Agency (DEA)**—The federal agency within the Department of Justice that is responsible for governing health services providers' use of controlled substances.

**drug rebates**—A requirement of the 1990 OBRA that drug manufacturers that wished to have their prescription drugs listed on state Medicaid formularies pay rebates to the Medicaid programs. The provisions were later extended to other federal programs, such as the Veterans Administration.

**dually entitled**—Individuals entitled to both Medicare and Medicaid coverage. See *crossover population*.

**durable medical equipment (DME)**—Medical supplies and items such as hospital beds and wheelchairs.

**durational rating**—A rating that initially offers a low rate of premium but then imposes large increases in subsequent years after the predictive effects of traditional medical screening begin to dissipate and workers are no longer protected under preexisting exclusion periods.

# E

**Economic Stabilization Program (ESP)**—A program established during the Nixon administration in the early 1970s that froze wages and prices in an effort to curb inflation and escalating costs. Although the ESP may have held down hospital wages and prices during its duration, those wages and prices climbed as soon as the program was suspended.

**Educational Commission for Foreign Medical Graduates (ECFMG)**—The body that certifies international medical graduates for entrance into graduate medical education in the United States.

**efficiency**—Technical efficiency is a measure of how close a given combination of resources is to producing a maximum amount of output. Allocative or economic efficiency is a measure of how close a given combination of resources is to yielding maximum consumer satisfaction.

**Emergency Maternal and Infant Child Care Program (EMIC)**—A World War II–era program that provided care to mothers and children of active-duty military personnel.

**Emergency Medical Treatment and Active Labor Act (EMTALA)**—A statute governing the treatment required for persons seeking care from an emergency department to ensure against "dumping" of uninsured patients.

**Emerson Report**—A report commissioned by the American Public Health Association in the late 1940s that identified six basic functions of state and local health departments: vital statistics, public health education, environmental sanitation, public health laboratories, prevention and control of communicable diseases, and hygiene of maternity, infancy, and childhood.

**employee assistance programs (EAP)**—Programs established to counsel employees who are dealing with alcoholism, other substance abuse, and mental health problems, and to aid them in seeking appropriate treatment.

**Employee Retirement Income Security Act (ERISA) of 1974**—Legislation established in response to concerns about pension fund mismanagement and designed to protect assets used for pensions and health services benefits packages. ERISA permits employers to self-fund their health insurance plans and exempts them from the provision of state-mandated health benefits.

**employer-sponsored health insurance**—Health insurance provided by an employer. It may be self-funded insurance, or the employer may obtain health insurance services from organized providers of such services.

**end result idea**—Ernest Codman's ideas, in the nineteenth century, for assessing quality of health care and accepting responsibility for the quality of care rendered.

**end-stage renal disease (ESRD)**—Irreversible kidney failure that requires either a kidney transplant or periodic kidney dialysis for patient survival. Persons with this disease, regardless of age, became eligible for Medicare benefits in 1972.

**entitlement programs**—Governmentally established programs in which the beneficiaries are entitled to all covered services. Programs such as Medicare and Medicaid are entitlement programs. Benefits are not capped, and these programs become open-ended in terms of their costs and expenditures.

**epidemiologic transition**—The change in focus on categories of disease as environmental and other disease agents are conquered. The epidemiologic transition has moved from a focus on communicable diseases to a focus on chronic diseases.

**equity**—A precept of social justice in which all classes can expect to be treated the same way in the same circumstances. Equity is often seen as a contrast to efficiency, the economic concept of the optimal use of resources.

**essential access community hospital (EACH)**—A hospital classification system intended to promote regionalization of health services in rural areas and improve access to hospital and emergency services.

**excess capacity**—The stage in a health system when the availability of personnel or facilities exceeds the need for them in the population.

**exclusive provider organization (EPO)**—A type of insurance plan popular in the early 1980s. Enrollees obtained their care from a closed (exclusive) panel of providers. The costs of services provided by nonpanel members might be covered only partially or not at all in a EPO plan.

**expenditure**—The amount spent for goods or services.

**expenditures caps**—Efforts to control costs and expenditures by placing limits on what can be spent for the provision of certain services. Some health insurance policies include lifetime expenditure caps. If an insured exceeds such a cap, he or she is involuntarily disenrolled and loses coverage from the plan.

**experience rating**—A method of setting health premiums for health services coverage in which insured persons in a group pay premiums based on risk-related characteristics, including prior claims history.

**experimental/investigational practice**—A new therapy or drug whose effectiveness has not yet fully been established; thus, insurance companies usually do not cover it. Examples include bone marrow transplantation for breast and some other cancers and the off-label use of a drug for purposes other than those for which the drug has FDA approval.

**Experimental Medical Care Review Organization (EMCRO)**—One of the earliest federal efforts, established in the early 1970s, to review and assess the quality of care provided to specific populations. Some of the early EMCRO work focused on the appropriateness of certain types of immunizations to specific populations.

**extra billing**—Billing insured persons for the amount above that paid by their insurer for a specific service. Under Medicare Part B, for example, physicians can choose to accept Medicare's payment schedule as payment-in-full for a service, which is called *assignment,* or they can choose to bill the Medicare beneficiary for the difference in their charge to Medicare and the payment they received from Medicare.

**F**

**faculty practice plan**—Faculties in medical schools and academic health centers provide direct patient care as part of their teaching responsibilities. Payments made for this care are used, in part, to support educational endeavors and to maintain the cutting-edge physical plant that permits this level of care to be offered.

**FDA premarket approval**—One in several levels of approval that a pharmaceutical company or device manufacturer must receive in the Food and Drug Administration's oversight of safety and clinical efficacy of new products (see Figure 10.3).

**FDA premarket notification**—See *FDA premarket approval.*

**Federal Employee Health Benefits Program (FEHBP)**—A national-level program of a broad range of health insurers and benefit packages from which federal employees may choose their coverage. Plans range from basic to extensive coverage, and the premiums range accordingly.

**federal match rate**—The rate of federal funds provided to states to operate state Medicaid programs. The minimum match is 50 cents of each dollar, and the current maximum match is 76.8 to the state of Mississippi. The match rate is determined by the state's per capita income.

**federal poverty level (FPL)**—Income guidelines established annually by the Department of Agriculture and other units of the federal government. Public assistance programs usually define income limits in relation to the FPL.

*Federal Register*—Publication that documents all actions related to the issuance of federal regulations, including notice of proposed rule making, draft, and final regulations.

**Federal Security Agency**—The executive agency at the federal level responsible for the nation's health programs. It was replaced by a cabinet-level agency in 1953—the U.S. Department of Health and Welfare. That department was renamed the U.S. Department of Health and Human Services in 1980.

**Federal Trade Commission Act**—Legislation that, among its many provisions, addresses unfair competition and has been used to examine hospital antitrust issues.

**fee-for-service reimbursement**—The health services payment system in which physicians and other providers bill for each unit of service they provide.

**Financial Accounting Standards Board Release 106**—This federal standard governs the ways in which employers must report and account for retiree health benefit plans.

**first-dollar coverage**—A practice by employers who sponsored health insurance to pay all costs of providing this insurance, including the full premium, requiring no deductible and little or no copayments or co-insurance. This practice was initiated in the automobile industry when labor unions were successful in negotiating strong benefit packages for their members, and employers saw it as more advantageous than increasing salaries. Once employers began to appreciate the full effects of paying all costs of providing health insurance, this practice ended.

**fiscal intermediaries**—Entities used by Medicare, and sometimes by Medicaid, to handle beneficiary claims and pay providers. Major insurance companies often successfully bid to serve as the fiscal intermediary for a geographic region.

**flat fee per medical case**—One of several types of provider reimbursement that is based on the entire episode of care rather than on a series of specific procedures and services.

**flat fee per patient**—A type of provider reimbursement in which payment is based on the number of patients enrolled in a system of care rather than on specific procedures and services provided to these patients.

**Flexner Report**—A 1910 report by Abraham Flexner on the state of medical education in the United States and Canada. Flexner found a wide range in the quality of education being provided, almost all of it outside the university setting, and recommended a standardized, university-based approach to physician training.

**Food and Drug Act of 1906**—The act that standardized drug strength and purity and prohibited drug adulteration and misbranding.

**Food, Drug, and Cosmetic Act (FDCA) of 1938**—One of the early pieces of consumer protection legislation enacted to prevent the disbursal of unregulated and harmful products.

**foreign medical graduate (FMG)**—See *international medical graduate (IMG)*.

**formal caregiver**—A recognized (and often licensed or certified) health professional who provides health services to a patient. This term in usually used in the context of long-term care (see *informal caregiver*).

**formularies**—A list of specific prescription drugs that an insurer will cover for its subscribers. The formulary may include both brand name and generic drugs.

**for-profit hospital (or other type of facility or organization)**—A facility that is financed by shareholders who expect some return on their investment. This type of facility is also referred to as a *proprietary facility*.

**forward integration**—A type of vertical integration in which a hospital, for example, extends its reach to capture and control more

services; forward integration aims that process toward the consumer of hospital services.

**frail elderly**—A term used to described that part of the population, usually Medicare eligible, who are not in an institutional setting but require a number of support services to maintain their health.

**fraud and abuse**—Intentional activities on the parts of providers of health services and others to defraud the payer by billing for services not rendered, by billing at a higher rate than is warranted, or other unethical practices.

**freestanding hospital**—A hospital unaffiliated with any other or with a hospital system.

**freestanding surgery centers**—Centers established outside the inpatient hospital setting, and often in competition with hospitals, for the provision of certain surgical services.

**functional status**—A determination of one's physical and mental capacity to perform routine functions of independent living.

## G

**gag rules**—Restrictions placed on providers of managed care that do not allow providers to fully inform their patients about the range of possible treatments available for their conditions as one way to contain costs. Some states have passed legislation that forbids systems of care from using gag rules.

**gatekeeping**—The use of a health services provider to screen access to specialists by enrollees in some types of managed care plans.

**general inflation**—Economy-wide inflation that covers all market baskets.

**generic drugs**—Prescription drugs, often developed by competitors after the developer's patent rights have expired, that are usually offered at lower prices than the original brand-name drug.

**genetic testing**—Screening, often based on blood sample testing, to determine the presence or absence of certain markers for disease or physical traits and characteristics that are transmissible from parents to their children.

**global budgeting**—A resource allocation method in which the full amount of financing for a particular budget cycle is prospectively determined. The recipient must manage this amount to cover all expected costs for the budget period. Canada uses a global budgeting method for its hospitals.

**graduate medical education (GME)**—Advanced training that an individual with a medical degree pursues in order to specialize in a particular area of medicine, such as surgery, internal medicine, or pediatrics.

**Graduate Medical Education National Advisory Committee (GMENAC)**—One of many bodies convened to address the issue of physician supply. GMENAC in 1981 issued a report on physician oversupply.

**Great Society**—The popular label for the administration of President Lyndon B. Johnson, whose leadership during the 1960s resulted in a mushrooming of publicly funded programs, including Medicare, Medicaid, Neighborhood Health Centers, Community Health Centers, Migrant Health programs, and capitation grants for professional education.

**gross domestic product (GDP)**—The total dollar value of all final goods and services (consumer, investment, and government) produced within the defined geographical boundaries of a country or nation.

**gross national product (GNP)**—The total dollar value of all final goods and services (consumer, investment, and government) produced not only within the defined geographical boundaries of a country or nation, but also such goods and services that are produced internationally by companies owned and operated by that particular country or nation.

**group health insurance**—Health insurance provided by an employer that offers a basic set of benefits to all enrolled employees. Group health insurance is less costly per covered life than is individual health insurance because the risk can be spread across more individuals.

**group model HMO**—A type or model of health maintenance organization in which the HMO contracts with an independent group practice to provide care for its members. The contractual arrangements are made usually on a per capita (capitation) basis.

**group purchasing consortia**—Organizations established by coalitions of health services facilities, such as hospitals or nursing homes, that purchase basic supplies in bulk, thus reducing the cost to all participants.

**guaranteed issue**—Requires insurers to offer plans to small employers.

**guaranteed renewal**—Requires insurers to renew coverage to small employers.

## H

**halfway technology**—A "bridging" technology used until a more complete technology can be developed and utilized. Some consider kidney dialysis to be a halfway technology because it keeps an individual alive and functioning until a more complete technology—kidney transplantation—can be implemented (if appropriate).

**health**—A complete state of physical, mental, and social well-being, and not merely the absence of disease or illness (World Health Organization definition); more specifically, a state characterized by anatomic integrity and the ability to perform personally valued family, work, and community roles while free from the risk of disease.

**health behavior model**—A model developed by Aday, Andersen, and Fleming in 1980 to explain care-seeking behavior.

**health belief model**—A model developed by Rosenstock in 1974 to explain care-seeking behavior.

**health care outcomes**—The results of treatments or interventions intended to improve health or ameliorate health status.

**health care reform**—Periodic efforts, usually at state and national levels, to change the way that health services are delivered and/or reimbursed.

**Health Insurance Flexibility and Accountability Initiative**—A 2001 initiative under the Bush administration that permits states greater flexibility in covering low-income uninsured persons through their Medicaid programs.

**Health Insurance Portability and Accountability Act of 1996 (HIPAA)**—National legislation enacted to correct some of the gaps in the health insurance industry—principally, the gap in insurance coverage when employees changed employers and had to experience a waiting period before their new coverage became effective. HIPAA was also enacted to address some of the limitations of small-business coverage. Its amendments address the need for confidentiality of patient and provider data in research and other activities.

**health insurance purchasing cooperative (HIPC)**—An insurance organization that acts as a broker between payers of health insurance (households, governments, businesses) and health services providers by setting standards for services and seeking competitive bids for these services.

**health maintenance organization (HMO)**—An organization that delivers and manages health services under a risk-based arrangement. HMOs usually receive a monthly premium or capitation payment for each enrollee that is based on a projection of what the typical patient will cost.

**Health Maintenance Organization Act, 1973**—Legislation established during the Nixon administration that required employers of a certain size to offer an HMO health insurance option to their workforces if such were available.

**HealthMarts**—A type of group health insurance purchasing arrangement offered in the 1990s to allow many smaller businesses to be treated as one larger entity in the purchase of health insurance benefits for employees.

**Health Plan Employer Data and Information Set (HEDIS®)**—A series of data collection instruments and resulting databases developed by the National Committee on Quality Assurance (NCQA) to allow employers and others to compare managed care plans on the basis of specific quality indicators.

**health planning**—The effort to define needs for health services, identify resources to meet those needs, assist or advise in the creation of programs to meet the needs, and monitor and evaluate plan implementation.

**health powers**—Constitutionally based authority, at the national or state level, that delegates to specific governmental units the authority to establish and regulate the offering of certain kinds of health services.

**health professional shortage area (HPSA)**—One of several types of federal designations used to attract health services providers to practice by offering financial incentives, including loan forgiveness for federal loans obtained to support their health professional training.

**health promotion**—Education and/or other supportive services that assist individuals or groups to adopt healthy behaviors and/or reduce health risks and increase self-care skills.

**health savings accounts**—A type of insurance product authorized by the 2003 Medicare Modernization Act (MMA) that may be offered by an employer. Employees can choose this high-deductible type of plan that allows them to own and control their health care spending and save for future health care costs with tax-free interest until retirement. Not to be confused with medical savings accounts.

**Health Security Act of 1993 (HSA)**—Legislation proposed by the Clinton administration that would have moved the U.S. health services system closer to a national health insurance system. The act was defeated, in part due to intense lobbying against it by the health insurance industry and others with vested interests in maintaining the status quo.

**health services**—The provision of services, therapies, drugs, devices, and other interventions aimed at improving the health of individuals and populations.

**health services technology**—All procedures, devices, equipment, and drugs used in the maintenance, restoration, and promotion of health.

**health status**—A measure of health that can incorporate physical, emotional, social, and role functioning; pain; and many other factors.

**Health Systems Agency (HSA)**—Local-level agencies created by the 1974 National Health Planning and Resources Development Act, HSAs were to assess local needs and develop plans to address those needs. These plans were provided to the State Health Planning and Development Agency for incorporation into a statewide plan that specified how the health facilities and services in a state were to be offered.

*Healthy People 2010* **objectives**—The most recent in a series of nationally established objectives that guide the public and private health systems in disease prevention, health promotion, and development of the delivery system.

**Hill-Burton program**—Established as the 1946 Hospital Survey and Construction Act by its two congressional supporters, Hill and Burton, to provide construction funds for the development of community hospitals and nursing homes throughout the nation.

**home- and community-based services (HCBS)**—An optional Medicaid benefit that allows states to design and implement services at a community level to deter or prevent more costly institutionalization for vulnerable populations.

**home health agency**—A public or private organization that provides skilled nursing and other therapeutic services in the patient's home and that meets certain conditions to ensure the health and safety of the individual.

**home health care or services**—Personal care, housekeeping, and chore services or health services provided in a patient's home. These services are furnished under a plan established and periodically reviewed by a physician and may include part-time or intermittent skilled nursing care; physical, occupational, or speech therapy; medical social services; medical supplies and appliances (other than drugs and biological); home health aide services; and services of interns and residents.

**horizontal integration**—Focuses on the development of a continuum of care, from health promotion to inpatient acute care to long-term and palliative care.

**hospice**—A public agency or private organization that is primarily engaged in providing pain relief, symptom management, and supportive services to patients who are certified to be terminally ill.

**hospital authority**—A provision in some state statutes whereby hospitals that were once part of a governmental system (state or local) may be relieved of burdensome governmental requirements for such functions as human resources administration and purchasing to increase their efficiency.

**hospital diploma nursing program**—One of the first educational processes for creating the registered nurse workforce. Nurses train in an on-the-job setting in inpatient hospitals, generally for a three-year period, and are then prepared to take their licensure exams for the profession.

**hospital insurance (HI)**—An insurance program (also known as Medicare Part A) that provides basic protection against the costs of hospital and related posthospital services for individuals who are age 65 or over and are eligible for retirement benefits under the Social Security or Railroad Retirement Systems, for individuals under age 65 who have been entitled for at least 24 months to disability benefits under the same systems, and for certain other individuals who are medically determined to have end-stage renal disease and are covered by the Social Security or Railroad Retirement Systems.

**hospitalist**—A physician, often a specialist in internal medicine, who focuses on the inpatient care of patients hospitalized by his or her practice group or managed care plan.

**hospital joint ventures**—Organizational and financial initiatives that link two or more hospitals for the provision of specific services.

**hospital mergers**—A movement, especially evident during the mid-1990s, in which individual hospitals or systems merged with others in order to protect and expand market share and maintain a competitive edge in a volatile industry.

**hospital planning councils**—Entities in the 1960s and 1970s that worked together to rationalize the acquisition of health care technology and the offering of services in an effort to avoid unnecessary duplication.

**hospital service contract**—An early form of health insurance in which the insurer guarantees payment for services provided to its subscribers directly to the hospital, and the payment often covered the full bill.

**Hospital Survey and Construction Act of 1946**—See *Hill-Burton program.*

**hospital system**—The organization of a number of hospitals, from several to many, into a system that provides direction and administrative services from a central office. Hospital systems can be regional or national in scope and can be structured as proprietary or not-for-profit.

**human genome research**—The study of the approximately 35,000 genes that humans possess, including the actions of single genes and the interactions of multiple genes with each other and with their environment.

**hybrid organization**—The result of the evolution going on among the various models of managed care. Once clear-cut and pristine models of care are metamorphosing into new variants as organizations focus on survival.

**I**

**iatrogenic illness**—An illness that results from the treatment received, such as a drug interaction.

**illness**—A relative term, generally used in the lay community, to represent an individual response to a set of psychologic and physiologic stimuli.

**indemnity health insurance**—A type of health insurance contract in which the insurer pays, usually on a fee-for-service basis, for care received up to a fixed amount per episode of illness.

**independent practice association (IPA)**—A type of HMO where the organization contracts with independent physician practices to provide healthcare for the enrollees. Providers are usually paid on a fee-for-service basis.

**Indian Health Services (IHS)**—The federal governmental unit, now located within the U.S. Department of Health and Human Services, that is responsible for the provision of or payment for care to certain indigenous populations who are entitled to this care by treaty rights.

**Indian Self-Determination Act of 1975**—Legislation that permitted American Indian and Alaska Native tribes, villages, pueblos, and other organizational units to directly manage resources to provide health and other services, rather than have services provided to them by federal governmental units.

**indirect medical education (IME) payments**—Payments made by Medicare to compensate teaching hospitals for the proportion of their higher costs due to increased diagnostic testing, greater number of procedures performed, higher staffing ratios, and increased record keeping associated with the educational process.

**individual health insurance policy**—Persons who are self-employed, unemployed, or do not have access to group health insurance coverage may, if they have the resources, purchase individual insurance policies. Such policies are likely to be much more limited in coverage and more expensive to obtain than is group health insurance.

**informal caregivers**—In the context of providing long-term care, those family members and friends who care for a patient in a home setting in the absence of the provision of care by trained providers.

**Institute of Medicine (IOM)**—A unit of the National Academy of Sciences that convenes expert panels to study and report on topical health services issues.

**instrumental activities of daily living (IADLs)**—A functional assessment scale that measures the ability of individuals to function independently by determining their ability to perform such activities as using the telephone, doing light housework, and managing money.

**insurance vouchers**—Similar to educational and other vouchers, insurance vouchers can be provided by an employer to employees, permitting employees to choose the level of insurance coverage they wish. A standard voucher amount is generally offered; all employees are then responsible for securing their own coverage.

**integrated delivery network system**—Integration of a variety of health services organizations to deliver a broad array of health services across the continuum of care in a cost-effective manner.

**integrated health care network**—A system of care in which hospitals, physicians' offices, and other types of services delivery (laboratory, X-ray, rehabilitation, and other services) are offered through a single entry point.

**Intermediate Care Facilities for the Mentally Retarded (ICFMR)**—Optional Medicaid service that provides residential care and services for individuals with developmental disabilities.

**international medical graduate (IMG)**—Formerly referred to as foreign medical graduates (FMGs), IMGs are physicians trained in medical schools outside the United States who seek graduate medical education (specialty training) in the United States. About one-quarter of the current U.S. physician workforce is composed of IMGs.

**Internet pharmacies**—Online pharmacies that sell prescription drugs at reduced prices, often with less regulatory oversight than would occur in a standard pharmacy, where only licensed pharmacists can dispense prescription drugs. Such pharmacies may vary in their requirements for a physician's prescription for such drugs.

**investigational device exemption**—Part of the review and approval process for device manufacturers seeking Food and Drug Administration approval (see Figure 10.3).

**investigational new drug (IND)**—A designation awarded by the Food and Drug Administration as one step in the prospective approval of a new drug (see Figure 10.3).

**investor-owned hospitals**—For-profit or proprietary hospitals. Investors expect a return on their investment in the form of dividends paid on stock holdings.

## J

**Jackson Hole group**—An organization of policy, economic, and health services leaders who meet periodically (initially in Jackson Hole, Wyoming) to deliberate on such issues as managed competition and to suggest changes in U.S. health services policy.

## L

**leveraged buyout (LBO)**—A type of facility (or other asset) acquisition used in the era of facility mergers and consolidations. Under an LBO, control of one corporation is purchased by another with substantial amounts of debt financing and the elimination of publicly held equity.

**life expectancy**—The average number of years of life remaining to a person at a particular age, based on a given set of age-specific death rates—generally, the mortality conditions in the period mentioned. May be determined by race, sex, or other characteristics.

**Longshoremen and Harbor Workers' Act**—A type of workers' compensation legislation enacted to protect maritime workers other than seamen.

**long-term care (LTC)**—Services that address the health, social, and personal care needs of individuals who have never developed or have lost the capacity for self-care on a permanent or intermittent basis.

**long-term care (LTC) insurance**—A type of insurance policy, usually an individual policy, that provides specified coverage for certain types of long-term care services, including nursing home care.

**loss leader**—An insurance term in which one line of business may be offered, even if it is marginally profitable or even unprofitable, in order to have available a full array of business lines. The theory is that a loss-leader line may attract a buyer, who then can be approached about purchasing other lines of business.

**loss ratio**—The ratio of premium received to benefit paid out by an insurer.

## M

**magnetic resonance imaging (MRI)**—One of several advances in the ability to "see" the human body from cross-sectional and other perspectives in order to better diagnose and treat disease.

**mail-order pharmacy**—Pharmaceutical services that provide prescription and other drugs to a purchaser by mail. This provides convenience to the user, particularly those with chronic diseases who take multiple medications.

**malpractice**—An incorrect or wrong medical intervention that results in an adverse event, ranging from a temporary injury to death, to a patient.

**managed care**—An umbrella term for a variety of health plans, each of which at some level integrates the financing and delivery of care to an enrolled population.

**managed care organization (MCO)**—An entity that provides or contracts for managed care. These include entities such as HMOs and PPOs.

**managed competition**—A purchasing strategy to obtain maximum value for both consumers and employers. A purchasing agent purchases coverage for a large group of subscribers and, in doing so, structures and adjusts the market to overcome attempts by insurers to avoid price competition.

**managed mental health services**—The provision of mental health services, often in a carve-out plan that separates them from the provision of other health services.

**management services organization (MSO)**—Organizations that buy the physical assets of their participating physicians, provide administrative services, and negotiate with managed care firms.

**mandated health insurance benefits**—The list of health benefits, maintained by the states' insurance commission, that the state's legislature mandates be included in any health insurance policy offered in the state. The offering of health insurance is controlled at the state government level. Most states have established insurance commissions that specify what an insurer must do, including the type(s) of plans that can be offered, in order to do business in that state. Self-funded insurers are exempt from the requirement to offer mandated benefits.

**maximum lifetime benefits**—The specification by an insurer of the total amount it will pay out to insured individuals over their lifetime. Insured individuals who experience a catastrophic event or a costly illness may be at risk of exceeding their lifetime benefit—in which case, the insurance policy could be cancelled. These uninsured individuals then might have difficulty obtaining other insurance because of a preexisting condition.

**McCarran-Ferguson Act**—The 1945 legislation that delegated the regulation of health insurance to states.

**means test**—An evaluation of an individual's economic circumstances in order to determine eligibility for certain governmental benefits. Medicaid employs a means test to determine whether an individual has too much income and/or assets to qualify for Medicaid services.

**Medicaid**—A joint federal/state entitlement program that pays for medical care on behalf of certain groups of low-income persons. Enacted in 1965 under Title XIX of the Social Security Act.

**Medicaid optional services**—All states that participate in the Medicaid program must offer a standard set of services to eligible populations, including inpatient and outpatient hospital services, physician services, laboratory and X-ray, and other specified services. Medicaid programs may also offer a wide range of optional services, including prescription drug coverage, and receive the same federal matching funds that they receive for required services.

**Medicaid waiver programs**—Medicaid law requires that Medicaid programs provide the same set of services on a statewide basis. If a Medicaid program identifies a special population that would benefit from a specific set of services available only to them and not the at-large group of Medicaid beneficiaries, it may request a waiver from the Centers for Medicare and Medicaid Services, requesting permission to offer a unique set of services to a subset of the population (e.g., a waiver to offer specific services to a group of Medicaid eligibles with traumatic brain injury).

**medical device**—Any item promoted for a medical purpose that does not rely on a chemical action to achieve its desired results.

**medical-industrial complex**—A term coined in the early 1970s to describe a health services system that was shifting from a cottage industry to an increasingly complex and commercial set of businesses.

**medical inflation**—The rate of inflation specifically linked to the medical market basket of goods and services. Medical inflation outpaces general inflation in most years.

**Medical Information Bureau**—An organization that centralizes and maintains data on negative answers to health screening questions asked on health and life insurance applications. Such data are then available to insurers as they make determinations about preexisting conditions.

**medically indigent**—Persons who, by virtue of limited economic means, are unable to pay for needed health services.

**medically needy**—Persons who meet Medicaid's categorical definition(s) of eligibility but who, at the present time, may have assets and/or income that exceed Medicaid's standards. Such individuals may spend-down their assets or income on the provision of health services in order to qualify for Medicaid.

**medically underserved area (MUA)**—One of several federal designations used to encourage health providers (through the provision of various incentives) to practice in such areas.

**medical practice act**—The generic name for the statute that most states have enacted to cover the licensure and practice of physicians, including osteopathic physicians, in that state.

**medical savings accounts**—A type of health insurance plan in which an insured may choose to have before-tax dollars placed into an account, to cover anticipated medical costs or to cover only catastrophic events. Medical savings accounts may be a complement to an existing insurance policy or serve as an individual's sole coverage. See *health savings accounts*.

**medical screening**—The requirement for individuals seeking health insurance to undergo a physical exam to determine their level of health risk, which will influence the amount of premium to be paid.

**Medicare**—A national program that provides health insurance protection to people 65 years of age and over, people entitled to Social Security disability payments for two years or more, and people with end-stage renal disease regardless of income. It consists of two separate but coordinated programs: hospital insurance (Part A), which is available to all beneficiaries, and supplementary medical insurance (Part B), which is optional coverage that Medicare beneficiaries may purchase.

**Medicare Catastrophic Care Act of 1988**—The act that expanded Medicare's services, including the addition of a prescription drug benefit. Many Medicare beneficiaries, however, were upset by certain provisions of the act. In the following year, Congress repealed parts of the act that were objectionable to some Medicare beneficiaries, and the prescription coverage was among those repealed provisions.

**Medicare+Choice plans**—Managed care plans established for Medicare beneficiaries by the 1997 Balanced Budget Act.

**Medicare hospital insurance (Part A)**—This coverage is available to all who qualify for Medicare benefits. It covers inpatient hospitalization, home health care, skilled nursing care, and hospice care. Beneficiaries pay a deductible. The number of inpatient days per hospitalization is limited to 60.

**Medicare Hospital Trust Fund**—The financing mechanism for the provision of inpatient hospital services. Both employers and employees pay into this fund because Medicare was established as a pay-as-you-go program. This fund is projected to go bankrupt sometime in the early part of the twenty-first century because the number of workers contributing to the fund will be a fraction of the number contributing when the fund was established, and the number of beneficiaries drawing from the fund will be the highest ever, with the baby boomers coming of Medicare age.

**Medicare/Medicaid facility certification**—A requirement by Medicare and Medicaid that services for which they reimburse must be provided in a health care facility that has been certified to meet their quality of care standards.

**Medicare Payment Advisory Commission (MedPAC)**—A national body that establishes and periodically reviews provider payment for the treatment of Medicare beneficiaries.

**Medicare Physician Payment Reform Program (PPRC)**—The body appointed to advise on payment for physician services to Medicare beneficiaries. The PPRC implemented and monitors the Resource-Based Relative Value Scale (RBRVS) for physician payment.

**Medicare Prescription Drug Improvement and Modernization Act of 2003 (MMA)**—Legislation that established outpatient prescription drug coverage for qualifying Medicare beneficiaries, starting January 1, 2006. This legislation also authorized other health-related programs and products, including health savings accounts.

**Medicare prospective payment system (PPS)**—Medicare in 1983 instituted a prospective payment system for hospitals, using a payment schedule based on diagnostic related groups (DRGs). Medicare established this system as one way to curtail the hospital's ability to shift costs of nonpaying patients to Medicare by billing Medicare for more than its fair share of costs.

**Medicare risk-sharing HMOs**—An early form of Medicare demonstration in which providers who accepted Medicare's payment for its beneficiaries were at risk to provide all needed services, even if the cost of doing so exceeded the agreed-to payment.

**Medicare SELECT**—A supplemental type of Medicare policy that functions like a preferred provider organization (PPO).

**Medicare supplementary medical insurance (Part B)**—The optional part of Medicare insurance. Beneficiaries may purchase this coverage for physician and outpatient care.

**Medicare trust funds**—The mechanisms whereby employer and employee contributions to Medicare are collected and reserved for the payment of services to Medicare beneficiaries. Because these trust funds were organized as a pay-as-you-go mechanism, and the number of workers that support each beneficiary is decreasing over time, the viability of these trust funds is periodically called into question, particularly in times of economic downturn.

**Medigap policies**—See *Medisup policies*.

**Medisup policies**—A range of ten types of private insurance policies that Medicare beneficiaries may purchase to cover Part B co-insurance, other deductible and premium costs, outpatient prescription drugs, and costs of other health services.

**mental health**—The state of being of an individual with respect to emotional, social, and behavioral maturity. In the U.S. system of care, mental health care remains largely separated from physical (somatic) health care.

**Mental Health Parity Act of 1996—**
Legislation enacted to try to ensure that coverage for mental health services was equivalent to coverage for other health services. The act expired in September 2001. Alternative legislation has not yet been passed.

**mental illness—**Impairment of one's mental health that may be organic in origin or induced by external factors.

**metropolitan statistical area (MSA)—**
A county or group of counties containing at least one city with a population of 50,000 or more plus adjacent counties that are metropolitan in character and are economically and socially integrated with the central city. Established by the U.S. Office of Management and Budget on the advice of the Federal Committee on Metropolitan Statistical Areas.

**midlevel practitioners—**Physician assistants, nurse practitioners, and other types of advanced practice nurses who function at a level below that of the physician but well above that of entry-level health services providers.

**Mountin Report—**A 1945 report on the availability of public health services and departments at the level of local government.

**multi-institutional systems—**Health care systems constituted of a range of like facilities (such as hospitals) that may be dispersed across geographic regions of various sizes.

**multiple-employer trusts (METs)—**A trust established by a sponsor, such as the Chambers of Commerce, that brings together a number of small, unrelated employers and businesses for the purpose of providing group medical coverage on an insured or self-funded basis.

**multiple-employer welfare arrangements (MEWAs)—**Arrangements that bring together, under a sponsor, a number of small, unrelated employers for the purpose of providing group medical coverage.

**N**

**National Health Accounts database—**The central repository for national data on health expenditures. Maintained by the Centers for Medicare and Medicaid Services (CMS) within the U.S. Department of Health and Human Services.

**national health insurance (NHI)—**
A countrywide system of health insurance coverage, in which all citizens have access to a basic set of health services; no one is uninsured. Canada has a national health insurance system.

**National Health Interview Survey (NHIS)—**A periodic national survey conducted by the CDC's National Center for Health Statistics that collects data on health status, utilization of services, expenditures, patient satisfaction, and other aspects of the U.S. health services system from a national sample.

**National Health Planning and Resources Development Act (PL 93-641)—**Legislation that established a system of Health Systems Agencies (HSAs), State Health Planning and Development Agencies (SHPDA), and Statewide Health Coordinating Councils (SHCCs) to plan and regulate the health services system. The legislation's intent was to reduce expenditures for unnecessarily duplicative services, but it foundered on issues of territoriality and "me-too" approaches to facility expansion and equipment acquisition.

**National Health Service Corps (NHSC)—**
A federally program established in the early 1970s that provides scholarship assistance or loan forgiveness to certain types of health professions (physicians, nurses, dentists, and pharmacists) in exchange for a specified term of practice in an underserved area. The hope of retaining these health professionals, once they were recruited to an underserved area, has not been realized for most placements.

**National Long-Term Care Survey—**
A periodic survey of long-term care facilities to determine capacity, occupancy, facility ownership, case mix, and other aspects of institutionalized populations.

**National Medical Expenditure Survey (NMES)—**A periodic survey conducted by the Agency for Healthcare Research and Quality (AHRQ) that provides data on costs of and expenditures for a range of health services, taking into account geographic and other variability.

**National Practitioner Databank—** A database maintained by the Health Resources and Services Administration within the U.S. Department of Health and Human Services that catalogs legal actions brought against physicians for adverse patient events.

**net cost of health insurance expenditures—** The difference between premiums collected and benefits paid out.

**network model HMO—**A network of two or more existing group practices that has contracted to care for the majority of patients enrolled in an HMO plan.

**new drug application (NDA)—**A step in the process of approval for a new drug by the Food and Drug Administration (see Figure 10.3).

**NIH Consensus Development Conference—**A technology assessment process in which the National Institutes of Health convenes an expert panel on an emerging technology or therapy, obtains testimony and evidence about this intervention, and issues a consensus report about the level of acceptability this intervention should receive (from experimental to therapeutic).

**nondurable medical equipment—**Medical supplies, generally of one-time usage.

**nonphysician clinicians (NPC)—**Providers of care, including advanced practice nurses, physician assistants, pharmacists, and many others, who are not trained in medicine (as medical doctors or osteopaths).

**nonphysician providers (NPP)—**See *nonphysician clinicians.*

**nosocomial infection—**An illness or infection contracted in a hospital setting and not the reason for initial hospitalization.

**not-for-profit hospitals—**Hospitals structured as 501(c)(3) organizations under the IRS code. Profits from operation, rather than being returned to shareholders, are reinvested in the organization.

**not-for-profit or nonprofit corporation—** An IRS designation that requires the profits from a 501(c)(3) corporation to be reinvested in the firm rather than disbursed to shareholders.

**"not-in-my-backyard" (NIMBY) position—** A term coined to describe neighborhood resistance to the placement of a facility or service that homeowners believe will devalue their private properties or introduce to their neighborhoods populations that they do not want to encounter (e.g., a community mental health center or group home).

**Nurse Practice Act—**The generic label for state statutes that govern the licensure and practice of the profession of nursing.

**nurse practitioner (NP)—**An advanced practice nurse, sometimes referred to as a midlevel practitioner.

**nursing home—**A generic name for one of several types of institutions that provide residential and medical and nursing care to patients who have, temporarily or permanently, lost their abilities to function independently.

## O

**off-label use—**The use of a prescription drug, either recommended by a clinician or adopted by a patient, for a purpose other than that for which it was specifically approved by the Food and Drug Administration.

**omnibus budget reconciliation act (OBRA)—**The annual budget bill prepared by Congress and signed by the president that specifies how federal funds, including those for health services, are to be allocated for a given year.

**opportunity costs—**The value of the alternative use of resources that was of highest valued but not selected.

**Oregon Death with Dignity Act of 1994—** Legislation in the state of Oregon that permits terminally ill patients to obtain a lethal dose of a prescription drug in order to choose the ending of their lives.

**Oregon Health Plan—**Oregon's expanded Medicaid program designed to increase all uninsured persons' access to a basic set of insured benefits.

**organized delivery system**—A system of care structured to deliver a defined set of services to a particular (and often enrolled) population. The system may be organized as for-profit or not-for-profit.

**orphan drugs**—Prescription drugs that are effective against conditions that affect only a small proportion of the population, usually fewer than 200,000 individuals. The drugs are costly to manufacture, and pharmaceutical companies feel particularly at risk for their production. The federal government may undertake the support of designated orphan drugs to ensure an available supply for the small population that requires them.

**osteopathic physician**—A physician whose training differs in emphasis from that of an allopathic physician. Osteopathic physicians are medical doctors, take the same board examinations, and are usually licensed by the same state entities as are allopathic physicians.

**outcome measurement**—In assessing quality of care, the measurement of the end result of an intervention. Other kinds of quality measurement, using Donebedian's construct, are structural and process measures.

**outcomes research**—A relatively recent field of inquiry that shifts the focus on measuring the quality of care from the structure and process of care to the final result of an intervention.

**outlier review**—The special review of cases of care that exceed the norm for payments set for Medicare's DRG payment system.

**outpatient care**—Medical and other services provided on an ambulatory, non-inpatient basis by a hospital or other qualified facility or supplier, such as a physician's office, mental health clinic, rural health clinic, X-ray mobile unit, or freestanding dialysis unit. Such services include outpatient physical therapy, diagnostic X-ray and laboratory tests, and X-ray or other radiation therapy.

**out-of-pocket payment**—The amount paid directly from personal resources for health services and goods not covered by any insurance plan. This may also include the amounts paid for insurance premiums, deductibles, copayments, and co-insurance.

**outsourcing**—Contracting with outside entities to perform certain organizational functions.

**over-the-counter (OTC) drugs**—Drugs that do not require prescriptions. A number of OTC drugs at one time required prescriptions but have been deemed effective and safe with personal administration.

## P

**palliative care**—Care provided at the end of life, regardless of the patient's age, to ease pain and suffering.

**patent medications**—Prior to the creation of the Food and Drug Administration to regulate the safety and efficacy of medications, substances that were concocted and sold by purveyors who often made outrageous claims in marketing their products.

**patient management categories**—One of several ways to assess patient health status and severity of illness in order to provide appropriate levels of care.

**patient outcome research team (PORT)**—A major program funded by the Agency for Healthcare Research and Quality (AHRQ) to encourage the focus on the outcomes of medical intervention rather than the processes.

**patient satisfaction**—An important measure of quality of care that often focuses on the process of care, which considers the interactions between patient and provider.

**patients' bill of rights**—Proposed legislation that would provide patients a larger role in decisions about their care and would permit them to bring legal action against managed care providers under select circumstances.

**pay for performance (P4P)**—A proposed method of reimbursing providers, based on the extent to which they meet predetermined outcomes for patients. P4P intends to focus on the outcomes more than the processes of care.

**payer of first/last resort**—A person with more than one type of health insurance, in submitting a claim, will generally have a priority order for the companies to which claims are submitted. Governmental insurance programs, such as Medicare, or vendor payment programs, such as Medicaid, are generally the payers of last resort, meaning that the bill must first be submitted to and rejected by other insurers before the governmental programs will consider them for payment.

**peer review organization (PRO)**—The successor to professional standard review organizations (PSROs) and the predecessor to quality improvement organizations (QIOs), Regardless of the name, these organizations have been established under federal law to assure the quality of care provided to Medicare beneficiaries. PROs and QIOs are organized on the basis of state boundaries, though some may include more than one state in their geographic areas.

**personal health care expenditures (PHCE)**—Health services goods and services purchased directly by or for individuals, such as inpatient and outpatient care, physician and other clinical services, prescription drugs, and long-term care. They exclude: public program administration costs, the net cost of private health insurance, research by nonprofit groups and government entities, and the value of new construction put in place for hospitals, nursing homes, and other facilities.

**Personal Responsibility and Work Opportunity Reconciliation Act of 1996 (PL 104-93)**—Often referred to as the Welfare Reform Act, this legislation abolished the Aid to Families with Dependent Children (AFDC) program, replacing it with the Temporary Assistance to Needy Families (TANF) program. Recipients of cash assistance, TANF, and Medicaid are required to obtain employment and to move off of welfare rolls as one way to reduce Medicaid expenditures.

**physician assistant (PA)**—A midlevel practitioner trained in the medical model of providing health services.

**physician-assisted suicide**—Terminally ill patients in the state of Oregon can legally end their lives thought the use of physician-prescribed fatal doses of certain medications.

**physician-hospital organization (PHO)**—A type of health services delivery system in which physicians ally with hospitals to form an integrated system of care. Some such organizations may have bypassed the health insurer as part of the delivery system. This model was seen most frequently in the mid-1990s and is less in evidence today.

**physician-induced demand**—In a health services delivery system in which the patient is dependent on a physician to diagnose, treat, prescribe, hospitalize, and control access to other services, the potential for the physician to have a financial as well as a clinical interest in referring the patient for certain services.

**physician practice variations**—The recognition that physicians practice care in different ways, often related to where they trained, the geographic site in which they practice, and other variables. Different practice in and of itself does not necessarily mean better or worse quality of care is being rendered.

**play or pay**—A slogan popular in the mid-1990s, when pressure was brought to bear on employers who did not provide health insurance for their employees. Proposals were floated that would require employers either to provide health insurance—to play—or to pay into a pool of funds from which insurance coverage could be provided.

**pluralistic health system**—A mix of public- and private-sector resources in the delivery of health services.

**point-of-service (POS) plan**—A health maintenance organization plan that allows its members to use providers not on the organization's rolls. Members must pay an added premium or out-of-pocket expense to access such providers at the point at which service is provided.

**portability of health insurance**—The ability of workers to transfer insurance coverage from one employer to another to avoid any periods in which they are not covered by health insurance.

**potentially ineffective care**—An inappropriate level of services provided to a patient with a terminal and untreatable illness or disorder and who is unlikely to return to a positive health status.

**poverty level**—An income level established by several U.S. governmental agencies that is based on family size and identifies the proportion of the population that may qualify for public assistance and other governmental services because of insufficient income.

**practice profiling**—The examination and delineation of a clinician's patterns of providing care in a managed care setting to encourage the most efficient use of resources.

**practice variations**—The differences in practice patterns among physicians in different geographic areas. Beginning in the 1970s, researchers, led by John Wennberg, began to examine practice variations, trying to determine the extent to which differences in practices of medicine indicated differences in the quality of care provided.

**preadmission screening or review**—The prospective evaluation of proposed elective hospital or nursing home admissions using acceptable medical criteria as the standard for determining the appropriateness of the site or level of care.

**precertification**—The result of a preadmission review process at which time the appropriateness of the procedure is evaluated and a proposed length of stay is assigned (in the case of a hospital), or the patient is assessed and deemed to meet the admissions criteria for a nursing home or other long-term care facility.

**preexisting condition**—A physical or mental condition for which an individual has been/is being diagnosed and treated that may preclude coverage by a new health insurance plan for a period of time, or in some cases permanently, because the individual is deemed to be a high risk (likely to have claims for care).

**preferred provider organization (PPO)**—An arrangement between a provider network and a health insurer or self-insured employer where providers accept payments less than traditional fee-for-service payments in return for a potentially greater share of the patient market. PPO enrollees are not required to use the preferred providers but are given financial incentives, such as reduced co-insurance and deductibles, to do so. Providers do not accept the financial risk for the management of care.

**premium**—A periodic, often monthly, fee paid by insurance enrollees (including Medicare) for their coverage. Employers who sponsor health insurance typically pay part of the premium.

**premium support**—A concept under discussion for the Medicare program in which Medicare, instead of paying for hospital and physician services, would provide to beneficiaries a fixed amount that they could use to pay for the premium of the health plan they chose.

**prepaid group practice (PGP)**—One of the earliest forms of managed care in which physicians, either of like specialty or of mixed specialties, offered their services to patients from a central location. Facilities and expenses were shared, common billing was used, referral among the group was important, and the intent was to provide one-stop shopping for the consumer.

**prepaid health plan (PHP)**—A type of insurance coverage in which a specific set of benefits is provided to an enrolled population for an agreed-to-in-advance payment, regardless of the amount of covered services an enrolled individual uses in a specific period.

**price**—Used in the noneconomic sense of the word to designate the charge for a service (such as an inpatient hospitalization) as opposed to the cost of providing this service.

**primary care**—Basic or general care, traditionally provided by family practice, pediatric, and internal medicine providers.

**primary disease prevention**—An intervention that reduces the risk of developing a disease or disorder.

**prior authorization**—The requirement by some insurers that prior authorization be obtained from a designated source before certain services or procedures are incurred. Failure to obtain this authorization may result in an insurance claim being only partially reimbursed or denied payment altogether.

**private health insurance**—May be group insurance or individually purchased insurance. Private insurance is distinguished from public or social health insurance, which is governmentally sponsored (e.g., Medicare).

**private sector**—The commercial, free-enterprise part of a political-economic system such as prevails in the United States.

**process measures**—A quality of care measure that studies the interactions between a care provider and a patient, looking particularly at the effectiveness of the communication that occurs.

**Producer Price Index for Prescription Drugs (PPI-DRUGS)**—A report prepared by the Bureau of Labor Statistics that reports drug price statistics.

**professional standards review organization (PSRO)**—The antecedent organization to the peer review organizations (PRO) and the quality improvement organization (QIO). PSROs were financed by Medicare and charged with monitoring the quality of inpatient care for Medicare beneficiaries.

**Program of All-Inclusive Care for the Elderly (PACE)**—A demonstration program sponsored by the Centers for Medicare and Medicaid Services (CMS) that incorporates the provision of medical, health, and social services to frail elders in an effort to keep them in independent, noninstitutional settings as long as possible.

**proposed rule making**—An early step in the development and issuance of regulations. At the federal level, a notice of proposed rule making is issued in the *Federal Register*.

**proprietary health organization**—A for-profit organization with shareholders who expect a return on their investments.

**proprietary hospital**—A hospital organized as a for-profit entity with shareholders.

**Prospective Payment Assessment Commission (PROPAC)**—The predecessor organization to the Medicare Payment Advisory Commission (MedPAC), with responsibilities for setting Medicare provider payment rates.

**prospective payment system (PPS)**—A reimbursement system whereby Medicare payment for inpatient services is made at a predetermined specific rate for each diagnosis, rather than on a reasonable-cost basis. Discharges are classified according to a list of diagnosis-related groups (DRGs). Rates exclude direct medical education costs, cost of bad debts for deductibles and co-insurance incurred by beneficiaries, and kidney acquisition costs, which continue to be reimbursed under a reasonable-cost-based system.

**provider assignment**—Physicians who agree to accept Medicare reimbursement as payment in full for their services and do not extra bill (i.e., bill the beneficiary for the amount of their charge that Medicare does not pay).

**provider service network (PSN)**—A service network that is operated by providers and that is funded in part by the capital contributions of its members. A PSN is designed to operate like an HMO but is exempt from being regulated as an insurance company.

**provider-sponsored organization (PSO)**—A type of managed care organization in which coalitions of providers, such as physicians and hospitals, organize, finance, and deliver care, often bypassing the health insurance system.

**public hospital**—A governmentally supported hospital, at the federal, state, or local level.

**public sector**—In a pluralistic health services system such as that of the United States, a public, or governmental sector exists, as does a private or commercial nongovernmental sector. The balance between the two sectors in the United States continues to shift toward the public sector.

**public/social health insurance**—Governmentally sponsored and supported health insurance. Medicare is the prime example of social health insurance.

**purchasing alliances**—Coalitions of providers that form for the purpose of achieving economies of scale by purchasing goods and services in volume and redistributing them at cost to the alliance members.

# Q

**Qualified Medicare Beneficiary (QMB)**—A low-income beneficiary who qualifies for some Medicaid services, based on 1988 amendments to Title XVIII, but who is not entitled to Medicaid prescription drug coverage.

**quality**—The degree to which health services for individuals and populations increase the likelihood of desired health outcomes and are consistent with current knowledge.

**quality-adjusted life years (QALYs)**—A measure of health status that takes into account not only life expectancy but also the quality of life of remaining years for an individual or a population.

**quality assessment**—Determining the extent to which an intervention or health service provides a certain level of quality of care.

**quality assurance**—A review process intended to ascertain that a certain level of quality of care results from an intervention or health service.

**quality of care**—The degree to which the process of medical care increases the probability of outcomes desired by patients and reduces the probability of undesired outcomes, given the state of medical knowledge.

**quality improvement**—A process of continuous review of the outcomes of an intervention or health service to provide evidence for needed change and to facilitate that change. Continuous quality improvement (CQI) does not blame or sanction; rather, it works toward refinement and improvement.

**quality improvement organizations (QIOs)**—Medicare-supported agencies to assess the quality of care received by Medicare beneficiaries, often through the support of research into the quality of care for specific diagnoses or conditions. QIOs formerly were called peer review organizations (PROs).

**quality of life**—The degree to which individuals can function with the level of independence possible for their health status and other circumstances.

**quasi-governmental organizations**—Organizations that perform a function of government, whether oversight or regulatory, but are not in and of themselves governmental organizations. Quality improvement organizations (QIOs) are examples of such organizations.

**quaternary care**—Advanced levels of high-technology services, such as burn units or other specialty care, usually offered by academic health centers or other teaching facilities.

# R

**RAND Health Insurance Experiment (HIE)**—A seminal health services research study funded in the late 1970s through the mid-1980s to examine the effects of cost sharing on care-seeking behavior and to compare costs and utilization between conventional fee-for-service and managed care plans.

**randomized clinical (controlled) trial (RCT)**—The current gold standard of research that reduces the potential for the effects of chance on an intervention and its interpretation.

**rationing**—The distribution of limited resources according to predetermined criteria.

**redlining**—A process that insurance companies use to exclude certain geographic areas or certain professions from purchasing health insurance coverage because of higher-than-expected risk.

**reengineering**—Restructuring an organization, including the personnel who work within it, to make it more responsive to current needs and the demand for services.

**regional medical program (RMP)—** A system of 56 federally funded programs developed in the early 1970s to reduce the amount of time between the reporting of research findings and their application at the bedside level. The program focused its efforts on heart disease, cancer, and stroke.

**regulation—**(1) A law or rule imposing government or government-mandated standards and significant economic responsibilities on individuals or organizations outside the government establishment; (2) the process of regulation as carried out by government or mandated agencies through such means as awarding licenses, certificates, and permits; setting or approving prices; setting quality levels; and discouraging discrimination.

**rehabilitative care—**Care provided after a major illness or accident to restore patients to their previous functional level or as close to that as possible. May include physical, speech, and occupational therapy.

**reinsurance—**Acceptance by an insurer (the reinsurer) to cover all or part of the loss underwritten by another insurer.

**reinvention of government initiatives—** A Clinton administration initiative to streamline public functions, reduce paperwork, and reduce the burden of reporting.

**report cards—**A report on the performance of select care indicators for managed care plans, hospitals, physicians, and other health services providers and facilities.

**resource-based relative value scale (RBRVS)—**A Medicare payment scale for physician and outpatient providers that replaced the usual/customary/reasonable scale with one based on weighted values for certain types of services. The RBRVS was intended to reduce inequities that were inherent in the former system, particularly the undervaluing of such physician services as history taking and physical exams, as well as consultations with patients.

**respite care—**Care available for short periods to an impaired person being cared for in a family setting. Respite care allows family members to get temporary relief from the constant demands of caring for an impaired individual.

**retention rate—**The amount of premium the insurer is able to retain as profit after paying out all eligible claims.

**retiree health insurance—**Health insurance benefits provided to qualifying retirees of some large employers that may cover them for services not provided by Medicare or until they become Medicare-eligible.

**retrospective review—**A review of the need for and appropriateness of a health service after it has been incurred. The intent is to provide insight into the quality of care provided and the appropriate use of resources.

**right to die—**The ethical issue of whether and when individuals may choose to end their life when their functional status is compromised or the pain from a terminal condition becomes unmanageable.

**risk—**Uncertainty as to loss. In health services, the loss can be due to the cost of medical treatment and other losses arising from illness.

**risk adjustment—**As used in health insurance, the review of the likely risk that could be incurred over the pool of insured persons and the establishment of a benefit package and premiums that guarantee the insurer a profit margin.

**risk assessment—**Evaluating the risk that certain behaviors or personal choices may have on health status. Also used to describe the evaluation of risk to the provider or an insurer inherent in the provision of health services to a defined population.

**risk factors—**Behaviors or conditions that, based on evidence or theory, are thought to directly influence the level of a specific health problem.

**risk pooling—**Spreading the risk of an adverse event such as an organ transplantation over a large group so that one or more such catastrophic events may be offset by limited or no use of services on the part of the majority of those insured.

**rural primary care hospital (RPCH)—** A type of hospital designation that may provide exemptions from certain licensure and certification requirements or make the hospital eligible for certain financial incentives. An RPCH hospital is a small (often with fewer than 75 beds) rural hospital that provides outpatient and short-term inpatient care needed to stabilize a patient before discharge or transfer to another facility for additional care.

## S

**safe harbor regulations—** Regulations that provide greater flexibility for physicians to refer patients to facilities (such as clinical laboratories) in which they have a financial interest.

**"safety-net" hospital—** Generally, a public hospital that provides care to individuals who are uninsured or underinsured.

**"safety-net" provider—** Typically refers to a hospital or other provider that accepts Medicaid enrollees and provides them a safety net against declining health status.

**"sandwich generation"—** Persons who are raising a family and caring for children at the same time they are providing care for older parents or other older family members who can no longer function independently.

**secondary care—** Specialist-referred care for conditions of a relatively low level of complication and risk. May be provided in an office or hospital and may be diagnostic or therapeutic.

**secondary disease prevention—** An intervention that slows the progress of a disease or disorder.

**second surgical opinion—** Requirement that patients must sometimes obtain a second or even a third consulting opinion for specified nonemergency surgical procedures.

**selection bias—** The tendency of individuals to choose the health insurance plan or other benefit that they anticipate using. If resources are available, the person with the poorest health status will likely choose the richest benefit package. When many individuals do this, the risk that such individuals pose is no longer spread over a larger group but is concentrated in one plan or benefit.

**selective contracting—** Permitting only those entities that meet certain standards to qualify to provide health services to certain populations.

**self-assessed health—** An individual's evaluation of his or her health status, usually as excellent, good, fair, or poor.

**self-funded/self-insured employers—** Employers who sponsor health insurance and who choose to finance and offer a benefit package without using a commercial insurer. Self-funded businesses are exempt from important provisions required by state insurance commissions.

**self-insured business—** A business that arranges for the provision of health benefits to employees without the use of a health insurance company. Self-insured businesses maintain appropriate reserves to pay for these services. They are exempt from many of the provisions that state health insurance commissions mandate of health insurance companies offering services in their states.

**self-referral—** The ability of an individual to identify and successfully arrange to see a provider without the intercession of an intermediary such as a gatekeeper.

**severity of disease—** Recognition that the state or stage of disease differs from one individual to another.

**shared services—** The group purchase of goods or services to take advantage of volume purchasing and lower unit costs.

**Shepherd-Towner Act—** A federal statute in effect from 1921 through 1929 that provided assistance to states to support maternal and child health programs.

**Sherman Act—** One of several major pieces of federal legislation that address antitrust.

**Sickness Impact Profile (SIP)—** One of several instruments to measure the intensity of illness.

**single payer system**—A reimbursement system in which there is a single payer or one dominant payer for all health services. Canada has a single payer system.

**single state agencies**—The requirement as per the Social Security Act that the state designate a single agency to administer or supervise administration of the state's Medicaid plan.

**skilled nursing facilities (SNFs)**—Institutions that have a transfer agreement with one or more participating hospitals, are primarily engaged in providing skilled nursing care and rehabilitative services to inpatients, and meet specific regulatory certification requirements.

**sliding-scale payments**—A fee-for-service payment system structured to permit an individual with limited resources to pay a proportion of the charge in lieu of the full charge.

**social health maintenance organization (SHMO)**—An organization that provides both medical and social services in an integrated delivery system to frail elderly persons.

**Social Security Act (SSA) of 1935 (PL 74-271)**—Federal legislation significant for its many health-related titles, including those for Medicare, Medicaid, and the State Children's Health Insurance Program.

**Social Security Disability Insurance (SSDI)**—The payment of cash support to impaired individuals who meet the Social Security Administration's definition of *disability*, which is more stringent than the definition required by Medicaid and some other programs.

**socioeconomic status (SES)**—The classification of individuals or populations based on income, education, and other measures.

**sole community hospital**—The only general hospital available in a service area. This designation provides some relief from certain Medicare regulatory requirements for hospitals.

**Special Supplemental Nutrition Program for Women, Infants and Children (WIC)**—A program sponsored by the U.S. Department of Agriculture that provides food supplements to low-income mothers and their children.

**spend-down**—The use of income and assets to pay for health services in order to achieve a level of means that makes one eligible for certain social and health services, particularly Medicaid services.

**spousal impoverishment**—A provision of the Medicaid regulations that protects a healthier spouse who is able to remain in a family home from immediate impoverishment when his or her spouse must be moved into a long-term care facility.

**staff model HMO**—A health maintenance organization whose practitioner staff are employees of the health plan and are paid on a salary rather than a fee-for-service basis.

**State Children's Health Insurance Program (SCHIP)**—Title XX of the Social Security Act that supports states in providing health insurance to qualifying children, either through new programs or as part of the state Medicaid program.

**state health insurance commission**—The entity within each state's executive structure that regulates the offering of health insurance plans and HMOs.

**state health insurance programs**—Programs offered by some states to individuals who, because of chronic conditions or other health problems are uninsured and may be considered uninsurable. Individuals must pay premiums and other costs for this coverage.

**State Health Planning and Development Agency (SHPDA)**—One of several organizational entities established by the 1974 National Health Planning and Resources Development Act. SHPDAs were to develop state health plans, using input from all health systems agencies in the state.

**Statewide Health Coordinating Council (SHCC)**—An organizational unit created by the 1974 National Health Planning and

Resources Development Act to oversee the development of the state health plan and to make other planning and regulatory decisions related to health services provided within a state.

**step-down unit**—An intermediate care unit in an inpatient hospital where patients receive skilled or intermediate nursing care while awaiting a bed in a long-term care unit. Often used as a transitional unit as a patient's condition improves or deteriorates.

**structural measures**—The first of three types of measures of quality of care. Structural measures consider such things as the physical plant of a health provider, physical access to these services, and their availability.

**supplemental medical insurance (SMI or Medicare Part B)**—A voluntary insurance program that provides insurance coverage for physician, outpatient hospital, and ambulatory services, and other medical supplies and services to Medicare beneficiaries who elect to enroll under the program in accordance with the provisions of Title XVIII of the Social Security Act. SMI is financed by enrollee premium payments (about 25 percent of the revenues) and general funds appropriated by the federal government (about 75 percent of revenues).

**Supplemental Security Income (SSI)**—A welfare program that provides cash assistance to low-income and disabled persons.

**surgeon general**—The top official of the U.S. Public Health Service.

**swing bed**—A bed in an inpatient hospital that is licensed to be utilized for acute care or for long-term care.

**T**

**Taft-Hartley Act**—One of several pieces of federal legislation that regulate issues of antitrust.

**tax credit**—As it applies to expenditures for health services, would permit an individual or a family to get a refund through the annual income tax filing process if their qualifying expenditures for health services exceeded a set threshold.

**Tax Equity and Fiscal Responsibility Act (TEFRA) of 1982**—The federal law that created the current risk and cost contract provisions under which health plans contract with the Centers for Medicare and Medicaid Services.

**tax expenditures**—A significant loss of revenue to the federal government related to the exemption from taxing of employer-paid health premiums and the deductibility of other health-related expenses.

**teaching hospital**—A tertiary or higher-level hospital, including academic health centers, that participates in the on-site training of physicians and other types of health personnel.

**technology assessment (TA)**—A comprehensive form of policy research that looks at technical, clinical, economic, and social consequences of the introduction and use of technology.

**Temporary Assistance for Needy Families (TANF)**—The program established by the 1996 Personal Responsibility and Work Opportunity Act to replace the welfare program Aid to Families with Dependent Children (AFDC) and to encourage adults on welfare to enter the workforce.

**TennCare**—Tennessee's Medicaid program implemented in the mid-1990s to expand Medicaid eligibility and control costs through the use of managed care plans.

**tertiary care**—Highly specialized care administered to patients who have complicated medical conditions or require high-risk pharmaceutical treatments or surgery by specialists and subspecialists in a setting that houses high-technology and intensive care services.

**tertiary disease prevention**—An intervention that may or may not slow the progress of a complicated disorder or disease but may ameliorate the individual's condition.

**third-party administrators (TPA)**—An individual or firm that provides the record keeping of insurance benefit utilization and may pay claims as well. TPAs may be engaged by businesses with self-funded insurance to help them with the administrative aspects of providing health insurance.

**third-party payer**—A private or governmental insurer that pays a medical provider for care given to a patient.

**tiered benefit design**—A redesign of benefit packages in which the subscriber's cost sharing increases in direct relationship to the extent of choice the subscriber desires. For example, tiered pharmacy benefits may provide a generic drug with little or no copayment, a brand-name drug for which no generic equivalent is available for a midrange copayment, or a brand-name drug for which a generic is available for the highest copayment.

**tier rating**—A type of medical underwriting that stratifies groups according to their members' particular health risks and their industry's claims experience.

**total quality management (TQM)**—An integrated system of assessing the process and the product (outcome) of an intervention and making efforts to improve the quality of both without focusing on sanctions or blame.

**transinstitutionalization**—The movement from one institution (e.g., a mental hospital) to another (e.g., a nursing home).

**transitional medical devices**—Those devices (such as renal dialysis machines) that provide a life-saving service until an organ transplant is available. May also be used to describe devices (such as the Jarvik heart) that serve as a bridge to an as-yet imperfect technology.

**TRICARE**—A system of managed care for military retirees and their dependants. Health services may be provided in military facilities or via contracts with civilian facilities and providers.

**triple option**—An employer who sponsors health insurance may offer three types of plans: indemnity plans, health maintenance organizations, and preferred provider organizations.

**triple threat**—A term used to describe a health services facility that provides patient care, trains health care providers, and serves as a clinical (and sometimes basic science) research center.

**turnover**—The tendency in any health plan for certain parts of the enrolled population to leave the plan and others to come in as new members. Some turnover is due to employers changing the health insurance plans that they provide for their employees.

## U

**unbundled services**—The disaggregation of units of health services so that each can be billed for separately.

**uncompensated care**—See *bad-debt care; charity care.*

**underwriting**—The process by which an insurer tries to determine the risk of insuring an individual or a group. Requiring physical exams before the issuance of a policy is one type of underwriting.

**uninsurable**—A person who, because of genetic heritage, poor health status, or a catastrophic health event, is unable to obtain group or individual health insurance.

**uninsured**—Individuals who possess neither public nor private health insurance.

**United States medical graduate (USMG)**—A U.S. citizen who trains as a physician and graduates from a foreign medical school.

**universal access or universal coverage**—Systems of health services in which all residents have access to services and/or have coverage for a basic package of health benefits.

**urgent care centers**—Freestanding, non-inpatient facilities that provide care for acute and emergent conditions.

**usual, customary, reasonable charge (UCR)**—An outdated form of Medicare reimbursement for physician and other outpatient services, based on charges by other area providers for comparable services.

**utilization management**—A set of techniques used by or on behalf of purchasers of health benefits to manage costs by influencing patient care decision making through case-by-case assessments of the appropriateness of care prior to provision.

**utilization review**—The review of care provided to an individual or a group of individuals to determine its appropriateness and quality.

**utilization of services**—A way to measure which populations are using particular health services (and, by elimination, which populations are not using services).

## V

**vendor payment program**—A program such as Medicaid that pays providers for a specific set of services to beneficiaries.

**vertical integration**—A type of delivery system integration wherein a hospital, for example, extends its reach to capture and control more services that lead to inpatient hospitalization.

**veterans nursing homes**—Long-term care facilities, supported by federal or state governments, that care for military veterans.

**viatical settlements**—The sale, often at a discounted rate, of life insurance policies by policy holders who have terminal illnesses. The purchaser of the policy can then claim the full benefit at the policy's termination point. Persons with AIDS have used this mechanism to help them finance health services when other resources had been exhausted.

**victim blaming**—When adverse health events happen to certain individuals or populations, the tendency to blame those populations for their reduced health status (e.g., smokers having compromised respiratory health).

**virtual integration**—Achieves coordination of health services on a contractual basis without the encumbrance of a large, salaried workforce or hierarchies or bureaucratic structures.

**volume performance standard**—A feature of the 1989 Medicare Physician Payment Reform legislation designed to restrain the annual rate of increase in Medicare physician payments.

**voluntary hospital**—A class of hospital initially supported by voluntary donations rather than tax revenues.

**voluntary sector**—The part of the U.S. health services system that has been organized, usually as not-for-profit entities, to focus on specific health conditions (e.g., heart disease, cancer, lung disease, and birth defects).

**vouchers**—In lieu of providing a health insurance policy, a payer provides a voucher for a fixed amount to all eligible persons to purchase the best health insurance coverage they can find for the face value of the voucher. Beneficiaries desiring more coverage than the value of the voucher must pay for the additional costs out of pocket.

## W

**Washington Basic Health Plan**—A health insurance plan sponsored by the state of Washington that offers a basic set of health benefits to low-income persons who cannot obtain other types of health insurance.

**watchful waiting**—When a course of action about a medical problem is unclear, the physician may engage in "watchful waiting" until circumstances make the course of appropriate intervention clearer.

**Welfare reform**—See *Personal Responsibility and Work Opportunity Reconciliation Act*.

**willing-provider laws**—A focus of state or federal laws or regulations that specifies that any qualified provider who wishes to participate in a health plan cannot automatically be excluded from participation.

**"woodwork" effect**—Describes the unexpected volume of people who emerge "from the woodwork" to take advantage of a service that heretofore had not been available to them. This term has frequently been used to describe the increasing volume of individuals who sought assistance from Medicaid's home- and community-based services once the services became established in a community.

**workers' compensation insurance**—State-developed and sponsored programs that use employer contributions to pay for health services and income loss to persons who are injured on the job.

# BIBLIOGRAPHY

## A

AcademyHealth. 2006. *State of the States: Finding Their Own Way.* Washington, DC: AcademyHealth.

———. 2002. *State of the States.* Washington, DC: AcademyHealth.

Adams, E. K., M. Meiners, and B. Burwell. 1993. "Asset Spend-Down in Nursing Homes." *Medical Care* 31 (1): 1–23.

Aday, L. A., R. Andersen, and G. V. Fleming. 1980. *Health Care in the U.S.: Equitable for Whom?* Thousand Oaks, CA: Sage Publications.

Agency for Health Care Policy and Research. 1994. *Growth in Health Care Expenditures for Children and Adults.* Bethesda, MD: Intramural Research Highlights: NMES, No. 37, AHCPR Pub. No. 94-0136.

Agency for Healthcare Research and Quality. 2001. *Annual Report of the National CPHPS® Benchmarking Database 2000.* Rockville, MD: AHRQ.

———. 2001. "Centers and Topics." [Online information; retrieved 7/15/02.] www.ahrq.gov/clinic/epc/.

Aiken, L. H., and M. E. Gwyther. 1995. "Medicare Funding of Education." *Journal of the American Medical Association* 273 (19): 1528–32.

Aiken, L. H., and M. E. Salmon. 1994. "Health Care Workforce Priorities: What Nursing Should Do Now." *Inquiry* 31 (3): 318–29.

Alliance for Human Reform. 1994. *The Doctor Track.* Washington, DC: AHR.

ALPHA Center. 1994. "New York Adopts Pure Community Rating—Other States Take Incremental Approach." State Initiatives in Health Care Reform, No. 7. New York: ALPHA Center.

Altman, S. H., and M. A. Rodman. 1988. "Halfway Competitive Markets and Ineffective Regulation: The American Health Care System." *Journal of Health Politics, Policy, and Law* 13 (2): 323–29.

American Association of Colleges of Nursing. 2004. "Nursing Shortage Fact Sheet." [Online information; retrieved 1/3/2006.] www.aacn.nche.edu/Media/Backgrounders/shortagefacts.htm.

American College of Healthcare Executives. 2003. "February Fact Sheet." Chicago: ACHE.

American Hospital Association. 2006. *2006 AHA Guide to the Health Care Field.* Chicago: AHA.

———. 1988. *Promoting Health Insurance in the Workplace: State and Local Initiatives to Increase Private Coverage.* Chicago: AHA.

American Medical Association. 2004. "International Medical Graduates: IMGS in the U.S." [Online information; retrieved 1/3/06.] www.ama-assn.org/ama/pub/category/211.html.

———. 1996. "National Institutes of Health Consensus Statement: Cochlear Implants in Adults and Children." *Technology News* 9 (2): 5, 7–8.

American Medical Association Council of Medical Service. 1986. "Quality of Care." *Journal of the American Medical Association* 256: 1032–34.

American Osteopathic Association. 2002. "College of Osteopathic Medicine." [Online information; retrieved 8/26/02.] www.aoa-net.org/students/colleges.htm.

American Public Health Association. 1992. *America's Public Health Report Card.* Washington, DC: APHA.

Anderson, G., R. Heyssel, and R. Dickler. 1993. "Competition vs. Regulation: Its Effect on Hospitals." *Health Affairs* 12 (1): 70–80.

Anderson, G., and J. R. Knickman. 1984. "Patterns of Expenditures among High Utilizers of Medical Care Services." *Medical Care* 22 (2): 143–49.

Anderson, O. W. 1968. *The Uneasy Equilibrium: Public and Private Financing of Health Services in the United States, 1875–1965.* New Haven, CT: College and University Press.

Angell, M. 1990. "Prisoners of Technology: The Case of Nancy Cruzan." *New England Journal of Medicine* 322 (17): 1226–28.

Asch, S. M., E. A. Kerr, J. Keesey, J. L. Adams, C. M. Setodji, S. Malik, and E. A. McGlynn. 2006. "Who Is at Greatest Risk for Receiving Poor-Quality Health Care?" *New England Journal of Medicine* 354 (11): 1147–56.

Association of American Medical Colleges. 1997. *Legislative and Regulatory Update.* Washington, DC: AAMC Office of Governmental Regulations.

Averill, R. F., N. I. Goldfield, M. E. Wynn, T. E. McGuire, R. L. Mullin, L. W. Gregg, and J. A. Bender. 1993. "Design of a Prospective Payment Patient Classification System for Ambulatory Care." *Health Care Financing Review* 15 (1): 71–100.

Ayanian, J. Z., J. S. Weissman, E. C. Schneider, J. A. Ginsburg, and A. M. Zaslavsky. 2000. "Unmet Health Needs of Uninsured Adults in the United States." *Journal of the American Medical Association* 284 (16): 2061–69.

**B**

Baker, D. W., J. J. Sudano, J. M. Albert, E. A. Borawski, and A. Dor. 2002. "Loss of Health Insurance and the Risk for a Decline in Self-Reported Health and Physical Functioning." *Medical Care* 40 (11): 1126–31.

Banta, H. D., and S. B. Thacker. 1990. "The Case for Reassessment of Health Care Technology: Once Is Not Enough."

*Journal of the American Medical Association* 264 (2): 235–40.

Barnes, P. M., E. Powell-Griner, K. McFann, and R. L. Nahin. 2004. "Complementary and Alternative Medicine Use among Adults, United States, 2002." *Advance Data from Vital and Health Statistics, No. 343.* Hyattsville, MD: Centers for Disease Control and Prevention (National Center for Health Statistics).

Barton, P. L., J. Bondy, and J. Glazner. 1993. *Colorado Medicaid Reform Study.* Denver: University of Colorado Health Sciences Center.

Barton P. L., J. Glazner, and C. Poole. 1995. *Final Report: Colorado Medicaid Reform Study, Phase II, Long-Term Care.* Denver, CO: University of Colorado Health Sciences Center.

Bazzoli, G. J. 2004. "The Corporatization of American Hospitals." *Journal of Health Politics, Policy and Law* 29 (4-5): 885–905.

Bazzoli, G. J., L. R. Brewster, G. Liu, and S. Kuo. 2003. "Does U.S. Hospital Capacity Need to Be Expanded?" *Health Affairs* 22 (6): 40–54.

Bazzoli G. J., L. Dynan, D. R. Burns, and R. Lindrooth. 2000. "Is Provider Capitation Working? Effects on Physician-Hospital Integration of Costs of Care." *Medical Care* 38 (3): 311–324.

Bednash, G. 2000. "The Decreasing Supply of Registered Nurses: Inevitable Future or Call to Action?" *Journal of American Medical Association* 283 (22): 2985–87.

Berk, M. L., and A. C. Monheit. 1992. "The Concentration of Health Expenditures: An Update." *Health Affairs* 11 (4): 145–49.

Berwick, D. M. 1996. "Part 5: Payment by Capitation and the Quality of Care." *New England Journal of Medicine* 335 (16): 1227–31.

Biles, B., and L. Simon. 1996. "Academic Health Centers in an Era of Managed Care." *Bulletin of the New York Academy of Medicine* 73: 484–89.

Blaum, C. S., J. Liang, and X. Liu. 1994. "The Relationship of Chronic Diseases and Health Status to the Health Services

Utilization of Older Americans." *Journal of American Geriatrics Society* 42 (10): 1087–93.

Blendon, R. J., M. Brodie, J. M. Benson, D. E. Altman, L. Levit, T. Hoff, and L. Hugick. 1998. "Understanding the Managed Care Backlash." *Health Affairs* 17 (4): 80–94.

Blewett, L. A., and V. Weslowski. 2000. "New Roles for States in Financing Graduate Medical Education: Minnesota's Trust Fund." *Health Affairs* 19 (1): 248–52.

Blocke, M. G., and F. Cournos. 1990. "Mental Health Policy for the 1990s: Tinkering in the Interstices." *Journal of Health Politics, Policy and Law* 15 (2): 387–411.

Blostin, A. P. 2003. "Tiered Hospital Plans. Compensation and Working Conditions Online." [Online information; retrieved 1/2/06.] www.bls.golv/opub/cwc/print/;cm20030715ar01p1.htm.

Blue Cross/Blue Shield Association. 1996. "Kassenbaum-Kennedy Review." (unpublished). Chicago: Blue Cross/Blue Shield Association.

Blumenthal D. 1996. "The Origins of the Quality-of-Care Debate." *New England Journal of Medicine* 335 (15): 1146–49.

Blumenthal, D., E. G. Campbell, and J. S. Weissman. 1997. *Understanding the Social Missions of AHCs.* New York: The Commonwealth Fund.

Blumenthal, D., and G. S. Meyer. 1996. "Academic Health Centers in a Changing Environment." *Health Affairs* 15 (2): 200–15.

———. 1993. "Using Academic Health Centers to Help Avoid Health Care's Next Crisis." *Journal of the American Medical Association* 269 (19): 2548–49.

Booth, A., B. Djulbegovic, B. Guthrie, M. Perleth, D. Sackett, S. Endersly, D. Jenkins, S. Richardson, C. Taylor, T. Dent, and M. Enkin. "What Proportion of Health Care Is Evidence-Based?" Resource Guide. [Online information; retrieved 12/15/05.] www.shef.ac.uk/ scharr/ir/percent.html.

Bowen, B. 1995. "The Practice of Risk Adjustment." *Inquiry* 32 (1): 33–40.

Brennan, T. A. 1996. "What Role for Hospitals in the Health Care Endgame?" *Inquiry* 32 (2): 106–09.

Breslow, L. 1990. "A Health Promotion Primer for the 1990s." *Health Affairs* 9 (2): 6–21.

Brigham and Women's Hospital. 2002. "Facts about Nurse Midwives." [Online information; retrieved 1/3/2006.] http://brighamandwomens.org/midwifery/Patient/facts.asp.

Brook, R. H. 1991. "Health, Health Insurance, and the Uninsured." *Journal of the American Medical Association* 265 (22): 2998–3002.

———. 1989. "Practice Guidelines and Practicing Medicine: Are They Compatible?" *Journal of the American Medical Association* 262 (21): 3027–30.

Brook, R. H., M. R. Chassin, A. Fink, D. H. Solomon, J. Kosecoff, and R. E. Park. 1986. "A Method for the Detailed Assessment of the Appropriateness of Medical Technology." *International Journal of Technology Assessment* 2 (1): 53–63.

Brook, R. H., E. A. McGlynn, and P. D. Cleary. 1996. "Part 2: Measuring Quality of Care." *New England Journal of Medicine* 335 (13): 966–70.

Brook, R. H., and K. N. Williams. 1976. "Effect of Medical Care on the Use of Injections: A Study of the New Mexico Experimental Medical Care Review Organization." *Annals of Internal Medicine* 85 (4): 509–15.

Buerhaus, P. I., and D. O. Staiger. 2000. "Implications of an Aging Registered Nurse Workforce." *Journal of the American Medical Association* 283 (22): 2948–54.

Butler, P. 2000. *ERISA Preemption Primer.* Washington, DC: ALPHA Center and National Academy for State Health Policy.

C

Canadian Institute for Health Care. 2002. "Health Care in Canada 2002." [Online information; retrieved 2/3/03.]

http://secure.cihi.ca/cihiweb/dispPage.
jsp?cw_page=AR_43_E&cw_topic=43.

Carlisle, D. M., B. D. Leake, and M. F. Shapiro. 1995. "Racial and Ethnic Differences in the Use of Invasive Cardiac Procedures among Cardiac Patients in Los Angeles County, 1986 through 1988." *American Journal of Public Health* 85 (3): 352–56.

Center for Health Economic Research. 1994. *The Nation's Health Care: Who Bears the Burden?* Waltham, MA: Center for Health Economic Research.

Centers for Disease Control and Prevention (CDC). 2002. "The National Nursing Home Survey: 1999 Summary." *Vital Health Statistics* 13 (152): 1–116.

Centers for Medicare and Medicaid Services (CMS). 2006. *Medicare and Medicaid Statistical Supplement, 2004.* Baltimore, MD: CMS.

———. 2005. "Highlights—National Health Expenditures 2004." [Online information; retrieved 1/12/2006.] http://cms.hhs.gov/statistics/nhe/historical/highlights.asp.

———. 2005. "Intermediate Care Facilities for the Mentally Retarded (ICFMR)." [Online information; retrieved 1/17/2006.] http://new/cms/hs.gov/CertificationandComplican/09_ICFRMs.asp.

———. 2005. *Medicare and Medicaid Statistical Supplement, 2003.* Pub. No. 03460. Baltimore, MD: CMS.

———. 2005. "Program of All-Inclusive Care for the Elderly (PACE)." [Online information; retrieved 1/9/2006.] www.cms.hhs.gov/PACE/.

———. "Welcome to the State Children's Health Insurance Program." [Online information; retrieved 10/13/05.] www.cms.hhs.gov/schip/about-SCHIP.asp.

———. 2004. *Medicare and Medicaid Statistical Supplement, 2002.* Baltimore, MD: CMS.

———. 2000. "Highlights, National Health Expenditures, 2000." [Online information; retrieved 2/17/03.]

http://cms.hhs.gov/statistics/nhe/historical/highlights.asp.

———. 2000. *Medicare and Medicaid Statistical Supplement 2000.* Pub No. 03424. Baltimore, MD: CMS.

———. 2000. "A Profile of Medicaid, 2000 Chartbook." [Online information; retrieved 3/28/02.] www.cms.gov.

Chaguturu, S., and S. Vallabhaneni. 2005. "Aiding and Abetting—Nursing Crises at Home and Abroad." *New England Journal of Medicine* 353 (17): 1761–63.

Chassin, M. R. 1996. "Part 3: Improving the Quality of Care." *New England Journal of Medicine* 335 (14): 1060–63.

Christakis, N. A., and J. J. Escarce. 1996. "Survival of Medicare Patients after Enrollment in Hospice Programs." *New England Journal of Medicine* 335 (3): 172–78.

Clement, J. P., and M. J. McCue. 1996. "The Performance of Hospital Corporation of America and Healthtrust Hospitals after Leveraged Buyouts." *Medical Care* 34 (7): 672–85.

Cohen, J. J., and E. K. Siegel. 2005. "Academic Medical Centers and Medical Research." *Journal of the American Medical Association* 294 (11): 1367–72.

Cohen, J. W., and W. D. Spector. 1996. "The Effect of Medicaid Reimbursement on Quality of Care in Nursing Homes." *Journal of Health Economics* 15 (1): 23–48.

Cohen, M. A., and A. K. Nanda Kumar. 1997. "The Changing Face of LTC Insurance in 1994: Profiles and Innovations in a Dynamic Market." *Inquiry* 34 (1): 50–61.

Commerce Clearing House Medicare and Medicaid Guide. 1995. "CBO Memorandum on Managed Care and Medicare." Internal Memorandum, Congressional Budget Office, April 26, Paragraph 43, 208.

Committee for the Study of the Future of Public Health of the Institute of Medicine. 1988. *The Future of Public Health.* Washington, DC: National Academy Press.

Commonwealth Fund, The. 2003. *Envisioning the Future of Academic Health Centers.* Pub. No. 600. New York: The Commonwealth Fund.

———. 1995. *Managed Care: The Patient's Perspective.* New York: The Commonwealth Fund.

Congressional Budget Office. 1992. *Economic Implications of Rising Health Care Costs.* Washington, DC: CBO.

———. 1992. *Projections of National Health Expenditures.* Washington, DC: CBO.

Congressional Research Service. 1993. *Medicaid Source Book: Background Data and Analysis (an Update).* Washington, DC: U.S. Government Printing Office.

Cooksey, J. A., K. K. Knapp, S. M. Walton, and J. M. Cultice. 2002. "Challenges to the Pharmacist Profession from Escalating Pharmaceutical Demand." *Health Affairs* 21 (5): 182–88.

Cooper, P. F., and B. S. Schone. 1997. "More Offers, Fewer Takers for Employment-Based Health Insurance: 1987 and 1996." *Health Affairs* 16 (6): 142–49.

Cooper, R. A. 1995. "Perspectives on the Physician Workforce to the Year 2020." *Journal of the American Medical Association* 274 (19): 1534–43.

Cooper, R. A., and S. J. Stoflet. 1996. "Trends in the Education and Practice of Alternative Medicine Clinicians." *Health Affairs* 15 (3): 226–38.

Cornwell, L. J., and A. C. Short. 2001. "Premium Subsidies for Employer-Sponsored Health Coverage: An Emerging State and Local Strategy to Reach the Uninsured." *Issue Brief: Findings from Health Systems Change, No. 47.* Washington, DC: The Center for Studying Health System Change.

Coughlin, T., J. Holahan, and L. Ku. 1994. *Medicaid Since 1980.* Washington, DC: The Urban Press.

Council on Accreditation of Nurse Anesthesia Programs. 2003. "Accredited Nurse Anesthesia Programs." [Online information; retrieved 3/27/03.] www.aana.com/coa/accreditedprograms.asp.

Council on Graduate Medical Education. 1995. *7th Report-COGME 1995 Physician Workforce Funding Recommendations for DHHS Programs.* Rockville, MD: COGME.

Cowan C. A., H. C. Lazenby, A. B. Martin, P. A. McDonnell, A. L. Sensenig, J. M. Stiller, L. S. Whittle, K. A. Kotova, M. A. Zezza, C. S. Donham, A. M. Long, and M. W. Stewart. 1999. "National Health Expenditures, 1998." *Health Care Financing Review* 21 (2): 165–210.

Cuellar, A. E., and P. J. Gertler. 2003. "Trends in Hospital Consolidation: The Formation of Local Systems." *Health Affairs* 22 (6): 77–87.

Culbertson, R. A., L. D. Goode, and R. M. Dickler. 1996. *Organizational Models: Medical School Relationships to the Clinical Enterprise.* Washington, DC: Association of American Medical Colleges.

Cunningham, R. 1997. "Hybrids Take Center Stage as New Phase in Cost War Looms." *Medicine and Health* 51 (14): S1–S4.

Cunningham III, R., and R. M. Cunningham, Jr. 1997. *The Blues: A History of the Blue Cross and Blue Shield System.* Dekalb, IL: Northern Illinois University Press.

**D**

Davies, A. R., and J. E. Ware. 1988. "Involving Consumers in Quality of Care Assessment." *Health Affairs* 7 (1): 33–48.

Davis, K., C. Schoen, and D. R. Sandman. 1996. "The Culture of Managed Care: Implications for Patients." *Bulletin of the NY Academy of Medicine* 73 (1): 173–83.

Davis, K., D. Rowland, D. Altman, K. S. Collins, and C. Morris. 1995. "Health Insurance: The Size and Shape of the Problem." *Inquiry* 32 (2): 196–203.

Delevan, S. M., and S. Z. Koff. 1990. "The Nursing Shortage and Provider Attitudes: A Political Perspective." *Journal of Health Politics, Policy and Law* 11 (1): 62–80.

Deming, W. E. 1986. *Out of Crisis.* Cambridge, MA: Massachusetts Institute of Technology.

Demkovich, L. 1997. "$24 Billion Question: Which Child Health Options Will States Choose?" *State Health Notes* 18 (264): 1, 6.

———. 1997. "CON and Managed Care: Can the Concepts Coexist?" *State Health Notes* 18 (249): 1–2

Desonia, R. A. 2004. "The Promise and the Reality of Long-Term Care Insurance." NHPF Background Paper. Washington, DC: National Health Policy Forum.

diGuiseppi, C., D. Atkins, and S. H. H. Woolf. 1996. *Clinical Preventive Services Report of the U.S. Preventive Services Task Force.* Alexandria, VA: International Medical Publishing.

Donabedian, A. 1989. "The End Results of Health Care: Ernest Codman's Contribution to Quality Assessment and Beyond." *The Milbank Quarterly* 67 (2): 322–61.

———. 1980. *Explorations in Quality Assessment and Monitoring. Vol. I. The Definition of Quality and Approaches to Its Assessment.* Chicago: Health Administration Press.

Drake, D. F. 1997. "Managed Care: A Product of Market Dynamics." *Journal of the American Medical Association* 227 (7): 560–63.

Duffy, S. Q., and D. E. Farley. 1993. "Intermittent Positive Pressure Breathing: Old Technologies Rarely Die." *Provider Studies Research Note #8.* Bethesda, MD: Agency for Health Care Policy and Research.

Dummit, L. A. 2005. "Specialty Hospitals: Can General Hospitals Compete?" *Issue Brief No. 804.* Washington, DC: National Health Policy Forum.

**E**

Eisenberg, J. M. 1994. "If Trickle-Down Physician Workforce Policy Failed, Is the Choice Now Between the Market and Government Regulation?" *Inquiry* 31 (3): 241–49.

Ellwood, P. M., and G. D. Lundberg. 1996. "Managed Care: A Work in Progress." *Journal of the American Medical Association* 276 (13): 1083–86.

Engquist, G., and P. Burns. 2002. "Health Insurance Flexibility and Accountability Initiative: Opportunities and Issues for States." *State Coverage Initiatives Issue Briefs* 3 (2): 1–6. Washington, DC: AcademyHealth.

Enthoven, A. C. 1993. "The History and Principles of Managed Competition." *Health Affairs* 12 (Supplement): 4–48.

———. 1993. "Why Managed Care Has Failed to Contain Health Costs." *Health Affairs* 12 (3): 27–43.

Etheredge, L., and S. B. Jones. 1997. "Consumers, Gag Rules, and Health Plans: Strategies for a Patient-Focused Market." Research Agenda Brief. Washington, DC: The George Washington University.

**F**

Fabini, S. 1996. "Not-for-Profits vs. For-Profits: Reading the Tea Leaves." *Healthcare Trends Reporter* 10 (4): 1–2.

Farley, D. 1985. *Sole Community Hospitals: Are They Different?* Pub. No. 85-3348. Washington, DC: USDHHS/NCHSR.

Faulkner & Gray. 1996. "'Excellence Centers' Bargains Sought." *Medicine and Health* 50 (16): 3.

———. 1996. "FTC Won't Ease Up on Mergers Creating Dominant Nonprofits." *Medicine and Health* 50 (46): 1.

———. 1996. "Interest in PHOs Wanes, Survey Says." *Medicine and Health* 50 (28): 3.

———. 1996. "More Nonprofit Hospital Mergers Predicted in Wake of FTC Defeat." *Medicine and Health* 50 (41): 3.

Feder, J., H. L. Komisar, and M. Niefeld. 2000. "Long-Term Care in the United States: An Overview." *Health Affairs* 19 (3): 40–56.

Fein, R. 1990. "For Profits: A Look at the Bottom Line." *Journal of Public Health Policy* 11 (1): 49–61.

Feldman, R., J. Kralewski, and B. Dowd. 1989. "Health Maintenance Organizations: The Beginning or the End?" *Health Services Research* 24 (2): 191–211.

Feldman, R., D. Wholey, and J. Christianson. 1989. "Economic and Organizational Determinants of HMO Mergers and Failures." *Inquiry* 33 (2): 118–32

Feldstein, P. J., and T. M. Wickizer. 1995. "Analysis of Private Health Insurance Premium Growth Rates: 1985–1992." *Medical Care* 33 (10): 1035–50.

Ferris, T. G., Y. Chang, D. Blumenthal, and S. D. Pearson. 2001. "Leaving Gatekeeping Behind—Effects of Opening Access to Specialists for Adults in a Health Maintenance Organization." *New England Journal of Medicine* 345 (18): 1312–17.

Finnegan, L. P. 1996. "The NIH Women's Health Initiative: Its Evolution and Expected Contributions to Women's Health." *American Journal of Preventive Medicine* 12 (5): 292–93.

Fisher, M. 1989. *Guide to Clinical Preventive Services: An Assessment of the Effectiveness of 169 Interventions.* Baltimore, MD: Williams & Wilkins.

Fleming, M. F., K. L. Barry, L. B. Manwell, K. Johnson, and R. London. 1997. "Brief Physician Advice for Problem Alcohol Drinkers: A Randomized Controlled Trial in Community-Based Primary Care Practices." *Journal of the American Medical Association* 277 (13): 1039–45.

Fletcher, K. E., W. Underwood, S. Q. Davis, R. S. Mangrulkar, L. F. McMahon, and S. Saint. 2005. "Effects of Work Hour Reduction on Residents' Lives: A Systematic Review." *Journal of the American Medical Association* 294 (9): 1088–1100.

Flynn, P. 1994. "COBRA Qualifying Events and Elections, 1987–1991." *Inquiry* 31 (2): 215–20.

Food and Drug Administration. 2006. [Online information; retrieved 1/17/2006.] www.fda.gov/cder/handbook/develop.htm.

Franks, P., C. M. Clancey, and M. R. Gold. 1993. "Health Insurance and Mortality." *Journal of the American Medical Association* 270 (6): 737–41.

Freed, M. J., and J. Grigsby. 2002. "Telemedicine and Remote Patient Monitoring." *Journal of the American Medical Association* 288 (4): 423–25.

Friedlob, A. 1993. "The Use of Physical Restraints in Nursing Homes and the Allocation of Nursing Home Resources." Ph.D. diss., University of Minnesota, Minneapolis.

Fries, B. E. 1992. *Update RUG-III Briefing Document.* Ann Arbor, MI: University of Michigan.

Fries, J. F., C. E. Koop, and C. E Beadle. 1993. "Reducing Health Care Costs by Reducing the Need and Demand for Medical Services." *New England Journal of Medicine* 329 (5): 321–25.

Frist, W. H. 2002. "Federal Funding for Biomedical Research." *Journal of the American Medical Association* 287 (13): 1722–24.

Fuchs, B., and J. A. James. 2005. "Health Savings Accounts: The Fundamentals." NHPF Background Paper. Washington, DC: National Health Policy Forum.

Fuchs, B., M. Merlis, and J. James. 2002. "Expanding Health Coverage for the Uninsured: Fundamentals of the Tax Credit Option." NHPF Background Paper. Washington, DC: National Health Policy Forum.

Fuchs, V. R. 1997. "Managed Care and Merger Mania." *Journal of the American Medical Association* 277 (11): 920–21.

———. 1990. "The Health Sector's Share of the Gross National Product." *Science* 247 (4942): 534–38.

Fuchs, W. R. 1988. "The 'Competition Revolution' in Health Care." *Health Affairs* 7 (3): 5–24.

**G**

Gabel, J. R., H. Whitmore, T. Rice, and A. T. LoSasso. 2004. "Employers' Contradictory Views about Consumer-Driven Health

Care: Results from a National Survey." *Health Affairs Web Exclusive* W4-210, April 21, 2004.

Gallin, J. I., and H. L. Smits. 1997. "Managing the Interface Between Medical Schools, Hospitals, and Clinical Research." *Journal of the American Medical Association* 277 (8): 651–54.

Galvin, R., and A. Milstein. 2002. "Large Employers' New Strategies in Health Care." *New England Journal of Medicine* 374 (12): 939–42.

Galvin, R. S., S. Delbanco, A. Milstein, and G. Belden. 2005. "Has the Leapfrog Group Had an Impact on the Health Care Market?" *Health Affairs* 24 (1): 228–33.

Gaskin, D. J., and J. Hadley. 1997. "The Impact of HMO Penetration on Hospital Cost Inflation, 1985–1993." *Inquiry* 34 (3): 205–16.

Gates, V. S. 2002. *State of the States: State Coverage Initiatives.* Washington, DC: Academy for Health Services Research and Health Policy.

Gauthier, A. K., J. A. Lamphere, and N. L. Barrand. 1995. "Risk Selection in the Health Care Market: A Workshop Overview." *Inquiry* 32 (1): 14–22.

Gauthier, A. K., and D. L. Rogal. 2001. *The Challenge of Managed Care Regulation: Making Markets Work?* Washington, DC: Academy for Health Services Research and Health Policy.

Gebbie, K. M., and R. Merrill. 2001. "Enumerations of the Public Health Workforce: Developing a System." *Journal of Public Health Management and Practice* 9 (60): 440–42.

Gill, T. M., and A. R. Feinstein. 1994. "A Critical Appraisal of Quality-of-Life Measurements." *Journal of the American Medical Association* 272 (8): 619–26.

Ginsburg, P. B. 2001. *Navigating a Changing Health System.* Washington, DC: Center for Studying Health System Change.

Ginsburg, P. D., and J. D. Pickreign. 1997. "Tracking Health Care Costs: An Update." *Health Affairs* 16 (4): 151–55.

Ginzberg, E. 1992. "Physician Supply Policies and Health Reform." *Journal of the American Medical Association* 268 (21): 3115–18.

———. 1990. "High Technology Medicine (HTM) and Rising Health Care Costs." *Journal of the American Medical Association* 263 (13): 1820–22.

———. 1988. "For Profit Medicine: A Reassessment." *New England Journal of Medicine* 319 (12): 757–61.

Ginzberg, E., and M. Ostow. 1997. "Managed Care—A Look Back and a Look Ahead." *New England Journal of Medicine* 336 (14): 1018–20.

Giordano, J., D. Boatwright, S. Stapelton, and L. Huff. 2002. "Blending the Boundaries: Steps Toward an Integration of Complementary and Alternative Medicine into Mainstream Practice. *Journal of Alternative and Complementary Medicine* 8 (6): 897–906.

Glazner, J., W. R. Braithwaite, and S. Hull. 1995. "The Questionable Value of Medical Screening in the Small-Group Health Insurance Market." *Health Affairs* 12 (2): 224–34.

Glenn, K. J. 1989. "Perspectives. Assessing Medical Technology." *McGraw-Hill's Medicine & Health* 43 (22): supplement 4p.

Goff, V. 2004. "Consumer Cost Sharing in Private Health Insurance: On the Threshold of Change." NHPF Issue Brief No. 798. Washington, DC: National Health Policy Forum.

Grady, M. L. 1992. *Summary Report, New Medical Technology: Experimental or State of the Art.* AHCPR Pub. No. 92-0057. Rockville, MD: Agency for Health Care Policy and Research.

Gray, B. H. 1986. *For-Profit Enterprise in Health Care.* Washington, DC: National Academy Press.

Greenberg, J., W. Leutz, and M. Greenlick. 1988. "The Social Health Maintenance Organization Demonstration: Early Experience." *Health Affairs* 7 (3): 66–79.

Greenfield, S., C. E. Lewis, S. H. Kaplan, and M. B. Davidson. 1975. "Peer Review by Criteria Mapping: Criteria for Diabetes

Mellitus." *Annals of Internal Medicine* 83 (6): 761–70.

Griffith, J. R. 1995. *The Well-Managed Health Care Organization*. Chicago: Health Administration Press.

Grob, G. N. 1992. "Mental Health Policy in America: Myths and Realities." *Health Affairs* 11 (3): 7–22.

Grossman, J. M., B. C. Strunk, and R. E. Hurley. 2002. "Reversal of Fortune: Medicare+Choice Collides with Market Forces." Issue Brief No. 52. Washington, DC: Center for Studying Health System Change.

Grumbach, K., S. H. Becker, and E. H. S. Osborn. 1995. "The Challenge of Defining and Counting Generalist Physicians: An Analysis of Physician Masterfile Data." *American Journal of Public Health* 85 (10): 1402–07.

Gudin, M. 1997. "Hospital Report Cards: Pass, Fail, or Incomplete?" *State Health Notes* 18 (254): 1, 6.

## H

Hackey, R. B. 1993. "New Wine in Old Bottles: Certificate of Need Enters the 1990s." *Journal of Health Politics, Policy and Law* 18 (4): 927–35.

Hall, M. A. 1992. "The Political Economies of Health Insurance Market Reform." *Health Affairs* 11 (2): 108–24.

Hall, M. A., and C. J. Conover. 2003. "The Impact of Blue Cross Conversions on Accessibility, Affordability, and the Public Interest." *The Milbank Quarterly* 81(40): 509-42.

Hall, M. A., E. K. Wicks, and J. S. Lawlor. 2001. "HealthMarts, HIPCs, MEWAs, and AHPs: A Guide for the Perplexed." *Health Affairs* 20 (1): 142–53.

Harrington C., C. Cassel, C. L. Estes, S. Woolhandler, and D. U. Himmelstein. 1991. "A National LTC Program for the U.S." *Journal of the American Medical Association* 266 (21): 3023–29.

Harrington C., S. Preston, L. Grant, and A. H. Swan. 1992. "Revised Trends in States' Nursing Home Capacity." *Health Affairs* 11 (2): 170–80.

Havighurst, C. C. 2004. "Star on the Corporatization and Commodification of Health Care: The Sequel." *Journal of Health Politics, Policy, and Law* 29 (4, 5): 947–67.

Health Care Authority. 2003. "Basic Health." [Online information; retrieved 4/21/03.] www.basichealth.hca.wa.gov/ bhhistory.shtml/.

Health Care Financing Administration. 2000. *Medicare and Medicaid Statistical Supplement*. Washington, DC: HCFA.

Health Insurance Association of America (HIAA). 2002. *Source Book of Health Insurance Data 2002*. Washington, DC: HIAA.

———. 1996. *Source Book of Health Insurance Data*. Washington, DC: HIAA.

———. 1992. *Source Book of Health Insurance Data*. Washington, DC: HIAA.

———. 1985. *Source Book of Health Insurance Data*. Washington, DC: HIAA.

Hellinger, F. J. 1995. "Selection Bias in HMOs and PPOs: A Review of the Evidence." *Inquiry* 32 (2): 135–42.

Henderson, T. M. 2000. Medicaid's Role in Financing Graduate Medical Education. *Health Affairs* 19 (1): 221–29.

Hill, L. D., and J. I. Madara. 2005. "Role of the Urban Academic Medical Center in U.S. Health Care." *Journal of the American Medical Association* 294 (17): 2219–20.

Himmelstein, J., and K. Rest. 1996. "Working on Reform: How Workers' Comp Medical Care Is Affected by Health Care Reform." *Public Health Reports* 111 (1): 12–24.

Hirsch, M. 1994. "Health Care of Vulnerable Populations Covered by Medicare and Medicaid." *Health Care Financing Review* 15 (4): 1–5.

Hocker, R. S., and L. E. Berlin. 2002. "Trends in the Supply of Physician Assistants and Nurse Practitioners in the United States." *Health Affairs* 21 (5): 174–81.

Hollingsworth, E. J. 1992. "Falling Through the Cracks: Care of the Chronically Mentally Ill in the U.S., Germany, and the United Kingdom." *Journal of Health Politics, Policy and Law* 17 (4): 899–928.

Hurley, A. C., and L. Voliar. 2002. "Alzheimer's Disease: 'It's OK, Mama, If You Want to Go, It's OK.'" *Journal of the American Medical Association* 288 (18): 2324–31.

Hurley, R. E., D. A. Freund, and J. E. Paul. 1993. *Managed Care in Medicaid: Lessons for Policy and Program Design.* Chicago: Health Administration Press.

Hurley, R. E., B. C. Strunk, and J. S. White. 2004. "The Puzzling Popularity of the PPO." *Health Affairs* 23 (2): 56–68.

**I**

Iglehart, J. K. 2002. "Changing Health Insurance Trends." *New England Journal of Medicine* 347 (12): 956–62.

———. 1996. "The National Committee for Quality Assurance." *New England Journal of Medicine* 335 (13): 995–99.

———. 1995. "Rapid Changes for AMCs. Part 2." *New England Journal of Medicine* 332 (6): 407–11.

———. 1994. "Rapid Changes for AMCs. Part 1." *New England Journal of Medicine* 331 (20): 1392–95.

———. 1992. "The American Health Care System: Private Insurance." *New England Journal of Medicine* 326 (25): 1715–20.

Indian Health Service. 2002. "Indian Health Service Introduction." [Online information; 3/27/03.] www.ihs.gov/PublicInfo/PublicAffairs/Welcome—Info/ThisFacts.asp.

Institute of Medicine. 2002. *Care Without Coverage: Too Little, Too Late.* Washington, DC: National Academy of Sciences Press.

Institute of Medicine. 2002. *Who Will Keep the Public Healthy?* Washington, DC: National Academy of Sciences Press.

Institute of Medicine. 1995. *Primary Care: America's Health in a New Era.* Washington, DC: National Academy Press.

**J**

Jaggar, S. F. 1995. Medicare and Medicaid: Opportunities to Save Program Dollars by Reducing Fraud and Abuse. GAO/

T-HEHS-95-110. Washington, DC: USGAO.

Jones, A. 2002. "The National Nursing Home Survey: 1999 Summary." *Vital Health Statistics* 13 (152): 1–116.

Jones, P. E., and J. F. Cawley. 1994. "Physician's Assistants and Health System Reform." *Journal of the American Medical Association* 271 (16): 1266–72.

**K**

Kahn, K. L., J. Kosecoff, M. R. Chassin, M. F. Flynn, A. Fink, N. Pattaphongse, D. H. Solomon, and R. H. Brook. 1988. "Measuring the Clinical Appropriateness of the Use of a Procedure: Can We Do It?" *Medical Care* 26 (4): 415–22.

Kane, N. M., N. C. Turnbull, and C. Schoen. 1996. *Markets and Plan Performance: Summary Reports on Case Studies of IPA and Network HMOs.* New York: The Commonwealth Fund.

Kane, R. A. 1995. "Expanding the Home Care Concept: Blurring the Distinctions among Home Care, Institutional Care, and Other Long-Term Care Services." *The Milbank Quarterly* (73) 2: 161–86.

Kane, R. L., C. Harrington, and R. Newcomer. 1991. "Social Health Maintenance Organizations' Services, Use, and Costs, 1985–89." *Health Care Financing Review* 12 (3): 37–52.

Kaplan, G. A., and T. Camacho. 1983. "A Nine-Year Follow-Up of the Human Population Laboratory Cohort." *American Journal of Epidemiology* 117 (3): 292–304.

Kassirer, J. P. 1997. "Is Managed Care Here to Stay?" *New England Journal of Medicine* 336 (14): 1013–14.

———. 1995. Managed Care and the Morality of the Marketplace. *New England Journal of Medicine* 333 (1): 50–52.

———. 1995. "Our Ailing Public Hospitals: Cure Them or Close Them?" *New England Journal of Medicine* 333 (20): 1348–49.

———. 1994. "The Use and Abuse of Practice Profiles." *New England Journal of Medicine* 330 (9): 634–35.

Kenney, G., and D. I. Chang. 2004. "The State Children's Health Insurance Program: Successes, Shortcomings, and Challenges." *Health Affairs* 23 (5): 51–62.

Kessler, D. A., S. M. Pape, and D. N. Sundwall. 1987. "The Federal Regulation of Medical Devices." *New England Journal of Medicine* 217 (6): 357–66.

Keyhani, S., M. Diener-West, and N. Powe. 2005. "Do Drug Prices Reflect Development Time and Government Investment?" *Medical Care* 43 (8): 753–62.

Kiplinger's Retirement Report. 2005. "Disappearing Retiree Health Benefits." [Online information; retrieved 1/17/06.] www.kiplinger.com/ retirementreport/ features/Cover_Dec21005_01.html.

Kogan, M. D., G. R. Alexander, M. A. Teitelbaum, B. W. Jack, M. Kotelchuck, and G. Pappas. 1995. "The Effect of Gaps in Health Insurance on Continuity of a Regular Source of Care among Preschool-Aged Children in the United States." *Journal of the American Medical Association* 274 (18): 1429–35.

Kohn, L. T., J. M. Corrigan, and M. S. Donaldson. 2000. *To Err Is Human: Building a Safer Health System.* Washington, DC: National Academy Press.

Kosecoff, J., M. R. Chassin, and A. Fink. 1987. "Obtaining Clinical Data on the Appropriateness of Care in Community Practice." *Journal of the American Medical Association* 258 (18): 2538–42.

Kronick, R. 1991. "Health Insurance, 1979–1989: The Frayed Connection Between Employment and Insurance." *Inquiry* 28 (4): 318–32.

Kudva, G. C., B. T. Collins, and F. R. Dunphy. 2001. "Thalidomide for Malignant Melanoma." *New England Journal of Medicine* 345 (16): 1214–15.

Kuttner, R. 1997. "The Kassenbaum-Kennedy Bill—the Limits of Incrementalism." *New England Journal of Medicine* 337 (1): 64–67

———. 1996. "Columbia/HCA and the Resurgence of the For-Profit Hospital Business (1st part)." *New England Journal of Medicine* 335 (5): 362–76.

## L

Lakdawalla, D., D. P. Goldman, J. Bhattacharya, M. D. Hurd, G. F. Joyce, and C. W. A. Panis. 2003. "Forecasting the Nursing Home Population." *Medical Care* 41 (1): 8–20.

LaRue, A., L Bank, L. Jarvik, and M. Hetland. 1979. "Health in Old Age: How Do Physicians' Ratings and Self-Ratings Compare?" *Journal of Gerontology* 34 (5): 687–91.

Lawrence, D. 2001. "Gatekeeping Reconsidered." *New England Journal of Medicine* 345 (18): 1342–43.

Lawrence, D. M., P. H. Mattingly, and J. M. Ludden. 1997. "Trusting in the Future: The Distinct Advantage of Nonprofit HMOs." *Milbank Quarterly* 75 (1): 5–10.

Leape, L. L. 2002. "Reporting of Adverse Events." *New England Journal of Medicine* 347 (20): 1633–38.

Lee, T. H., and K. Zapert. 2005. "Do High-Deductible Health Plans Threaten Quality of Care? *New England Journal of Medicine* 353(12): 1202–04.

LePlante, M. P., G. E. Hendershot, and A. J. Moss. 1992. "Assistive Technology Devices and Home Accessibility Features: Prevalence, Payment, Need, and Trends." *Advance Data* 217 (September 16): 1–11.

Levit, K., C. Smith, C. Cowan, H. Lazenby, and A. Martin. 2002. "Inflation Spurs Health Spending in 2000." *Health Affairs* 21 (1): 172–81.

Levit, K. R., and C. A. Cowan. 1991. "Businesses, Households, and Governments: Health Care Costs, 1990." *Health Care Financing Review* 12 (2): 83–93.

Levit, K. R., H. C. Lazenby, and L. Sivarajan. 1996. "Health Care Spending in 1994: Slowest in Decades." *Health Affairs* 15 (2): 130–44.

Levit, K. R., G. L. Olin, and S. W. Letsch. 1992. "Americans' Health Insurance

Coverage, 1980–1991." *Health Care Financing Review* 14 (1): 31–57.

Lewin, L. S., T. J. Eckels, and L. B. Miller. 1988. "Setting the Record Straight: The Provision of Uncompensated Care by Not-for-Profit Hospitals." *New England Journal of Medicine* 318 (18): 1212–15.

Lichtveld, M. Y., J. P. Cioffi, E. L. Baker, Jr., K. Gebbie, J. V. Henderson, D. L. Jones, R. F. Kurz, S. Margolis, K. Miner, L. Thielen, and H. Tilson. 2001. "Partnership for Front-Line Success: A Call for a National Action Agenda on Workforce Development. *Journal of Public Health Management and Practice* 7 (4): 1–7.

Light, D. W. 1992. "The Practice and Ethics of Risk-Rated Health Insurance." *Journal of the American Medical Association* 267 (18): 2503–08.

Liska, D. W., N. J. Brennan, and B. K. Bruen. 1998. *State-Level Databook on Health Care Access and Financing,* 3d ed. Washington, DC: Urban Institute.

Litman, T. J. 1997. *Health Politics and Policy,* 3d ed. New York: Delmar.

———. 1992. "Appendix." In *Health Politics and Policy,* 2d edition, by T. J. Litman and L. S. Robins. New York: Delmar Publishers.

Litman, T. J., and L. S. Robins. 1991. *Health Politics and Policy,* 2d ed. New York: Delmar.

Lohr, K. N. 1990. *Medicare: A Strategy for Quality Assurance.* Washington, DC: National Academy Press.

Lohr, K. N., N. A. Vanselow, and D. E. Detmer (eds.). 1996. *The Nation's Physician Workforce: Options for Balancing Supply and Requirements. Summary.* Washington, DC: National Academy Press.

Luce, B. R., and R. E. Brown. 1995. "The Use of Technology Assessment by Hospitals, HMOs, and Third Party Payers in the U.S." *International Journal of Technology Assessment in Health Care* 11 (1): 79–92.

Ludmerer, K. M. 1985. *Learning to Heal— the Development of American Medical Education.* New York: Basic Books

Luft, H. S. 1996. "Compensating for Biased Selection in Health Insurance." *The Milbank Quarterly* 64 (4): 566–91.

———. 1986. "Compensating for Biased Selection in Health Insurance." *The Milbank Quarterly* 64 (4): 566–91.

———. 1981. *Health Maintenance Organizations: Dimensions of Performance.* New York: John Wiley.

———. 1980. "The Relation between Surgical Volume and Mortality: An Exploration of Causal Factors and Alternative Models." *Medical Care* 18 (9): 940–59.

Lurie N., W. G. Manning, and C. Peterson. 1987. "Preventive Care: Do We Practice What We Preach?" *American Journal of Public Health* 77 (7): 801–04.

## M

Maciejewski, M., and M. Chapko. 2002. "Community-Based Outpatient Clinics Improve Access to Care and Patient Satisfaction, HSR&D Evaluation Shows." *Forum* (October): 4, 8.

Mann, J. M., G. A. Melnick, and A. Bamezai. 1997. "A Profile of Uncompensated Hospital Care, 1983–1995." *Health Affairs* 16 (4): 223–32.

Manning, W., A. Leibowitz, G. A. Goldberg, W. H. Rogers, and J. P. Newhouse. 1984. "A Controlled Trial of the Effect of a Prepaid Group Practice on the Use of Services." *New England Journal of Medicine* 310 (23): 1505–10.

Manton, K. G., L. S. Corder, and E. Stallard. 1993. "Estimates of Change in Chronic Disability and Institutional Incidence and Prevalence Rates in the U.S. Elderly Population from the 1982, 1984, and 1989 National Long-Term Care Survey." *Journal of Gerontology* 48 (4): S153–S166.

Marchetta, M., and D. Rogal. 2005. "Health Savings Accounts as a Tool for Market Change." Changes in Health Care Financing & Organization Issue Brief No. 4. Washington, DC: Academy Health.

Matherlee, K. 2002. "Managing Advanced Illness: A Quality and Cost Challenge to Medicare, Medicaid, and Private

Insurers." National Health Policy Forum Issue Brief No. 779. Washington, DC: George Washington University.

May, L. A. 1993. "The Physiologic and Psychological Bases of Health, Disease, and Care Seeking." In *Introduction to Health Services,* 4th ed., edited by S. J. Williams and P. Torrens, 31–45. New York: Delmar.

McCall, N., T. Rice, J. Boismier, and R. West. 1991. "Private Health Insurance and Medical Care Utilization: Evidence from the Medicare Population." *Inquiry* 28 (3): 276–87.

McCormack, L. A., J. R. Gabel, N. D. Berkman, H. Whitmore, K. Hutchinson, W. L. Anderson, J. Pickreign, and N. West. 2002a. "Retiree Health Insurance: Recent Trends and Tomorrow's Prospects." *Health Care Financing Review* 23 (3): 17–34.

McCormack, L. A., J. R. Gabel, H. Whitmore, W. L. Anderson, and J. Pickreign. 2002b. "Trends in Retiree Health Benefits." *Health Affairs* 21 (6): 169–76.

McKinley, J. B. 1981. "From 'Promising Report' to 'Standard Procedure': Seven Stages in the Career of a Medical Innovation." *The Milbank Memorial Fund Quarterly* 59 (3): 374–411.

McLaughlin, C. G., and K. Mortensen. 2003. "Who Walks Through the Door: The Effect of the Uninsured on Hospital Use." *Health Affairs* 22 (6): 143–55.

McNeil, B. J. 2001. "Hidden Barriers to Improvement in the Quality of Care." *New England Journal of Medicine* 345 (22): 1613–20.

Mechanic, D. 1994. "Managed Care: Rhetoric and Realities." *Inquiry* 31 (2): 124–28.

———. 1989. "Medical Sociology: Some Tensions among Theory, Method, and Substance." *Journal of Health and Social Behavior* 30(2):147–60.

———. 1987. "Correcting Misconceptions in Mental Health Policy: Strategies for Improved Care of the Seriously Mentally Ill." *Milbank Quarterly* 65 (2): 203–30.

Mechanic, D., M. Schlesinger, and D. D. McAlpine. 1995. "Management of Mental Health and Substance Abuse Services: State of the Art and Early Results." *Milbank Quarterly* 73 (1): 19–55.

Mechanic, R. E., and A. Dobson. 1996. "The Impact of Managed Care on Clinical Research: A Preliminary Investigation." *Health Affairs* 15 (3): 72–89.

Medical Study News. 2005. "Impact of Medicare Drug Law on Retiree Health Benefits." [Online information; retrieved 12/16/05.] www.news-medical.net/ print_article.asp?id=15005.

Medicine and Health. 2006. "Pay for Performance Not Reaching Small Physician Practices." *Medicine and Health* 60 (2): 1,4. Washington, DC: Health Care Information Center.

Melski, J. W. 1992. "Price of Technology: A Blind Spot." *Journal of the American Medical Association* 267 (11): 1516–18.

Merritt, D. (ed.). 1997. "State Notes Update: Assisted Suicide." *State Health Notes* 18 (259): 3.

Merson, M. H., R. E. Black, and A. J. Mills. 2001. *International Public Health: Diseases, Programs, Systems, and Policies.* Gaithersburg, MD: Aspen Publications.

Meyer, J. A. 1985. *Incentives vs. Controls in Health Policy.* Washington, DC: American Enterprise Institute for Public Policy Research.

Miller, R. H., and H. S. Luft. 2002. "HMO Plan Performance Update: An Analysis of the Literature, 1997–2001." *Health Affairs* 21 (4): 63–86.

———. 1997. "Does Managed Care Lead to a Better or Worse Quality of Care?" *Health Affairs* 16 (5): 7–25.

———. 1994. "Managed Care Plan Performance Since 1980: A Literature Analysis." *Journal of the American Medical Association* 271 (19): 1512–19.

Moloney, T. W., and D. E. Rogers. 1979. "Medical Technology—A Different View of the Contentious Debate over Costs." *New England Journal of Medicine* 301 (26): 1413–19.

Monheit, A. C., and M. L. Berk. 1992. "The Concentration of Health Expenditures: An Update." *Health Affairs* 11 (4): 145–49.

Monheit, A. C., L. M. Nichols, and T. M. Selden. 1996. "How Are Net Health Insurance Benefits Distributed in the Employment-Related Insurance Market?" *Inquiry* 32 (4): 379–91.

Monheit, A. C., and C. L. Schur. 1989. *National Medical Expenditure Survey: Health Insurance Coverage of Retired Persons.* Washington, DC: National Center for Health Services Research.

Moon, M. 1996. *Long-Term Care in the U.S.* New York: The Commonwealth Fund.

Moore, J. 1996. *The Pharmaceutical Industry.* Washington, DC: National Health Policy Forum.

Morrissey, J. P., R. P. Harris, J. Kincade-Norburn, C. McLaughlin, J. M. Garrett, A. M. Jackman, J. S. Stein, C. Lannon, R. J. Schwartz, and D. L. Patrick. 1995. "Medicare Reimbursement for Preventive Care: Changes in Performance of Services, Quality of Life, and Health Care Costs." *Medical Care* 33 (4): 315–31.

Morrissey, M. A., J. Alexander, and L. R. Burns. 1996. "Managed Care and Physician/Hospital Integration." *Health Affairs* 15 (4): 62–73.

Moses, H., E. R. Dorsey, D. H. M. Matheson, and S. O. Their. 2005. "Financial Anatomy of Biomedical Research." *Journal of the American Medical Association* 294 (11): 1333–42.

Moses, H., S. O. Their, D. H. M. Matheson. 2005. "Why Have Academic Medical Centers Survived?" *Journal of the American Medical Association* 293 (12): 1495–1500.

Mullan, F., R. M. Politzer, and C. H. Davis. 1995. "Medical Migration and the Physician Workforce: International Medical Graduates and American Medicine." *Journal of the American Medical Association* 273 (19): 1521–27.

Murtaugh, C. M., P. Kemper, and B. C. Spillman. 1990. "The Risk of Nursing Home Use in Later Life." *Medical Care* 28 (10): 952–62.

**N**

National Association of City and County Health Officials (NACCHO). 2002. "About NACCHO." [Online information; retrieved 8/26/02.] www.nacho.org/about.cfm.

National Association of State Budget Officers. 2004. "The Fiscal Survey of States: April 2004." [Online article or information; retrieved 12/28/05.] www.nasbo.org/publications/fiscsurvey/2004/fsapril2004.pdf.

National Committee on Quality Assurance. 2001. "The State of Managed Care Quality." [Online information; retrieved 7/15/02.] www.ncqa.org/somc2001/.

National Health Policy Forum (NHPF). 2002. "Too Few? Too Many? The Right Kind? Physician Supply in an Aging and Multicultural Society." Washington, DC: NHPF meeting announcement. September 10.

———. 2001. *Reconsidering Medicare+Choice: What Options Remain?* Washington, DC: The George Washington University.

———. 1997. *The Medicare Risk Contract Game: What Rules Should PSOs Play By?* Issue Brief No. 702. Washington, DC: The George Washington University.

———. 1996. *Eligibility for Medicaid in Nursing Homes: Coverage for Indigent or Well-off Older Americans?* Washington, DC: The George Washington University.

———. 1996. *Trends in Health Network Development: Community and Provider Incentives in a Managed Care Environment.* Issue Brief No. 690. Washington, DC: The George Washington University.

National Hospice and Palliative Care Organization. 2003. "NHPCO Facts and Figures." [Online information; retrieved 5/7/03.] www.nhpco.org/public/articles/index.cfm?cat=11.

National Institutes of Health. 2006. "Institutes, Centers, and Officers." [Online information; retrieved 6/3/06.] www.nih.gov/icd.

———. 1998. "Diagnosis and Treatment of Attention Deficit Hyperactivity Disorder (ADHD)." *NIH Consensus Statement* 16 (2): 1–37.

———. 1997. "Management of Hepatitis C." *NIH Consensus Statement* 15 (3): 1–41.

———. 1995. "Physical Activity and Cardiovascular Health." *NIH Consensus Statement* 13 (3): 1–33.

———. 1994. "Optimum Calcium Intake." *Journal of the American Medical Association* 272 (24): 1942–48.

National Viatical Association. 1996. *National Viatical Association Information Booklet.* Washington, DC: National Viatical Association.

Neuman, P. 2004. *The State of Retiree Health Benefits: Historical Trends and Future Uncertainties.* Washington, DC: The Kaiser Family Fund Foundation.

Newcomer, L. N. 1990. "Defining Experimental Therapy: A Third Party Payer's Dilemma." *New England Journal of Medicine* 323 (24): 1702–04.

Newhouse, J. P. 1993. *Free for All? Lessons from the RAND Health Insurance Experiment.* Cambridge: Harvard University Press.

Newschaffer, C. J., and J. A. Schoenman. 1990. "Registered Nurse Shortages: The Road to Appropriate Public Policy." *Health Affairs* 9 (1): 98–106.

Nichols, L. 1996. *Nonphysician Health Care Providers: Uses of Ambulatory Services, Expenditures, and Sources of Payment.* AHCPR Pub. No. 96-0013. National Medical Expenditure Survey Research Findings, 27. Rockville, MD: Public Health Service/Agency for Health Care Policy and Research.

Norton, E. C., and J. P. Newhouse. 1994. "Policy Changes for Public Long-Term Care Insurance." *Journal of the American Medical Association* 271 (19): 1520–24.

O

Oberg, C., and C. Polich. 1988. "Medicaid: Entering the Third Decade." *Health Affairs* 7 (4): 83–96.

O'Donnell, J. W., and J. H. Taylor. 1990. "The Bounds of Charity: The Current Status of the Hospital Property-Tax Exemption." *New England Journal of Medicine* 322 (1): 65–68.

Office of Technology Assessment. 1992. *Does Health Insurance Make a Difference? A Background Paper.* OTA-BP-H-99. Washington, DC: U.S. Government Printing Office.

Okie, S. 2005. "Physician-Assisted Suicide— Oregon and Beyond." *New England Journal of Medicine* 352 (16): 1627–30.

Okpaku, S., A. Silbukin, and C. Schenzler. 1994. "Disability Determinations for Adults with Mental Disorders: Social Security Administration vs. Independent Judgments." *American Journal of Public Health* 84 (11): 1791–95.

Olshanksy, S. J., and A. B. Ault. 1986. "The Fourth Stage of Epidemiologic Transition: The Age of Delayed Degenerative Diseases." *The Milbank Memorial Fund Quarterly* 64: 335–91.

Olson, M. K. 2004. "Explaining Reductions in FDA Drug Review Times: PDUFA Matters." *Health Affairs Web Exclusive.* [Online article; posted 1/30/04.] http://content.healthaffairs.org/cgi/content/full/hlthaff.w4.s1v1/DC1.

Omran, A. R. 1971. "The Epidemiologic Transition." *The Milbank Memorial Fund Quarterly* 49: 509–38.

O'Neil, E., and T. Riley. 1996. "Health Workforce and Education Issues During System Transition." *Health Affairs* 15 (1): 105–12.

P

Park, R. E., A. Fink, R. H. Brook, M. R. Chassin, K. L. Kahn, N. J. Merrick, J. Kosecoff, and D. H. Solomon. 1986. "Physician Ratings of Appropriate Indications for Six Medical and Surgical

Procedures." *American Journal of Public Health* 76 (7): 766–72.

Patrick, D. L., and P. Erickson. 1993. *Health Status and Health Policy.* New York: Oxford University Press.

Pauly, M. V. 1993. "U.S. Health Care Costs: The Untold True Story." *Health Affairs* 12 (3): 152–29.

Peden, E. A., and M. S. Freeland. 1995. "A Historical Analysis of Medical Spending Growth, 1960–1993." *Health Affairs* 14 (2): 235–47.

Penchansky, R., and J. W. Thomas. 1981. "The Concept of Access: Definition and Relationship to Consumer Satisfaction." *Medical Care* 19 (2): 127–40.

Pew Memorial Trust. 1995. *Critical Challenges: Revitalizing the Health Professions for the 21st Century. Third Report.* Philadelphia: Pew Memorial Trust.

Pham, H. H., K. J. Devers, S. Kus, R. Berenson. 2004. "Health Care Market Trends and the Evaluation of Hospitalists and Roles." *Journal of General Internal Medicine* 20: 101–07.

Potter, M. A., and B. B. Longest, Jr. 1994. "The Divergence of Federal and State Policies on the Charitable Tax Exemption of Nonprofit Hospitals." *Journal of Health Politics, Policy, and Law* 19 (2): 393–419.


**R**

Rasell, M. E. 1995. "Cost-Sharing in Health Insurance: A Reexamination." *New England Journal of Medicine* 332 (17): 1164–68.

Reed, M. C., and S. Trude. 2002. "Who Do You Trust? Americans' Perspectives on Health Care, 1997–2001." Tracking Report No. 3. Washington, DC: Center for Studying Health System Change.

Reichard, J. 1997. "Study Says Medigap May Become Unaffordable to Oldest, Sickest." *Medicine and Health* 51 (35): 2.

Reinhardt, U. E. 2003. "Is There Hope for the Uninsured?" *Health Affairs Web Exclusive,* August 27, 2003.

http://content.healthaffairs.org/cgi/reprint/hlthaff.w3.376v1.pdf

———. 1996. "Perspective: Our Obsessive Quest to Gut the Hospital." *Health Affairs* 15 (2): 145–54.

———. 1994. "Planning the Nation's Workforce: Let the Market In." *Inquiry* 31 (3): 250–63.

———. 1993. "Reorganizing the Financial Flows in American Health Care." *Health Affairs* 12 (Supplement): 172–93.

Relman, A. S. 1980. "The New Medical Industrial Complex." *The New England Journal of Medicine* 303 (17): 963–70.

Rettig, R. A. 1994. "Medical Innovation Duels Cost Containment." *Health Affairs* 13 (3): 7–27.

Rivo, M. L., H. L. Mays, and J. Katzoff. 1995. "Managed Health Care: Implications for the Physician Workforce and Medical Education." *Journal of the American Medical Association* 274 (9): 712–15.

Robert Wood Johnson Foundation. 2004. "Kaiser/HRET Employer Benefits Survey as Reported in Robert Wood Johnson Foundation." In *About Coverage: Health Insurance in the United States.* Princeton, N.J.: Robert Wood Johnson Foundation.

———. 2004. *State Coverage Initiatives: About Coverage: Health Insurance in the United States.* Princeton, NJ: Robert Wood Johnson Foundation.

———. 1996. *Chronic Care in America: A 21st Century Challenge.* Princeton, NJ: RWJ Foundation.

Robinson, J. C. 2005. "Health Savings Accounts—The Ownership Society in Health Care." *New England Journal of Medicine* 353 (12): 1199–1202.

———. 2001. "The End of Managed Care." *Journal of the American Medical Association* 285 (20): 2622–78.

———. 1996. "Decline in Hospital Utilization and Cost Inflation under Managed Care in California." *Journal of the American Medical Association* 276 (13): 1060–64.

Robinson, J. C., and L. P. Casalino. 1996. "Vertical Integration and Organizational Networks in Health Care." *Health Affairs* 15 (1): 7–22.

Robinson, J. C., and L. B. Gardner. 1995. "Adverse Selection among Multiple Competing Health Maintenance Organizations." *Medical Care* 33 (12): 1161–75.

Roemer, M. I. 1991. *National Health Systems of the World, Vol. I.* New York: Oxford University Press.

———. 1985. *National Strategies for Health Care Organization: A World Overview.* Chicago: Health Administration Press.

———. 1984. "Analysis of Health Services Systems—A General Approach." In *Reorienting Health Services,* edited by C. O. Pannenborg, A. van der Werff, G. B. Hirsch, and K. Barnard, 47–59. New York: Plenum Press.

Rohrer, J. E. 1987. "The Political Development of the Hill-Burton Program: A Case Study in Distributive Policy." *Journal of Health Politics, Policy, and Law* 12 (1): 137–75.

Rosenblatt, A. 2004. "The Underwriting Cycle: The Rule of Six." *Health Affairs* 23 (6): 103–06.

Rosenstock, I. M. 1974. "Historical Origins of the Health Belief Model." *Health Education Monograph* 2: 344.

Rosenthal, M. B., R. G. Frank, L. Zhonghi, and A. M. Epstein. 2005. "Early Experience with Pay for Performance: From Concept to Practice." *Journal of the American Medical Association* 294 (14): 1788–93.

Ross, J., J. Ratner, and H. Fein. 1991. *U.S. Health Care Spending: Trends, Contributing Factors, and Proposals for Reform.* GAO/HRD 91–102. Washington, DC: USGAO.

Russell, L. B. 1989. *Medicare's New Hospital Payment System: Is It Working?* Washington, DC: The Brookings Institute.

Ryan, J. M. 2002. "SCHIP Turns 5: Taking Stock, Moving Ahead." National Health Policy Forum Issue Brief No. 781. Washington, DC: The George Washington University.

**S**

Salsberg, E. S., and G. J. Forte. 2002. "Trends in the Physician Workforce, 1980–2000." *Health Affairs* 21 (5): 165–81.

Schactman, D., and S. Altman. 1995. *Market Consolidation, Antitrust, and Public Policy in the Health Care Industry.* Princeton, NJ: The Robert Wood Johnson Foundation.

Schactman, D., S. H. Altman, E. Eilat, K. E. Thorpe, and M. Doonan. 2003. "The Outlook for Hospital Spending." *Health Affairs* 22 (6): 12–26.

Schlesinger, M. 1997. "Countervailing Agency: A Strategy of Principled Regulation under Managed Competition." *The Milbank Quarterly* 75 (1): 35–87.

Schlesinger, M. J., B. H. Gray, and K. M. Perreira. 1997. "Medical Professionalism under Managed Care: The Pros and Cons of Utilization Review." *Health Affairs* 16 (1): 106–24.

Schroeder, S. A. 1994. "Managing the U.S. Health Care Workforce: Creating Policy Amidst Uncertainty." *Inquiry* 31 (3): 266–75.

———. 1992. "Physician Supply and the U.S. Medical Marketplace." *Health Affairs* 11 (1): 235–43.

Schroeder, S. A., and L. G. Sandy. 1993. "Specialty Distribution of U.S. Physicians—The Invisible Driver of Health Care Costs." *New England Journal of Medicine* 328 (13): 961–63.

Schwartz, A., P. B. Ginzburg, and L. B. LeRoy. 1993. "Reforming Graduate Medical Education: Summary Report of the Physicians Payment Review Commission." *Journal of the American Medical Association* 270 (9): 1079–82.

Schwartz, W. B., and D. M. Mendelson. 1994. "Eliminating Waste and Inefficiency Can Do Little to Contain Costs." *Health Affairs* 13 (1): 224–38.

———. 1990. "No Evidence of an Emerging Physician Surplus." *Journal of the American Medical Association* 263 (14): 557–60.

Shaneyfelt, T. M. 2001. "Building Bridges to Quality." *Journal of the American Medical Association* 286 (20): 2600–01.

Sheils, J., and R. Haught. 2004. "The Cost of Tax-Exempt Health Benefits in 2004." *Health Affairs Web Exclusive,* W4-106-112, February 25, 2004.

Sheils, J., and P. Hogan. 1999. "Cost of Tax-Exempt Health Benefits in 1998. *Health Affairs* 18 (2): 176–81.

Sherertz, R. J., and S. A. Streed. 1994. "Medical Devices: Significant vs. Nonsignificant Risk." *New England Journal of Medicine* 272 (12): 955–56.

Shonick, W. 1995. *Government and Health Services.* New York: Oxford University Press.

Short, P. F., and T. J. Lair. 1994/95. "Health Insurance and Health Status: Implications for Financing Health Care Reform." *Inquiry* 31 (4): 425–37.

Shortell, S. M. 1997. "Restructuring AHCs: Values, Leadership, and Strategies." Presentation to the Association of Academic Health Centers, Washington, DC. Unpublished.

Shortell, S. M., R. R. Gillies, and D. A. Anderson. 1996. *Remaking Health Care in America: Building Organized Delivery Systems.* San Francisco: Jossey-Bass, Inc.

Shortell, S. M., R. R. Gillies, D. A. Anderson, J. B. Mitchell, and K. L. Morgan. 1993. "Creating Organized Delivery Systems: The Barriers and the Facilitators." *Hospital and Health Services Administration* 38 (4): 447–66.

Shortell, S. M., R. R. Gillies, and K. J. Devers. 1995. "Reinventing the American Hospital." *The Milbank Quarterly* 73 (2): 131–60.

Shortell, S. M., J. L. O'Brien, J. M. Carman, R. W. Foster, E. F. Hughes, H. Boerstler, and E. J. O'Connor. 1995. "Assessing the Impact of Continuous Quality Improvement/Total Quality Management: Concept vs. Implementation." *Health Services Research* 30 (2): 377–401.

Siegel, B. 1996. *Public Hospitals— A Prescription for Survival.* New York: Commonwealth Fund.

Siu, A. L., E. A. McGlynn, H. Morgenstern, and R. H. Brook. 1991. "A Fair Approach to Comparing Quality of Care." *Health Affairs* 10 (2): 62–75.

Smith, B. M., and S. Rosenbaum. 1999. "Potential Effects of the 'Premium Support' Proposal on the Security of Medicare." *New England Journal of Medicine* 282 (10): 1760–63.

Sochalski, J. 2002. "Nursing Shortage Redux: Turning the Corner on an Enduring Problem." *Health Affairs* 21 (5): 157–73.

Spilker, B. A. 2002. "The Drug Development and Approval Process." [Online information; retrieved 4/1/03.] www.pharma.org/newmedicines/newmedsdb/phases.pdf.

Spillman, B. C. 2004. "Changes in Elderly Disability Rates and the Implications for Health Care Utilization and Cost." *The Milbank Quarterly* 82 (1): 157–94.

———. 1992. "The Impact of Being Uninsured on Utilization of Basic Health Care Services." *Inquiry* 29 (4): 457–66.

Spillman, B. C., and J. Lubitz. 2002. "New Estimates of Lifetime Nursing Home Use: Have Patterns of Use Changed?" *Medical Care* 40 (10): 965–75.

Sprague, L. 2002. "Contracting for Quality: Medicare's Quality Improvement Organizations." National Health Policy Forum Issue Brief No. 774. Washington, DC: The George Washington University.

Sprague, L. 2001. "Primary Care Case Management: Lessons for Medicare?" National Health Policy Forum Issue Brief No. 768. Washington, DC: National Health Policy Forum.

Staines, V. S. 1993. "Potential Impact of Managed Care on National Health Spending." *Health Affairs* 12 (Supplement): 248–57.

Starr, P. 1982. *The Social Transformation of American Medicine.* New York: Basic Books, Inc.

Stauffer, M. 1997. *Point of Service.* Washington, DC: National Conference of State Legislatures, Policy Training Service.

Stearns, S. C., and T. A. Mroz. 1996. "Premium Increases and Disenrollment from State Risk Pools." *Inquiry* 32 (4): 392–406.

Stoddard, J. J., R. F. St. Peter, and P. W. Newacheck. 1994. "Health Insurance Status and Ambulatory Care for Children." *New England Journal of Medicine* 330 (20): 1421–25.

Strunk, B. C., P. B. Ginsburg, and J. R. Gabel. 2001. "Tracking Health Care Costs." *Health Affairs Web Exclusives,* September 26.

Strunk, B. C., and D. J. Reschovsky. 2002. "Kinder and Gentler: Physicians and Managed Care, 1997–2001." Tracking Report, No. 5. Washington, DC: Center for Studying Health System Change.

Sullivan, C. B., M. Miller, R. Feldman, and B. Dowd. 1992. "Employer-Sponsored Health Insurance in 1991." *Health Affairs* 11 (4): 172–85.

Swartz, K. 1994. "Dynamics of People Without Health Insurance: Don't Let the Numbers Fool You." *Journal of the American Medical Association* 271 (1): 64–66.

**T**

Tarlov, A. R. 1995. "Estimating Physician Workforce Requirements: The Devil Is in the Assumptions." *Journal of the American Medical Association* 274 (19): 1558–60.

TennCare. 2003. "What Is TennCare?" [Online information; retrieved 2/5/03.] www.state.tn.us/tenncare/whatis.

Thomas, J. W., and M. L. Ashcraft. 1991. "Measuring Severity of Illness: Six Different Systems and Their Ability to Explain Cost Variations." *Inquiry* 28 (1): 39–55.

Thorpe, K. E. 1992. "Inside the Black Box of Administrative Costs." *Health Affairs* 11 (2): 41–55.

"Three Years into SCHIP, State Spending Rises." 2001. *New Federalism Policy Research and Resources, Issue 12.* Washington, DC: Urban Institute.

TRICARE. 2002. "Stakeholders' Report, Volume IV." [Online information; retrieved 6/19/02.] www.TRICARE.osd.mil/onestop/index.html.

**U**

U.S. Bipartisan Commission on Comprehensive Health Care. 1990. *A Call for Action: The Pepper Commission Final Report.* Washington, DC: U.S. Government Printing Office.

U.S. Bureau of the Census. 2005. *Income, Poverty, and Health Insurance Coverage in the United States, 2004.* Washington, DC: U.S. Department of Commerce.

———. 2002. "Older Americans Month Celebrated in May." [Online article or information (CB02-FF.07); retrieved 1/19/06.] www.Census.gov/Press-Release/www.releases/archives/facts_for_features_special_editions.

U.S. Department of Commerce. 2001. *Statistical Abstract of the United States, 2001.* Washington, DC: U.S. Government Printing Office.

———. 2000. *Statistical Abstract of the United States.* Washington, DC: U.S. Government Printing Office.

———. 1995. *Statistical Abstract of the United States, 1995.* Washington, DC: U.S. Government Printing Office.

———. 1992. *Statistical Abstract of the United States.* Washington, DC: U.S. Government Printing Office.

U.S. Department of Health and Human Services. 2006. *Medicare and Medicaid Statistical Supplement.* Pub. No. (PHS) C3-24-07. Baltimore, MD: USDHHS.

———. 2006. "USDHHS Organizational Chart." [Online information; retrieved 5/2/06.] www.dhhs.gov/about/orgchart.html.

———. 2005. *Health, United States, 2005.* Pub. No. (PHS) 2005-1232. Hyattsville, MD: USDHHS.

———. 2005. *Health, United States, 2005.* Pub. No. 05-1232. Hyattsville, MD: USDHHS. [Online information accessed in 2005 and 2006.] www.aacn.nche.edu/Media/Backgrounders/shortagefacts.htm.; www.ama-assn.org/ama/pub/category/1550.html.; www.aoa-net.org/

students/college.htm.;
http://brighamandwomens.org/
midwifery/Patient/facts.asp.;
www.aana.com/coa/
accreditedprograms.asp.

———. 2005. *Medicare and Medicaid Statistical Supplement 2003.* Pub. No. (PHS) 03460. Baltimore, MD: USDHHS.

———. 2004. *Health, United States, 2004.* Pub. No. (PHS) 2004-1232. Hyattsville, MD: USDHHS.

———. 2003. *Medicare and Medicaid Statistical Supplement.* Pub. No. (PHS) 03386. Baltimore, MD: USDHHS.

———. 2002. *Health, United States, 2002.* Pub. No. (PHS) 2002–1232. Hyattsville, MD: USDHHS.

———. 2001. *Health, United States, 2001.* Pub. No. (PHS) 2001–1232. Hyattsville, MD: USDHHS.

———. 2001. *Medicare and Medicaid Statistical Supplement.* Baltimore, MD: USDHHS.

———. 2000. *Healthy People 2010: National Health Promotion and Disease Prevention Objectives.* Washington, DC: U.S. Government Printing Office.

———. 2000. *Medicare and Medicaid Statistical Supplement, 2000.* Pub. No. (PHS) 03386. Baltimore, MD: USDHHS.

———. 1996. *Medicare and Medicaid Statistical Supplement.* Baltimore, MD: USDHHS.

———. 1995. *Health, United States, 1995.* Pub. No. (PHS) 96-1232. Hyattsville, MD: USDHHS.

———. 1995. *Medicare and Medicaid Statistical Supplement, 1995.* Pub. No. (PHS) 03386. Baltimore, MD: USDHHS.

———. 1993. *Morbidity and Mortality of Dialysis: NIH Consensus Statement.* Bethesda, MD: National Institutes of Health.

———. 1991. *Healthy People 2000: National Health Promotion and Disease Prevention Objectives.* Pub. No. (PHS) 91-50212. Washington, DC: U.S. Government Printing Office.

———. 1990. *Seventh Report to the President and Congress on the Status of Health Personnel in the United States.* Pub. No. HRS-P-OD-90-3. October. Washington, DC: USDHHS.

U.S. Department of Health and Human Services/Bureau of Health Professions. 1996. "Health Workforce." *Newslink* 2 (1): 1–12.

U.S. Department of Health and Human Services/Health Care Financing Administration. 1990. *Health Care Financing Program Statistics: Medicare and Medicaid Databook, 1990.* HCFA Pub. No. 03314. Baltimore, MD: USDHHS/HCFA.

U.S. Department of Health and Human Services/Health Resources and Services Administration. 1994. *Physician's Assistants in the Health Workforce.* Washington, DC: USDHHS.

U.S. Department of Health, Education, and Welfare. 1979. *Healthy People: The Surgeon General's Report on Health Promotion and Disease Prevention.* Pub. No. (PHS) 79-55071. Washington, DC: DHEW.

U.S. Department of Labor. 2004. "Occupation and Employment." [Online information; retrieved 1/3/2006.] http://stats.bls.gov/oes/2004/may/oes 291111.htm.

U.S. Government Accountability Office (formerly the U.S. General Accounting Office). 2005. *Defense Health Care: Implementation Issues for New TRICARE Contracts and Regulatory Structure.* GAO-05-773. July. Washington, DC: USGAO.

———. 2005. *FDA: Limited Available Data Indicate That FDA Has Been Meeting Some Goals for Review of Medical Device Applications.* GAO-05-1042. September. Washington, DC: USGAO.

———. 2005. *Indian Health Service; Health Care Services Are Not Always Available to Native Americans.* GAO-05-789. August. Washington, DC: USGAO.

———. 2005. *Long-Term Care Financing: Growing Demand and Cost of Services Are Straining Federal and State Budgets.* GAO-05-564T. Washington, DC: USGAO.

———. 2005. *Medicaid Managed Care: Access and Quality Requirements Specific to Low-Income and Other Special Needs Enrollees.* GAO-05-44R. December 2004. Washington, DC: USGAO.

———. 2005. *Nonprofit, For-Profit, and Government Hospitals: Uncompensated Care and Other Community Benefits.* USGAO-05-743T. May. Washington, DC: USGAO.

———. 2004. *Health Coverage Tax Credit: Simplified and More Timely Enrollment Process Could Increase Participation.* GAO-04-1029. September. Washington, DC: USGAO.

———. 2004. *Internet Pharmacies: Some Pose Safety Risks for Consumers.* GAO-04-820. Washington, DC: USGAO.

———. 2004. *Undocumented Aliens: Questions Persist about Their Impact on Hospitals' Uncompensated Care Costs.* USGAO-04-472. May. Washington, DC: USGAO.

———. 2003. *Long-Term Care: Federal Oversight of Growing Medicaid Home- and Community-Based Waivers Should Be Strengthened.* GAO-03-576. September. Washington, DC: USGAO.

———. 2003. *Medicare: Modest Eligibility Expansion for Critical Access Hospital Program Should Be Considered.* USGAO-03-948. September. Washington, DC: USGAO.

———. 2003. *Private Health Insurance: Federal and State Requirements Affecting Coverage Offered by Small Businesses.* GAO-03-1133. Washington, DC: USGAO.

———. 2002. *Long-Term Care: Availability of Medicaid and Home- and Community-Based Services for Elderly Individuals Varies Considerably.* GAO-02-1121. Washington, DC: USGAO.

———. 2002. *Long-Term Care: Baby Boom Generation Increases Challenge of Financing Needed Services.* GAO-01-563T. Washington, DC: USGAO.

———. 2002. *Medigap: Current Policies Contain Coverage Gaps, Undermine Cost Control Incentives.* GAO-02-533T. March. Washington, DC: USGAO.

———. 2001. *Higher Expected Spending and Call for New Benefits Underscore Need for Meaningful Reform.* GAO-01-539T. Washington, DC: USGAO.

———. 2001. *Retiree Health Insurance: Gaps in Coverage and Availability.* GAO-02-178T. November. Washington, DC: USGAO.

———. 2000. *Mental Health Parity Act: Despite New Federal Standards, Mental Health Benefits Remain Limited.* GAO/HEHS-00-95. Washington, DC: USGAO.

———. 1997. *Medicaid Managed Care: Challenge of Holding Plans Accountable Requires Greater State Effort.* GAO/HEHS-97-86. Washington, DC: USGAO.

———. 1997. *Medicaid: Sustainability of Low 1996 Spending Growth Is Uncertain.* GAO/HEHS-97-128. June. Washington, DC: USGAO.

———. 1997. *Medicare HMO Enrollment: Area Differences Affected by Other Than Payment Rates.* GAO/HEHS-97-37. Washington, DC: USGAO.

———. 1997. *Private Health Insurance: Continued Erosion of Coverage Linked to Cost Pressures.* GAO/HEHS-97-122. July. Washington, DC: USGAO.

———. 1996. *Medical Device Regulation: Too Early to Assess European System's Value as Model for FDA.* USGAO/HEHS-96-65. March. Washington, DC: USGAO.

———. 1996. *VA Health Care: Better Data Needed to Effectively Use Limited Nursing Home Resources.* GAO/HEHS-97-27. Washington, DC: USGAO.

———. 1995. *Community Health Centers: Challenges in Transitioning to Prepaid Managed Care.* USGAO/HEHS-95-138. Washington, DC: USGAO.

———. 1995. *Defense Health Care: Despite TRICARE Procurement Improvements, Problems Remain.* GAO/HEHS-95-142. August. Washington, DC: USGAO.

———. 1995. *Durable Medical Equipment: Regional Carriers' Coverage Criteria are Consistent with Medicare Law.* USGAO/HEHS-95-185. September. Washington, DC: USGAO.

———. 1995. *Employer-Based Health Plans: Issues, Trends, and Challenges Posed by ERISA.* GAO/HEHS-95-167. July. Washington, DC: USGAO.

———. 1995. *Health Care: Employers and Individual Consumers Want Additional Information on Quality.* GAO/HEHS-95-201. Washington, DC: USGAO.

———. 1995. *Health Care Shortage Areas: Designations Not a Useful Tool for Directing Resources to the Underserved.* GAO/HEHS-95-200. September. Washington, DC: USGAO.

———. 1995. *Health Insurance Portability: Reform Could Ensure Continued Coverage for Up to 25 Million Americans.* GAO-HEHS-95-257. September. Washington, DC: USGAO.

———. 1995. *LTC: Current Issues and Future Directions.* GAO/HEHS-95-109. Washington, DC: USGAO.

———. 1995. *Medical Devices: FDA Review Time.* GAO/PEMD-96-2. October. Washington, DC: USGAO.

———. 1995. *Medicare: Excessive Payments for Medical Supplies Continue Despite Improvements.* USGAO/HEHS-95-171. August. Washington, DC: USGAO.

———. 1995. *Prescription Drug Prices: Official Index Overstates Producer Price Inflation.* USGAO/HEHS-95-90. April. Washington, DC: USGAO.

———. 1995. *Testimony on Employer Association Health Plans.* GAO/HEHS-96-59R. December. Washington, DC: USGAO.

———. 1994. *Access to Health Insurance: Public and Private Employers' Experiences with Purchasing Cooperatives.* GAO/HEHS-94-142. May. Washington, DC: USGAO.

———. 1994. *Blue Cross and Blue Shield: Experiences of Weak Plans Underscore the Role of Effective State Oversight.* GAO/HEHS-94-71. April. Washington, DC: USGAO.

———. 1994. *Health Care: Federal and State Antitrust Actions Concerning the Health Care Industry.* USGAO/HEHS 94-220. August. Washington, DC: USGAO.

———. 1994. *Health Care Reform: Considerations for Risk Adjustment under Community Rating.* GAO-HEHS-94-173. September. Washington, DC: USGAO.

———. 1994. *Health Professions Education: Role of Title VII/VIII Programs in Improving Access to Care Is Unclear.* HEHS-94–164. Washington, DC: USGAO.

———. 1994. *Medicare: Graduate Medical Education Payment Policy Needs to Be Examined.* USGAO/HEHS-94-33. May. Washington, DC: USGAO.

———. 1994. *Medicare: Technology Assessment and Medical Coverage Decisions.* USGAO/HEHS-94-195FS. July. Washington, DC: USGAO.

———. 1994. *Prescription Drugs: Spending Controls in Four European Countries.* USGAO/HEHS-94-30. May. Washington, DC: USGAO.

———. 1993. *Health Insurance: How Health Care Reform May Affect State Regulation.* GAO/T-HRD-94-55. November. Washington, DC: USGAO.

———. 1993. *Long-Term Care Insurance: High Percentage of Policyholders Drop Policies.* GAO/HRD-93-129. August. Washington, DC: USGAO.

———. 1993. *Nonprofit Hospitals: For-Profit Ventures Pose Access and Capacity Problems.* USGAO/HRD 93-124. July. Washington, DC: USGAO.

———. 1992. *Access to Health Insurance: State Efforts to Assist Small Businesses.* GAO/HRD-92-90. May. Washington, DC: USGAO.

———. 1992. *Employer-Based Health Insurance: High Costs, Wide Variation Threaten System.* USGAO/HRD-92-125. September. Washington, DC: USGAO.

———. 1992. *Health Insurance: Vulnerable Payers Lose Billions to Fraud and Abuse.* USGAO/HRD-92-69. Washington, DC: USGAO.

———. 1991. Medicaid Expansions: Coverage Improves but State Fiscal Problems Jeopardize Continued Progress. GAO/HRD-91-78. Washington, DC: USGAO.

———. 1991. *Private Health Insurance: Problems Caused by a Segmented Market.* GAO/HRD-91-114. July. Washington, DC: USGAO.

———. 1991. *Rural Hospitals: Federal Efforts Should Target Areas Where Closures Would Threaten Access to Care.* USGAO/HRD 91-41. Washington, DC: USGAO.

———. 1990. *Rural Hospitals: Factors That Affect Risk of Closure.* USGAO/HRD-90-134. June. Washington, DC: USGAO.

United Seniors Health Cooperative. 1995. *1995 Medigap Update and Medicare Summary.* Washington, DC: United Seniors Health Cooperative Newsletter.

**V**

Varmus, H. 1995. "Shattuck Lecture: Biomedical Research Enters the Steady State." *New England Journal of Medicine* 333 (12): 811–15.

Vladek, B. C. 2001. "Learn Nothing, Forget Nothing—the Medicare Commission Redux." *New England Journal of Medicine* 345 (6): 456–58.

**W**

Wachter, R. M., and L. Goldman. 2002. "The Hospitalist Movement 5 Years Later." *Journal of the American Medical Association* 287 (4): 487–94.

———. 1996. "The Emerging Role of 'Hospitalists' in the American Health Care System." *New England Journal of Medicine* 335 (7): 514–17.

Wallack, S. S., K. C. Skwara, and J. Cai. 1996. "Redefining Rate Regulation in a Competitive Environment." *Journal of Health Politics, Policy and Law* 21 (3): 489–510.

Ward, D., and B. Berkowitz. 2002. "Arching the Flood: How to Bridge the Gap Between Nursing Schools and Hospitals." *Health Affairs* 21 (5): 42–52.

Warshawsky, M. J. 1994. "Projections of Health Care Expenditures as a Share of the GDP: Actuarial and Macroeconomic Approaches." *Health Services Research* 29 (3): 293–313.

Watt, J. M., R. A. Derzon, and S. C. Renn. 1986. "The Comparative Economic Performance of Investor-Owned Chains and Not-for-Profit Hospitals." *New England Journal of Medicine* 314 (2): 89–96.

Weil, A. 1997. *The New Children's Health Insurance Program: Should States Expand Medicaid? New Federalism Issues and Options for States.* Series A, No. A-13. Washington, DC: The Urban Institute.

Weiner, J. P. 1994. "Forecasting the Effects of Health Reform on U.S. Physician Workforce Requirements: Evidence from HMO Staffing Patterns." *Journal of the American Medical Association* 272 (3): 222–40.

Weiner, J. P., and G. de Lissovoy. 1993. "Razing a Tower of Babel: A Taxonomy for Managed Care and Health Insurance Plans." *Journal of Health Politics, Policy and Law* 18 (1): 75–103.

Weinstein, R. A., J. D. Siegel, and P. J. Benjamin. 2005. "Infection-Control Report Cards—Securing Patient Safety." *New England Journal of Medicine* 353 (3): 225–27.

Weissert, W. G., C. M. Cready, and J. E. Pawalek. 1988. "The Past and Future of Community-Based Long-Term Care." *The Milbank Quarterly* 66 (2): 309–88.

Weissman, J. 2005. "The Trouble with Uncompensated Hospital Care." *New England Journal of Medicine* 352 (12): 1171.

Weissman, J., and A. M. Epstein. 1992. "The Relationships among Insurance Coverage, Access to Services, and Health Outcomes: A Critical Review and Synthesis of the Literature." Contractor paper prepared for the Office of Technology Assessment. Washington, DC: U.S. Congress.

Wennberg, J., and A. Gittelsohn. 1982. "Variations in Medical Care among Small Areas." *Scientific American* 246 (4): 120–34.

———. 1973. "Small Area Variations in Health Care Delivery." *Science* 192 (4117): 1102–08.

Wennberg, J. E., J. P. Bunker, and B. Barnes. 1980. "The Need for Assessing the Outcome of Common Medical Practices." *Annual Review of Public Health* 1: 277–95.

Wennberg, J. E., D. C. Goodman, R. F. Nease, and R. B. Keller. 1993. "Finding Equilibrium in U.S. Physician Supply." *Health Affairs* 12 (2): 89–103.

Whelen, G. P., N. E. Gary, J. Kostes, J. R. Boulet, and J. A. Hallock. 2002. "The Changing Pool of International Medical Graduates Seeking Certification Training in U.S. GME Programs." *Journal of the American Medical Association* 288 (9): 1079–84.

Wickizer, T. M., and P. J. Feldstein. 1995. "The Impact of HMO Competition on Private Health Insurance Premiums, 1985–1992." *Inquiry* 32 (3): 241–51.

Wilensky, G. 2001. "Medicare Reform: Now Is the Time." *New England Journal of Medicine* 345 (6): 458–62.

———. 1996. "Presentation to Kaiser Founder's Day Dinner." Unpublished presentation, Denver, CO. November.

Wilensky, G., P. J. Farley, and A. K. Taylor. 1984. "Variations in Health Insurance Coverage: Benefits vs. Premiums." *The Milbank Quarterly* 62 (1): 53–81.

Wolf, D. A., K. Hunt, and J. Knickman. 2005. "Perspectives on the Recent Decline in Disability at Older Ages." *The Milbank Quarterly* 83 (3): 365–95.

Wolinsky, F. D., and R. J. Johnson. 1992. "Perceived Health Status and Mortality in Older Men and Women." *Journal of Gerontology* 47 (6): 5304–12.

Woolhandler, S., and D. U. Himmelstein. 1995. "Extreme Risk—The New Corporate Proposition for Physicians." *New England Journal of Medicine* 333 (25): 1706–08.

———. 1991. "The Deteriorating Administrative Efficiency of the U.S. Health Care System." *New England Journal of Medicine* 324 (18): 1253–38.

World Health Organization/Health Promotion. 1999. "Ottawa Charter for Health Promotion." [Online information; retrieved 1/27/03.] www.who.int/hpr/archive/docs/ottawa.html.

**Y**

Young, C. 2001. "Recent Research Findings on Medicare+Choice." The Monitoring Medicare+Choice Project of Mathematica Policy Research, Inc., No. 6., November. Washington, DC: Mathematica Policy Research, Inc.

**Z**

Zellers, W. K., C. G. McLaughlin, and K. D. Frick. 1992. "Small Business Health Insurance: Only the Healthy Need Apply." *Health Affairs* 11 (1): 174–80.

Zerhouni, E. H. 2005. "U.S. Biomedical Research—Basic, Translational, and Clinical Sciences." *Journal of the American Medical Association* 294 (11): 1352–58.

Zimmerman, D. L. 1994. *Medical Technology and Health Reform: Devising Policy for the Medical Device Market.* Washington, DC: National Health Policy Forum.

Zuvekas, S. H., and S. C. Hill. 2004. "Does Capitation Matter? Impacts on Access, Use, and Quality." *Inquiry* 41 (3): 316–335.

Zwanziger, J., and G. A. Melnick. 1996. "Can Managed Care Plans Control Health Care Costs?" *Health Affairs* 15 (2): 185–99.

# Index

Page numbers in *italics* identify illustrations. An italic *t* next to a page number (e.g., 241*t*) indicates information that appears in a table. An italic *n* and number next to a page number (e.g., 241*n*1) indicate information that appears in an end-of-chapter note.

"A" agencies, 98

AARP, 89

Abuse, impact on health care expenditures, 197

Academic health centers: defined, 405; distinguishing features, 406–7; policy issues for, 407–10

Acceptability of care, 70*n*1

Accessibility of care, 70*n*1

Access to care: dimensions of, 47–49, 69–70*n*1; government-provided, 59–61; impact of Medicare cuts, 234; impact on costs and utilization, 9, 47–48; major factors affecting, 49–52; managed care impact, 443; for mental illness, 430–32; out-of-pocket payment and, 57; palliative, 417–18; primary care services, 345–49; private insurance and, 52–54, 55–56; public insurance and, 55–57, 58*t*; relation of adverse outcomes to, 61–62; secondary medical treatment, 357–59; trends for, 502–3; for uninsured population, 61–62, 63–68. *See also* Health insurance; Uninsured population

Accommodation of care, 70*n*1

Accreditation, 103, 105

Accreditation Council for Graduate Medical Education (ACGME), 233

Achievable benchmarks, 482

Acquisitions: among HMOs, 457; hospital, 280–81; nursing home, 390

Activities of daily living, 367–68, 391

Activity limitations, *354*

Acute care focus, 198–99

Acute mental illness, 424

Adjusted average per capita cost, 208, 459

Administration for Children and Families, 84

Administration of health services: as career, 250–51; elements of, 100–101; growth in spending on, 188, 196–97; sources of funding for, *192*

Administrative data, 478

Administrative load, 134

Administrative Procedures Act, 103

Administrative services only agreements, 133

Administrators, role in hospitals, 266

Advanced practice nurses, 241–42, 344

Adverse events, 482, 504

Adverse outcomes, 61–62

Adverse selection, 112, 461–62

Affordability of care, 70*n*1

Age: activity limitations by, *354*; ambulatory care visits by, *356*; average length of stay by, *362*; general relation to utilization, 27–28; home health care utilization by, *39*, *389*; hospice care by, 416–17; physician visits by, 32, *33*, *37*, *38*, *346*, *347*; primary care visits by, *344*; private insurance coverage by, *53*, *55*, 118*t*; serious psychological distress by, 424; uninsured population by, *64*

Age-adjusted death rates, 22, 24*t*

Agency for Health Care Policy and Research, 307, 480

Agency for Healthcare Research and Quality: basic functions, 480–81, 503–4; origins, 307; overview, 84; provider payment standards, 204

Aging populations, impact on health care expenditures, 195

AIDS: halfway technologies for treating, 306; impact on drug review process, 298; prevention costs, 333*t*; viatical settlements resulting from, 154

Aid to Families with Dependent Children (AFDC), 57, 145

Alcoholism prevention costs, 333*t*

Allied health workers, 237

Almshouses, 12, 259, 427

Alternative medicine providers, 237, 251, 252*t*

Alzheimer's disease, 370

# ABOUT THE AUTHOR

Phoebe Lindsey Barton, Ph.D., is a professor in the School of Medicine at the University of Colorado at Denver and Health Sciences Center. She is director of the Master of Science in Public Health (MSPH) program and teaches courses in health care systems and health services research. Prior to coming to Colorado, she was on the faculty of the School of Public Health at the University of California, Los Angeles and was a consultant with the RAND Corporation. Dr. Barton has been an administrator in two state health and human services departments. Her health services research interests include the financing and delivery of health services and programs, including Medicaid; technology assessment in areas of telemedicine and organ transplantation; community-based participatory research related to health promotion; and health issues among incarcerated populations.